W0106429

The Diabetic Pancreas

The Diabetic Pancreas

Edited by
Bruno W. Volk
*Isaac Albert Research Institute, Brooklyn, New York
and University of California, Irvine, California*

and
Klaus F. Wellmann
*Isaac Albert Research Institute, Brooklyn, New York
and Beekman Downtown Hospital, New York*

Plenum Press · New York and London

Library of Congress Cataloging in Publication Data

Main entry under title:

The Diabetic pancreas.

Includes bibliographical references and index.
1. Diabetes. 2. Islands of Langerhans. I. Volk, Bruno W. II. Wellmann, Klaus F.
[DNLM: 1. Diabetes mellitus. 2. Islands of Langerhans—Physiopathology. WK810
V916d]
RC660.D57   616.4'62   77-7321
ISBN-13: 978-1-4684-2327-3   e-ISBN-13: 978-1-4684-2325-9
DOI: 10.1007/978-1-4684-2325-9

© 1977 Plenum Press, New York
 Softcover reprint of the hardcover 1st edition 1977
A Division of Plenum Publishing Corporation
227 West 17th Street, New York, N.Y. 10011

All rights reserved

No part of this book may be reproduced, stored in a retrieval system, or transmitted,
in any form or by any means, electronic, mechanical, photocopying, microfilming,
recording, or otherwise, without written permission from the Publisher

Contributors

Charles H. Best   University of Toronto, Ontario, Canada

Lennart Boquist   University of Umea, Umea, Sweden

John E. Craighead   University of Vermont, Burlington, Vermont

Werner Creutzfeldt   Medizinische Klinik und Poliklinik der Universität, Göttingen, West Germany

William E. Dulin   The Upjohn Company, Kalamazoo, Michigan

Sture Falkmer   University of Umea, Umea, Sweden

Willy Gepts   Universitair Ziekenhuis Brugmann, Vrije Universiteit Brussel, Brussels, Belgium

Orion D. Hegre   University of Minnesota, Minneapolis, Minnesota

Claes Hellerström   University of Uppsala, Uppsala, Sweden

Paul E. Lacy   Washington University, St. Louis, Missouri

Arnold Lazarow   Late of the University of Minnesota, Minneapolis, Minnesota

Philip M. LeCompte   Formerly Faulkner Hospital and Harvard Medical School, Boston, Massachusetts

Rachmiel Levine   City of Hope National Medical Center, Duarte, California

Arthur A. Like   University of Massachusetts, Worcester, Massachusetts

Auguste Loubatières   Late of the Faculté de Médecine de Montpellier, Montpellier, France

Lelio Orci   Institute of Histology, Medical School, University of Geneva, Geneva, Switzerland

Yngve Östberg   University of Umea, Umea, Sweden

Alain Perrelet   Institute of Histology, Medical School, University of Geneva, Geneva, Switzerland

M. G. Soret   The Upjohn Company, Kalamazoo, Michigan

Bruno W. Volk   Isaac Albert Research Institute of the Kingsbrook Jewish Medical Center, and Downstate Medical Center, State University of New York, Brooklyn, New York. Present address: University of California, Irvine, California

Klaus F. Wellmann   Isaac Albert Research Institute of the Kingsbrook Jewish Medical Center, and Downstate Medical Center, State University of New York, Brooklyn, New York. Present address: Beekman Downtown Hospital, New York, New York

Foreword

I consider it an honor to have been asked to write the Foreword for *The Diabetic Pancreas*. Although I have been involved in the study of the pancreas since 1921, my interest goes back even further to the time, in 1918, that my father's sister, a nurse who had trained at the Massachusetts General Hospital, developed diabetes, lost weight, and died in diabetic coma. This sad event made a deep impression on me and was certainly partly responsible for my choosing to join the Department of Physiology of the University of Toronto to begin a career in research into diabetes.

This is not the place to describe in detail the wide-ranging research and study of the diabetic pancreas in which I have engaged in the past 56 years. Suffice it to say that I am familiar enough with the subject area to be able to predict a great future for this book. The editors have undertaken a very ambitious and worthwhile project, and their efforts have been supported and strengthened by contributors who are respected authorities in their fields, thus ensuring a successful presentation of this major work.

From my constant study of pertinent books and journals—and particularly from reading the accounts of the many seminars held on the fiftieth anniversary of the discovery of insulin—I know the awesome extent of the literature that the editors and contributors to this volume had to review in order to prepare their chapters. This book, then, will fill a great need, and medical scientists and chemists from all over the world will profit from it. But ultimately, of course, it is the diabetic patient who is the beneficiary when a splendid source of information like *The Diabetic Pancreas* is added to the literature and made available to researchers and practitioners in the field.

Charles H. Best

Preface

Since the publication of the monograph by Lazarus and Volk on *The Pancreas in Human and Experimental Diabetes* in 1962, important progress has been made in various fields of diabetes research, which contributed considerably to a better understanding of this disease. The significant advances in morphologic techniques such as quantitative and qualitative histochemistry, staining with fluorescent antibodies, electron microscopy, and others, applied to human and experimental diabetes, have contributed to a more fundamental appreciation of the physiological processes occurring in the islets of Langerhans. Particularly, the growing field of research in various animal species which exhibit spontaneous or hereditary disturbances of carbohydrate metabolism has remarkably widened the scope of our knowledge of diabetes.

Various studies have contributed to the present-day concepts concerning the secretion of insulin and the importance of the A cells in blood sugar homeostasis and also to the clarification of the function of the D cells. Moreover, the availability of various drugs such as the sulfonylureas, streptozotocin, and others have immeasurably aided in the study of the islet physiology. As a result of these and other newly developed techniques, such as the isolation of islets, it became possible to better evaluate the physiology involved, particularly of the B cells of the islets of Langerhans.

Because of the increasingly broad interest in diabetes mellitus and its complications, several handbooks and proceedings of various symposia dealing with this subject have been published in the past decade. However, there are few volumes which deal almost exclusively with the pancreatic changes in human and experimental diabetes. The aim of this book is to present a more integrated approach to the correlation between morphologic alterations and the various metabolic aspects of diabetes. Furthermore, the editors have attempted to integrate the more recent concepts of the pathogenesis of this disease which resulted from new fundamental physiological and experimental observations.

The authors contributing to this monograph are recognized authorities in the various fields dealing with comparative morphology, pathology, and pathophysiology of the endocrine pancreas. It is therefore hoped that these combined efforts have produced a source book which is readable and thoroughly referenced. As this volume goes to press new areas of research are still being investigated. Although many are promising, they are not as yet sufficiently understood or developed. Experimental and clinical evidence indicates that the diabetic syndrome is more complex than originally thought.

The chronologic aspects which have been incorporated in this volume are considered to be of importance to the evolution of our knowledge of the pathology and pathophysiology of the endocrine pancreas and its many interrelationships with other hormonal glands involved in carbohydrate metabolism. However, these considerations have been kept to a minimum, in keeping with the principal purpose of this monograph which deals primarily with the morphologic aspects of the diabetic pancreas.

There will be unavoidable overlaps of certain observations and ideas in various chapters. However, it appears to us that the incorporation of some similar material in different parts of this volume will help to elucidate the presented facts. The editors are indebted to Mrs. Renee Brenner and Mrs. Sarah Ginsberg for reviewing and typing the manuscripts and to Mr. Herbert A. Fischler, Chief Medical Photographer of the Isaac Albert Research Institute, who prepared some of the microphotographs. We gratefully acknowledge the cooperation of Plenum Publishing Corporation in making this book possible.

Brooklyn, N.Y.   B.W.V.
                                                                                                          K.F.W.

Contents

Introduction

By asking me to write the introduction to their book, the editors have given me the inestimable benefit of compelling me to learn about the newest findings and to refresh my mind about the more established data, involving the pancreas as an endocrine organ. For this I thank them most sincerely.

The present volume is concerned in a thorough and careful manner with about 1.5 grams of tissue, consisting of specialized cells, a network of thin nerve fibrils, and an abundance of small blood vessels. In the average, adult, healthy human being, this tiny heap of living tissue exists subdivided into about one million specks, each one by itself a fully functioning multihormonal endocrine system, sensing and responding to chemical gradients and neural impulses in an integrated and homeostatic fashion.

In 1851 Bouchardat, professor of hygiene in Paris, proficient in chemistry and an adept practitioner of clinical research, ventured the opinion that the severe diabetes of the lean (diabète maigre) had an etiologic relationship to the pancreas. He did this on the basis of autopsy findings on his own cases, which were carefully followed. Some other clinicians with experience in diabetes corroborated his findings and shared his views. However, two circumstances prevented acceptance of such an opinion. Many individuals in whom diabetes had been diagnosed during life showed normal-appearing pancreatic glands postmortem. This was particularly true when no distinction was made between "lean" diabetes and "obese" diabetes (diabète gras).

In addition, two preeminent nineteenth century physiologists, Bernard and Schiff, produced profound atrophy of the pancreas in experimental animals without causing a diabetic state (hyperglycemia and/or glycosuria).

These circumstances delayed the discovery of the pancreas (or one of its parts) as a gland of internal secretion for some thirty years, until the work of Mering and Minkowski in 1889. It is ironic that their first pancreatic ablations were done not because of a presumed relationship of the gland to diabetes, but primarily in order to study probable deviations in fat absorption.

From that point on, interest in, and study of, the islets of Langerhans (so named in 1893) has never flagged. One result is the present compendium which describes the current state of the art, by a detailed analysis of the structure and function of the endocrine system residing (in most animals) within the body of the pancreas.

It should be remembered that Minkowski immediately sensed the physiological import of his chance observation, and established the regulatory function of the pancreas in carbohydrate metabolism. He did this by showing that a small, surviving portion of the pancreas prevented the expected hyperglycemia, until the time that it degenerated *in situ.* His work was immediately confirmed by others (especially Hedon). Thus, the first steps were taken (1891–1893) in showing that an "internal secretion" was produced by the gland which was essential for the control of the blood sugar level and glycogen deposition. Structural and developmental studies of the gland began with Laguesse (1893), who designated the scattered secretory cell aggregates as the "islands of Langerhans." It became then evident why the severe pancreatic atrophy produced by Claude Bernard and by Schiff was not followed by diabetes. Obstruction of the pancreatic ducts led to degeneration of the exocrine system, while the "tenant" islands of endocrine cells were preserved; since the "tenant" occupied only 1–2% of the pancreatic volume it could easily be overlooked.

The initial assumption that the islets elaborated and secreted a single hormone (named "insulin" long before its successful extraction) held sway for many years, despite the clear and convincing findings by histologists from 1899 onward (Tschasownikow, Diamare, Sobolev, and Lane) that there were at least two distinct secretory cells in the islets. It was Lane who named them A and B (or beta) in 1907; Bensley added the agranular C cell (1911), and Bloom described a granular D cell in 1931. We will come back to the latest views concerning the separate secretory products thought to be associated with the distinct cell types further on.

For many years the secretory product of the second most numerous cell type of the islets (A) was unknown, and almost as long a period was needed to understand the findings of Murlin and of Buerger, who detected an initial *hyperglycemic* effect of intravenously injected insulin (1923–1926). The *h*yperglycemic, *g*lycogenolytic *f*actor (HGF) was rediscovered in 1945, purified and chemically identified by 1957, and rechristened glucagon. A series of both indirect and direct studies in comparative morphology and immunological detection techniques established that glucagon was the secretory product of cells belonging to the A type. Thus the two research paths finally crossed.

The research direction in diabetes has never proceeded in as straight a line as it might have. Observations were frequently made which went unnoticed and unsung and had to be rediscovered at a more propitious time. Thus even strong indications that the gastrointestinal tract was probably involved in blood sugar regulations (notably MacCallum in 1932) were shunted aside for many years. In the last ten to fifteen years these attitudes have changed completely owing to the development of knowledge of the endocrinology of the gut. The gastro-entero-pancreatic peptide hormone systems are achieving ever more recognition physiologically and biochemically.

Even though we cannot as yet pinpoint the pathways accurately, there is no doubt that in man and some other mammals carbohydrate and protein food ingestion by contact with certain enteric cells releases a chemical signal or signals which lead to a discharge of insulin from the B cell of the pancreas. This occurs before there has been sufficient glucose or amino acid absorption to cause a rise in their blood levels and thus be the direct stimulus to insulin secretion.

In some instances, specifically identifiable endocrine cell types associated with the pancreatic islets may be found in the gastric or intestinal mucosa. "Glucagon" cells (type A_2) are ensconced in the stomach; they elaborate and secrete what is essentially "pancreatic" glucagon. Another cell type found both in the gastrointestinal tract and in the pancreas is A_1 (or D in the older nomenclature), which is known to produce somatostatin. In cases with functional tumors one can identify some insulinomas arising along the gut, as well as gastrinomas within the pancreas.

Exciting developments in the physiology of the regulation of foodstuff digestion, absorption, and distribution are to be expected presently and for some time into the future. The roles played by each one of the entero-pancreatic peptides are still largely unknown.

Carbohydrate absorption rates are probably stimulated by glucagon and suppressed by somatostatin. There are hints that gastrin is not only the stimulator of gastric acid secretion, but that it is an insulin antagonist. Which of the gastrointestinal peptides is *the* insulin secretion stimulus? And what of the newest recruit—pancreatic polypeptide? It has a cellular site (the PP cell in the pancreas), and is a polypeptide—but what function does it subserve?

At this point it might be instructive to look at the pancreatic islet from the vantage point of 1977, insofar as it is possible, both as to structure and function.

The B cell produces proinsulin, splits it into free insulin and C-peptide, packages both into the beta granule, and releases the contents in conformity with a variety of interlocking stimuli. A still unidentified enteric peptide stimulates insulin secretion when food is ingested. Is this a direct effect or is it transmitted by a localized provision of glucagon from the A_2 cell via a tight junction? The ultrastructural evidence tempts one to propose this type of control by hormonal action at short distances, *in situ*. Are the gap junctions between these cells part of the mechanism for accurate neural control of the islets? We know at least that α-adrenergic activity serves to inhibit insulin secretion and that vagal impulses can modulate insulin release.

The A_1 (or the old D) cell produces somatostatin whether it is located in the gastrointestinal mucosa or in the pancreas. The electron microscopic evidence would again favor the view that this peptide acts, in the main, locally and serves to moderate glucagon release.

The latest recruit to the pancreatic islet population of regulatory substances is GABA (gamma amino-butyric acid), found in rather high concentrations in the islets. In the central nervous system, of course, GABA serves as an inhibitory neurotransmitter.

This shortened and still very incomplete picture of the islet shows the great potential for ongoing research that modern histological and electron microscopic techniques are providing. Such studies, combined with our ever increasing information concerning the enteric hormonal peptides, will give us bit by bit

the understanding needed for the rational subdivision of the various disturbances now bracketed together as diabetes mellitus.

These are some reflections generated in one reader by the assembled
chapters of this book. But much more may be found in these contributions, an
abundance of material for study and enlightening thought:

- What are the possible etiologic factors in juvenile onset diabetes? Viruses and
immune factors operating on a background of proliferative stimuli seem to
be at present favored candidates. The whole pancreas becomes small and
atrophic in the juvenile onset form. Why? Do the acinar cells depend upon
endocrine regulation by the islets?
- In juvenile onset diabetes and in many of the syndromes of the spontaneous
disease in animals, hyperplasia of the islets may be noted early in the
progress of the disease. Does this point to an extrapancreatic hormonal or
neuroendocrine push preceding a viral and/or immune process?
- There are some indications that the functional relations already found
between the enteric and the pancreatic hormones point to a common origin
of many of the secretory cell types. The acronym APUD has been suggested
for the cells which elaborate diverse peptides but which have in common the
property of *a*mine *p*recursor *u*ptake and *d*ecarboxylation. It has been
theorized, but not yet shown, that these cells may have a common origin
from the neural crest, and that their regulatory effects, seemingly diverse,
may well fit together in regard to an overall system directing the conserva-
tion and correct routing of the foodstuffs to their metabolic destinations.

It would be tempting to go on and point to other nuggets of information in
this book, but then this would no longer be an introduction. I hoped simply to
provide a suitable developmental framework for the details of the structure of
the pancreatic islets in all of its complexity, which is the proper province of this
book itself.

Rachmiel Levine

Chapter 1

Historical Review

Klaus F. Wellmann and Bruno W. Volk

In a statement attributed to Allen, it has been said that the history of diabetes mellitus can be divided into four chronological sections.[1] The first of these, the ancient period, gave us the clinical description of the disease. Much later, during the diagnostic period which is associated with names such as Willis, Dobson, and Cawley, a first understanding of the nature of this affliction began to blossom. Then followed the period of empiric treatment initiated by Rollo. Finally, Claude Bernard ushered in the experimental period that has persisted to this day. There are literally hundreds of names for any of these four stages that could and should be mentioned in a comprehensive review of the history of diabetes. Obviously, this is quite impossible within the confines of the limited number of pages allotted to this chapter. Instead, an attempt will be made to retrace selectively some of the historical developments that led up to the present state of knowledge in this field, especially as they pertain to the various topics discussed in this book.

The term "diabetes," which is Ionic Greek and means "to run through a siphon," was coined by Aretaeus of Cappadocia (about A.D. 81–138), who noted that a large amount of urine "runs through" the kidneys in this disease. He was one of the first to provide a fairly complete clinical description of diabetes, but the phenomenon of polyuria had been observed at a much earlier time since it is mentioned in several of the ancient papyri, including the papyrus Hearst and the papyrus of Brugsch.[1] The very first reference to what might have been diabetes is contained in the papyrus Ebers which has been dated to around 1500 B.C. and was found at Luxor in Egypt in 1872[1–4]; this papyrus contains a medical prescription on how to stop polyuria. Writing earlier than Aretaeus, Celsus[5] believed that diabetics excrete more fluid with the urine than they take in, and he advised that such patients eat as little as possible. While all of these allusions may, indeed, refer to diabetes, it is well to remember that polyuria, as such, can also be found in several other conditions and need not be diabetic in origin.

Klaus F. Wellmann and Bruno W. Volk • Isaac Albert Research Institute of the Kingsbrook Jewish Medical Center, and Downstate Medical Center, State University of New York, Brooklyn, New York. Present address of K. F. W.: Beekman Downtown Hospital, New York, New York. Present address of B. W. V.: University of California, Irvine, California.

Japanese and Chinese physicians of the second and third centuries knew about the sweet taste and the abnormally large quantities of the diabetic urine. They observed that diabetics tend to develop furunculosis, and they spoke about "the malady of thirst."[6] Old Sanskrit texts from India refer to the "urine of honey," as do Indian physicians of the fifth and sixth centuries; they also noted that diabetes occurred more often in overweight persons and in those who consumed large quantities of starchy food, rice, and sugar. Later, during the ninth, tenth, and eleventh centuries, the disease was studied and described by several eminent Arab physicians. Foremost among them was Avicenna, or Ibn Sina, who lived from 960 to 1037 and observed such diabetic symptoms as abnormal appetite, sweetness of urine, gangrene, and loss of sexual function.[7] Avicenna also distinguished between primary and secondary diabetes, as did Aretaeus before him. There are few European references to diabetes during the Middle Ages until Aureolus Theophrastus Bombastus von Hohenheim, or Paracelsus (1493–1541), evaporated the urine of a diabetic patient and obtained a white, powdery residue which he mistook for salt.[8] Johann Baptista van Helmont (1574–1644) provided the first account of diabetic lipemia.[9]

Then, during the seventeenth century, Thomas Willis (1621–1675) ushered in the "diagnostic period" in the history of this disease. Apart from rediscovering the sweetness of the diabetic urine, Willis[10] was the first to separate diabetes mellitus from diabetes insipidus, the latter lacking glycosuria. He, as well as Dobson[11] one century later, stated that in diabetes, sugar appears first in the blood, then in the urine, and he prescribed undernourishment and limewater as therapeutic measures. The fact that glycosuria is a characteristic and constant feature of the disease became generally accepted so that William Cullen (1710–1790) added the qualifying adjective "mellitus" to "diabetes" in order to distinguish this affliction from diabetes insipidus.[12]

John Rollo, in 1797, inaugurated the period of empirical treatment of diabetics by prescribing an exclusive diet of meat.[13] The therapeutic effect of such a low-carbohydrate, high-protein diet probably also resulted from partial starvation. In addition, Rollo recorded diabetic cataract and compared the acetone-induced odor of diabetic patients to that of decaying apples. A second major step in the preinsulin treatment of diabetics was taken by Apollinaire Bouchardat (1806–1886), who observed that during the siege of Paris in the Franco-Prussian war of 1870/71 all his diabetic cases improved. Bouchardat devised specific dietary schedules in which carbohydrates were replaced by fats; he emphasized the importance of caloric restriction and introduced days of fasting and physical exercise.[14] Earlier, in 1835, he had been able to prove that the sugar in the urine of diabetics is grape sugar, i.e., glucose, and that it could be detected with the help of the polariscope and copper solutions. His compatriot, Claude Bernard, determined that grape sugar is an indispensible ingredient of the animal organism and is stored in the liver in the form of glycogen.[15,16] He is also credited with the discovery that puncture of the floor of the fourth ventricle of the dog renders this animal temporarily diabetic.[17]

It was not until late in the nineteenth century that diabetes and the pancreas began to be linked in the developing concept of this disease. Galen, for instance, believed that diabetes resulted from an injury to the kidneys; Paracelsus and Willis implicated the blood, Rollo the stomach, and Cullen the nervous system, while Claude Bernard placed the disturbance in the liver.[1] The first allusion to the pancreas as a separate organ has been attributed to Herophilus of Chalkidon during the first half of the third pre-Christian century.[4] Rufus of Ephesus who lived 200 years later is credited with having coined the term "pancreas" (pan = all, kreas = flesh).[1,18] This name was adopted by later anatomists who favored it over Galen's term "callicreas" (kallos = good). The ancient Hebrews customarily performed autopsies on ill animals considered by law not suitable to be eaten, and, as the Talmud attests, they knew about the pancreas which they called "finger of the liver." The organ attracted little attention during the Middle Ages until it was mentioned again near the end of the thirteenth century in Mondino de Luzzi's *Anathomia.*[19] The first thorough descriptions of the pancreas stem from the sixteenth century and are those of Andreas Vesalius (1514–1564) and of Gabriele Fallopio (1523–1562), his student.[20] Although Mondino de Luzzi had already mentioned the major pancreatic duct, it remained for Georg Wirsung, in 1642, to record this structure in detail.[21] Exactly 100 years later, in 1742, Giovanni Domenico Santorini followed with his description of the accessory duct of the gland.[22] Thomas Wharton (1610–1673) noted the structural similarity of the pancreas and the salivary glands.[23] The earliest systematic experiments on the external secretion of the pancreas were those of Regnier de Graaf (1641–1673), who collected pancreatic juice from a dog by means of a temporary fistula and recorded its "acid" reaction.[24]

While Thomas Cawley is usually credited with having been the first to associate diabetes with the pancreas,[1,4] a careful reading of his account[25] shows that he, like Galen (whom he quotes extensively), favored the kidneys, and not the pancreas, as the primary seat of this disorder (he concluded: "I take the proximate cause of diabetes to consist in a morbid dilatation of the uriniferous tubes of those organs, whereby they become pervious to the nutritious matter . . ."). Even though he did not make the connection, Cawley was the first to describe a case of pancreatogenic diabetes secondary to chronic calcifying pancreatitis. His patient was a 34-year-old man "accustomed to free living and strong corporeal exertions in the pursuit of country amusements," a phrase that makes one wonder whether he might perhaps have acquired his pancreatitis as a consequence of alcoholism. Actually, it was not until well in the nineteenth century that pancreatic lesions were unequivocally linked to diabetes by observers such as Lancereaux[26] and Frerichs.[27] Theoretically, the association could have been made as early as 1683 when Johann Conrad Brunner (1653–1727) succeeded in removing the pancreases of dogs and keeping the animals alive.[28] He noted that they displayed polydipsia and polyuria, but he failed to recognize these symptoms as being caused by diabetes, and his observations were soon forgotten. It remained for von Mering and Minkowski to repeat this experiment in 1889 and to establish, beyond any doubt, that total pancreatectomy in dogs causes diabetes.[29] From that date on, diabetes was linked closely to the pancreas, and for a long time all research in this field centered upon that organ.

Initially, it was believed that the external pancreatic secretion played a role in maintaining normal blood sugar levels. But when Hédon,[30] in 1893, observed that diabetes was absent in pancreatectomized dogs as long as a pancreatic transplant remained intact (in a situation in which external secretion could not occur), attention was drawn to the possibility that an internal, rather than an external, secretory function was instrumental in blood sugar homeostasis. During the same year of 1893, Laguesse[31] suggested that the islets of Langerhans (a name he proposed) were the anatomic substrate of the postulated internal secretion. These cells had first been described by Paul Langerhans (1849–1888) in his doctoral thesis of 1869.[32] Langerhans observed at low magnification tiny, intensely yellow spots, measuring 0.1 or 0.2 mm, in rabbit pancreas left for 2 or 3 days in Müller's fluid. He also identified these areas in the fresh gland and in glands stained for several days in iodinated serum, and found them to be composed of small, regular, polygonal translucent cells measuring 9 to 12 μm in diameter. Langerhans called these formations "Zellhaufen" (clusters of cells) and confessed his ignorance about their function, although he perceived "certain connections" with the nervous system since he had observed nerve fibers and ganglion cells in close proximity to such islet cells. Von Ebner, in 1872, confirmed the presence of these structures in the pancreas of the rabbit and frog but did not elaborate on their possible function.[33] Renaut,[34] in 1879, and Kühne and Lea,[35] 3 years later, suggested that these cell clusters were lymphatic follicles of a special nature, a view shared by many subsequent investigators.[36–45] Other authors, however, differed with this interpretation. Podwyssotski[46] denied that the cell clusters were lymphatic in origin; he called them "pseudo-follicles" without ascribing a specific function to them. Heidenhain and Luchsinger[47] adopted the name "intertubuläre Zellen," but they, too, failed to explain their nature. Others considered them modified[48] or exhausted[49] acinar cells or embryonic rests.[50]

The discovery of the pancreatic islets by Langerhans[32] in 1869 and the suggestion, advanced 24 years later by Laguesse,[31] that these structures are the anatomical counterpart of the internal secretory function of the organ were followed by studies that corroborated the existence of a relationship between the islets and carbohydrate metabolism, a relationship also claimed by Schäfer[51] and Diamare.[52] Both Dieckhoff[53] and Ssobolew,[54] for example, recorded the complete absence of islets in some cases of diabetes. In animal experiments, Ssobolew,[55] Dewitt,[56] and MacCallum[57] showed that pancreatic duct ligation is followed by atrophy of the exocrine parenchyma, whereas the islets survive and diabetes does not ensue. MacCallum[57] also demonstrated that the removal of such a duct-ligated organ will induce a diabetic state.

Soon after the turn of the century, several authors recorded a number of histologic alterations in the islets of Langerhans of diabetic individuals. In 1901, Opie[58,59] described hyalinization and sclerosis of the islets as well as interacinar fibrosis and parenchymal atrophy of the exocrine pancreas. During the same year, Weichselbaum and Stangl[60] found a reduction in islet number and size and a vacuolization of islet cells, the latter termed "hydropic degeneration." Other investigators, among them Lemoine and Lannois[30] and Hoppe-Seyler,[61] emphasized the frequent occurrence of arteriosclerotic lesions in such diabetic patients and suggested that pancreatic fibrosis (called "pancreatitis interstitialis angiosclerotica" by Hoppe-Seyler) as well as sclerosis of the pancreatic islets, with ensuing diabetes, were related to the impairment of the blood supply induced by vascular sclerosis. These authors and others[62-67] concluded that the islets of Langerhans and insular lesions such as the ones mentioned played an important, if not an exclusive, role in the causation of human diabetes. However, it soon became apparent that such alterations could also be observed in nondiabetic persons; for instance, Ohlmacher,[68] in 1904, and Saltykow,[64] 5 years later, recorded hyalinization of the islets in the absence of this disease, while Sauerbeck[69] encountered islet cell vacuolization in some nondiabetic subjects. Furthermore, it was realized that there are many diabetic pancreases which fail to display any islet lesion demonstrable by histologic examination,[69,70] a state of affairs that led to the exploration of extrapancreatic factors as possible causes—or partial causes—of the diabetic syndrome.

Foremost among such extrapancreatic factors were disorders of several endocrine glands known to affect carbohydrate metabolism. In 1886, Pièrre Marie first described a case of acromegaly associated with diabetes,[71] and 1 year later Minkowski recorded the presence of an eosinophilic adenoma of the pituitary in this disease.[72] Much later, the discovery that basophilic adenomas of the pituitary gland may cause Cushing's syndrome and the glycosuria often accompanying it[73] served to reemphasize the fact that a diabetic state can be induced by extrapancreatic lesions. In 1901, both Blum[74] and Zuelzer[75] observed cases of hyperglycemia caused by adrenalin, while Helly, in 1913, reported the association of hypertension and glycosuria in a patient with a medullary tumor of the adrenal gland.[76] However, the belief that a disturbance of adrenal medullary secretion might constitute the basic cause of diabetes collapsed when it was shown that adrenal medullectomy did not modify the clinical course of the disease in diabetic individuals.[77] The adrenal cortex, too, became implicated in diabetes after it was demonstrated that cortical adrenal tumors or hyperplasia can be associated with a disturbed carbohydrate metabolism.[78] Observations on hormone-induced hyperglycemia, such as those recorded here, led to the realization that in certain cases of diabetes, patients can be segregated from the general category of diabetics and placed within a group of diabetic patients with known extrapancreatic etiology. The present status of the role of extrapancreatic, diabetogenic hormonal agents has been explored in Chapters 11 and 18.

In the meantime, the histology of the pancreatic islets became a field for extensive study. Diamare,[52] in 1899, and Schulze,[79] 1 year later, were the first to realize that the islets of Langerhans contain more than one cell type. Other authors[55,80] soon confirmed these observations. In 1906, Tschassownikow[81] devised a method that permitted the tinctorial differentiation of the two cell types then known. Further progress in fixation and staining technology as applied to the pancreatic islets was achieved in 1907 by Lane,[82] who also introduced the designations "A cell" and "β cell," and by his teacher Bensley,[83] who changed Lane's term "β cell" to "B cell." Silver impregnation methods contributed further to the delineation of the pancreatic islet cells ever since Piazza,[84] in 1911, first reported that silver-positive cells do occur in this organ.

A third cell type, the D cell, was identified in 1931 by Bloom.[85] Thomas, in 1937, investigated the pancreases of 41 mammalian species and found that A, B, and D cells were present in all of them.[86]

Once an understanding of the basic facets of both the morphology and the function of the islet cells, and of their role in human diabetes, had been achieved, it became desirable to obtain further insight into the etiology and pathogenesis of diabetes by attempting to produce the disease in experimental animals. Various approaches were tried to that end. In the earliest experiments, conducted in 1913 by Allen[87] and slightly later by Homans,[88,89] up to 90% of the pancreatic parenchyma of dogs and cats was removed. Diabetes promptly ensued, and both investigators recorded hydropic degeneration and the eventual destruction of the B cells in the remaining portion of the organ. These changes were interpreted as the effect of exhaustion of this cellular system owing to excessive demands on its function.

The first experimental induction of diabetes by hormone action was accomplished in 1927 by Johns and his co-workers,[90] who caused dogs to become hyperglycemic after short-term injections of extracts from the anterior lobe of the pituitary gland. These results were confirmed by other investigators,[91,92] including Houssay,[93-98] who also established the existence of an antagonistic relationship between the functions of the anterior pituitary gland and the islets of Langerhans. Somewhat later, Young extended these experiments and demonstrated that prolonged daily injections in dogs of crude extracts from the anterior pituitary lobe will cause diabetes that persists indefinitely even after the injections have been discontinued.[99] Histologically, the B cells of such animals display degranulation and hydropic degeneration, and ultimately they become necrotic and disappear.[100,101] The changes are thus identical with those induced by subtotal pancreatectomy and were interpreted in a similar vein, i.e., as sequelae of functional B cell exhaustion brought on by the diabetic state. In 1936, Long and Lukens[102] were able to show that diabetes in adrenalectomized–depancreatized cats receiving daily injections of adrenocortical extract was much less intense than in animals subjected to pancreatectomy alone. Since that time, the induction of hyperglycemic states by 11-oxysteroid compounds has been repeatedly accomplished.[103-108]

Another avenue for the experimental production of diabetes opened up in 1943 when Dunn *et al.*[109] observed for the first time that alloxan causes selective necrosis of the pancreatic B cells and severe diabetes in rabbits. Additional chemical compounds capable of inducing permanent diabetes by destruction of B cells have since been discovered and tested. Foremost among these is streptozotocin; its diabetogenic properties were first recorded in 1963 by Rakieten *et al.*[110]

Harris,[111] in 1899, was the first to report a case of diabetes quickly following mumps. Similar observations in subsequent years[112,113] caused Gunderson,[113] in 1927, to suggest viral etiology for human diabetes. In recent years, it has been possible to test this hypothesis by experimental means following the demonstration, in 1966 by Craighead,[114] that the M variant of the encephalomyocarditis virus specifically attacks the B cells in the islets of Langerhans. It should be noted in this connection that insular inflammatory lesions (though not necessarily infectious in origin), termed "insulitis" by von Meyenberg,[115] had already been observed by Opie[59] in 1901 and by Schmidt[116] 1 year later. Renold *et al.,*[117] in 1964, were the first to experimentally induce insulitis in cows injected with crystalline bovine and porcine insulin in Freund's adjuvant, and in 1965 Lacy and Wright[118] did the same in rats subjected to guinea pig antiserum directed against bovine insulin. Observations such as those on virus-induced islet lesions and other types of "insulitis" contributed, in part, to the intense burgeoning of interest presently seen in the field of immunology (including autoimmune mechanisms) as it relates to diabetes mellitus (see Chapter 15).

The successful isolation of the blood-sugar-lowering hormone of the islets of Langerhans by Banting and Best,[119] in 1921, represents an important landmark in the history of diabetes. Other investigators[120–126] had tried to accomplish the same but had failed, either on account of technical difficulties or because the extracts they had obtained proved to be far too toxic to permit clinical trials in experimental animals or in human patients. Banting and Best prepared their extracts from both normal and duct-ligated canine pancreases as well as from adult beef pancreas and fetal calf pancreas, the latter being the most potent preparation. When administered to depancreatized dogs, these extracts resulted in a rapid amelioration of the diabetic state in many of these animals. When given to human diabetics, the effects were erratic at first, but the extracts were eventually purified by Collip, who succeeded in producing a preparation that was less toxic and more effective. As Papaspyros[1] relates, Banting and Best had first named the newly isolated hormone "isletin"; but at the insistence of Macleod, in whose laboratory the two young researchers worked, it came to be known as "insulin," a term that had already been proposed by de Mayer,[127] in 1909, and also by Sharpey-Schafer,[1] in 1916. Abel,[128] in 1926, obtained insulin in crystalline form, and Scott[129] established that zinc is indispensible for the crystallization of this hormone. The production of long-acting protamine zinc insulin by Hagedorn and his co-workers,[130] in 1936, initiated a new phase in the successful treatment of diabetics with insulin. The first direct demonstration of the hormone within the pancreatic B cells was accomplished with the fluorescent antibody technique by Lacy and Davies[131] in 1957.

Almost as soon as the first insulin preparations began to be administered for the treatment of diabetic patients, it was observed that these substances induced unexpected though transient hyperglycemia before lowering the blood sugar. In 1923, Murlin and his co-workers[132,133] suggested that the unknown hyperglycemic factor was a second pancreatic hormone which they called "glucagon." Its chemical characterization, initiated by Bürger and Brandt[134] in 1935, eventually lead to the isolation and crystallization of this protein by Staub and co-workers[135] in 1953. The first pivotal experiments demonstrating that it is the pancreatic A cell that manufactures, stores, and secretes glucagon were performed by Gaede *et al.*[136] and by Bencosme and co-workers.[137] From 1951 on, the availability of chemical agents which selectively damage the pancreatic A cells provided an additional means for research in this field; among the first ones utilized were cobaltous chloride, by van Campenhout and Cornelis,[138] sodium diethylthiocarbamate and potassium ethylxanthate, by Kadota and Midorikawa,[139] and Synthalin A, by Davis.[140] In 1962, Baum et al.[141] provided the first direct evidence for the production of glucagon in the A cells of the bovine pancreas by means of immunofluorescent techniques.

The elucidation of the function of the pancreatic D cells, which had remained a mystery for a long time, began when Alberti et al.,[142] in 1973, demonstrated that somatostatin, a growth hormone release-inhibiting polypeptide first isolated 2 years earlier by Vale and his co-workers,[143] lowers the basal plasma insulin levels in healthy human subjects by suppressing insulin release. These observations were soon confirmed and extended by other investigators. Moreover, it was established by several groups of workers and with different techniques that somatostatin is normally present in the mammalian pancreas and that it is the D cell of the islets of Langerhans that makes, stores (in the form of granules), and secretes this polypeptide hormone[143-150] (see Chapter 4).

During the purification of chicken insulin, Kimmel et al.,[151,152] in 1968, detected a straight-chain peptide with 36 amino acids which they named avian polypeptide (APP). Later, APP was found in pancreatic extracts of birds and reptiles.[153,154] Most recently, Larsson and co-workers[155-158] established by light- and electron-microscopic immunocytochemical studies in chicken and several mammals, including man, that pancreatic polypeptide (PP) is stored in insular and extrainsular pancreatic cells (PP cells) distinct from A, B, and D cells. The physiologic role of this newly identified class of pancreatic polypeptide hormones is still under investigation.

Recent research has clarified some of the many steps involved in the biosynthesis, storage, and release of insulin. It appears to be established that insulin is released from the B cell into the blood stream by emiocytosis, as first proposed in 1959 by Lacy and Hartroft[158] and recently confirmed by Orci et al.[159] in ultrastructural freeze-etching studies on isolated islets, a method that greatly facilitates the evaluation of events occurring on the cell surface (see Chapter 7). In 1968, Lacy and his co-workers[160] demonstrated the existence of an "internal cytoskeleton" in the B cell, and they suggested that the insulin-containing secretory granules are being translocated to the cell surface by and along the units of this microtubular–microfilamentous system which is thought to be responsive to high-energy intermediates of glucose. Since it has been shown that calcium is essential for insulin secretion,[161,162] Lacy,[163] in 1970, expanded his original model of B cell secretion by proposing that

> . . . calcium may be the trigger which would initiate contraction or a change in physical conformation of microtubules or microfilaments attached to the membrane around beta granules. This would result in the rapid displacement of the granules to the cell surface and liberation of these granules in tandem at specific loci on the plasma membrane.

Studies on biosynthesis, storage, and release of insulin, such as the ones mentioned, were considerably facilitated when Moskalewski,[164] in 1965, demonstrated that intact islets could be removed from the normal guinea pig

pancreas after incubation of the pancreatic tissue with collagenase; Moskalewski's original technique was subsequently modified and refined by Lacy and
his co-workers.[165,166]

Another line of investigation that promises to provide new insights into
normal and deranged functional states of pancreatic islet cells concerns itself
with the ultrastructure of their membranous systems. In 1975, Orci and
Unger[167] pointed out that insulin-producing B cells, glucagon-producing A
cells, and somatostatin-producing D cells are not randomly placed within the
islets. Since somatostatin inhibits the secretion of both insulin and glucagon, a
process apparently facilitated by the presence of certain surface membrane
modifications such as gap junctions between cells of different types,[168] an
ordered structural arrangement of A, B, and D cells would seem to have
important functional implications indeed.

In large measure, diabetes mellitus is determined by genetic and environmental factors. These factors are difficult, if not impossible, to control in
human populations. In 1950, Ingalls *et al.*[169] first described a new mutation in
the mouse characterized by the presence of diabetes and obesity. Since then, it
has become feasible to study the impact of genetic and environmental variables
on the disease within tightly controlled groups of experimental animals. By
1967, it was possible to draw up a list of 13 mutations, inbred strains, and
species lines that display a tendency for the spontaneous development of
diabetes.[170]

Tumors often exaggerate both normal and abnormal functional properties
of the nonneoplastic cells from which they arise and thus become suitable
objects for study. Wilder *et al.*,[171] in 1927, were the first to record the blood-
glucose-lowering effect of extracts obtained from endocrine pancreatic tumors.
As detailed in Chapter 22, several types of endocrine tumors, distinguishable
both by morphological criteria and by the hormonal compounds they produce,
can now be demonstrated in the pancreas. A method destined to facilitate
research in this field has been the successful experimental induction of such
tumors in laboratory animals. While islet cell neoplasms can be, and have been,
induced in some cases by irradiation[172] or by the injection of certain plant-
derived pyrrolizidin alkaloids,[173] a high-yield method involving the administration of streptozotocin and nicotinamide in the rat was devised in 1971, through
serendipity, by Rakieten *et al.*[174]; in two recorded series, 49%[175] and 64%[174] of
the rats so treated developed pancreatic islet cell tumors.

Two decades after the isolation of insulin by Banting and Best, another
landmark in the history of diabetes was the incidental discovery of the hypoglycemic effect of certain sulfonamide derivatives in the middle of World War II.
Samples of the first of these preparations, *p*-aminobenzenesulfonamidoiso-
propylthiodiazole, synthesized in Germany in 1941 by Kimmig[176] under the
designation VK 57, were tested (under the name 2254 RP) in France 1 year
later by Janbon *et al.*[177,178] in patients with typhoid fever. When Janbon and his
colleagues noted the occurrence of convulsions and coma in some of the
patients so treated (three of them actually died from these unexpected side
effects), they turned to Auguste L. Loubatières, who then studied the mechanism of action of this oral hypoglycemic agent. Loubatières quickly established

that the new drug failed to lower the blood sugar in depancreatized dogs, and he concluded that it stimulates the pancreas to increase the output of insulin.[179-182] Because of the conditions prevailing during the second half of World War II, Loubatières' work remained virtually unknown, and its potential for the treatment of diabetic patients was not realized for more than a decade. Then, between 1951 and 1953, history repeated itself when investigators in East Germany, among them Haack,[183,184] rediscovered the hypoglycemic effect of another, newly synthesized sulfonylurea compound; once more, several patients died before the drug was withdrawn. And again, the abnormal situation during the postwar years in the divided country prevented the dissemination of the newly gained knowledge. Thus, it was only after the third independent discovery, in 1955, of the hypoglycemic action of a sulfonylurea compound by a West German clinician, J. Fuchs (who had taken the drug himself), that systematic trials with diabetic patients were carried out and the era of oral diabetes treatment was initiated.[176,185-188]

Initially, it was believed that the sulfonylurea derivatives lower the blood sugar level by damaging the pancreatic A cells.[185-187] However, as early as 1946, Chen and co-workers[189] had already established that sulfanilamidocyclopropyl-thiadiazole is ineffective in the absence of pancreatic B cells since it fails to reduce the blood glucose concentrations in severely alloxan-diabetic rabbits. These results were confirmed in numerous studies from 1956 on, and it is generally agreed that the hypoglycemic sulfonylurea derivatives exert their effect by a reversible depletion of the insulin stores of the pancreatic B cells.[190]

In addition to insulin treatment and the administration of oral hypoglycemic agents, the transplantation of islets, first suggested as early as 1902 by Ssobolew,[55] has been attempted in an effort to ameliorate diabetes and retard the development of its complications. The numerous difficulties inherent in this procedure, and the various techniques applied, are discussed in Chapter 21. The first successful transplantation of isolated islets has been recorded in 1972 by Ballinger and Lacy,[191] who demonstrated that placement of islets into the peritoneal cavity or into muscle pouches appreciably alters the course of streptozotocin-induced diabetes in the rat.

References

1. Papaspyros, N. S.: *The History of Diabetes Mellitus.* 2nd Ed. Georg Thieme Verlag, Stuttgart, 1964.
2. Bryan, C. P.: *The Papyrus Ebers.* Bles, London, 1930.
3. *The Papyrus Ebers, The Greatest Egyptian Medical Document.* Translated by B. Ebbell. Copenhagen, 1937.
4. Lazarus, S. S., and Volk, B. W.: *The Pancreas in Human and Experimental Diabetes.* Grune & Stratton, New York, 1962, p. 1.
5. Celsus, A. A. C.: *De Medicina.* With an English Translation by W. G. Spencer; 3 Vol. London, 1935–1938.
6. Wong, K. C., and Wu, Lien-Teh: *History of Chinese Medicine.* Tientsin Press, Tientsin, 1932.
7. Avicenna (Ibn Sina): *A Treatise on the Canon of Medicine, Incorporating a Translation of the First Book,* by O. C. Gruner. London, 1930.

8. Paracelsus, Aureolus Philippus Theophrastus: *Sämtliche Werke.* 4 Vol. G. Fischer, Jena, 1926–1932.

9. Van Helmont, J. B.: *Ortus Medicinae.* L. Elzevir, Amsterdam, 1648.

10. Willis, T.: *Opera Omnia.* 2 Vol. Geneva, 1676–1680.

11. Dobson, M.: *Med. Obs. Inq.,* **5**:298, 1776.

12. Cullen, W.: *The First Lines of the Practice of Physic.* Edinburgh, 1787.

13. Rollo, J.: *An Account of Two Cases of the Diabetes Mellitus.* London, 1797.

14. Bouchardat, A.: *De la Glycosurie ou Diabète Sucré; Son Traitment Hygiènique.* Paris, 1875.

15. Bernard, C.: *Arch. Gen. Méd. (Paris),* **18**:303, 1848.

16. Bernard, C.: *C. R. Acad. Sci. (Memoires),* **41**:461, 1855.

17. Bernard, C.: *C. R. Soc. Biol.,* **1**:60, 1850.

18. Rufus of Ephesus: 1st French Ed. by C. Daremberg and C. E. Ruelle, Paris, 1879.

19. Wickersheimer, E.: *Anatonies de Guido de Vigevano et de Mondino dei Luzzi.* E. Droz, Paris, 1926.

20. Schwarz, I.: *Sudhoffs Arch. Gesch. Med.,* **3**:403, 1909/10.

21. Wirsung, G.: In: *Geschichte und Bibliographie der anatomischen Abbildung.* R. Weigel, Leipzig, 1852.

22. Santorini, G. D.: *Observationes Anatomicae.* J. B. Recurti, Venice, 1724.

23. Wharton, T.: *Adenographia Sive Glandularum Totus Corporis Descriptio.* London, 1656.

24. De Graaf, R.: *Disputatio Medica de Natura et Usu Succi Pancreatici.* Leyden, 1664.

25. Cawley, T.: *London Med. J.,* **9**:286, 1788.

26. Lancereaux, E.: *Union Méd.,* **29**:161, 1880.

27. Frerichs, F. T.: *Über den Diabetes.* Hirschwald, Berlin, 1884.

28. Brunner, J. C.: *Experimenta Nova circa Pancreas.* H. Wetstenium, Amsterdam, 1683.

29. Von Mering, J., and Minkowski, O.: *Arch. Exp. Pathol. Pharmacol.,* **26**:371, 1890.

30. Hédon, E.: *Arch. Physiol. Norm. Pathol.,* **5**:154, 1893.

31. Laguesse, E.: *C. R. Soc. Biol.,* **5**:819, 1893.

32. Langerhans, P.: Beiträge zur mikroskopischen Anatomie der Bauchspeicheldrüse. Inaugural-Dissertation, G. Lange, Berlin, 1869.

33. Von Ebner, V.: *Arch. Mikr. Anat.,* **8**:481, 1872.

34. Renaut, J.: *C. R. Acad. Sci.,* **89**:247, 1879.

35. Kühne, W., and Lea, A. S.: *Unters. aus dem Physiol. Inst. d. Univ. Heidelberg,* **2**:448, 1882.

36. Sokoloff, B.: Über die Bauchspeicheldrüse in verschiedenen Phasen ihrer Tätigkeit. Inaugural-Dissertation, M. I. Lumsch, St. Petersburg, 1883.

37. Krause, W.: *Die Anatomie des Kaninchen.* Engelmann, Leipzig, 1884.

38. Ellenberger, W.: *Grundriss der vergleichenden Histologie der Haussäugetiere.* Parey, Berlin, 1887.

39. Lemoine, G., and Lannois, M.: *Arch. Med. Exp. Anat. Pathol.,* **3**:33, 1891.

40. Dieckhoff, C.: Beiträge zur pathologischen Anatomie des Pankreas, mit besonderer Berücksichtigung der Diabetes-Frage. Inaugural-Dissertation, Rostock, 1894.

41. Mouret, M.: *C. R. Soc. Biol.,* **46**:731, 1894.

42. Kasahara, M.: *Arch. pathol. Anat.,* **143**:111, 1896.

43. Pugnat, C. A.: *C. R. Soc. Biol.,* **3**:1017, 1896.

44. Osawa, G.: *Arch. Mikr. Anat.,* **51**:481, 1898.

45. Orru, E.: *Monit. Zool. Ital.,* **11**:119, 1900.

46. Podwyssotski, W.: *Arch. Mikr. Anat.,* **21**:765, 1882.

47. Heidenhain, R., and Luchsinger, B.: *Handbuch der Physiologie.* Vol. 5, part 1. F. C. W. Vogel, Leipzig, 1879–1882.

48. Lewaschew, S. W.: *Arch. Mikr. Anat.,* **26**:453, 1885/86.

49. Dogiel, A.: *Arch. Anat. Entw. Gesch.,* p. 118, 1893.

50. Gibbes, H.: *Quart. J. Microsc. Sci.,* **24**:183, 1884.

51. Schäfer, E. A.: *Lancet,* **2**:321, 1895.

52. Diamare, V.: *Int. Mschr. Anat. Physiol.,* **16**:155, 1899.

53. Dieckhoff, C.: Beiträge zur pathologischen Anatomie des Pankreas mit besonderer Berücksichtigung der Diabetes-Frage. In: *Beiträge zur wissenschaftlichen Medizin, Festschrift für Theodor Thierfelder.* Leipzig, 1895.

54. Ssobolew, L. W.: *Zbl. Allg. Path. Path. Anat.,* **11**:202, 1900.

55. Ssobolew, L. W.: *Virchows Arch. Pathol. Anat.,* **168**:91, 1902.
56. Dewitt, L. M.: *J. Exp. Med.,* **7**:193, 1906.
57. MacCallum, W. G.: *Bull. Johns Hopkins Hosp.,* **20**:264, 1909.
58. Opie, E. L.: *J. Exp. Med.,* **5**:397, 1901.
59. Opie, E. L.: *J. Exp. Med.,* **5**:527, 1901.
60. Weichselbaum, A., and Stangl, E.: *Wien. Klin. Wochenschr.,* 14:968, 1901.
61. Hoppe-Seyler, G.: *Dtsch. Arch. Klin. Med.,* **52**:171, 1893.
62. Herzog, M.: *Virchows Arch. Pathol. Anat.,* **168**:83, 1902.
63. Von Halasz, A.: *Orvosi Hetilap,* **47**:723, 1903.
64. Saltykow, O.: *Corresp. Blatt Schweiz. Ärzte,* **39**:625, 1909.
65. Simmonds: *Dtsch. Med. Wochenschr.,* **38**:1020, 1912.
66. Fischer, B.: *Frankf. Z. Pathol.* **17**:218, 1915.
67. Lubarsch, O., and Wolff, E.: *Jahresk. Ärztl. Fortb.,* **16**:2, 1925.
68. Ohlmacher, J. C.: *Amer. J. Med. Sci.,* **128**:287, 1904.
69. Sauerbeck. E.: *Virchows Arch. Pathol. Anat.,* **177**:1, 1904.
70. Sauerbeck, E.: *Erg. Allg. Path. Path. Anat.,* **8**:538, 1902.
71. Marie, P.: *Rev. Méd.,* **6**:297, 1886.
72. Minkowski, O.: *Berl. Klin. Wochenschr.,* **24**:371, 1887.
73. Cushing, H.: *Bull. Johns Hopkins Hosp.,* **50**:137, 1932.
74. Blum, F.: *Dtsch. Arch. Klin. Med.,* **71**:146, 1901.
75. Zuelzer, G.: *Berl. Klin. Wochenschr.,* **38**:1209, 1901.
76. Helly, K.: *Münch. Med. Wochenschr.,* **60**:1811, 1913.
77. Grollman, A.: *The Adrenals.* William & Wilkins, Baltimore, 1936.
78. Achard, C., and Thièrs, J.: *Bull. Acad. Méd. (Paris),* **86**:51, 1921.
79. Schulze, W.: *Arch. Mikr. Anat.,* **56**:491, 1900.
80. Mankowski, A.: *Arch. Mikr. Anat.,* **59**:286, 1902.
81. Tschassownikow, S.: *Arch. Mikr. Anat.,* **67**:758, 1906.
82. Lane, M. A.: *Amer. J. Anat.,* **7**:409, 1907.
83. Bensley, R. R.: *Amer. J. Anat.,* **12**:297, 1911.
84. Piazza, C.: *Anat. Anz.,* **39**:127 & 167, 1911.
85. Bloom, W.: *Anat. Rec.,* **49**:363, 1931.
86. Thomas, T. B.: *Amer. J. Anat.,* **62**:31, 1937/38.
87. Allen, F. M.: *Studies Concerning Glycosuria and Diabetes.* W. M. Leonard, Boston, 1913.
88. Homans, J.: *J. Med. Res.,* **30**:49, 1914.
89. Homans, J.: *J. Med. Res.,* **33**:1, 1915.
90. Johns, W. S., O'Mulvenny, T. O., Potts, E. G., and Laughton, N. B.: *Amer. J. Physiol.,* **80**:100, 1927.
91. Evans, H. M., Meyer, K., Simpson, M. E., and Reichert, F. L.: *Proc. Soc. Exp. Biol. Med.,* **29**:857, 1932.
92. Baumann, E. J., and Marine, D.: *Proc. Soc. Exp. Biol. Med.,* **29**:1220, 1932.
93. Houssay, B. A., Biasotti, A., and Rietti, C. T.: *C. R. Soc. Biol.,* **111**:479, 1932.
94. Houssay, B. A., and Biasotti, A.: *Rev. Soc. Argent. Biol.,* **6**:8, 1930.
95. Houssay, B. A., Biasotti, A., di Benedetto, E., and Rietti, C. T.: *C. R. Soc. Biol.,* **112**:494, 1933.
96. Houssay, B. A., Biasotti, A., and Rietti, C. T.: *Rev. Soc. Argent. Biol.,* **9**:489, 1933.
97. Houssay, B. A., and Foglia, V.: *Rev. Soc. Argent. Biol.,* **12**:237, 1936.
98. Houssay, B. A.: *Endicrinology,* **30**:884, 1942.
99. Young, F. G.: *Lancet,* **2**:372, 1937.
100. Richardson, K. C., and Young, F. G.: *Lancet,* **1**:1098, 1938.
101. Richardson, K. C.: *Proc. Roy. Soc. London, S. B.,* **128**:153, 1940.
102. Long, C. N. H., and Lukens, F. D. W.: *J. Exp. Med.,* **63**:465, 1936.
103. Hausberger, F. X., and Ramsay, A. J.: *Endocrinology,* **53**:423, 1953.
104. Hausberger, F. X., and Ramsay, A. J.: *Endocrinology,* **56**:533, 1955.
105. Kobernick, S. D., and More, R. H.: *Proc. Soc. Exp. Biol. Med.,* **74**:602, 1950.
106. Lazarus, S. S., and Bencosme, S. A.: *Proc. Soc. Exp. Biol. Med.,* **89**:114, 1955.
107. Lazarus, S. S., and Bencosme, S. A.: *Amer. J. Clin. Pathol.,* **26**:1146, 1956.
108. Volk, B. W., and Lazarus, S. S.: *Amer. J. Pathol.,* **34**:121, 1958.

109. Dunn, J. S., Sheehan, H. L., and McLetchie, N. G. B.: *Lancet,* **1**:484, 1943.
110. Rakieten, N., Rakieten, M. C., and Nadkarni, M. V.: *Cancer Chemother. Rep.,* **29**:91, 1963.
111. Harris, H. F.: *Boston Med. Surg. J.,* **140**:465, 1899.
112. Patrick, A.: *Brit. Med. J.,* **2**:802, 1924.
113. Gunderson, E.: *J. Infect. Dis.,* **41**:197, 1927.
114. Craighead, J. E.: *Amer. J. Pathol.,* 48:375, 1966.
115. Von Meyenberg, H.: *Schweiz. Med. Wochenschr.,* **21**:554, 1940.
116. Schmidt, H. B.: *Münch. Med. Wochenschr.,* **49**:51, 1902.
117. Renold, A. E., Soeldner, J. S., and Steinke, J.: *Immunological Studies with Homologous and Heterologous Pancreatic Insulin in the Cow.* Edited by M. P. Cameron and M. O'Connor. Ciba Foundation Colloquium, Churchill, London, Vol. 15, 1964, p. 122.
118. Lacy, P. E., and Wright, D. H.: *Diabetes,* **14**:634, 1965.
119. Banting, F. G., and Best, C. H.: *J. Lab. Clin. Med.,* **7**:464, 1921/22.
120. Gley, E.: *C. R. Soc. Biol.,* **87**:1322, 1922.
121. Rennie, J., and Fraser, T.: *Biochem. J.,* **2**:7, 1906.
122. Scott, E. L.: *Amer. J. Physiol.,* **29**:306, 1911/12.
123. Murlin, J. R., and Kramer, B.: *J. Biol. Chem.,* **15**:365, 1913/14.
124. Kleiner, I. S.: *J. Biol. Chem.,* **40**:153, 1919.
125. Zuelzer, G.: *Berl. Klin. Wochenschr.,* **44**:474, 1907.
126. De Witt, L.: Quoted by Papaspyros (1).
127. De Mayer, J.: *Arch. Fisiol.,* **7**:96, 1909.
128. Abel, J. J.: *Proc. Nat. Acad. Sci.,* **12**:132, 1926.
129. Scott, D. A.: *Biochem. J.,* **28**:1592, 1934.
130. Hagedorn, H. C., Jensen, B. N., Krakup, N. N., and Wodstrup, I.: *J. Amer. Med. Assoc.,* **106**:177, 1936.
131. Lacy, P. E., and Davies, J.: *Diabetes,* **6**:354, 1957.
132. Murlin, J. R., Clough, H. G., Gibbs, C. B. F., and Stokes, A. M.: *J. Biol. Chem.,* **56**:253, 1923.
133. Kimball, C. P., and Murlin, J. R.: *J. Biol. Chem.,* **58**:337, 1923.
134. Bürger, M., and Brandt, W.: *Z. Gesamte Exp. Med.,* **96**:375, 1935.
135. Staub, A., Sinn, L., and Behrens, O. K.: *Science,* **117**:628, 1953.
136. Gaede, K., Ferner, H., and Kastrup, H.: *Klin. Wochenschr.,* **28**:388, 1950.
137. Bencosme, S. A., Liepa, E., and Lazarus, S. S.: *Proc. Soc. Exp. Biol. Med.,* **90**:387, 1955.
138. Van Campenhout, E., and Cornelis, G.: *C. R. Soc. Biol.,* **145**:933, 1951.
139. Kadota, I., and Midorikawa, O.: *J. Lab. Clin. Med.,* **38**:671, 1951.
140. Davis, J. C.: *J. Pathol. Bacteriol.,* **64**:575, 1952.
141. Baum, J., Simon, B. E., Jr., Unger, R. H., and Madison, L. L.: *Diabetes,* **11**:371, 1962.
142. Alberti, K. G. M. M., Christensen, N. J., Christensen, S. E., Hansen, A. P., Iversen, J., Lundbaek, K., Seyer-Hansen, K., and Ørskov, H.: *Lancet,* **2**:1299, 1973.
143. Vale, W., Brazeau, P., Rivier, C., Brown, M., Boss, R., Rivier, J., Burgus, R., Ling, N., and Guillemin, R.: *Rec. Progr. Horm. Res.,* **31**:365, 1975.
144. Hökfelt, T., Efendic, S., Hellerström, C., Johansson, O., Luft, R., and Arimura, A.: *Acta Endocrinol. Suppl.,* 200:5, 1975.
145. Arimura, A., Sato, H., Dupont, A., Nishi, N., and Schally, A. V.: *Science,* **189**:1007, 1975.
146. Pelletier, G., Leclerc, R., Arimura, A., and Schally, A. V.: *J. Histochem. Cytochem.,* **23**:699, 1975.
147. Dubois, M.: *Proc. Nat. Acad. Sci. USA,* **72**:1340, 1975.
148. Orci, L., Baetens, D., Dubois, M. P., and Rufener, C.: *Horm. Metabl. Res.,* **7**:400, 1975.
149. Polak, J., Pearse, A. G. E., Grimelius, L., Bloom, S. R., and Arimura, A.: *Lancet,* **1**:1220, 1975.
150. Goldsmith, P. C., Rose, J. Arimura, A., and Ganong, W. F.: *Endocrinology,* **97**:1061, 1975.
151. Kimmel, J. R., Pollock, H. G., and Hazelwood, R. L.: *Endocrinology,* **83**:1323, 1968.
152. Kimmel, J. P., Pollock, H. G., and Hazelwood, R. L.: *Fed. Proc.,* **30**:1318, 1971.
153. Langslow, D. R., Kimmel, J. R., and Pollock, H. G.: *Endocrinology,* **93**:558, 1973.
154. Hazelwood, R. L., Turner, S. D., Kimmel, J. R., and Pollock, H. G.: *Gen. Comp. Endocrinol.,* **21**:485, 1973.
155. Larsson, L. I., Sundler, F., Håkanson, R., Pollock, H. G., and Kimmel, J. R.: *Histochemistry,* **42**:377, 1974.
156. Larsson, L. I., Sundler, F., and Håkanson, R.: *Cell Tissue Res.,* **156**:167, 1975.

157. Larsson, L. I., Sundler, F., and Håkanson, R.: *Diabetologia,* **12**:211, 1976.
158. Lacy, P. E., and Hartroft, W. S.: *Ann. N.Y. Acad. Sci.,* **82**:287, 1959.
159. Orci, L., Amherdt, M., Malaisse-Lagae, F., Rouillier, C., and Renold, A. E.: *Science,* **179**:82, 1973.
160. Lacy, P. E., Howell, S. L., Young, D. A., and Fink, C. J.: *Nature (London),* **219**:1177, 1968.
161. Grodsky, G. M., and Bennett, L. I.: *Diabetes,* **15**:910, 1966.
162. Milner, R. D. G., and Hales, C. W.: *Diabetologia,* **3**:47, 1967.
163. Lacy, P. E.: *Diabetes,* **19**:895, 1970.
164. Moskalewski, S.: *Gen. Comp. Endocrinol.,* **5**:342, 1965.
165. Lacy, P. E., and Kostianovsky, M.: *Diabetes,* **16**:35, 1967.
166. Lacy, P. E., Young, D. A., and Fink, C. J.: *Endocrinology,* **83**:1155, 1968.
167. Orci, L., and Unger, R. H.: *Lancet,* **2**:1243, 1975.
168. Orci, L., Malaisse-Lagae, F., Ravazzola, M., Rouiller, D., Renold, A. E., Perrelet, A., and Unger, R. H.: *J. Clin. Invest.,* **56**:1066, 1975.
169. Ingalls, A. M., Dickie, M. M., and Snell, G. D.: *J. Hered.,* **41**:317, 1950.
170. Renold, A. E., and Dulin, W. E.: *Diabetologia,* **3**:63, 1967.
171. Wilder, R. M., Allan, F. N., Power, M. H., and Robertson, H. E.: *J. Amer. Med. Assoc.,* **89**:348, 1927.
172. Boschetti, A. E., and Moloney, W. C.: *Lab. Invest.,* **15**:565, 1966.
173. Schoental, R., Fowler, M. E., and Coady, A.: *Cancer Res.,* **30**:2127, 1970.
174. Rakieten, N., Gordon, B. S., Beaty, A., Cooney, D. A., Davis, R. D., and Schein, P. S.: *Proc. Soc. Exp. Biol. Med.,* **137**:280, 1971.
175. Volk, B. W., Wellmann, K. F., and Brancato, P.: *Diabetologia,* **10**:37, 1974.
176. Kimmig, T., quoted by Schadewaldt, H.: *Dtsche. Med. Wochenschr.,* **100**:2653, 1975.
177. Janbon, M., Chaptal, J., Vedel, A., and Schap, J.: *Montpellier Méd.,* **21–22**:441, 1942.
178. Janbon, M., Lazergues, P., and Metropolitanski, J. H.: *Montpellier Méd.,* **21–22**:489, 1942.
179. Loubatières, A., Goldstein, L., Metropolitanski, J., and Schaap, J.: In: *43 ième Congrés Médecins Aliénistes et Neurologistes de France et des Pays de Langue Française.* Montpellier, Masson, Paris, 1942, p. 415.
180. Loubatières, A.: *C. R. Soc. Biol.,* **138**:766, 1944.
181. Loubatières, A.: Physiologie et Pharmacodynamie de Certains Dérivés Sulfamides Hypoglycémiants. Thesis, Montpellier. Causse, Graille & Castelnau, Montpellier, 1946.
182. Loubatières, A.: *Arch. Int. Physiol.,* **54**:174, 1946.
183. Haack, E.: Discussion remark during the meeting of the Thuringian Pediatric Society, Jena, Germany, April 21, 1951.
184. Haack, E., quoted by Kleinsorge, H.: *Dtsche. Med. Wochenschr.,* **101**:467, 1976.
185. Franke, H., and Fuchs, J.: *Dtsch. Med. Wochenschr.,* **80**:1449, 1955.
186. Achelis, J. D., and Hardebeck, K.: *Dtsch. Med. Wochenschr.,* **80**:1452, 1955.
187. Bertram, F., Bendfeldt, E., and Otto, H.: *Dtsch. Med. Wochenschr.* **80**:1455, 1955.
188. Schadewaldt, H.: *Geschichte des Diabetes Mellitus.* Springer-Verlag, Berlin/Heidelberg/New York, 1975.
189. Chen, K. K., Anderson, R. C., and Maze, N.: *Proc. Soc. Exp. Biol. Med.,* **63**:483, 1946.
190. Lazarus, S. S., and Volk, B. W.: *The Pancreas in Human and Experimental Diabetes.* Grune & Stratton, New York, 1962, Chap. 22, p. 240.
191. Ballinger, W. F., and Lacy, P. E.: *Surgery,* **72**:*175, 1972.*

Chapter 2

Comparative Morphology of Pancreatic Islets in Animals

Sture Falkmer and Yngve Östberg

About 5 years ago the comparative endocrinology of the pancreatic islets was analyzed in two reviews from our laboratory,[1,2] when we tried to cover most of the relevant literature in that field published before 1971. Since then, remarkable advances have been made in the understanding of pancreatic islet hormone formation, secretion, molecular structure, and membrane receptor sites.[3,4] The intimate relationship that was found both phylogenetically and ontogenetically between the islet parenchyma and the endocrine cells of the gastrointestinal (GI) tract[1,2] has been further substantiated structurally,[5] as well as biochemically, physiologically, and clinically.[6-10] Moreover, the APUD (amine precursor uptake and decarboxylation) concept has become so well established that it is now obvious that the islet and GI endocrine cells belong to one and the same system.[11-14] As a matter of fact, the whole field of peptide endocrinology seems to become neuroendocrinology,[13] and a completely new approach has been offered to solve some crucial problems in the pathology of endocrine neoplasms in general and of so-called islet cell tumors in particular.[11,12] Recently, new aspects have also come to light on the production sites in the pancreas and the GI tract of somatostatin,[15,16] gastrin,[17,18] the newly discovered pancreatic polypeptide (PP),[19-21] and other hormones of the gastro-entero-pancreatic (GEP) endocrine system.[5,8-14] The methods for the structural analysis of GEP cells have been critically scrutinized,[22] improved, and standardized,[11,12] and, as a result, there has been rapid progress in the understanding of the cellular composition of the islet parenchyma in various kinds of neoplasia and hyperplastic conditions in man.[20,23-26] The islet cells, appearing in these pathologic states—but only rarely observed in normal human islets—seem to be (at least structurally) related to those parenchymal cells that occur in the endocrine pancreas of lower vertebrates, offering opportunities for comparisons between neo- (or hyper-)plastically dedifferentiated and phylogenetically immature islet cells.[26] This gives further reasons for a continued and intensified research on the comparative morphology of the pancreatic islets, particularly in lower animals.

Sture Falkmer and Yngve Östberg. • University of Umea, Umea, Sweden.

Against this background it is obvious that the preceding reviews[1,2]—and even a few more recent ones from our laboratory[27,28]—should be supplemented by an updated and revised edition, comprising the whole GEP endocrine system.

Taxonomy

As in preceding reports from our laboratory,[1,2,27,28] we have in the present review also tried to follow Karl Grobben's taxonomic classification of the animal kingdom, where two evolutionary lines are distinguished above the coelenterates (jellyfish, sea anemones, etc.), viz., the protostomian and the deuterostomian (Fig. 1). The former consists primarily of annelids, molluscs, and arthropods, but contains a considerable number of additional phyla, subphyla, classes, and orders (which have only been faintly outlined by three open lines in Fig. 1), forming the quantitatively predominating group. The deuterostomian line of evolution comprises all the vertebrates and those invertebrates that during their embryonic life have some features in common with the vertebrates, viz. (among others), the cephalochordate amphioxus and other protochordates, such as tunicates. The echinoderms also belong to these invertebrates. Among the vertebrates the cyclostomes (or Agnatha) are considered to be a sister group to all the gnathostomian vertebrates, possibly with a common Precambrian ancestor.[27]

The primary justification for this subdivision is embryological. It has been criticized and modified several times. We have previously given a brief account of its main features,[27] which are the formation of the mouth and anus, the method of coelom and mesoderm formation, and the localization of the nervous system, the occurrence of bilateral symmetry, and other developmental aspects.

Methods

In addition to the recent progress outlined in the introduction, there has also been some advance during the last 5 years with reference to the terminology of the GEP endocrine cells, notably the use of the so-called revised Wiesbaden classification as nomenclature.[29] Moreover, immunocytochemical and fluorescence histochemical characterizations of hormone-producing cells have both become more widely used than previously, owing to refined procedures[30-34] and to increased insight into the molecular composition of some islet hormones in lower vertebrates.[28,35] Notwithstanding, much work remains to be done here before the definitions of all the different GEP endocrine cells have been ultimately settled. For the present review at least some kind of operational definition is needed, employing histotechnical procedures that are fairly widely used and found to be reliable in the structural analysis of the endocrine pancreas of higher vertebrates.[1,12,22] It must be emphasized—as properly done

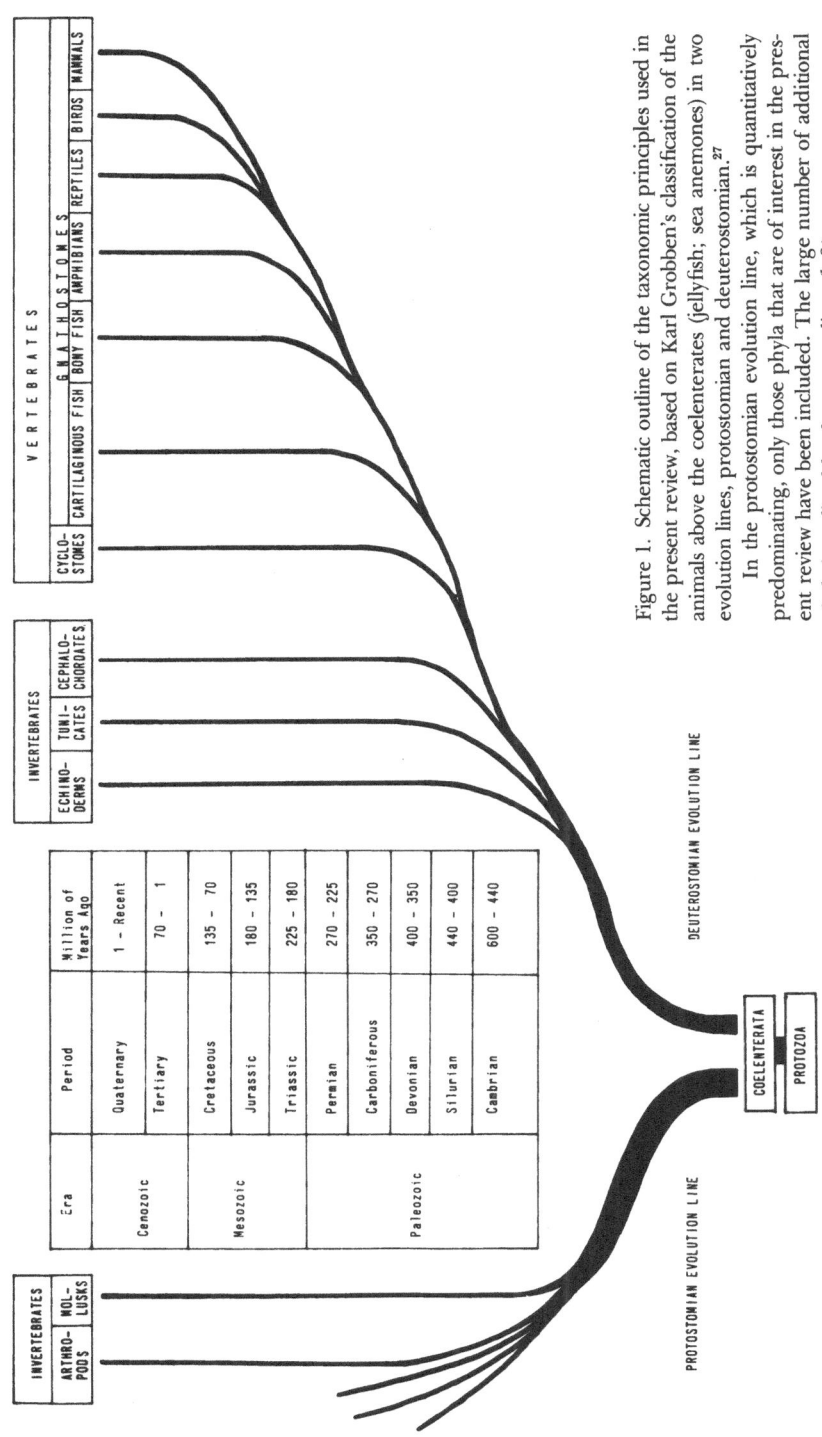

Figure 1. Schematic outline of the taxonomic principles used in the present review, based on Karl Grobben's classification of the animals above the coelenterates (jellyfish; sea anemones) in two evolution lines, protostomian and deuterostomian.[27]

In the protostomian evolution line, which is quantitatively predominating, only those phyla that are of interest in the present review have been included. The large number of additional phyla is outlined by three open lines (left).

The deuterostomian evolution line comprises both invertebrates and vertebrates. Among the former, echinoderms (starfish, sea urchins, etc.), tunicates (sea squirts), and the cephalochordate amphioxus are found. They all show several features in common with the vertebrates during embryonic life. Among the vertebrates (craniates), the cyclostomes (or Agnatha: hagfish and lampreys) form a sister group to all the gnathostomes (those equipped with jaws), possibly with a Cambrian or Precambrian ancestor.

by Lange in his excellent survey[22]—that the methods (particularly the histological ones) often have to be modified in several respects before they can be successfully applied to the GEP endocrine cells of nonmammalian species.

Conventional Histology

The principal histological methods used by us[1,36] and by others[12,22] are as follows*: (1) Lead hematoxylin to show the presence of endocrine cells in general; (2) aldehyde fuchsin (Af), chrome hematoxylin, and/or pseudoisocyanin (PIC) to detect insulin-producing cells (B cells); (3) Grimelius' silver nitrate stain for revealing glucagon-producing cells (A cells) in the pancreatic islets, enteroglucagon-producing cells (EG cells) of the GI mucosa, the D_1 (type IV) cells of the endocrine pancreas and the GI mucosa, the gastrin-producing cells (G cells)—and apparently also some other endocrine cells—of the GI mucosa; (4) the Hellerström–Hellman modification of the Davenport procedure to visualize the A_1 cells, which in most respects are synonymous with the somatostatin-containing, ultrastructurally defined D cells (see below) and possibly also some of the small-granulated islet cells; (5) the Masson–Hamperl method (or Singh modification) to detect argentaffin or enterochromaffin cells (EC cells), mainly occurring in the intestinal mucosa.

As stated previously,[1] the staining sequence of Epple (using some of these procedures), supplemented with Grimelius' silver nitrate staining method, gives a differentiation that is quite sufficient for many light-microscopical studies of comparative nature.

Specific Cytochemistry

For a more complete light-microscopical characterization of alleged endocrine cells, the conventional histological methods are as a rule supplemented by cytochemical procedures, essentially formaldehyde-induced fluorescence of biogenic amines and amine precursor uptake experiments, i.e., so-called APUD-FIF cytochemistry. Also, the fluorescamine-induced fluorescence procedure is used.

The histochemical procedures for detecting the presence of heavy metals, notably zinc, and proteins rich in tryptophan (particularly glucagon) have come to be less often applied, as they do not seem to contribute much to the differentiation of the various GEP cells.[1]

Immunocytochemistry

As mentioned in the introduction, recent years have seen rapid advances in the immunofluorescence and immunoperoxidase techniques, due to the fact that, surprisingly enough, antisera to mammalian polypeptide hormones have

---

*References to the original publications, where the procedures are described and the results are interpreted, are as a rule given in earlier reviews.[1,12,22,36]

been found to be reactive specifically with corresponding hormones of the lowest vertebrates[27,28] and even with those of protostomian invertebrates.[37] This fact has also opened up the possibility of using highly sensitive and specific radioimmunological procedures to check the immunocytochemical results by direct hormonal assays, as recommended previously when working with tissues of remotely related species.[1] A fairly large number of antisera are now available, but mistakes can still be made, owing to the fact that reactions with the antisera are not absolutely specific and that cross-reactions with other hormones or polypeptides cannot be excluded.[9] This is easily understood for the GI endocrine system, where the hormones of the gastrin group [cholecystokinin (CCK) caerulein, and various gastrins] and those of the secretin–glucagon family [secretin, glucagon, vasoactive intestinal peptide (VIP), gastric inhibitory peptide (GIP)] show great similarities in the sequences of their amino acid residues.[6-10] Moreover, for comparative purposes it is imperative to remember that only positive results are significant.[12]

Transmission Electron Microscopy (TEM)

It should also be stressed that specific immunocytochemistry will usually be unsuccessful unless there is ultrastructural evidence of the presence of at least a few secretion granules in the cells investigated.[11,12] Consequently, an ultrastructural analysis, usually by means of TEM, is required. Another reason is that some information on the structure of the storage granules must be available in order to classify the cells according to the revised Wiesbaden nomenclature.[29] The granule ultrastructure may be so characteristic that it is diagnostic.[12]

Identification of Hormone Production of Different Cell Types

Ideally, identification of hormone-producing cells should rest on immunocytochemistry at an ultrastructural level[30,31] or, at least, on the analysis of serial sections, where immunofluorescence in a semithin section is matched precisely with the results of a TEM study of an adjacent section in the series.[32] Unfortunately, fixation allowing preservation of the antigen/antibody reaction is suboptimal for TEM, implying that correlations may often be difficult.[9] Usually, however, a plausible interpretation is possible by this procedure.[40]

Definitions

Since the revised Wiesbaden classification[29] was published in 1973, the research front has been advanced so rapidly that a new revision seems necessary.[40] Therefore, some minor modifications have been made in this review, based on the methods described in the preceding paragraph. In accordance with the revised Wiesbaden nomenclature[29] and well-established practice in European literature,[23] the Latin alphabet is used for the cells and the Greek alphabet for the granules.

A Cells

In the pancreatic islet parenchyma, this cell type is clearly defined (by microdissection and direct hormonal assays) as the production site of pancreatic glucagon.[28] It is easily detected by Grimelius' silver nitrate procedure; it is of APUD type; it gives bright immunofluorescence with antisera against pancreatic glucagon; and its secretion granules are of astonishingly similar type throughout the gnathostomian vertebrate series,[2] although their size can differ considerably.[22] This cell type is synonymous with the A_2 or α_2 cells of other authors.[1]

Considering the recent discoveries in the mammalian stomach mucosa of the production of a polypeptide hormone identical to pancreatic glucagon ("stomach glucagon") by the so-called A-like ("AL") cells of closed[5] type, possessing also all the other criteria of pancreatic A cells,[38,39] it is now clear that these AL cells are true A cells. The consequences of these observations, and of our own phylogenetic studies in lower vertebrates,[36] are that the ancestors to pancreatic glucagon cells are in the gut. The EG cells of open type in the mammalian intestinal mucosa are, however, not true A cells, since they lack some A cell characteristics and produce a mixture of several peptides ("glucagoids," called enteroglucagon or "intestinal glucagon").[9,39] Consequently, they should be called EG cells and not A cells.

B Cells

The B cells are so well known that no detailed account needs to be given of the definitions used in our phylogenetic studies in addition to those given previously.[1] No other endocrine cells have been so comprehensively studied. Suffice it to say that the B cells are nonargyrophil (and consequently also nonargentaffin) APUD cells with secretion granules, giving typical reactions with Af and PIC. The granules vary considerably between species but are, nevertheless, as a rule typical enough to permit easy identification.[1]

Islet C Cells ("Agranular" Cells)

In contrast, the light-microscopically chromophobic, clear, ultrastructurally "agranular" or only sparsely granulated islet parenchymal cells[1,41] are rather poorly known and often neglected in classifications of CEP cells. Obviously, this mostly depends on the fact that they actually are only immature precursor cells to the granular islet parenchymal cells, apparently without any specific hormone production of their own.[41] To judge from observations made in neoplastically immature islet parenchyma in man and states of regeneration and islet hyperplasia,[23,41–44] they may in the maturation process to A, B, or D cells pass through a stage in which they appear as D_1 cells ("type IV cells"), a hypothesis that can explain why they sometimes are said to be argyrophil by Grimelius' procedure.[23] Otherwise, their most characteristic feature is their inability to give any "positive" light-microscopical staining reactions or cyto-chemical characteristic features at all.[36,41–44] Consequently, they can only be completely defined by a concomitant comprehensive ultrastructural study.[42] As further specified in subsequent sections, it may then be obvious that many of these allegedly agranular C cells are actually granulated parenchymal cells (A, B, D, or D_1)[5,23] and that their light-microscopical characteristics are only fixation artifacts[22] or are due to the fact that their granule content is too low to give any visible reactions.[11,12] Nevertheless, in studies of the comparative morphology of the endocrine pancreas and in experimental diabetes research, as well as in the analysis of islet-cell neoplasms and hyperplasias, they are a reality which cannot be neglected.[41] Particularly, the differentiation between real islet C cells and degranulated B cells can give rise to considerable practical problems that may lead to serious misinterpretations. Therefore, the essential differences between light-microscopically agranular islet C cells of precursor type and so-called degranulated B cells, as they appear in ordinary histological sections and in electron micrographs, have been summarized in Table 1, based on earlier reports from our laboratory.[41–44]

In recent monographs and reviews that have included the C cells in their classifications of the islet cell types,[22,45] the identification pitfalls have as a rule been clearly outlined, particularly the fact that the storage granules of the D cells may be so poorly fixed by OsO_4 that the cells may appear agranular. Moreover, the importance of cutting several thin sections from each block with agranular cells is emphasized since one thin section only can accidentally hit an agranular part of an elsewhere granulated cell.[45]

D Cells

The D cells form another highly controversial issue in the definition and classification of GEP endocrine cells. Their existence as a separate cell type has even been denied[1] (see also Chapter 3). Now there is general agreement that the D cells actually form a separate unit,[46] but it is still not clear whether or not the originally light-microscopically defined A_1 cells really are completely synon-ymous with the D cells. The A_1 cells (and the D cells) are granular parenchymal cells of APUD type that are argyrophil by the Hellerström–Hellman modifica-tion of the Davenport procedure but usually nonargyrophil by Grimelius' silver nitrate method. It has been found, however, that, exceptionally, a small fraction of the A_1 cells in man are argyrophil by both procedures.[26] In cases of persistent neonatal hypoglycemia[24,25] and in some islet cell neoplasms[23,26] this minor fraction seems to increase markedly, apparently consisting of the so-called D_1 (or "type IV") cells[23–26] which obviously can be slightly argyrophil by Grimelius' procedure (see below). It has been claimed that the A_1 cells in normal islets in man correspond to D cells + D_1 cells.[47,48] As the D_1 cells are only seldom found in normal mammalian pancreatic islets (see below), this means that for all practical purposes, the A_1 cells are synonymous with the D cells. Moreover, if some immature precursor cells[23] (slightly more differentiated than the islet C

Table 1. *Summary of the Essential Differences between Light-Microscopically "Agranular" Cells of Precursor Type and "Degranulated" B Cells as They Appear in Ordinary Histological Sections and in Electron Micrographs*

Areas of occurrence and histo-pathological and ultrastructural features	"Agranular" cells of precursor type, i.e., C cells	"Degranulated" B cells
Occurrence in states of islet cell regeneration and new formation	Frequent	Variable
Occurrence in acute insulin deficiency	Rare	Frequent
Occurrence in chronic diabetic states	Variable	Variable
Location in pancreas	Close to ductules, often as buds from the epithelium; varying location in the islets	Distinctly localized to B cell areas in the islets; no relationship to ductular epithelium.
Tinctorial characteristics in B cell staining procedures	"Chromophobe" reaction	"Chromophobe" reaction or weakly positive
Tinctorial characteristics in staining procedures for A and D cells	Usually a chromophobe reaction only	Sometimes a slight greenish color in sections stained according to Grimelius
Size and appearance in routine sections	Variable, but often large and clear	Variable, but often large and clear
Hydropic degeneration	Never	Often
Ultrastructural features: Nucleus	Rounded, usually central	Rounded, sometimes peripheral
Nucleolus	Moderately large	Large
Cytoplasm	Low electron density	Low electron density
Endoplasmic reticulum	Poorly developed	Prominent, often lamellar
Free ribosomes	Few	Numerous
Golgi apparatus	Moderately developed	Prominent
Secretion granules	None, or only a few small immature granules located close to the Golgi complex	Mainly "mature" granules (complete degranulation does not occur!)
Mitotic figures	Fairly frequent	Infrequent

cells) (Fig. 2) with structural and tinctorial similarities to the D_1 cells occur in the islet parenchyma, then the identity between A_1 and D cells can be considered as complete.

The hormone production of the D cells is another problem which is still not finally solved. In a preceding review[1] the D cells were supposed to produce gastrin. This statement was based on reports of the results of immunofluorescence studies. Later on, these results were seriously questioned,[17] and it was concluded that the islet D cells do not produce gastrin. Recently, it has been clearly established that the D cells contain somatostatin,[15,16] but, surprisingly enough, it has also been observed that the D cells may contain some kind of gastrin hormone as well.[46] Whether they not only contain but actually also produce somatostatin is still far from established in most species, but recent observations in bony fish indicate that the D cells really produce somatostatin.[49]

The D cells are nonargentaffin, and they occur in the GI mucosa as well,[5,9] where they also have been found to contain somatostatin.[15] Their secretion granules are typically large, of low electron density with a slightly granular core, as further described elsewhere in this volume (Chapter 6), usually offering no identification problems in comparative studies.

Small-Granulated Islet Cells: D₁ Cells (Type IV Cells), "PP-Cells" (F Cells)

The islet cells with small secretion granules are still incompletely understood and partly controversial. They consist of D_1 cells and PP cells[21] and possibly also some immature cells (see above). The D_1 cell was originally described in the islets of Langerhans in patients with persistent neonatal hypoglycemia with hyperinsulinism[50] and, later on, also in normal islets of children of neonatal age.[48] Recently, the D_1 cells (and the small-granulated immature islet cells) have been found to occur in considerable numbers in all kinds of islet cell tumors.[23] The D_1 cells were originally called "type III"[50] and later on "type IV" cells.[48] According to the revised Wiesbaden classification it has been claimed that the type IV cells of endocrine pancreas are synonymous with the D_1 cells that originally were described in the GI mucosa.[29] Their histological and cytochemical properties are not well known. As mentioned above, their principal characteristics are that they can be slightly argyrophil by Grimelius' procedure[21,23] and sometimes also by the Hellerström–Hellman technique as well.[24,40] Otherwise, they may appear like C cells light-microscopically.[23] Also ultrastructurally, they may be mistaken for C cells. Their secretion granules are so small that they can be overlooked due to improper fixation. Recent results of cytochemical studies and immunocytochemical investigations indicate that cells that (to judge from the ultrastructure of their secretion granules) can be D_1 cells have APUD characteristics[20] and show immunofluorescence with antisera against the newly discovered avian and human pancreatic polypeptide (PP).[19,20] In other reports it is explicitly denied that the D_1 cells and PP cells are identical.[21] Instead, it is claimed that the PP cells are the previously described F cells (type V cells; X cells).[21] Of particular interest are the observations that these "PP cells" can be unreactive or only weakly stained (light brown) with Grimelius' procedure—but not with the Hellerström–Hellman technique for argyrophilia[21]—and that they occur in locations where islet cell neoformation can be supposed to occur, viz., in the epithelium of small and medium-sized ducts, in the interstitial parts of the acinar parenchyma, and in the periphery of the islets of Langerhans.[21] Moreover, they seemed to be most numerous in fetuses and young patients.[21] Of particular interest with regard to their presence in all kinds of islet cell tumors[23] is the recent observation that PP

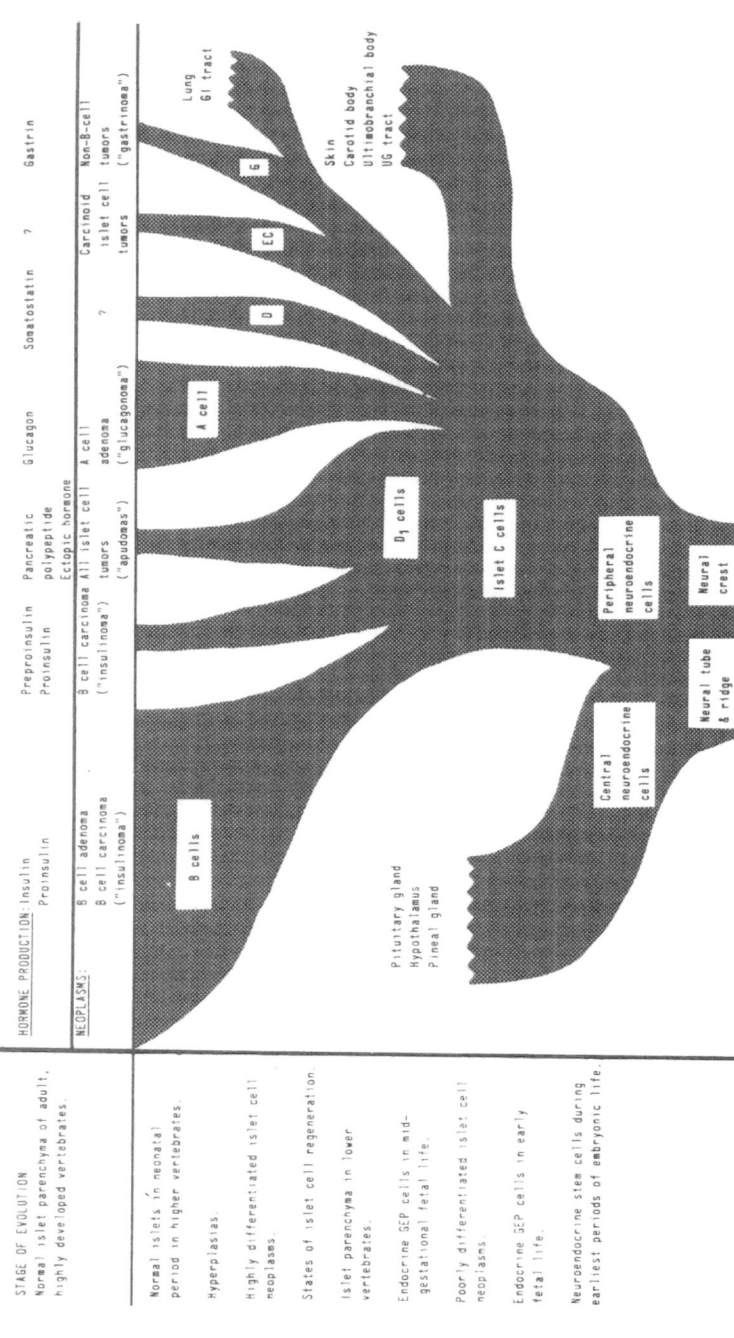

Figure 2. A schematic presentation of the hypothetic interrelationship, development, and cellular differentiation of the gastro-entero-pancreatic (GEP) endocrine cells in higher vertebrates, particularly the cells of the pancreatic islets, forming the background of the present review. The scheme also tries to coordinate phylogenetic and ontogenetic aspects with those of the pathology of GEP endocrine cells, notably states of islet cell regeneration, hyperplasias, and actual neoplasms of various differentiation. It is based on our interpretations of Pearse's APUD concept and its application in neuroendocrine pathology[11,12] and on Creutzfeldt's hypothesis on the role of cells of D_1 type in the development and differentiation of pancreatic endocrine tumors,[23] as well as on earlier phylogenetical and histopathological observations and working hypotheses from our own laboratory.[1,26,41-44]

The schematic presentation does not lay claim to be accurate in regard to the time periods and sequences for the "branching off" of the mature islet parenchymal cells from the immature precursor cells, nor does it aim to give an absolutely correct picture of the relative frequencies of various cell types during the maturation process, but is simply an attempt to illustrate our lines of thinking in our phylogenetic works.

The development of endocrine (and nonendocrine) cells outside the endocrine pancreas has also been indicated (by broken ramifications) in this scheme.

occurs in addition to other hormones in extracts of several kinds of pancreatic endocrine tumors and also from the surrounding pancreas. Moreover, PP-immunoreactive tumor cells occur intermingled with tumor cells immunoreactive to other GEP hormones.[20,51] All these observations—as well as reports that more or less permanently ascribe the production of other GEP hormones (GIP, VIP, somatostatin) to the D_1 cells[9,40]—can be said to conform with the hypothesis that these small-granulated islet cells represent a rather heterogeneous population, consisting not only of D_1 cells and PP cells but also of precursor cells to several GEP endocrine cells.[23] Thus, the islet C cells and the small-granulated islet cells may belong to the same category of precursor cells, where the C cells represent the most immature stage and the D_1 cells and PP cells are so differentiated that they have attained some ability to produce some kind of hormone.[23] Against this background it is reasonable to expect the occurrence of both C and small-granulated islet cells of D_1 type in the phylogenetically presumably less highly differentiated GEP endocrine system of lower vertebrates.[26]

The working hypothesis we have used in our phylogenetic studies conforms to those formulated by Pearse[11-13] and Creutzfeldt.[23] It is schematically outlined in Fig. 2.

Intermediate Islet Cells ("Mixed" or "Amphiphil" Cells)

In connection with the account given above of the origin and various developmental stages of the GEP endocrine cells, the controversy of the alleged occurrence of acinoinsular and other intermediate islet cells should be clarified since the interrelationship between the exocrine and endocrine parenchyma in the pancreas is of great interest in the comparative morphology of the pancreatic islet in animals, as emphasized in the preceding review from our laboratory.[1] Here, some new aspects have recently been offered by the results obtained in a series of careful and comprehensive ultrastructural and experimental studies in some vertebrates, mainly mammals.[52,53] To judge from the electron micrographs of these reports, taken from material fixed by immersion only, intermediate (acinar-B; acinar-A; acinar-D; A-B; A-D; B-D) cells would exist also in normal pancreatic islets. They are claimed to be widespread, and their frequency of occurrence is said to be "inversely proportional to the degree of separation of the exocrine and endocrine elements."[52] This statement is supported phylogenetically by the frequent occurrence of so-called amphiphil islet cells in the pancreas of amphibians and cartilaginous fish.[1,52] Hybrid cells of this kind can be explained by the existence of a functional polarity in the Golgi complex, analogous to that observed in the Golgi apparatus of blood granulocytes capable of packing different types of specific granules.[53] The acinar-B cells are found in the exocrine parenchyma immediately outside the islets of Langerhans, and their existence explains some unsolved problems of the effects of secretin upon the secretion of insulin in the blood and the pancreatic juice.[53]

These recent observations on the occurrence of various intermediates of A, B, and D cells give further support to the working hypothesis that some endocrine pancreatic cells are omnipotent and able to differentiate in various directions after their origin from the neural crest (Fig. 2). The finding of intermediate exocrine–endocrine cells is, however, more difficult to understand. Are they artifacts only, or products of the fusion of two or more cells?[54] It has been emphatically claimed that intermediate cells only are found after immersion fixation and never after adequate fixation by perfusion.[145] (See also below.) Are exocrine acinar cells, equipped with zymogen granules, also derived from the neural crest, or do the islet parenchymal cells originate from the endoderm of the foregut, after all, like the rest of the glands of the GI tract? The lack of any convincing answers to these questions illustrates the need of intensified ontogenetic and phylogenetic studies of GEP endocrine cells. The whole problem has been carefully analyzed in the light of the APUD concept in an ontogenetic study of the GEP endocrine cells.[54]

Other Kinds of Islet Parenchymal Cells

Apart from these new aspects on the D cells, the small-granulated cells, and the intermediate cells, there have not been any major changes in the definitions and the terminology of islet parenchymal cells since the earlier review[1] was given. Except for the EC cells, all the other allegedly occurring kinds of islet parenchymal cells (e.g., E and W cells) still lack functional characterization.[40,45]

Invertebrates and Protochordates

In the earlier review of the comparative endocrinology of the pancreatic islets[1] the section on invertebrates and protochordates could give an account of some discoveries—that were rather new at that time—where extrainsular insulin-producing cells had been found in the GI mucosa of several invertebrates, both protostomian and deuterostomian. Two new principles were offered by these observations, viz: (a) that insulin was not a hormone restricted to the vertebrates only, and (b) that the islet B cells were closely related to the mucosa of the GI tract.[1] Whether glucagon-producing and/or other GI endocrine cells also existed in invertebrates was more equivocal at that time, but there were some reports on the occurrence of endocrine cells (EC cells) in the GI tract of some protochordates.[1] Since then, practically no progress with regard to the occurrence of GEP cells in invertebrates—particularly the existence of insulin-producing B cells in the GI mucosa—had been made for almost 5 years,[27,28] until quite recently, when several most interesting reports suddenly appeared.

First of all, it was clearly shown by combined cytochemical and immunofluorescence investigations of the intestinal mucosa of the pelecypode mollusc, *Mytilus edulis* (the common edible mussel) that cells with insulin-like immunoreactivity were localized to the area where B cells had been supposed to occur according to earlier correlated light-microscopical studies, a brief ultrastructural report, and the results of insulin assays of the GI mucosa.[1,37] This observation further illustrates the close interrelationship that exists between the islet parenchymal cells and the endocrine cells of the GI tract and shows that molluscan insulin shares antigenic sites with mammalian insulin.[37] No argyrophil cells were found and no positive immunofluorescence results were obtained with antisera against caerulein and mammalian gastrin, pentagastrin, and glucagon.[37] Notwithstanding, gastrin has recently been isolated from the GI tract of two other species of mollusc.[55] Also of interest was the finding that these intestinal B cells did not show the APUD characteristics[37]; similar observations have recently been made in the GI endocrine cells of the most primitive vertebrates (see below).

Further support for a localization to the GI mucosa of the insulin production in species below the vertebrates, where no separate islet organ exists,[1] was given in a preliminary report[56] on the GI mucosa of the cephalochordate *Branchiostoma lanceolatum* (the amphioxus), where the previously observed, fine-grained cells of open type, stained by Af and PIC,[57,58] were found to contain an insulin-like substance by immunofluorescence, using antisera against mammalian insulin. The cells were nonargyrophil. They responded by degranulation and release of Af-positive material into the gut to immersion of the amphioxus for 24 hr in 100 mg/100 ml glucose seawater.[59] Ultrastructurally, they corresponded to one of three kinds of granulated cells of endocrine type, described a couple of years previously in the gut.[60] In addition, scattered argyrophil (Grimelius' procedure) cells of open type were observed,[56] different from these intestinal B cells; they were immunofluorescent with antisera to mammalian gastrin and glucagon and corresponded to one of the two remaining, ultrastructurally defined cell types.[60] Probably the gastrin and glucagon reactivity occurred in one and the same cell,[56] an interesting finding in view of analogous observations made in the most primitive vertebrates[36] (as further described in the subsequent section). It may be assumed that the third ultrastructural type of endocrine cell corresponded to the light-microscopically observed EC cells, described 15 years ago.[61] Meanwhile, further proofs had been obtained that insulin (and proinsulin) actually is produced by a pelecypode mollusc,[62] and that even mammalian insulin can exert physiological effects in a mollusc by decreasing the blood glucose level and increasing the glycogen content of skeletal musculature.[63]

Consequently, additional circumstantial evidence has now been gained that there actually is a close evolutionary connection between the islet parenchymal cells and the mucosa of the GI tract. Thus, concepts, such as "the enteroinsular axis" and the "GEP endocrine system" have a sound and solid phylogenetical background.[36]

Considering the recent observation that insulin seems to affect glucose uptake even in the Protozoa,[64] one may question whether insulin—and perhaps also other GEP hormones—may be even more widespread than previously thought.[1] Some support for such a possibility has recently been obtained from both brief reports and more comprehensive works, reporting an insulin-like hormone in protein extracts of insects[65,66] and glucagon-like activity in an insect[67] and a crustacean.[68] The cells producing these islet hormones have not been described. However, of particular interest for the hypothesis that islet cells are derived from the neural crest[13] is that the insulin-like and glucagon-like hormones were found in the insect neurosecretory system.[65] Thus, it may be that in the insects studied (diverging from the deuterostomian-vertebrate-mammalian line approximately 900 million years ago[67]) (Fig. 1) the islet hormones have retained their neurosecretory character, as postulated in the APUD theory.[11-13] It is also well known that in another large group of arthropods, viz., the crustaceans, the hyperglycemic hormone from the eyestalk is of typical neurosecretory character.[69]

Of additional interest in this connection is the fact that both insulin and glucagon seem to show a remarkable "stability" in their molecular structure throughout evolution. Observations made in a current functional evolution analysis of insulin in our laboratory[28,35] indicate that the amino acid sequence and three-dimensional structure of the hormone in the most primitive verte-

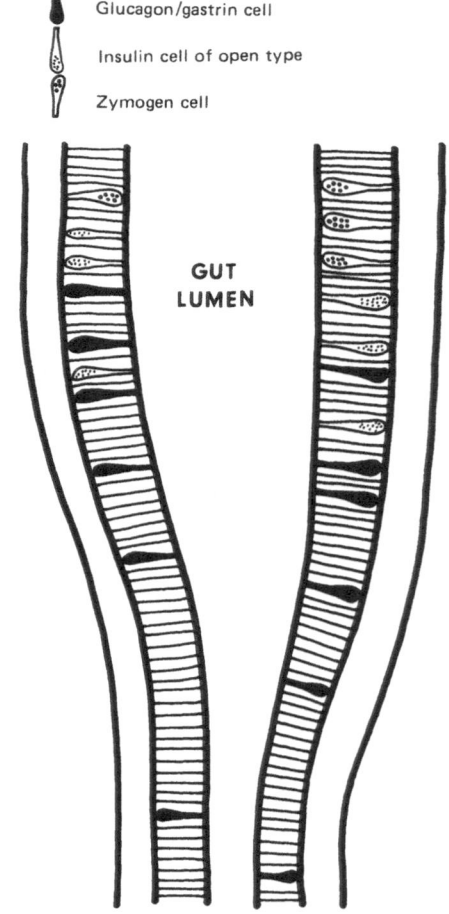

Glucagon/gastrin cell

Insulin cell of open type

Zymogen cell

GUT
LUMEN

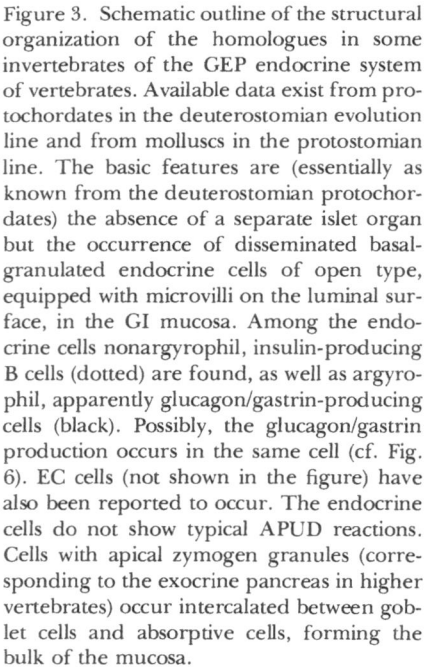

Figure 3. Schematic outline of the structural organization of the homologues in some invertebrates of the GEP endocrine system of vertebrates. Available data exist from protochordates in the deuterostomian evolution line and from molluscs in the protostomian line. The basic features are (essentially as known from the deuterostomian protochordates) the absence of a separate islet organ but the occurrence of disseminated basal-granulated endocrine cells of open type, equipped with microvilli on the luminal surface, in the GI mucosa. Among the endocrine cells nonargyrophil, insulin-producing B cells (dotted) are found, as well as argyrophil, apparently glucagon/gastrin-producing cells (black). Possibly, the glucagon/gastrin production occurs in the same cell (cf. Fig. 6). EC cells (not shown in the figure) have also been reported to occur. The endocrine cells do not show typical APUD reactions. Cells with apical zymogen granules (corresponding to the exocrine pancreas in higher vertebrates) occur intercalated between goblet cells and absorptive cells, forming the bulk of the mucosa.

brates differ astonishingly little from those in pig insulin despite evolution lines being divergent for several hundred million years (Fig. 1). The fact that insulin from invertebrates[70] and primitive vertebrates[71] is of low biological potency in mammalian test systems, and vice versa,[70] may depend on evolutionary differences in the insulin receptors rather than on the presence of large amounts of proinsulin, as suggested previously.[7] Whether differences exist also with regard to the actual numbers of receptors is unknown. Glucagon is more incompletely known in this respect, but available data from mammals and birds indicate that the structure of this hormone also has been unexpectedly well preserved during evolution.[65,67] Thus, it may be that the islet hormones are of essential character for all forms of animal life. Here, continued and intensified comparative studies with correlated structural and biochemical techniques are obviously urgently needed.

To summarize: The morphology of the endocrine system in invertebrates, homologous to the GEP endocrine cells in vertebrates, is not yet well known. Some information is available on echinoderms,[1] tunicates,[1] the amphioxus (among the deuterostomes),[56-61] and some molluscs (among the protostomes).[1] Recent ultrastructural studies of the GI epithelium in a tunicate[72] have clearly shown that the basal-granulated endocrine cells that occur are all of open type, equipped with microvilli on the luminal surface. Against this background and considering other data given above, the structural features of the homologues in deuterostomian invertebrates of the GEP endocrine system in vertebrates have been tentatively summarized in Fig. 3, using available information about these cells in amphioxus[56-61] as a model.

Vertebrates

As shown in earlier reviews from our laboratory on the phylogeny of the islet parenchyma,[1,2,27,28] the GEP endocrine system of lower vertebrates offer the most interesting aspects from an evolutionary point of view. This has been confirmed by some recent overviews from other laboratories[9,73] where, in particular, investigations of the cyclostomes are emphasized to be of fundamental importance because the cyclostomes represent the most ancient of surviving vertebrate groups.[9,36] Consequently, we have focused our attention primarily on the cyclostomes and secondarily on the lower groups in gnathostomian vertebrates (Fig. 1), viz., cartilaginous and bony fish, whereas the amphibians, reptiles, and birds have been treated more superficially. Their pancreatic islets do not show too many principal differences from those of mammals.[1] The histochemistry and ultrastructure of mammalian islet parenchyma is reviewed elsewhere in this volume (Chapter 6).

Cyclostomes (Agnatha)

In addition to review a couple of years ago, covering the whole endocrine system of the cyclostomes,[74] two rather extensive works have been published in

1976, partly from our laboratory, on the GEP endocrine systems in cyclostomes in general[75] and in the Atlantic hagfish, *Myxine glutinosa,* in particular.[36] Moreover, a comprehensive review was given 4 years ago on the exocrine and endocrine pancreas and intestine of the lamprey,[76] and quite recently the islet cytology of the sea lamprey, *Petromyzon marinus,* has been thoroughly revised,[73,77] and some interesting evolutionary correlations of islet histophysiology have been given, particularly in lower vertebrates. As a consequence, there have been considerable advances during these last 5 years in our knowledge of the GEP endocrine system in both hagfish and lampreys—at least of those of the northern hemisphere.[78] This applies both to the morphology and to the biochemistry of the insulin production.[35] As a result, *Myxine* insulin is, next to pig insulin, the best known of all insulins located so far. These biochemical and physiological aspects,[35,71] which are outside the scope of this work, have to some extent been the subject of a separate recent review.[28]

As partly outlined above (Fig. 1), the hagfish (Myxinoidea) and the lampreys (Petromyzontia) form two evolutionary lines, separate from all the other vertebrates (the gnathostomes)—and also from each other—for more than 500 million years (possibly with a common Cambrian or Precambrian ancestor). Their endocrine system can be regarded as the most primitive and original in the whole vertebrate series.[36,74,75] There is no stomach[9] in the hagfish, just a straight intestinal tube, and no organized exocrine pancreatic gland.[76,78] The islet parenchyma forms a grossly visible organ,[1] often containing large cystic cavities, looking rather similar to the follicles of the thyroid gland.[74] The hagfish is apparently the most primitive animal to have a separate islet organ although, admittedly, some of its peculiar features may be adaptations to the special way of life and/or neotenous characters of the hagfish (see below).

In the hagfish, *M. glutinosa,* the islet organ occurs as a whitish swelling at the junction of the common bile duct with the gut[26] (Fig. 4). In the river

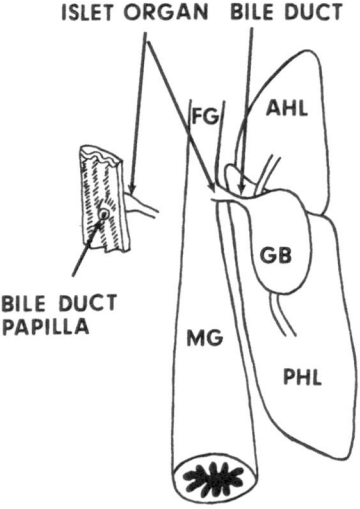

Figure 4. Schematic presentation of that part of the gastrointestinal tract of the hagfish *(Myxine glutinosa)* that is of particular interest in the present review, viz., the foregut (FG), midgut (MG), anterior hepatic lobe (AHL), posterior hepatic lobe (PHL), and gallbladder (GB). The islet organ, surrounding the distal part of the bile duct, is partly embedded in the gut connective tissue and is close to the bile duct papilla, protruding into the gut lumen.

lamprey, *Lampetra fluviatilis*, it is split up into three gross portions, partly embedded in the intestinal wall, and extending into the dorsal surface of the liver.[74] Excellent, illustrated descriptions of the gross aspects in the lamprey have recently been given.[76,79]

The typical cyclostomian islet organ is a lobular or follicular gland, consisting of multiple lobules of large sheets of polygonal parenchymal cells, mainly B cells, surrounded by strands of collagenous connective tissue (Fig. 5). Usually, no nerves and no vessels are found inside the lobules. There are three principal microscopic features of this islet parenchyma that need particular attention, where marked progress has been made during the last 5 years, viz.:

1. *The follicular cavities* in this islet parenchyma[27,28,36,74,75,80] have recently been found by TEM and SEM* to be of two kinds, viz., one smooth-surfaced type of degenerative nature (Fig. 5A) and another with rough inner surface, being surrounded by agranular cells, equipped with microvilli and antennulae microvillares, indicating an absorptive and storing function.[75] The latter kind of cavities predominate.[80] The cavities are particularly numerous in the Atlantic hagfish, *M. glutinosa*. This has been interpreted as a result of a long period of adaptation to the uniformity of deep-sea environment with low insulin demands.[75] Such cavities are more rare in the islet parenchyma of lampreys and other kinds of hagfish, all of which are more exposed to environmental changes.[75] Fundamentally, however, these cavities of nondisintegrative nature seem to belong to the same category as other cysts in endocrine organs, not only of cyclostomes[77] but also of higher vertebrates, including mammals,[74] viz., an expression of an inherent lumen-forming tendency of the epithelium from which the endocrine parenchymal cells originate.[42] This concept is illustrated by recent observations of cysts, cystic hamartomas, and actual islet cell tumors (insulomas) in both *M. glutinosa*[27,74,81] and *L. fluviatilis*,[82] and *P. marinus*.[77] It is also well known that islet cell tumors in man often show tubular structures.[26] As shown in Fig. 5B, and as reviewed previously,[27] it is now clearly established that the content in the rough-surfaced cavities is not insulin, proinsulin, or pre-proinsulin. The content of the smooth-surfaced cavities is just cellular débris,[27] explaining why positive reactions may sometimes be obtained with Af and PIC[1] (Fig. 5A).

2. *The cellular composition* of the islet parenchyma differs only in some respects between hagfish and lampreys.[1,74] Common to all cyclostomian species investigated so far is the absence of acinar pancreatic epithelium and ducts, that no direct innervation seems to exist,[77] that there seem to be no glucagon-producing A cells in the islet parenchyma, and that—at least in the hagfish—the B cells predominate (Fig. 5).[1,74] However, some granular cells of non-B-cell nature have also previously been observed,[1,74] and have now been reinvestigated, both in the hagfish[36] and in the lamprey.[77]

In the sea lamprey, *P. marinus*, not less than four types of acidophil non-B-cells were found light microscopically[73] and ultrastructurally.[77] Interestingly, it

---

*Scanning electron microscopy.

could be shown that all of these lamprey islet cells were, at least in some respect, related to the B cells, indicating a common origin. The tinctorial features of their secretion granules showed, however, that they obviously contained some polypeptide(s) different from insulin.[77] It was not stated whether any of these non-B-cells were argyrophil by Grimelius' procedure, whether they showed APUD characteristics, or whether they were immunoreactive with any antisera to the common GEP hormones. No hormonal assays were made.

So far, these cells have been observed during the latest stage of the life cycle only (of *P. marinus*), indicating that the cyclostomian islet parenchyma may be secondarily simple, due to neotenous factors.[83] This seems particularly plausible for the islet organ of *M. glutinosa*. This scavenger feeder apparently lives a stationary wormlike life in darkness at almost constant temperature,

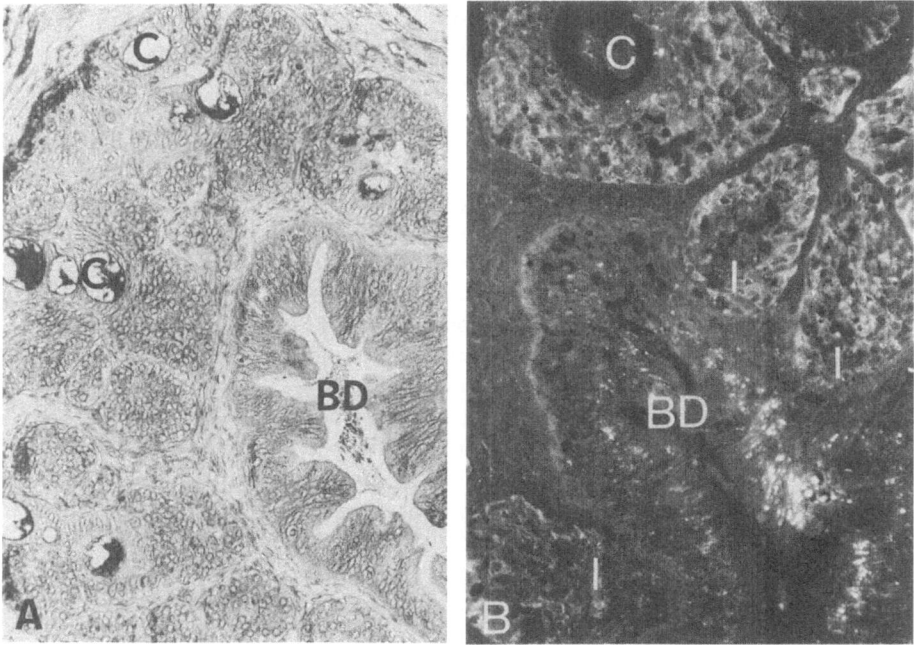

Figure 5. Low-power photomicrographs of parts of the common bile duct (BD) and the islet organ in *Myxine glutinosa*, as they appear in a histological section stained with aldehyde fuchsin (Af) (Fig. 5A) and in an immunofluorescence section after application of anti-human-insulin serum (Fig. 5B). The close association between some of the islet lobules (I) and the bile duct mucosa is obvious: Two islet lobules are budding off (Fig. 5B). There is no exocrine acinar pancreatic parenchyma. The cavities (C) of some of the islet lobules contain Af-positive material (Fig. 5A), but this does not give immunofluorescence with antiinsulin serum (Fig. 5B). These cavities are presumably of degenerative nature. It is obvious from both photomicrographs that practically all the parenchymal cells in the islet lobules are insulin-producing B cells. There are no endocrine cells in the bile duct mucosa in these particular sections. (The bright parts in the bile duct mucosa in Fig. 5B represent nonspecific autofluorescence.) ×260 (5A) and ×480 (5B).

darkness, and salinity.[74,75] Neotenous characters are known to occur in animals living under similar shielded conditions (cf. the axolotl). It may even be so that *M. glutinosa* (and other extant cyclostomes as well?) represents the second larval stage of the now extinct Ostracoderms.[83]

In the Atlantic hagfish the cells that differed in their ultrastructure from the typical B cells were also found to be somehow related to the development of the B cells. Whereas the typical hagfish β granules were markedly poikiloform, showing so-called connective tissue secretion by an emiocytotic process,[36,84] the secretion granules of this second type of hagfish islet cells were essentially spherical[83] and in some respects reminiscent of those of the D_1 cells of higher vertebrates. However, the cells were nonargyrophil. They were of closed type and showed cytochemical characteristics of APUD cells.[84,85] They occurred mainly in the mucosa of the bile duct epithelium but also in the islet parenchyma. The cells were not immunofluorescent with antisera against human insulin.[84,85] It could clearly be shown that the hagfish islet parenchyma originates from precursor cells in the bile duct mucosa[85] (Fig. 5B), where also typical, mature, B cells occur as cells of "closed" type. The non-insulin-immunoreactive APUD cells with spherical secretion granules were more numerous in this location than the typical B cells. Moreover, intermediate forms between these cells and the typical B cells were observed in the bile duct mucosa. They also contained more annulate lamellae than the typical B cells, a feature which is common in cells of all tissues during the early stages of differentiation.[36] All these observations indicated that the cells with spherical secretion granules were—at least partly—precursors to the typical B cells,[36] possibly related to the D_1 cells (Fig. 2). However, in a current project* on the occurrence of somatostatin-producing D cells in the GEP endocrine system of lower vertebrates and in that of invertebrates we have observed in our laboratory the presence of somatostatin (8 ng/mg wet wt.) in extracts of excised islet organs with the bile duct mucosa of the Atlantic hagfish, *M. glutinosa*. By immunofluorescence, somatostatin-containing cells have also quite recently been found in locations corresponding well to the major portion of these non-insulin-immunoreactive APUD cells with spherical secretion granules.[86] A still open question is whether or not some of the insulin-containing cells of intermediary type contain both insulin and somatostatin. By personal communication (J. Stewart†) we have been informed that also in the Pacific hagfish *(Eptatretus stouti)* somatostatin has been found not only in the brain and spinal cord but also in the islet body and intestine.

3. In regard to *the interrelationship between the islet parenchyma and the GI endocrine cells,* it has recently been confirmed that neither the hagfish,[36] nor the adult lamprey[87,88] has any B cells in the mucosa of the primitive intestinal tube.

---

*Together with Dr. Robert P. Elde, Dept. of Anatomy, University of Minnesota, Minneapolis, and Drs. Claes Hellerström and Birger Petersson, Dept. of Histology, University of Uppsala.

†Work by Jennifer Stewart, Ph.D., at the Harborview Medical Center, Seattle, Wash., together with Drs. D. Koerker, C. J. Goodner, and A. Gorbman.

In the larval lamprey, however, the B cells indubitably develop as buds from the base of the gut mucosa at the junction of the esophagus and the intestine,[74-76] Immunoreactive insulin is present in the developing follicles at this stage.[87,88] Moreover, it has been shown, both in the lamprey and the hagfish, that scattered argyrophil (Grimelius' procedure) endocrine cells of basal-granulated, open type occur. These cells showed no, or only faint, APUD characteristics but were found to be equipped with spherical secretion granules,[88-90] in some respects looking rather like those observed in A and EG cells of higher vertebrates. In immunofluorescence studies, using a large number of antisera against GEP hormones, it was found, again in both the lamprey and the hagfish, that the GI cells were immunoreactive with gastrin and pancreatic glucagon and that one and the same cell obviously contained both hormones.[36,88,89] The number of secretion granules increased during fasting.[90] There were no cells of this kind in the bile duct mucosa or in the islet parenchyma.

To summarize: The morphology of the GEP system in the cyclostomes is now fairly well known in both of the extant orders of this diphyletic class, viz., the hagfish and the lampreys. It can be said to form the first step in the evolution of a separate islet organ, occurring even before the development of an exocrine pancreas. However, in the hagfish it is only the B cells and B cell precursors (islet C cells and D_1 cells?)—and obviously also the D cells—that have left the gut, now being restricted to the bile duct and the adjacent islet parenchyma, where they appear as endocrine cells of closed type. Glucagon/gastrin-producing endocrine cells of open type, with no or only faint APUD characteristics, are still found only in the gut mucosa. The structure and interrelationship of the various components of the GEP system in the cyclostomes have been schematically summarized in Fig. 6. The sketchy presentation is based on recent data obtained from studies in the Atlantic hagfish, *M. glutinosa.*[36]

The working hypothesis, put forward in earlier reviews from our laboratory,[1,2,27,28,74] that cyclostomian islet tissue represents some kind of an evolutionary link between the gut-connected dispersed insulin-producing parenchyma of invertebrates and the islets of Langerhans of higher vertebrates, thus seems to be correct.

Gnathostomes

The most primitive islet parenchyma of the six classes, constituting the main subphylum of the vertebrates, viz., those equipped with jaws (Fig. 1), is known to occur in the cartilaginous fish.[1,91] Recent studies in some bony fish have shown, however, that primitive exocrine–endocrine relationships, similar to those in cartilaginous fish, exist also in the pancreas of this class,[73] which previously has been looked upon as highly developed.[1] Consequently, in order to show the islet evolution more clearly, and to avoid unnecessary repetitions in this review, cartilaginous and bony fish have been brought together in the same section (Fig. 7).

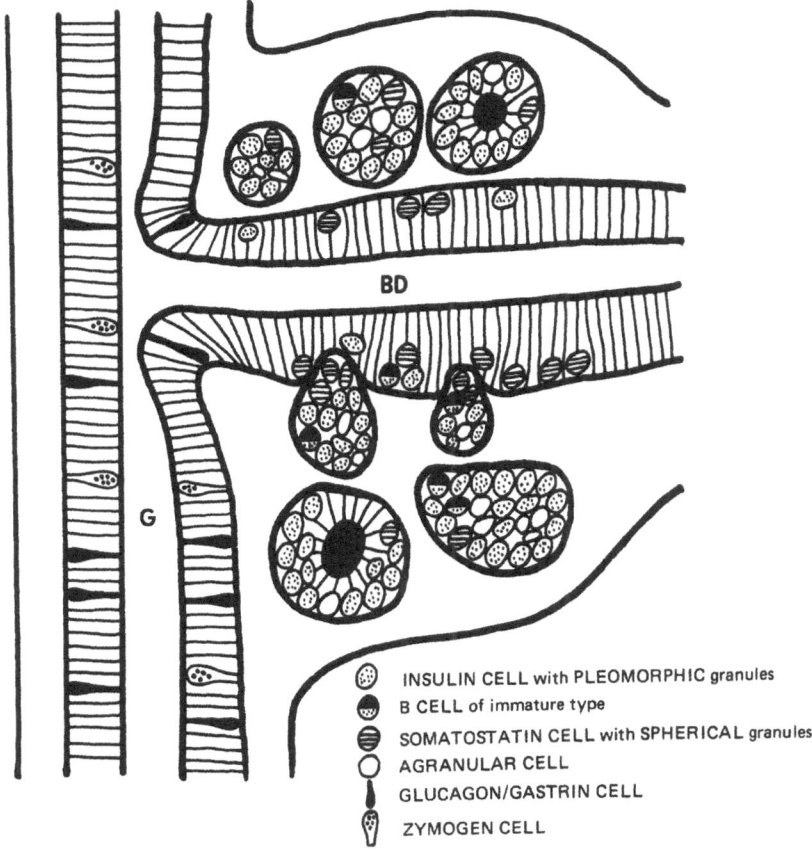

INSULIN CELL with PLEOMORPHIC granules
B CELL of immature type
SOMATOSTATIN CELL with SPHERICAL granules
AGRANULAR CELL
GLUCAGON/GASTRIN CELL
ZYMOGEN CELL

Figure 6. Schematic outline of cells, constituting the Atlantic hagfish's enteroinsular endocrine organ and the hagfish homology of mammalian exocrine pancreatic parenchyma (zymogen cells). In the gut (G) mucosa, scattered, slender, flask-shaped (black) argyrophil glucagon/gastrin immuno-reactive cells and single, intercalated cells with apical zymogen granules are present. In the basal portion of the bile duct (BD) mucosa, and occasionally in the islet parenchyma, nonargyrophil APUD cells (striped) are found. These cells are ultrastructurally characterized by spherical secretion granules and have recently been observed to produce somatostatin. Also, insulin-containing B cells (dotted) are present in the bile duct mucosa and in groups and buds of cells with a close relation to the bile duct epithelium. The buds mature into islet lobules in the surrounding connective tissue.

Pisces

Cartilaginous fish. The class Chondrichthyes is subdivided into two sub-classes, viz., the Elasmobranchii, consisting of sharks, skates, and rays, and the Holocephali, the ratfish[1] (Fig. 7). In regard to the morphology of the GEP endocrine system, only minor advances have been made in these two subclasses since the earlier review from our laboratory,[1] as far as we have been able to find.

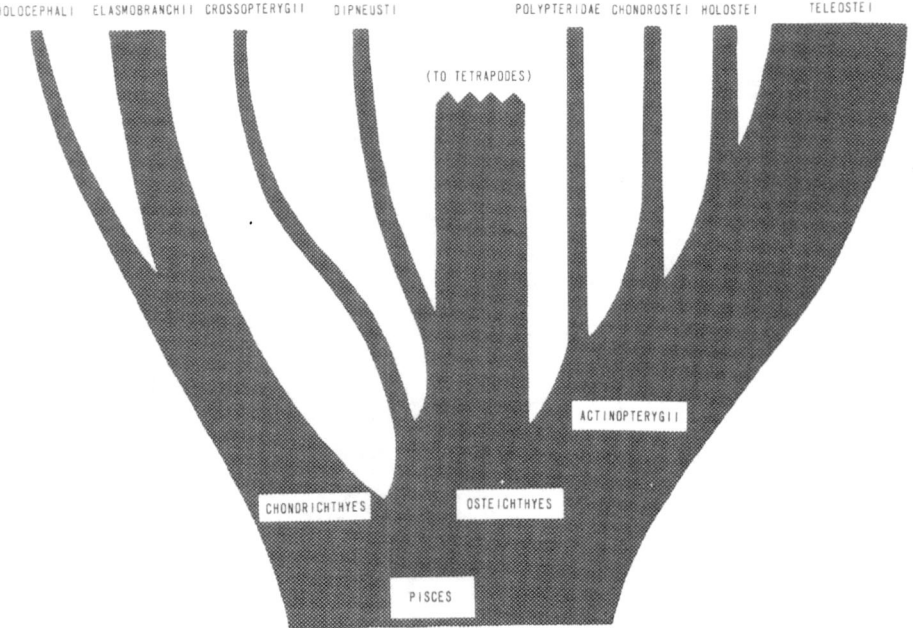

Figure 7. Schematic illustration of the interrelationship between those subclasses of cartilaginous and bony fish that are included in this review.

Grossly, the chondrichthyean pancreas is a compact gland of mammalian type, where the endocrine parenchyma is disseminated as something like islets of Langerhans in the large acinar gland. In elasmobranchs the gland is a bilobed structure, consisting of a dorsal and a ventral part. In the ratfish, however, it is just a single-lobed compact gland, attached to the liver cranially and to the spleen at its caudal end.[1]

Light-microscopically, the most conspicuous feature in both subclasses is the close association of the islet cells with the epithelium of the pancreatic ducts.[1] Often the endocrine cells occur as an outer layer around the ductal epithelium. Several of the ducts, even the larger ones, contain endocrine cells, apparently both of closed and open type, interspersed among the epithelial cells. Isolated endocrine cells can also be scattered in the interstitium of the acinar parenchyma and at the bases of the larger ducts. In some species actual islets of Langerhans are formed, often with a central slotlike lumen, containing cellular debris of similar kind as in the smooth-surfaced islet cavities of the cyclostomian islet lobules (see above). In the holocephalans the size of the pancreatic islets can vary from a few cells only to islets larger than 1 mm in diameter.[1] In contrast to the cyclostomian islet organ(s), the chondrichthyean islets are innervated.[73]

It is clear that both in the elasmobranchs and in the holocephalans A, B, and D cells are found, but additional cell types occur in both subclasses.[1] Thus, "amphiphils" have been observed in elasmobranch endocrine pancreas, and so-called X cells occur in holocephalans.[1] The latter are defined light-microscopically. They are granular cells with some A and D cell staining features, being argyrophil both by the Hellerström–Hellman and the Grimelius procedures.[1] Otherwise, they are not well known. Preliminary immunocytochemical observations (S. Van Noorden, personal communication) indicate that the A, B, and D cells contain insulin, glucagon, and somatostatin, respectively. The X cells did not react with any of these three antisera. Also the amphiphils are not well known immunocytochemically. The X cells constitute not less than 50% of the holocephalan islet cells, whereas the amphiphils comprise only a minor fraction of the elasmobranchian islet parenchyma.[1] Roughly, the relative frequencies are: B cells, 30–40% (in elasmobranchs even up to 70%), A cells, 15–25% (in elasmobranchs sometimes even up to 60%); and D cells, about 5%.[1]

Ultrastructurally,[1,92] the A, B, and D cells in cartilaginous fish islets do not seem to deviate much from the fine structure of the corresponding cell types in mammals (Fig. 8).* Thus, the A cell granules have the characteristic spherical form with marked electron density and fairly closely apposed granule membrane (Fig. 8A), the B cells often show rod-shaped crystalline cores of their secretion granules (Fig. 8B), and the D cells have secretion granules of low electron density with slightly wrinkled, moderately closely apposed granule membranes[1] (Fig. 8D). The δ granules are, however, rather small. In addition, cells are occasionally found, equipped with small, electron-dense, spherical granules (Fig. 8C). These cells might correspond to the mammalian D_1 (type IV) or PP cell. The secretion granules of the X cells of the ratfish (Fig. 8E) are large, often even larger than the β granules. Otherwise, they show some similarities to the α granules. Thus, in the ratfish, the islet parenchymal cells can be grouped in order of (decreasing) size of their secretion granules as follows: X, B, A, D, and D_1 (PP) cells. In addition, some granulated cells are occasionally found which are difficult to classify (Fig. 8F). They may represent the chondrichthyean amphiphils, EC cells, intermediate X-A cells, or even invaded blood granulocytes.[36] Considering the facts (see below) that in the reptilian islet A cells the secretion granules can be as large as zymogen granules and that in the islet parenchyma of teleosts the tinctorial features of the A cells and the fine structure of the α granules can vary so much that two different kinds of A cells were supposed to occur, a plausible working hypothesis seems to be that the holocephalan islet X cells may be related to the A cells (as the X cells of the islet parenchyma of the horse ultimately turned out to be; see below). However, such a working hypothesis has obtained no support from the results of immunocytochemical studies so far (see above).

From one of several comprehensive light-microscopical studies of the GEP endocrine system in poikilothermic vertebrates performed by Gabe and Martoja it is known that at least two or three kinds of GEP endocrine cells (EC, EC-like, and G cells) occur in the mucosa of the GI tract of cartilaginous fish.[93] They

---

*The information given in this paragraph and the illustrations in Fig. 8 of the ultrastructure of the ratfish islets have been generously provided by Dr. Gregory J. Patent, University of Montana, Missoula. A more detailed report is presently being published.[92]

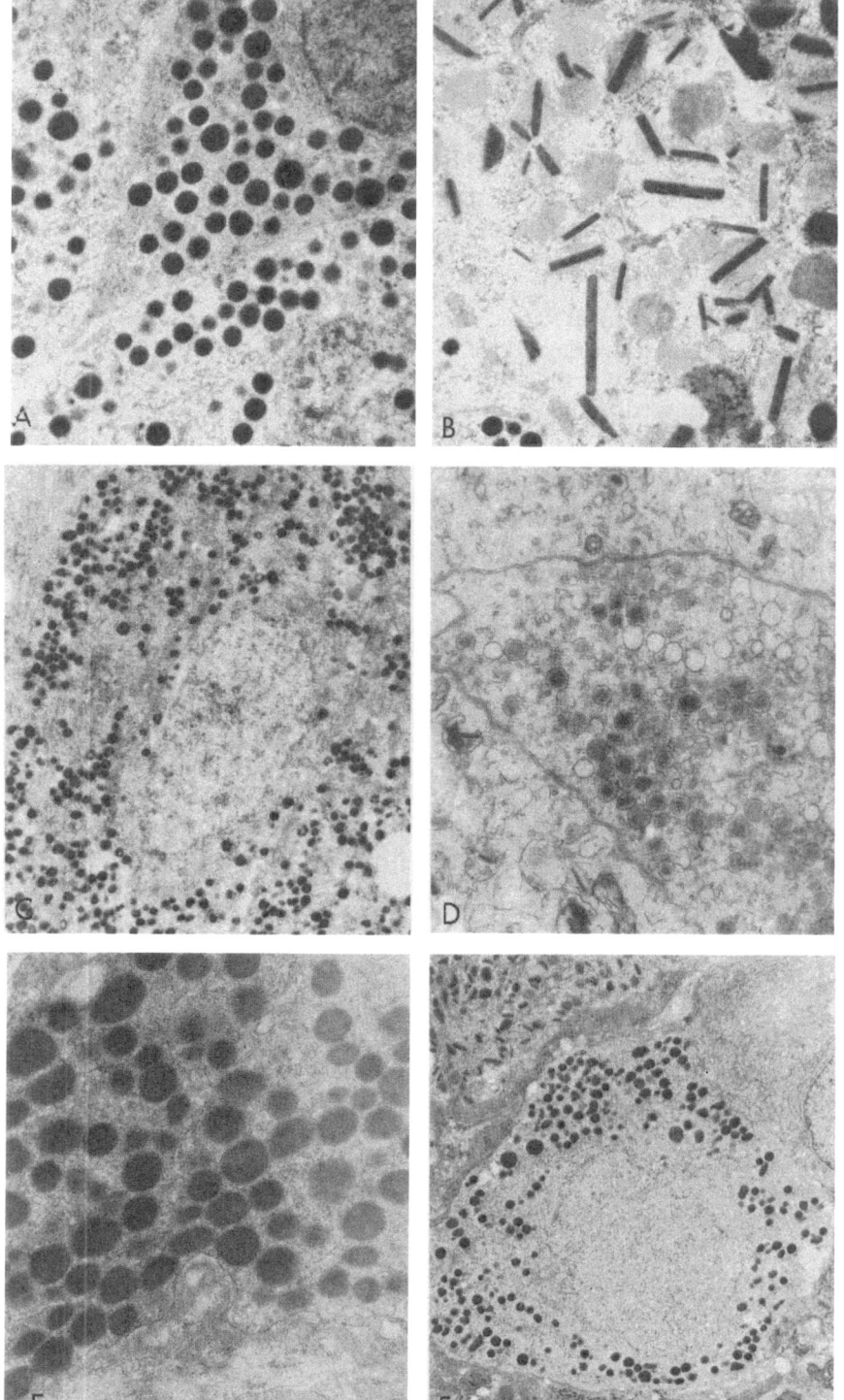

seem to be of both open and closed type.[93] Hormonal assays have shown the presence of several of the common GI hormones (gastrin, secretin, and possibly also CCK and VIP) in extracts of the GI mucosa of both cartilaginous and bony fish.[9,94] Whether endocrine cells also are present in the bile duct mucosa is unknown. The immunocytochemical characteristics of the endocrine cells in the pancreatic duct epithelium are also unknown. Similarly, the nature of the slitlike cavities in some islets is an unexplored territory.

Notwithstanding all these hypothetical aspects, the morphology of the chondrichthyean GEP endocrine system has been tentatively summarized in Fig. 9. It is of particular interest in the phylogeny of the GEP endocrine system, since this is the first time in the phylogeny of extant vertebrates that (a) not only the B and D cells but also some of the glucagon-producing A cells have left the gut mucosa to join the islets, and (b) the islet parenchyma has become closely associated with the exocrine pancreatic gland. The GEP endocrine system of cartilaginous fish thus really deserves continued and intensified structural and functional studies.

Bony fish. The class Osteichthyes is usually subdivided (Fig. 7) into three major subclasses, viz.; Dipneusti (lungfishes), Crossopterygii (fringe fins), and Actinopterygii (ray fins). Both the lungfish and the fringe fins are from a quantitative point of view small subclasses only, where—with a few exceptions—no major advances have been made in the morphology of the GEP system during the last 5 years. Nevertheless, they are of great phylogenetical interest.[73] We have only been able to find a brief histological and ultrastructural report of the islet tissue in a lungfish[95] and a light-microscopical reinvestigation in two additional kinds of lungfish and in *Latimeria chalumnae* (the "living fossil"), the only extant representative of the suborder Coelacanthini of the Crossopterygii.[73] At the same time, some serious histological mistakes in earlier reports in both subclasses were corrected.[73]

Earlier reports[1] were confirmed. Thus, it was clearly established that the *Latimeria* islet parenchyma is located in a compact pancreas and that it appar-

---

Figure 8. Electron micrographs (generously provided by Dr. G. J. Patent, University of Montana, Missoula) of islet parenchymal cells in the holocephalan ratfish,[92] essentially showing their secretion granules. Those of the A cells (A) are of moderate size, electron dense, and spherical with fairly closely apposed granule membranes; thus showing all the characteristic features of the α granules of mammalian islet cells. The β granules (B) are large, often with rod-shaped crystalline cores. The smallest secretion granules are found in cells showing some similarities to the mammalian "PP cells" ("F cells") or D_1 (type IV) cells (C). Only slightly larger are the diameters of the secretion granules of the somatostatin-containing D cells (D). Except for this surprisingly small size, the fine structure of the δ granules conforms to that of the δ granules in the pancreatic islets of higher vertebrates.

The X cells (E) are unique to this subclass. Their secretion granules are largest of all. Except for their size, they show some similarities to the A cells, although no glucagon production has been observed immunocytochemically. In addition, occasional, granulated cells occur, difficult to classify (F). They may represent the chondrichthyean amphiphils, EC cells, intermediate X-A cells, or even granulocytes from the blood.

Glutaraldehyde fixation followed by postfixation in osmium tetroxide. Reproduced at 70%. Original magnifications: × 12,500 (A, B); ×8500 (C); ×17,100 (D); ×13,000 (E); ×5300 (F).

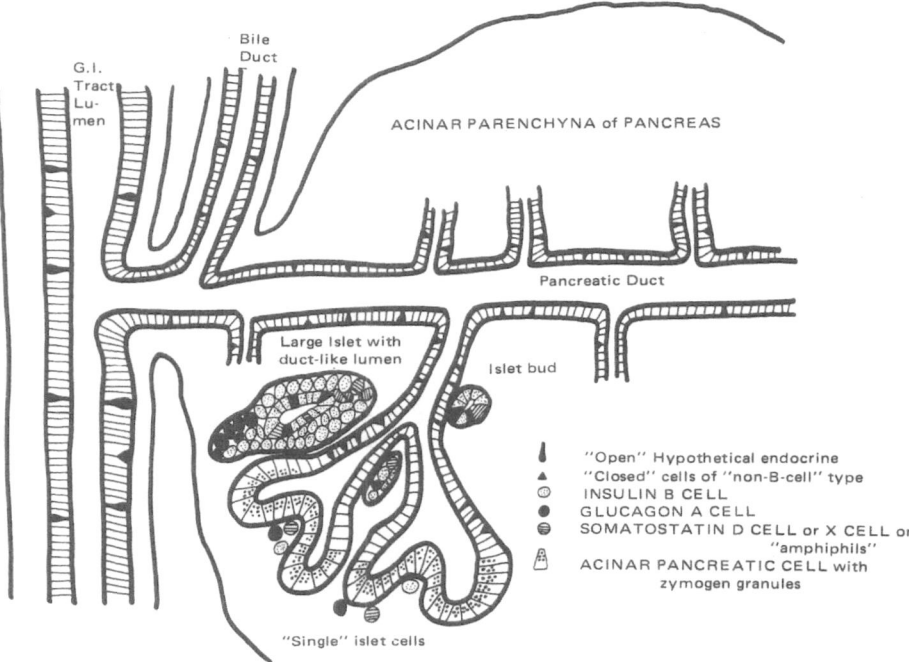

Figure 9. Schematic outline of the GEP endocrine system in an elasmobranchian cartilaginous fish (and in some primitive bony fish as well) and its relationship to the mucosa of the GI tract, the bile duct, and the compact pancreatic gland with its ducts. Due to the fact that only sparse information is available, the presentation is to a large extent highly hypothetical. Thus, it is not clear whether actually any endocrine cells of closed or open type occur in the mucosa of the bile duct. It has been shown, however, that hormones belonging to both the gastrin group and the secretin–glucagon family are produced in the GI tract of some elasmobranchs, and both EC, EC-like, and G cells have been found in the GI mucosa. It is well known that endocrine cells of islet type occur in the epithelium of both large and small pancreatic ducts and are scattered between the acinar cells, but practically no data are available on their ultrastructure and immunocytochemical properties. However, the presence of A, B, and D cells is definitely established, as well as the close association of the islet cells with the ducts. In the islets slit-like ductular structures can be found fairly frequently, in some respects reminding of the follicular cavities of the cyclostomian islet parenchyma.

This is the first time in vertebrate evolution when not only the B cells but also some of the glucagon-producing A cells have left the gut mucosa to join the islets, and when the islet parenchyma has become closely associated with the exocrine pancreatic gland.

ently shows all the typical features known of the primitive gnathostomian GEP system occurring in the cartilaginous fish.[73] However, the observations were based on conventional light microscopy only and, consequently, any detailed information of the GEP endocrine system in Crossopterygii is not available.

The most conspicuous feature of the pancreas in lungfish is that it is a compact, intraintestinal gland, situated inside the dorsal wall of the foregut.[1] It is marked grossly by a particularly strong and even distribution of melanophores.[73] The islets are few and usually separated from the exocrine parenchyma by a thick capsule of collagenous connective tissue. Thus, in some respects they may look rather similar to small Brockmann bodies ("principal islets") of the kind occurring in some ray fins (Fig. 10). Both light-microscopically and ultrastructurally it has now been clearly established that they contain typical A cells[95] in addition to the previously found B and D cells.[1] Whether or not any other kinds of cells also occur is still unknown, and the same holds true for the presence or absence of endocrine cells in the GI tract.

The Actinopterygii (ray fins) form quantitatively the completely predominating subclass among the bony fish. They, in turn, are dominated by one large group, viz., the teleosts (the common bony fish) (Fig. 7). There are, however, some additional minor groups here also, which recently have been studied with regard to their pancreatic islets, viz., the Polypteridae (bichirs and reedfish), the Chondrostei (sturgeons and paddlefish), and the Holostei (gars and bowfins).[73] As emphasized previously,[1] the latter group is of particular interest in diabetes research, owing to the fact that insulin from the pancreas of one of its representatives, the bowfin, *Amia calva,* has interesting immunological properties, combined with a remarkably low potency in a mammalian test system.[70] In the earlier review[1] it was stated that the islet cytology in Chondrostei and Holostei was essentially unknown (that of the Polypteridae was not mentioned at all).

The recent reinvestigation[73] showed that in all three groups the pancreas is widely scattered in the abdominal cavity, accompanying the branches of the portal vein and the bile ducts, also when they enter the liver parenchyma. Except for some large islets in the intrahepatic portion of the pancreas,[73] there are no gross islet accumulations with the formation of any structures like the Brockmann bodies ("principal islets") of some teleost fish.[1] Instead, the islets are rather of mammalian type, widely scattered throughout the exocrine pancreatic parenchyma.[73] The cytological composition of the islet parenchyma of the Chondrostei is still poorly known, but in some species of Polypteridae and Holostei it has been clearly established by correlated light and electron microscopy that at least four different kinds of islet parenchymal cells occur, viz., A, B, and D cells and a fourth type, obviously the same kind of cell that is present in the islet parenchyma of most of the teleosts (see below). Thus, except for the occurrence of partly intrahepatic pancreatic islets, often closely associated with the bile ducts, no fundamentally different or peculiar features have been found in the islet parenchyma of Polypteridae, Chondrostei, and Holostei when compared with that of other ray fins. We have been unable to find any reports—and have no data of our own to offer—in regard to the occurrence of endocrine cells in the GI tract of the Polypteridae, Chondrostei, and Holostei.

In the common bony fishes (Teleostei), ample information is available on the histophysiology of the islet parenchyma,[1] and some aspects have also been studied on the GI endocrine cells.[94,96] Consequently, there are a few teleost species where at least something is known about the whole GEP system. Considerable progress has been made in the morphology of the pancreatic islets in teleosts during the last 5 years, particularly in regard to the cytological composition of the islet parenchyma, where methodological errors, leading to previously made, false interpretations, have been clarified.[95] Moreover, the teleosts are still the only class outside the mammals where "spontaneous" diabetes mellitus has been discovered and histopathologically analyzed.[97]

The gross features of the endocrine pancreas of teleosts are often characterized by the presence of one, two, or even multiple Brockmann bodies—also called principal islets (Fig. 10)—in addition to small islets of Langerhans,

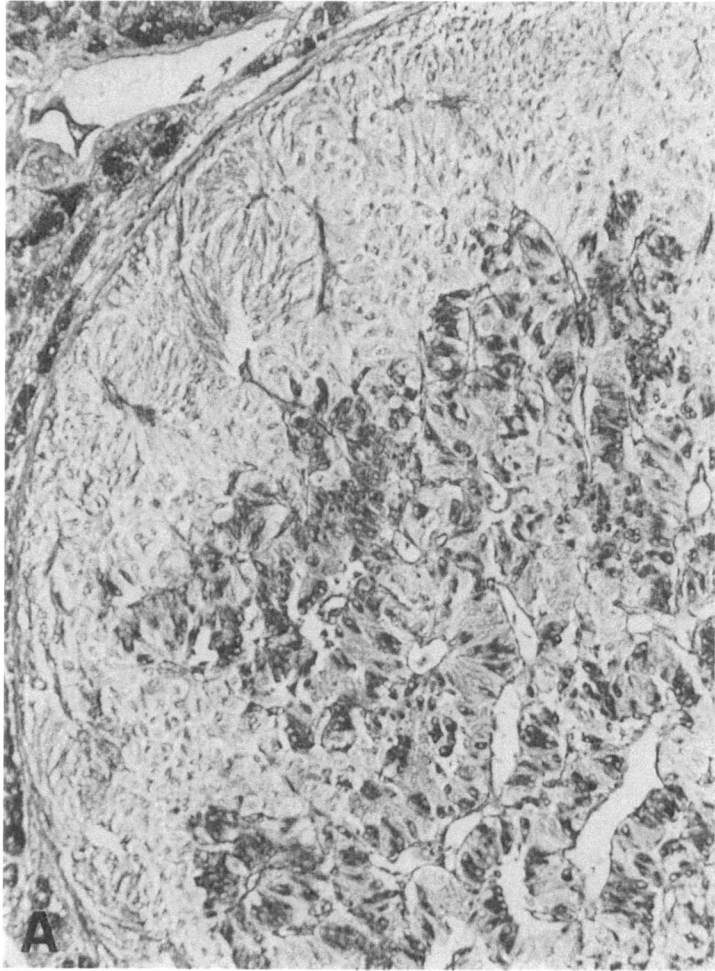

Figure 10. Medium-power photomicrographs of approximately one quadrant of a Brockmann body ("principal islet") of the teleost fish, *Cottus scorpius* (the daddy sculpin). Bouin's fixative has been used which implies that a "dark" central region and a "light" periphery can be distinguished in Fig. 10A, where the section is stained with Af. The thin capsule of collagenous connective tissue is also clearly seen (left). Outside the capsule there is exocrine acinar pancreatic parenchyma (dark) (upper and lower left corners) with a large vessel. In the central region two kinds of cells occur, viz., insulin-producing B cells (black) and somatostatin-producing D cells (dark gray). In addition, there are large amounts of thin-walled blood vessels (empty spaces) but practically no supporting stroma. In the peripheral region all the cells appear uniformly light-grayish in the photomicrograph. ×320.

occurring in a more or less compact pancreatic gland or widely disseminated in the mesenterial fat, usually associated with thin strands of exocrine pancreatic parenchyma.[1,98-100] Two things must be emphasized,[73] viz.: (a) that the arrangement with Brockmann bodies is far from regular in common bony fish and that it tends to occur only in "higher" teleosts (essentially the Ctenosquamata among Euteleostei), whereas all other teleost groups have a "disseminated" or "diffuse"

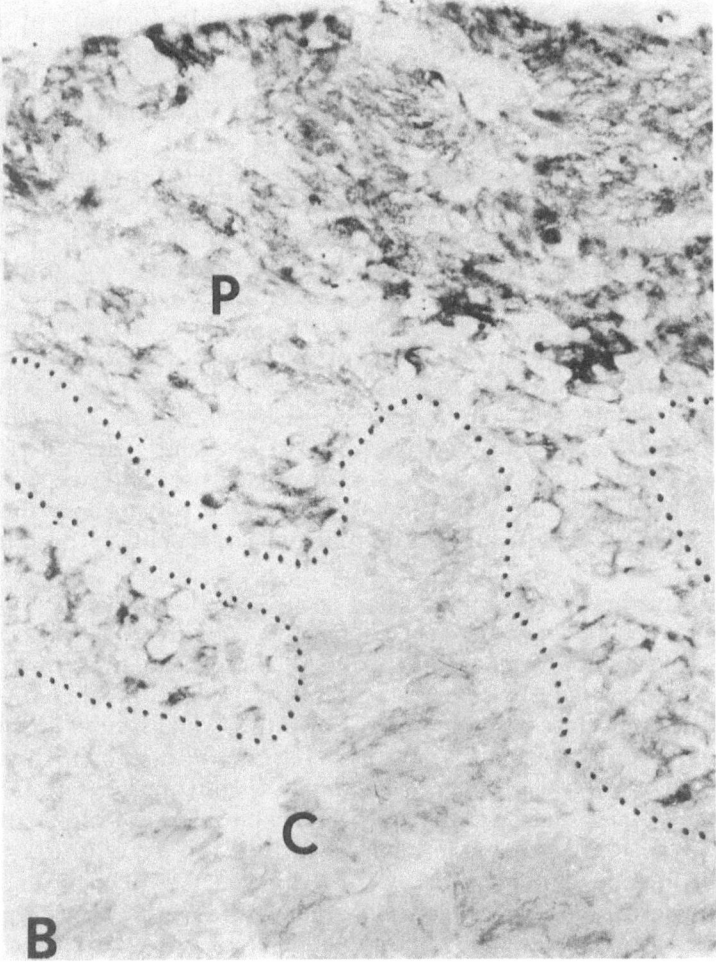

Fig. 10B shows a similar sector of the Brockmann body after staining by Grimelius' silver nitrate procedure, and the central region (C) is barely discernible (no counterstain has been used), whereas the periphery (P) stands out distinctly, due to its content of argyrophil, glucagon-producing A cells (black). There are, however, both in the central region and in the peripheral one, cells that give a faint argyrophilia. They may be D_1 cells, previously interpreted as "agranular" C cells.

The high degree of vascularity and the sparse occurrence of supporting stroma explains why teleost islet parenchyma of this kind is particularly prone to obtain artifacts during manipulations and fixation procedures.[95] ×400.

pancreas with small, grossly invisible, widely scattered islets of Langerhans[73,98]; and (b) that even when Brockmann bodies of "high purity" occur (i.e., those containing no strands of exocrine, acinar pancreatic parenchyma inside the surrounding capsule of collagenous connective tissue) as in, for instance, *Cottus scorpius* (the daddy sculpin) (Fig. 10), *Scorpaena scropha* (scorpion fish), *Lophius piscatorius* (the angler fish), and *Xiphophorus helleri*,[1,99,100] no complete separation of these giant accumulations of islet tissue from exocrine pancreas has occurred, although the two parts may be separated by a capsule of connective tissue.[100] Of phylogenetical interest is the frequently seen close association of these Brockmann bodies with the gallbladder and bile ducts.[73] Also, when the endocrine and exocrine pancreas is of "diffuse" or "disseminated" type, there is an intimate topographical relationship to the bile ducts, even when they enter the liver. Thus, even in teleosts an "intrahepatic" pancreas can occur.[73]

The fact that no principal differences exist between the Brockmann bodies and the smaller islets of Langerhans, disseminated in the exocrine pancreas and/or the mesentery, is further supported by the cellular composition and the distribution of the parenchymal cells (Fig. 11). Although the relative frequencies of islet cells can vary rather widely between islets of different size,[99] the general pattern is practically constant, not only for one and the same species but also for the whole subgroup of teleosts. As a matter of fact, it is possible to discern some almost regularly recurring features in the general outline of the large and small islets of all higher teleosts, as previously suggested from our laboratory.[57] Here, however, some corrections of preceding reports must be made after the recent discovery of methodological errors made in the morphological analysis of teleostean islet parenchyma, particularly the Brockmann bodies.[22,95]

Owing to the fact that these giant islets—often as large as a pea[1]—have only little connective tissue stroma to support the tissue and are highly vascularized with a high fluid content (Fig. 10), dicing—to provide uniform exposure to the fixative—even with the sharpest instruments results in considerable cellular damage.[95] Moreover, it has long been known that some fixatives (usually those with a poor protein-precipitating capacity) are notorious for their inability to preserve the cells in the peripheral region of teleostean islets[99]; a fact that has caused some misinterpretations of early experimental results in diabetes research in fish.[101] When modern ultrastructural preparation techniques are applied in the morphological analysis of the islet parenchyma of bony fish, using intravascular perfusion techniques and paraformaldehyde–glutaraldehyde fixatives, with and without postfixation in osmium tetroxide, it has convincingly been shown that all[95]—or at least most of—teleostean islet cells, previously interpreted as "agranular" islet C cells,[1,41] are actually granulated parenchymal cells of a fourth (or even fifth) type.[22,95,100]

Since the preceding review a fairly large amount of work has been published on the light-microscopic and ultrastructural appearance of the teleostean islet parenchyma[77,91,95,96,100,103–106] but only one group[100] has used most of the procedures needed for a complete structural analysis, as described above (in Methods). Moreover, only one has comprised the whole GEP endocrine system.[96] Nevertheless, the conclusions of the reports have so many features in

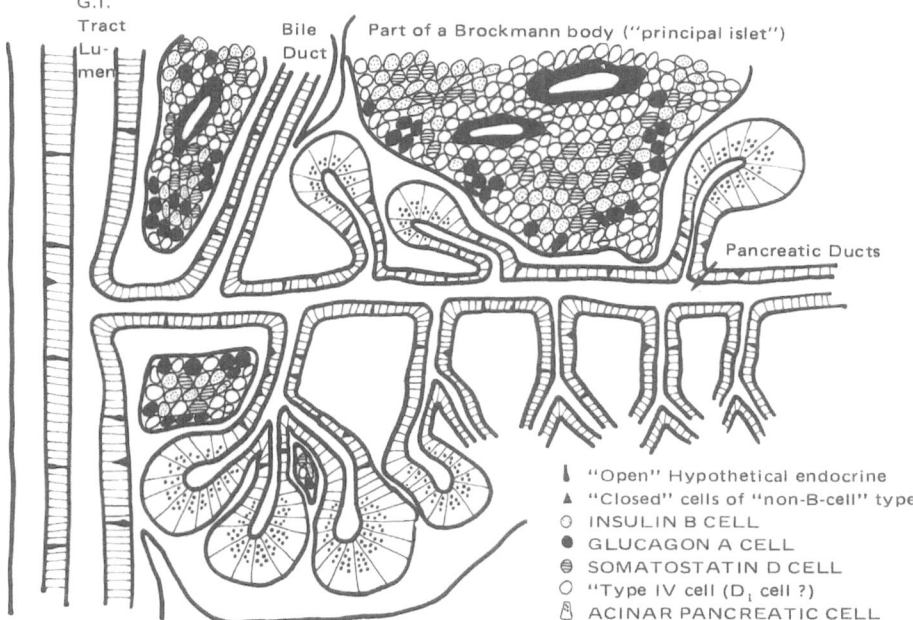

G.I. Tract Lumen

Bile Duct

Part of a Brockmann body ("principal islet")

Pancreatic Ducts

⌇ "Open" Hypothetical endocrine
▲ "Closed" cells of "non-B-cell" type
○ INSULIN B CELL
● GLUCAGON A CELL
⊖ SOMATOSTATIN D CELL
○ "Type IV cell (D_1 cell ?)
⌂ ACINAR PANCREATIC CELL

Figure 11. Schematic outline of the GEP endocrine system in bony fish, essentially as it appears in highly developed teleosts, and its relationship to the mucosa of the GI tract, the bile duct, and the more or less disseminated pancreas with its ducts. Due to the fact that only sparse information is available on the extrainsular endocrine cells, the presentation is to a large extent highly hypothetical. Thus, it is not known whether any endocrine cells of closed or open type actually occur in the bile duct mucosa and in the pancreatic duct epithelium. In the GI mucosa, however, open and closed endocrine cells of the same type as in cartilaginous fish (Fig. 9) are known to occur, viz., at least G and EC cells.

Although the predominating amounts of islet parenchyma occur in the Brockmann bodies ("principal islets"), there are, in addition, always smaller islets of mammalian type, associated with the exocrine acinar pancreas and its ducts. Moreover, even the most "pure" Brockmann bodies contain some exocrine parenchyma, at least outside the connective tissue capsule. The principal islets are usually situated close to the gallbladder and bile ducts, but in lungfishes the large islets are located so intimately to the gut that they are almost "intraintestinal."

The cellular composition is essentially the same in the giant and small islets, consisting of insulin-producing B cells and somatostatin-producing D cells in the central region of the islets and glucagon-producing A cells and (PP producing???) D_1 cells, mainly in the periphery (cf. Fig. 10).

common that it seems possible to try some generalizations and to form a tentative opinion of the general pattern of the GEP endocrine system in higher teleost fish (Fig. 11).

It is clearly established that typical B cells occur, mainly in the central region of the islets, often intermingled with A_1 (or D) cells.[99] In the peripheral parts glucagon-producing A cells are present, giving all the characteristic reactions met with in higher vertebrates, although in some species[100,104] the ultrastructural appearance of the secretion granules shows more marked variability than was supposed to occur previously.[1] As far as the A and B cells are concerned, the light-microscopical tinctorial features, the histochemical characteristics, and the fine structure of the secretion granules—i.e., all the parameters that usually form the basis of the islet cell classifications—have only been checked by immunofluorescence in a single report.[100] As to the A_1 (or D) cells, no such immunocytochemical investigations have been published.

Here, however, we have some still unpublished results of current research to offer.* In the daddy sculpin *(C. scorpius)*, where preceding light-microscopical studies showed the presence of A_1 cells in the central region of the principal islets (Fig. 10),[99] high concentrations (210 ng/mg wet wt.) of somatostatin were found by radioimmunological assays of acid–ethanol extracts of these Brockmann bodies. Previously, hormonal assays of extracts of sculpin principal islets failed to show the production of gastrin.[1] Similar results have been obtained in immunocytochemical investigations (by the unlabeled-antibody-peroxidase-antiperoxidase procedure) of the principal islets of the angler fish *(L. piscatorius)* and the channel catfish *(Ictalurus punctata)*, where the ratio of immunoreactive insulin/somatostatin/glucagon cells in the principal islets was found to be 9/6/4 in both species.[107]

Data available on the relative frequencies of occurrence of A, B, and D cells and other islet parenchymal cells in teleost fish vary somewhat. Common figures are: A cells, 25–40%; B cells, 30–50%; D cells, 15–20%; and chromophobic, clear cells (C and/or D_1 cells), 10–20%.[1,99,106] In diabetic fish the number of chromophobic, clear cells (C and/or D_1 cells) increases considerably,[97,104] again indicating their precursor character[1,41] (Fig. 2).

The most comprehensive ultrastructural and immunofluorescence studies of teleostean principal islets have been performed in *X. helleri*, where observations of great comparative interest were made.[100] Here it has been confirmed that several kinds of fixatives are needed in order to perform a correct structural analysis of teleostean Brockmann bodies, particularly of the clear, chromophobe cells. When this had been accomplished, and a correlated light-microscopic and ultrastructural technique had been applied, it was found that the glucagon-immunoreactive A cells showed a duality not described previously in any vertebrate islet parenchyma. One nonacidophil A cell type with rhombo-dodecahedral crystalline cores of the secretion granules was suggested to be a more mature form than another kind of A cell of more conventional type,[2] being acidophil and containing spherical secretion granules with electron-dense noncrystalline cores. The A cells of the allegedly more mature type were situated more centrally in the islets. This could be interpreted so that the cell renewal and the maturation process occurs from the periphery of teleostean principal islets towards the central region, as previously suggested from our laboratory.[1] The crystalline state of the cores of the α-granules was not anything typical for just glucagon; crystals were observed in the cores of some secretion granules of B cells, as well.[100] There is, however, good evidence that the cores of these α-granules are identical to dried glucagon rhombic dodecahedral crystals, implying that these granules contain trimers, as found by recent X-ray analyses of crystals of pig glucagon.[102]

*See first footnote on p. 33.

It was determined that the clear cells (fifth type) observed explicitly do not represent an immature precursor cell, or an intermediary form, or cells in a "resting state" of any of the A, B, or D cells; this was concluded by others as well.[104,105] To judge from the electron micrographs,[100] the clear cells seemed to contain secretion granules of several different types. The possibility that they might represent D_1 (type IV) cells was not discussed. It was not stated whether they showed APUD characters and, obviously, they were not argyrophil by Grimelius' procedure. No hormonal assays were made. Of particular interest is the statement that no intermediary cells of acino-insular type occurred.[100] By careful TEM studies it could be shown that special "neuroglandular" junctions existed in all kinds of islet parenchymal cells, giving good proofs for the interpretation that a direct nervous regulation of the synthesis and release of teleostean islet hormones exists. Autoradiographically, the nerve endings were obviously not adrenergic. They were supposed to be either serotoninergic or cholinergic.[100] These observations on the islet innervation essentially conform to those made in the principal islets of other teleosts,[106] and it has been suggested that the rarity of similar nerve endings in the islet parenchyma of other vertebrates indicates that they are unique to the teleosts.[73,106]

Except for the light-microscopic studies in *Mugil auratus*[96] and *Ictalurus nebulosus*,[95] practically nothing is known of the presence or absence of endocrine cells in the GI tract of teleost fish. From comparative studies[9,108–110] it has, however, been observed that in the GI mucosa of some species of teleosts there are hormones belonging to both the gastrin group (CCK) (108) and the secretin family,[110] the latter factor(s) resembling VIP more closely than secretin.[109] In the gastric mucosa of *M. auratus* apparently both "closed" and "open" cells of A type were found in the cardial zone, whereas the gizzard and the pyloric appendages contained typical EC cells.[96] In current histological and immuno-fluorescence investigations* in pilot studies from our laboratory we have also observed argyrophil cells in the pyloric appendages of *C. scorpius*, showing immunoreactivity with antisera to mammalian gastrin. Moreover, a large number of argyrophil cells were found by Grimelius' procedure throughout the entire GI tract.

A schematic outline of the GEP endocrine system in highly developed teleosts is given in Fig. 11. The scheme is to some extent highly hypothetical, particularly considering the fact that apparently nothing is known about the presence or absence of endocrine cells in the bile duct mucosa and in the mucosa of the larger pancreatic ducts.

Tetrapoda

There are several gross and microscopic features that are common to the endocrine pancreas and the whole GEP endocrine system of amphibians, reptiles, birds, and mammals.[1,2] They all seem to have a compact pancreatic gland, equipped with disseminated islets of Langerhans.[1,22] In the GI mucosa several kinds of endocrine cells occur.[94] In the pancreatic islets A, B,

*See first footnote on p. 33.

and D cells are regularly found, although their relative frequencies can vary considerably. Thus, among the four subclasses of tetrapods there are more quantitative rather than qualitative variations in the morphology of the islet parenchyma, implying that it can be accounted for rather briefly.

Amphibians. Being already previously a classical experimental object in diabetes research,[111] the amphibian has, during the last few years, stimulated renewed interest in GEP endocrinology, owing to the discoveries of all the interesting, biologically active polypeptides that are present in the skin of *Anura* (frogs and toads) that have mammalian counterparts,[9] usually located in cells of the mucosa of the GI tract.[112] Examples of such hormonal substances in the frog skin are the caerulein group of peptides, bearing a striking resemblance to CCK with an almost identical amino acid sequence in the active region; the physalae-min-type peptides, closely related to substance P; the bradykinin-like peptides, corresponding to mammalian plasma kinins; and now also the bombesin family, in which no mammalian counterpart has yet been established, although cells specifically stained with antibodies to bombesin have been found in endocrine cells of non-EC type, being widely distributed in the human GI mucosa.[113] All these observations can be considered as a further support to the neuroectoder-mal origin of GEP endocrine cells.[112]

In the three main extant subclasses of the amphibians, viz., the Urodela, the Apoda, and the Anura, the pancreatic islets are, as a rule, small, with a marked predominance of the B cells; for some time it was even claimed that the urodele islets would have no A cells.[2] Common figures for the relative frequen-cies of different islet cells are in anuran islets: 50–75% B cells, 10–25% A cells, and 10–25% D cells.[22] Excellent schematic illustrations of the gross anatomy of amphibian (and reptilian) pancreas have been given in a preceding review,[111] showing close anatomical connections with the bile ducts, in particular, but also with the duodenum and the spleen. In the splenic portion of the pancreas the islets increase in number and size (as in most other tetrapods). In addition to the A, B, and D cells, amphiphil cells have been found,[22] apparently corresponding to intermediary cells of acinoinsular type.[1,52,114] It can be assumed that also D_1 cells occur, considering the reports that in apodan islets some A cells have been found, giving faint argyrophilia also by the Hellerström–Hellman procedure,[2] and that in anuran islets some cells with β and α granules and others with δ and α granules have been observed,[114] as well as light-microscopically agranular cells.[115] As in teleost islets, the B cells occupy a central position in the islets.[22] Their granule cores are often crystalline.[22,114]

The occurrence of GI endocrine cells in amphibians has recently been investigated light-microscopically in 16 species of all the three major extant subclasses[116] and by TEM in one anuran species.[117] Four cell types were regularly found light-microscopically, two in the stomach (EC-like and G cells) and two (EC cells and A cells?) in the duodenum,[116] whereas at least six types were observed ultrastructurally of which five were identified as EC, EC-like, A, G, and S cells.[117] Most cells were of open type, equipped not only with microvilli but also with a single cilium of 8+1 axoneme pattern, suggesting a sensory nature of the cell.[117]

Consequently, not only the islet parenchyma but also the whole GEP endocrine system in most amphibians is similar to that in mammals.[116,117] Exceptions are the islet tissues of some low-order Urodela, viz., *Necturus* (the American "mudpuppy") and *Cryptobranchidae* (giant salamanders; the "hellbender"), which show similarities to the most primitive gnathostomian islet parenchyma.[73] Also as to the islet innervation, the similarities to mammalian islet parenchyma are striking. There is particularly a well-developed parasympathetic innervation.[118]

Reptiles. All the three main extant subclasses of the reptiles—Chelonia (turtles and tortoises), Squamata (snakes and lizards), and Crocodilia (alligators and crocodiles)—have, since the preceding reviews,[1,2] been the subject of several studies of their GEP endocrine system. Thus, Gabe, in the last works of his life, made two most comprehensive light-microscopical investigations of the endocrine cells in the stomach of not less than 42 reptilian species,[119] and in 21 of them he also studied the endocrine cells of the duodenum.[120] Moreover, the facts that the β granules of the islet parenchyma of some Squamata are especially large and equipped with crystalline cores have made the snakes and lizards particularly attractive as experimental animals in studies on various modes of intravital crystallization of insulin and/or proinsulin[22,121] and on the relationships between β granule morphology and B cell function,[122,123] including emiocytosis.[124]

The gross aspects of the compact reptilian pancreas has recently been most instructively illustrated in a review, comprising all the main subclasses.[111] Particularly interesting from a comparative point of view is the tendency of the islets to become larger but fewer in the splenic portion with the occasional occurrence of giant islets without exocrine parenchyma in the spleen, forming a structure homologous to a Brockmann body of teleosts in some species.[1,125] As to the quantitative aspects of the reptilian islet parenchyma, preceding statements that there is a marked predominance of A cells[1,2] have been confirmed. Thus, in two species of lizards the relative frequencies of the three main islet cells have been given as: A cells, 45–50%; B cells, 40%; and D cells, 10–15%,[122,126] whereas in *Varanus niloticus* the A cells have been found to constitute even more than 70% in the largest islet (a Brockmann body homologue), with B cells around 10%, whereas D cells, agranular C cells, and intermediate acinoinsular cells make up the rest.[125] These figures can be compared with those of preliminary results from our laboratory* of radioimmunoassays of the contents of glucagon, insulin, and somatostatin in pancreas of seven specimens of the snakes *Natrix natrix* and *Vipera berus*. They were 50, 70, and 20 ng/mg wet wt., respectively.

The reptilian islet C cells (as observed in *V. niloticus*) were of three types, viz.: (a) those budding out from the epithelium of the small ducts; (b) those located close to the adjacent acinar parenchyma, together with intermediate acinoinsular cells; and (c) those situated inside the islet parenchyma.[125] Their precursor characters become evident from the observation that they—as well as the intermediate acinoinsular cells—increased in number during the spawning

*See first footnote on p. 33.

season when the islets grow rapidly, and that some of them contained zinc (presumably B cell precursors), whereas others could be slightly argyrophil by the Hellerström–Hellman procedure (presumably D_1 cells or D cell precursors).[125] By SEM, combined with an X-ray microdiffraction procedure, the β granules were found to contain ample amounts of zinc but no cobalt or manganese.[125] The A cells contained no zinc at all.[125]

These recent observations give support to the working hypothesis that the crystal-like β granules of the pancreatic islets of some Squamata are actually zinc–insulin crystals of dodecahedral shape.[22,121] The size of the β granules decreases after long-term insulin administration,[123,126] as well as after glucose loading,[122] parallel to a decrease in the insulin content of the pancreas.[123] In stimulated insulin release from lizard pancreatic islets, perifused *in vitro*, emiocytosis of β granules was observed, but not in nonstimulated islets, nor in islet B cells from an intact lizard.[124]

The marked predominance of A cells in reptilian pancreatic islets has been supposed to be responsible for a rather high fasting blood glucose level and for the observations that some reptiles become hypoglycemic rather than hyperglycemic after pancreatectomy.[127] This is a situation that becomes more obvious in the closely related birds[1,2] (see below). The α granules are usually remarkably large but otherwise uniform in most reptiles studied,[22,122,125,126] whereas the diameter of the δ granules can vary considerably. Their basic structure is, nonetheless, essentially the same throughout the gnathostomian vertebrate series.[126]

Reptilian pancreas has a uniform distribution of nerve fibers, and the islets seem to show a well-balanced ratio between adrenergic and cholinergic innervation.[128] Possible exceptions to this rule are said to be found in Chelonia and Crocodilia.[73] Neuroglandular junctions occur only occasionally in reptiles.[128] In the cytoplasm of both A and B cells a nonnervous acetylcholinergic activity has been observed.[128]

Although in an earlier study no gastrin was found in the islet parenchyma of some snakes,[1] it is reasonable to expect not only gastrin-producing cells but also a well-developed GI endocrine system in general in reptiles, because both EC cells and non-EC, endocrine, argyrophil cells have been found light-microscopically in the GI mucosa of a large number of reptile species.[119–120]

Birds. The birds are often brought together with the reptiles into one large subclass, Sauropsida,[2] and this is sometimes also done when the phylogeny of the GEP endocrine system is reviewed.[73,119,129] The birds have been of great importance in diabetes research and in the comparative endocrinology of GEP hormones, due to some anatomical and physiological peculiarities of these animals.[1,2] Some of the first observations linking the production of glucagon with the A cells were made in birds,[1] as well as the ultimate light-microscopical subdivision of the "α cells" into A and D cells.[2] Still, they are playing an important role in GEP endocrinology, due to the recent discovery of PP[19–21] that was originally made in birds ("avian pancreatic polypeptide"), where its physiological and biochemical characteristics and cytological localization are best known.[21,129,130] Most information available on the GEP endocrine system in birds stems from the results of investigations in fowls (the Phasianidae) only,[1,2] and it is not known to what extent observations in fowls may be applicable to feral birds also. Great variations probably occur (A. Epple, personal communication).

Grossly, the compact avian (fowl) pancreas is subdivided into four lobes: a ventral, a dorsal, a third, and a splenic lobe. The latter is often contiguous with the spleen and is so small that in some species it measures only about 5 mm³.[131] Its relationship to the Brockmann bodies of some bony fish and their homologues in reptiles (see above) is illustrated by the fact that about 50% of this lobe consists of islet parenchyma.[131]

The classical concept is that in birds there is a segregation of A and B cells into "dark" and "ligh" islets, respectively.[1,2,131,132] The "dark" A islets are large, irregularly shaped, and located exclusively to the third and splenic lobes, whereas the "light" B islets are small (in cross sections seldom consisting of more than 30 cells), spherical, and evenly distributed in all four lobes.[131] In addition, ordinary islets of Langerhans occur, called islets of "mixed type."[132] From the results of light-microscopical investigations it has been claimed that the avian endocrine pancreas should be particularly rich in D cells,[1,2] but recent ultrastructural studies have not confirmed these statements.[131,132] Although it is difficult to give any overall figures for the relative frequencies of the different cell types, it seems clear from the results of correlated light-microscopic and ultrastructural studies that, in addition to the markedly predominating A, B, and D cells, also small-granulated islet cells of D_1 (and F?) type as well as agranular islet C cells occur, and that probably some of the small-granulated cells might previously have been interpreted as argyrophil D cells, thus accounting for the allegedly high frequency of occurrence of these cells.[131] However, it has recently been shown by immunofluorescence that the avian pancreas, particularly that of young birds, contains abundant amounts of somatostatin,[133,134] again indicating a rich supply of D cells.[134] Also intermediate acinoinsular cells, both of A and B type, have been found.[52] In the large, "dark" A islets not only A cells and irregularly disseminated D cells occur, but there are also a few B cells, as well as occasional D_1 and agranular C cells.[131,132] Mostly the D cells are located peripherally.[133] In the small, "light" B islets the predominating B cells occupy the central parts of the islets, whereas the D cells occur in the periphery together with a few A cells.[131,132] D_1 cells and agranular C cells occur only seldom in the B islets, viz., one or two cells per islet.[131] The general rule seems to be that the A cells in the B islets are not as frequent as the B cells in the A islets.[132]

Although the average diameters of the secretion granules of avian A, B, and D cells have been reported to be about 500 nm for all the three cell types,[131] there is a fairly wide variation within each type. Thus, in the domestic fowl the following values have recently been given for the mean diameters of the secretion granules and their ranges[132]: A cells, 410 (310–570) nm; B cells, 580 (350–960) nm; D cells, 470 (280–700) nm; D_1 cells, 240 (170–430) nm. The morphology of the maturation process of the secretion granules has also been described in detail in this species,[132] essentially supporting the working hypothesis for the differentiation of islet cells put forward in preceding sections of this review (Fig. 2). Avian D_1 cells are characterized by the presence of cytoplasmic secretion granules of rod-shaped or biconcave profiles with usually a higher electron density than that of the δ granules.[131] Emiocytosis has been observed in A, B, and D cells.[132]

Widely diverging opinions exist as to the innervation of the avian pancreatic islets. Whereas some reports state that the endocrine pancreas of birds is equipped with abundantly occurring autonomous innervation of sympathetic fibers, probably with axon terminals,[132,135] other works (in other species) explicitly deny the presence of islet innervation in birds, stating that there is exclusively a hormonal control of the secretion of avian islet hormones.[131,136] If so, the endocrine pancreas of birds would, in this respect, differ form all other kinds of tetrapod vertebrate islet parenchyma except for that of some reptiles.[73] The reason for this controversy is unclear but may be due to species differences or to the posibility that vasomotoric innervation has been misinterpreted as islet innervation.

As to the GI endocrine cells, the birds are obviously equipped with all the main hormone-producing cells of the GI tract occurring in mammals, possibly except for GIP.[94,119,120,137,138] This statement is based on the results of light-microscopical[119,129] and correlated immunocytochemical and ultrastructural investigations[133,136,137] in a fairly large number of species and individuals. Thus, it has recently been shown that PP cells (F cells?) occur in the upper duodenum of birds.[138] Moreover, the ontogeny of the GEP endocrine system is well known as a result of several comprehensive studies in chick embryos.[139–143] Of particular interest for the working hypothesis that also B cells may occur in the GI mucosa[1] is the observation in one of these reports that an insulin-like substance was discovered from the developing chick duodenal mucosa.[140] Also, the recent observation that complete pancreatectomy in the chicken does not abolish circulating insulin in the blood[144] points toward the presence of an extrapancreatic source of insulin production in birds.

Mammals. Detailed and comprehensive reviews of the morphology and ontogeny of the pancreatic islets in some mammals are given in Chapters 3 and 6 of this monograph. Handbooks on this subject usually deal with the endocrine pancreas of primates (monkeys, apes, man), carnivores (e.g., cats, dogs), lagomorphs (rabbits), and rodents (e.g., mice, rats, hamsters, guinea pigs), as well as with some notes on insectivores (hedgehogs, moles), Chiroptera (bats), and perissodactylan (horses) and artiodactylan (e.g., pigs, cattle) species.[1] Although some peculiarities can be found—and have been further clarified (see below) since the preceding reviews[1,2]—still no fundamental differences seem to exist in this major group. It is called Eutheria (Placentalia) and comprises some 24 subgroups. Among the more primitive mammals, such as the Metatheria (Marsupialia) and the Prototheria (egg-laying mammals), no major progress has been made since the preceding reviews[1,2] of the morphology of the GEP endocrine system. Still, it is essentially unknown. Likewise, no informative studies seem to have been made during the last 5 years of the islet morphology in mammals living under extreme climatic conditions (e.g., arctic and desert rodents).[1]

There are, however, a few recent reports on mammalian islet morphology that are of some comparative interest. An enigma for a long time was the so-called X cell in the central region of the islets of the horse. It has now been clarified that these "X cells" are nothing but ordinary glucagon-producing A cells, and that in the periphery of the horse islets not only B and D cells occur, but also occasional G cells and a cell type (called "S cells") with small granules.[145] To judge from the electron micrographs, it seems possible that these "S cells" might be F cells, capable of secreting PP. Intermediate cells were only seen after immersion fixation and not after perfusion fixation. Consequently, they were looked upon as simple artifacts.[145]

The peculiar topographical distribution of the different parenchymal cells in the horse islets gets some explanation from the results of recent studies of the microcirculation in horse pancreas.[146] Here, it was found that the afferent artery to the horse islets enters in the middle of the islet, instead of from the periphery as in most mammalian islets.[146] Moreover, it was found that the exocrine acinar pancreatic parenchyma receives its blood supply by the efferent vessels from the islets via an insuloacinar portal system.[146] This anatomical arrangement facilitates a direct hormonal action,[91] not only by the islet cells on the exocrine pancreatic parenchyma, but also as a direct influence of the A cells on the D cells and the A and D cells on the B cells.[146] As a matter of fact, it seems to be a rule that in the tetrapod pancreatic islets—and in Brockmann bodies of higher teleosts as well (see above)—the afferent blood vessels first reach the A and D cells and then pass to the B cells, thus allowing modifying effects of glucagon and somatostatin on the insulin release. This insuloacinar portal system also explains the so-called periinsular halos ("Zymogenhöfe") in the acinar parenchyma around the islets,[146] where somatostatin, in particular, has recently been proposed to play a major role.[83]

The GI endocrine cells are well known in eutherian mammals and have recently been reviewed several times.[8-14] They form the principal endocrine organ in the mammalian body, both in magnitude and in the variety of its products.[94]

Also, the innervation of the islet parenchyma in mammals is well known, and here some interesting observations have recently been made in the dog pancreas.[147] Structural modifications of the Schwann cells were found, indicating that they may play a role in the neural control of islet function.

Summarizing Conclusions

The phylogeny of the GEP endocrine cells offers several kinds of support for an embryological origin of these polypeptide-hormone-producing cells from the neuroectoderm. An obvious example is the recent isolation of insulin-like and glucagon-like hormones from typical neurosecretory glands in some arthropods.

Later on (when the possibly neural-crest-derived cells have settled down in the primitive GI mucosa), a close evolutionary connection obviously arises between the prospective islet parenchymal cells and the mucosa of the GI tract. As a matter of fact, insulin-producing B cells—in addition to glucagon-producing A cells, somatostatin-containing D cells, and some of the more conventional GI endocrine cells—are present in the GI mucosa of protostomian and deuterostomian invertebrates. Consequently, all the islet cells have their ancestors in the GI mucosa and represent a further specialization of them. Concepts such as "GEP endocrine system" and "enteroinsular axis" thus have a solid phylogenetical background.

The first time in evolution that a separate islet organ appears in extant species is in the most primitive vertebrates, viz., the cyclostomes (lampreys and hagfish). In the Atlantic hagfish the islet lobules bud off from the endocrine cells in the bile duct mucosa. Both B cells and D cells occur in the bile duct mucosa and the islet parenchyma, but no A cells occur in either location. Thus, B and D cells probably left the gut earlier in evolution than the A cells, forming a separate islet organ even before the development of an exocrine pancreas. The cyclostomian islet organ has, however, retained some primitive features, such as the occurrence of large cystic cavities, the (possible) absence of nerves and vessels inside the islet lobules, and the presence of so-called connective-tissue hormone secretion.

In all gnathostomian vertebrates the islet parenchyma is intimately associated with the exocrine acinar pancreas, and the islets contain not only B and D cells but also A cells. Thus, it is obvious that the cyclostomian islet parenchyma forms an evolutionary connecting link between the gut-associated A, B, and D cells of some invertebrates and the islets of Langerhans disseminated in the pancreatic gland of gnathostomian vertebrates.

No fundamental differences seem to exist between the major subclasses of the gnathostomian vertebrates in regard to the morphology and cellular composition of the GEP endocrine system. Considerable quantitative variations occur, however, Likewise, the ultrastructure of the secretion granules of all the islet cells is surprisingly uniform throughout the gnathostomian series despite large variations in their size.

In cartilaginous fish and in several of the more primitive bony fish the islet cells are markedly duct associated with ample amounts of A cells and the appearance of the peculiar X cells, as well as small-granulated islet cells (D_1 cells?) and amphiphils (intermediate cells). This islet parenchyma is in many respects similar to that observed in early fetal life of mammals.

In highly developed teleosts the giant principal islets, called Brockmann bodies, are the most characteristic features, containing about equal amounts of A, B, D, and chromophobic, clear, small-granulated (and/or agranular?) cells (D_1 and/or C cells?). They are, however, still associated with the exocrine pancreas, where also small islets of Langerhans usually occur.

In amphibians the islets are small and widely disseminated with a marked predominance of B cells. As in most gnathostomes, the β granules often have crystalline cores. Intermediary cells of acinoinsular type are said to be rather common.

In some reptiles the islets in the splenic part of the pancreas can be so large that they form homologues to the teleostean Brockmann bodies. There is a marked predominance of A cells, and their secretion granules are often as large as zymogen granules.

Also in birds the islets in the splenic lobe of the pancreas are few but large, constituting as much as 50% of the volume of this lobe with a predominance of A cells. Dark "A islets" and light "B islets" occur together with ordinary islets of mixed type. Neither the "A islets" nor the "B islets" contain one cell type only. There are always D cells and usually other islet parenchymal cells, as well. The A cells in the B islets are, however, not as numerous as the B cells in the A islets.

With the possible exception of the islet parenchyma of some birds and reptiles, the islet cells of all the gnathostomian vertebrates appear to be innervated. The vascularization seems to be arranged so as to allow a direct hormonal action of the A and D cells upon the B cells and a subsequent direct influence of all the islet hormones upon the adjacent acinar exocrine parenchyma.

In order to adequately characterize the GEP endocrine cells of both invertebrate and vertebrate species, it is necessary to use several fixation procedures (particularly for the Brockmann bodies), followed by more or less modified modern differential granule staining techniques, combined with immunofluorescence microscopy and TEM. Whenever possible, direct hormonal assays must also be performed in order to check the morphological observations, to get quantitative aspects on the hormone production, and to avoid failing immunological cross-reactivity.

The results of these phylogenetical studies give further support to the working hypothesis that the islet C cells, and apparently also some of the small-granulated islet cells, are more or less immature precursor cells to the A, B, and D cells. They appear in states of hyperplasia and regeneration as well as in the growth zone of the islet parenchyma of low-order vertebrates and are common in poorly differentiated islet cell tumors.

Thus, it can definitely be agreed that "those experiments which Nature has carried out are properly the province of the pathologist."[12] Phylogenetically and neoplastically immature islets obviously have several biological features in common.

Acknowledgments

Investigations of the authors and their collaborators, providing part of the background of this review, were supported by grants from the Swedish Diabetes Association, the Swedish Medical Research Council (Project No. 12X-718), and the Kroc Foundation, U.S.A.

References*

1. Falkmer, S., and Patent, G. J.: In: *Handbook of Physiology,* Vol. 1, *The Endocrine Pancreas.* Edited by D. F. Steiner and N. Freinkel. Williams & Wilkins, Baltimore, 1972, p. 1.
2. Falkmer, S., and Marques, M.: In: *Glucagon: Molecular Physiology, Clinical and Therapeutic Implications.* Edited by P. J. Lefebvre and R. H. Unger. Pergamon Press, Oxford, 1972, p. 343.
3. Lacy, P. E.: *Amer. J. Pathol.,* **79**:170, 1975.
4. Gerich, J. E., Charles, M. A., and Grodsky, G. M.: *Ann. Rev. Physiol.,* **38**:353, 1976.
5. Fujita, T. (ed.): *Gastro-Entero-Pancreatic Endocrine System. A Cell Biological Approach.* Georg Thieme, Stuttgart, 1974, p. 1.
6. Weinstein, B.: *Experientia,* **28**:1517, 1972.
7. Track, N.S.: *Comp. Biochem. Physiol.,* **45B**:291, 1973.
8. Grossman, M. I.: In: *Peptide Hormones.* Edited by J. A. Parsons. Macmillan, London, 1976, p. 105.
9. Barrington, E. J. W., and Dockray, G. J.: *J. Endocrinol.,* **69**:299, 1976.
10. Pfeiffer, E. F., Raptis, S., and Ziegler, R.: *Z. Gastroenterol.,* **14**:70, 1976.
11. Pearse, A. G. E., and Polak, J. M.: *Med. Biol.,* **52**:3, 1974.
12. Pearse, A. G. E.: *Z. Krebsforsch.,* **84**:1, 1975.
13. Pearse, A. G. E., and Takor Takor, T.: *Clin. Endocrinol.,* **5**, *Suppl.,* 229, 1976.
14. Fujita, T.: In: *Chromaffin, Enterochromaffin and Related Cells.* Proc. Naito Internat. Symp., 1975, Gifu, Japan. Edited by R. E. Coupland and T. Fujita. Elsevier, Amsterdam, 1976, p. 191.
15. Polak, J. M., Grimelius, L., Pearse, A. G. E., and Bloom, S. R.: *Lancet,* **1**:1220, 1975.
16. Hökfelt, T., Efendić, S., Hellerström, C., Johansson, O., Luft, R., and Arimura, A.: *Acta Endocrinol. 80, Suppl.,* **200**:1, 1975.
17. Lotstra, F., van der Loo, W., and Gepts, W.: *Diabetologia,* **10**:291, 1974.
18. Larsson, L. -I., Rehfeld, J. F., Sundler, F., and Håkanson, R.: *Nature (London)* **262**:609, 1976.
19. Heitz, P., Polak, J. M., Bloom, S. R., and Pearse, A. G. E.: *Gut,* **17**:755, 1976.
20. Heitz, P., Polak, J. M., Bloom, S. R., Adrian, T. E., and Pearse, A. G. E.: *Virchows Arch. B Cell Pathol.,* **21**:259, 1976.
21. Larsson, L. -I., Sundler, F., and Håkanson, R.: *Diabetologia,* **12**:211, 1976.
22. Lange, R. H.: In: *Handbuch der Histochemie,* Vol. VIII, part 1, *Histochemistry of the Islets of Langerhans.* Gustav Fischer, Stuttgart, 1973, p. 1.
23. Creutzfeldt, W.: *Israel J. Med. Sci.,* **11**:762, 1975.
24. Klöppel, G., Altenähr, E., Reichel, W., Willig, R., and Freytag, G.: *Diabetologia,* **10**:245, 1974.
25. Søvik, O., Vidnes, J., and Falkmer, S.: *Acta Pathol. Microbiol. Scand.,* **83A**:155, 1975.
26. Falkmer, S., and Boquist, L.: *Horm. Metab. Res., Suppl.,* **6**:55, 1976.
27. Falkmer, S., Emdin, S., Havu, N., Lundgren, G., Marques, M., Östberg, Y., Steiner, D. F., and Thomas, N. W.: *Amer. Zool.,* **13**:625, 1973.
28. Falkmer, S., Cutfield, J. F., Cutfield, S. M., Dodson, G. G., Gliemann, J., Gammeltoft, S., Marques, M., Peterson, J. D., Steiner, D. F., Sundby, F., Emdin, S. O., Havu, N., Östberg, Y., and Winbladh, L.:*Amer. Zool.,* **15**, *Suppl.,* **1**:255, 1975.
29. Solcia, E., Pearse, A. G. E., Grube, D., Kobayashi, S., Bussolati, G., Creutzfeldt, W., and Gepts, W.: *Rend. Gastroenterol.,* **5**:13, 1973.
30. Nakane, P. K.: *Acta Endocrinol. Suppl.,* **153**:190, 1972.
31. Moriarty, G. C., Moriarty, C. M., and Sternberger, L. A.: *J. Histochem. Cytochem.,* **21**:825, 1973.
32. Polak, J. M., Pearse, A. G. E., and Heath, C. M.: *Gut,* **16**:225, 1975.
33. Larsson, L. -I, Sundler, F., and Håkanson, R.: *Histochemistry,* **44**:245, 1975.
34. Larsson, L. -I., Sundler, F., and Håkanson, R.: *J. Histochem. Cytochem.,* **23**:873, 1975.
35. Peterson, J. D., Steiner, D. F., Emdin, S. O., and Falkmer, S.: *J. Biol. Chem.,* **250**:5183, 1975.
36. Östberg, Y.: The Entero-Insular Endocrine Organ in a Cyclostome, *Myxine glutinosa.* A light and fluorescence microscopical, histochemical, and ultrastructural study, aiming to give some

---

*The survey of the literature was concluded in October, 1976. References are mainly given to recent reviews and other larger articles, where the original works can be found in the list of reference.

evolutionary aspects on the origin of islet parenchymal cells and the entero-insular axis. *Umeå Univ. Med. Diss.,* **15**:1–41, 1976.

37. Fritsch, H. A. R., Van Noorden, S., and Pearse, A. G. E.: *Cell Tiss. Res.,* **165**:365, 1976.
38. Larsson, L. -I., Holst, H., Håkanson, R., and Sundler, F.: *Histochemistry,* **44**:281, 1975.
39. Grimelius, L., Capella. C., Buffa, R., Polak, J. M., Pearse, A. G. E., and Solcia, E.: *Virchows Arch. B Cell Pathol.,* **20**:217, 1976.
40. Solcia, E., Capella, C., Buffa, R., and Frigerio, B.: In: *Chromaffin, Enterochromaffin and Related Cells.* Edited by R. E. Coupland and T. Fujita. Elsevier, Amsterdam, 1976, p. 209.
41. Boquist, L., and Falkmer, S.: In: *The Structure and Metabolism of the Pancreatic Islets. A Centennial of Paul Langerhans' Discovery.* Edited by S. Falkmer, B. Hellman, and I. -B. Täljedal. Pergamon Press, Oxford, 1970, p. 25.
42. Edström, C.: Effects of Duct Ligation on the Endocrine Pancreas of the Rat. A light microscopical, microangiographic, and ultrastructural study, including glucose tolerance tests and experiments with alloxan administration. *Umeå Univ. Med. Diss.,* **10**:1–43, 1972.
43. Edström, C.: *Acta Pathol. Microbiol. Scand. Sect. A,* **81**:21, 1973.
44. Edström, C., and Boquist, L.: *Acta Pathol. Microbiol. Scand. Sect. A,* **81**:47, 1973.
45. Watari, N.: In: *Gastro-Entero-Pancreatic Endocrine System. A Cell-Biological Approach.* Edited by T. Fujita. Georg Thieme, Stuttgart, 1974, p. 71.
46. Erlandsen, S. L., Hegre, O. D., Parsons, J. A., McEvoy, R. C., and Elde, R. P.: *J. Histochem. Cytochem.,* **24**:883, 1976.
47. Deconinck, J. F., Potvliege, P. R., and Gepts, W.: *Diabetologia,* **7**:266, 1971.
48. Deconinck, J. F., Van Assche, F. A., Potvliege, P. R., and Gepts, W.: *Diabetologia,* **8**:326, 1972.
49. Noe, B. D., Weir, G. C., and Bauer, G. E.: *Proc. Natl. Acad. Sci.,* 1977 (in press).
50. Misugi, K., Misugi, N., Sotos, J., and Smith, B.: *Arch. Pathol.,* **89**:208, 1970.
51. Polak, J. M., Adrian, T. E., Bryant, M. G., Bloom, S. R., Heitz, P., and Pearse, A. G. E.: *Lancet,* **1**:328, 1976.
52. Melmed, R. N., Benitez, C. J., and Holt, S. J.: *J. Cell Sci.,* **11**:449, 1972.
53. Melmed, R. N., Turner, R. C., and Holt, S. J.: *J. Cell Sci.,* **13**:279, 1973.
54. Pearse, A. G. E., Polak, J. M., and Heath, C. M.: *Diabetologia,* **9**:120, 1973.
55. Straus, E., Yalow, R. S., and Gainer, H.: *Science,* **190**:687, 1975.
56. Van Noorden, S., and Pearse, A. G. E.: In: *The Evolution of Pancreatic Islets,* Proc. Sympos., Leningrad, Sept. 15–18, 1975. Edited by T. A. I. Grillo, L. Leibson, and A. Epple. Pergamon Press, Oxford, 1976, p. 163.
57. Falkmer, S.: *Excerpta Med. Int. Congr. Ser.,* **172**:55, 1969.
58. Winbladh Biuw, L., and Hulting, G.: *Z. Zellforsch.,* **120**:546, 1971.
59. Polyakova, T. I., and Plisetskaya, E. M.: *J. Evolu. Biochem. Physiol.,* **12**:184, 1976.
60. Kataoka, K., and Fujita, H.: *Arch. Histol. Jap.,* **36**:401, 1974.
61. Gerzeli, G.: *Nature (London),* **189**:237, 1961.
62. De Martinez, N. R., García, M. C., Salas, M., and Candela, J. L. R.: *Gen. Comp. Endocrinol.* **20**:305, 1973.
63. Marques, M., and Falkmer, S.: *Gen. Comp. Endocrinol.* **29**:522, 1976.
64. Csaba, G., and Lantos, T.: *Experientia,* **31**:1097, 1975.
65. Tager, H. S., Markese, J., Kramer, K. J., Speirs, R. D., and Childs, C. N.: *Biochem. J.,* **156**:515, 1976.
66. Meneses, P., and de los Angeles Ortíz, M.: *Comp. Biochem. Physiol.,* **51A**:483, 1975.
67. Tager, H. S., Markese, J., Spiers, R. D., and Kramer, K. J.: *Nature (London),* **254**:707, 1975.
68. Maier, V., Kroder, A., Groner, E., Keller, R., and Pfeiffer, E. F.: *Acta Endocrinol. (Kbh.), Suppl.,* **193**:41, 1975.
69. Kleinholz, L. H.: *Amer. Zool.,* **16**:151, 1976.
70. Falkmer, S., and Wilson, S.: *Diabetologia,* **3**:519, 1967.
71. Emdin, S. O., Gammeltoft, S., and Gliemann, J.: *J. Biol. Chem.,* **252**:602, 1977.
72. Burighel, P., and Milanesi, C.: *Cell Tiss. Res.,* **158**:481, 1975.
73. Epple, A., and Brinn, J. E., Jr.: *Gen. Comp.Endocrinol.,* **27**:320, 1975.
74. Falkmer, S., Thomas, N. W., and Boquist, L.: *Chem. Zool.* **8**:195, 1974.
75. Winbladh, L.: *Endocrine Pancreas in Cyclostomes.* Thesis, Univ. Stockholm, p. 1–24, 1976.

76. Barrington, E. J. W.: In: *The Biology of Lampreys.* Edited by M. W. Hardisty and I. C. Potter. Vol. 2. Academic Press, London/New York, 1972, p. 135.
77. Brinn, J. E., Jr., and Epple, A.: *Cell Tiss. Res., 171*:317, 1976.
78. Strahan, R., and Maclean, J. L.: *Austral. J. Sci., 32*:54, 1969.
79. Hardisty, M. W., Zelnik, P. R., and Moore, I. A.: *Gen. Comp. Endocrinol., 27*:179, 1975.
80. Winbladh, L., and Hörstedt. P.: *Acta Zool. (Stockholm), 56*:213, 1975.
81. Falkmer, S., Emdin, S. O., Östberg, Y., Mattisson, A., Johansson Sjöbeck, M. -L., and Fänge, R.: *Progr. Exp. Tumor. Res., 20*:217, 1976.
82. Hardisty, M. W.: *J. Zool. (London), 178*, 1976 (in press).
83. Epple, A., and Brinn, J. E., Jr.: In: *The Evolution of Pancreatic Islets.* Proc. Sympos., Leningrad, Sept. 15–18, 1975. Edited by T. A. I. Grillo, L. Leibson, and A. Epple. Pergamon Press, Oxford, 1976, p. 83.
84. Östberg, Y., Van Noorden, S., and Pearse, A. G. E.: *Gen. Comp. Endocrinol., 25*:274, 1975.
85. Östberg, Y., Boquist, L., Van Noorden, S., and Pearse, A. G. E.: *Gen. Comp. Endocrinol., 28*:228, 1976.
86. Van Noorden, S., Östberg, Y., and Pearse, A. G. E.: *Cell Tiss. Res., 177*:281, 1977.
87. Van Noorden, S., Greenberg, J., and Pearse, A. G. E.: *Gen. Comp. Endocrinol., 19*:192, 1972.
88. Van Noorden, S., and Pearse, A. G. E.: *Gen. Comp. Endocrinol., 23*:311, 1974.
89. Östberg, Y., Van Noorden, S., Pearse, A. G. E., and Thomas, N. W.: *Gen. Comp. Endocrinol., 28*:213, 1976.
90. Östberg, Y., and Boquist, L.: *Acta Zool. (Stockholm), 57*:41, 1976.
91. Epple, A., and Lewis, T. L.: *Amer. Zool., 13*:567, 1973.
92. Patent, G. J.: In: *The Evolution of Pancreatic Islets,* Proc. Sympos., Leningrad, Sept. 15–18, 1975. Edited by T. A. I. Grillo, L. Leibson, and A. Epple. Pergamon Press, Oxford, 1976, p. 131.
93. Gabe, M., and Martoja, M.: *Arch. Anat. Microsc. Morphol. Exp., 61*:17, 1972.
94. Falkmer, S., and Östberg, Y.: In: *Proc. 5th Int. Congr. Endocrinol., Hamburg, July 18–24, 1976.* Edited by V. H. T. James. *Excerpta Med. Int. Congr. Ser.,* 1976 (in press).
95. Brinn, J. E., Jr.: *Amer. Zool., 13*:653, 1973.
96. Gabe, M., and Martoja, M.: *Arch. Anat. Microsc. Morphol. Exp., 60*:219, 1971.
97. Nakamura, M., Yamada, K., and Yokote, M.: *Experientia, 27*:75, 1971.
98. Epple, A.: In: *Fish Physiology.* Edited by W. S. Hoar and D. J. Randall. Academic Press, New York, 1969, p. 275.
99. Falkmer, S.: *Acta Endocrinol., 37, Suppl. 59*:1, 1961.
100. Klein, C.: Étude Ultrastructurale et Cytochimique du Pancréas Endocrine d'un Poisson Téléostéen, *Xiphophorus helleri H.* Thesis, Univ. Louis Pasteur, Strasbourg, France, 1975, p. 1–143.*
101. Mosca, L.: *Quart. J. Exp. Physiol., 42*:49, 1957.
102. Sasaki, K., Dockerill, S., Adamiak, D. A., Tickle. I. J., and Blundell, T.: *Nature (London), 257*:751, 1975.
103. Kudo, S., and Takahashi, Y.: *Z. Zellforsch., 146*:425, 1973.
104. Kobayashi, K., and Takahashi, Y.: *Gen. Comp. Endocrinol. 23*:1, 1974.
105. Thomas, N. W.: *Gen. Comp. Endocrinol., 26*:496, 1975.
106. Brinn, J. E.: *Cell Tiss. Res., 162*:357, 1975.
107. Johnson, D. E., Torrence, J. L., Elde, R. P., Bauer, G. E., Noe, B. D., and Fletcher, D. J.: *Amer. J. Anat., 147*:119, 1976.
108. Barrington, E. J. W., and Dockray, G. J.: *Gen. Comp. Endocrinol., 19*:80, 1972.
109. Dockray, G. J.: *Gen. Comp. Endocrinol., 23,* 340, 1974.
110. Dockray, G. J.: *Gen. Comp. Endocrinol., 25*:203, 1975.
111. Penhos, J. C., and Ramey, E.: *Amer. Zool., 13*:667, 1973.
112. Pearse, A. G. E.: In: *Peptide Hormones.* Edited by J. A. Parsons. Macmillan, London, 1976, p. 33.

*Subsequent reports, essentially based on the observations made in this work, have recently been published, viz.: Klein, C., and Lange, R. H.: *Cell Tiss. Res., 176*:529, 1977; Klein, C., and Streicher, D.: *C. R. Acad. Sci., Paris,* 1976 (in press); and Klein, C.: *Int. Rev. Cytol.,* 1977 (in press).

113. Polak, J. M., Bloom, S. R., Hobbs, S., Solcia, E., and Pearse, A. G. E.: *Lancet,* **1**:1109, 1976.
114. Kobayashi, K.: *Gunma J. Med. Sci.,* **17/18**:60, 1969.
115. Khanna, S. S., and Kumar, S.: *Acta Anat.,* **86**:524, 1973.
116. Gabe, M.: *Arch. Histol. Jap.,* **35**:51, 1972.
117. Kataoka, K.: In: *Gastro-Entero-Pancreatic Endocrine System. A Cell-Biological Approach.* Edited by T. Fujita. Georg Thieme, Stuttgart, 1974, p. 39.
118. Trandaburu, T., and Leonte, E.: *J. Neur. Transm.* **36**:143, 1975.
119. Gabe, M.: *Arch. Anat. Micr. Morphol. Exp.,* **61**:175, 1972.
120. Gabe, M.: *Acta Anat.,* **85**:434, 1973.
121. Lange, R. H.: *J. Ultrastr. Res.,* **46**:301, 1974.
122. Rhoten, W. B.: *Gen. Comp. Endocrinol.,* **17**:203, 1971.
123. Rhoten, W. B.: *J. Exp. Zool.,* **184**:313, 1973.
124. Rhoten, W. B.: *Amer. J. Anat.,* **138**:481, 1973.
125. Théret, C., Alliet, J., Comlan, G., and Gourdier, D.: *C. R. Acad. Sci., Paris,* **280**:2125, 1975.
126. Rhoten, W. B.: *Gen. Comp. Endocrinol.,* **20**:474, 1973.
127. Khanna, S. S., and Kumar, S.: *Acta Anat.* **88**:67, 1974.
128. Trandaburu, T.: *J. Anat.* **117**:575, 1974.
129. Hazelwood, R. L., Turner, S. D., Kimmel, J. R., and Pollock, H. G.: *Gen. Comp. Endocrinol.,* **21**:485, 1973.
130. Kimmel, J. R., Hayden, L. J., and Pollock, H. G.: *J. Biol. Chem.,* **250**:9369, 1975.
131. Smith, P. H.: *Anat. Rec.,* **178**:567, 1974.
132. Watanabe, T., Paik, Y. K., and Yasuda, M.: *Arch. Histol. Japon.,* **38**:259, 1975.
133. Orci, L., Baetens, D., Dubois, M. P., and Rufener, C.: *Horm. Metab. Res.* **7**:400, 1975.
134. Weir, G. C., Goltsos, P. C., Steinberg, E. P., and Patel, Y. C.: *Diabetologia,* **12**:129, 1976.
135. Dahl, E.: *Z. Zellforsch.,* **136**:501, 1973.
136. Trandaburu, T.: *Gegenbaurs Morphol. Jahrb.,* **129**:888, 1974.
137. Polak, J. M., Pearse, A. G. E., Adams, C., and Garaud, J. -C.: *Experientia,* **30**:564, 1974.
138. Larsson, L. -I., Sundler, F., Håkanson, R., Rehfeld, J. F., and Stadil, F.: *Cell Tiss. Res.,* **154**:409, 1974.
139. Kalliecharan, R., and Gibson, M. A.: *Can. J. Zool.,* **50**:265, 1972.
140. Baxter-Grillo, D. L., Amakawa, T., and Ito, R.: *Histochemie,* **33**:281, 1973.
141. Dieterlen-Lièvre, F., and Beaupain, D.: *Gen. Comp. Endocrinol.,* **22**:62, 1974.
142. Beaupain, D., and Dieterlen-Lièvre, G.: *Gen. Comp. Endocrinol.,* **23**:421, 1974.
143. Andrew, A.: *Gen. Comp. Endocrinol.,* **26**:485, 1975.
144. Colca, J. R., and Hazelwood, R. L.: *Gen. Comp. Endocrinol.,* **28**:151, 1976.
145. Forssmann, A.: *Cell Tiss. Res.,* **167**:179, 1976.
146. Fujita, T.: *Arch. Histol. Japon.,* **35**:161, 1973.
147. Smith, P. H.: *Amer. J. Anat.,* **144**:513, 1975.

Chapter 3

Growth Pattern of Pancreatic Islets in Animals

Claes Hellerström

The efficiency with which the pancreatic islet organ maintains the blood sugar homeostasis is determined both by the total islet mass and the hormonal release of individual islet cells in response to changes in the blood sugar concentration. Alterations in islet mass caused by cell loss or proliferation may well lead to disturbances in hormone production which will contribute to the development of either diabetes mellitus or hypoglycemic states. Factors which cause damage or loss of various islet cell types have attracted much attention in the past, and studies of this kind have greatly expanded our knowledge on the pathogenesis of diabetes. In comparison, little is known so far about the kinetics and regulation of islet cell proliferation and the significance of this process for the manifestations of the diabetic syndrome. The following review is an attempt to summarize the relevant literature in this latter field with regard to the growth of the islet organ both in normal conditions and in spontaneous and experimental diabetes.

The Cell Types of the Pancreatic Islets

The islet organ is composed of several distinct cell types with widely different functions, and a stimulus causing the proliferation of one type of cell does not necessarily affect the others. An understanding of the morphological and functional characteristics of the different islet cell types is, therefore, of decisive importance for our knowledge of the regulation of islet cell growth. It is the purpose of this section to review briefly the function and light-microscopic properties of the different islet cell types in mammals and to define the nomenclature which will be used throughout this chapter. Only those cell types which have well-defined staining properties or can be regarded as functional entities have been included. The ultrastructural organization of the islet cells is thoroughly dealt with in Chapter 6 of the present volume.

Claes Hellerstrom • University of Uppsala, Uppsala, Sweden.

Despite a great deal of research in recent years there is still some disagreement as to the denomination of some of the islet cell types. This, of course, is true only for the non-B cells and may be ascribed to the chronic lack of knowledge concerning the function of these cells. However, the discovery of several new peptides, presumably of hormonal nature, and their immunohistochemical localization to the islets has recently elucidated the function of several cell types of hitherto unknown significance. It is, therefore, now possible to classify the great majority of islet cells with respect to both light-microscopic properties and production of well-defined polypeptides.

The A_1 or D Cell

The A_1 cell or the D cell contains somatostatin or a compound with somatostatin-like immunoreactivity[1-3] (Fig. 1). The occurrence in these cells also of a material cross-reacting with antibodies toward gastrin has been claimed by some authors,[4-7] but has been denied by others.[8-10] The A_1 (D) cells usually comprise less than 10% of the islets of laboratory animals[11-15] but seem to be considerably more common in human islets.[16-18] In the light microscope the cells are characterized by a positive reaction with the Hellerström–Hellman[19] silver impregnation procedure (Fig. 2). In 1960, the latter authors introduced the designation of A_1 cell to distinguish this cell type from the larger group of A

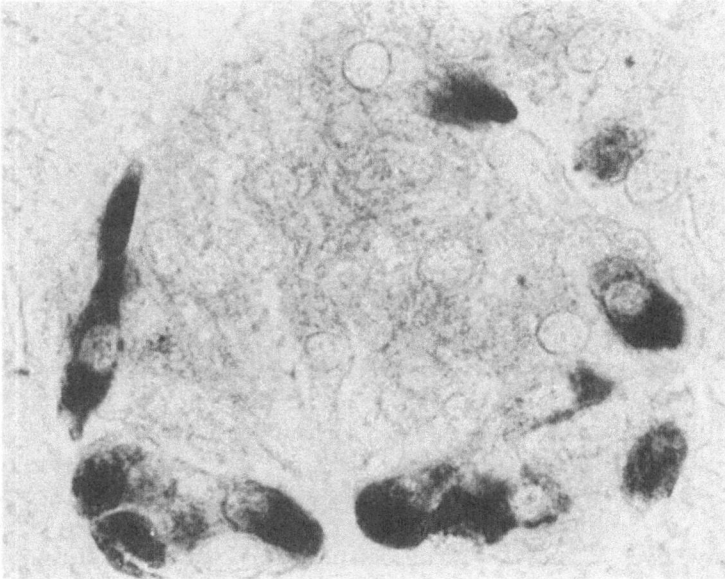

Figure 1. A small islet in a Bouin-fixed section of a human pancreas incubated with somatostatin antiserum and processed according to the immunoperoxidase technique. The specific (dark-brown) staining is localized in A_1 cells with a polymorphic, sometimes markedly elongated, shape. ×1000.

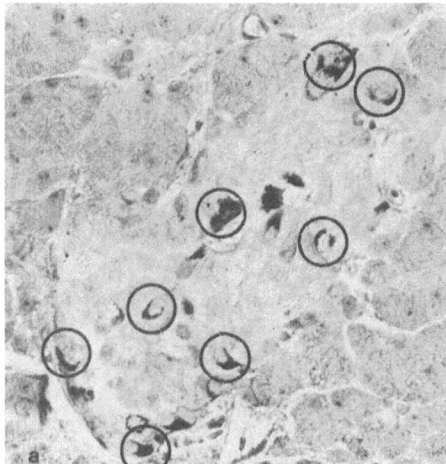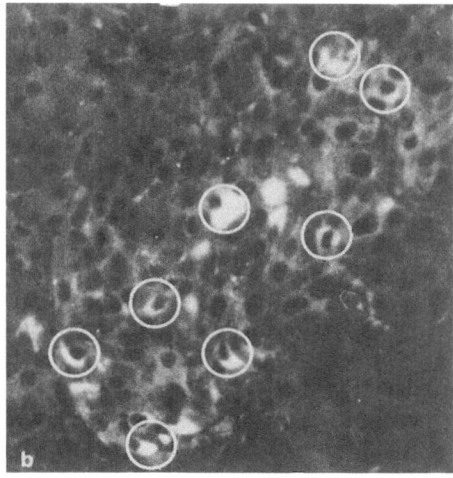

Figure 2. Section of a human pancreas fixed in formaldehyde vapor and subsequently stained with (a) Hellerström–Hellman's[19] argyrophil technique for A_1 cells followed by (b) an indirect immuno-fluorescence method[1] using antibodies to synthetic somatostatin. The argyrophil cells correspond precisely to those cells showing positive immunofluorescence. ×365, reduced 17% for reproduction. The original micrographs have been published in *Lancet*[1] and were generously placed at the author's disposal by Dr. L. Grimelius, University of Uppsala, Sweden. (Reproduced with permission of *Lancet*.)

cells, which at that time constituted a heterogeneous class of cells.[19] In a series of studies it was conclusively shown that the A_1 cell could be classified as a separate cell type from tinctorial, structural, and functional points of view.[20,21] Subsequent studies suggested that this cell type in most, but not all, species[18,22] corresponded to the D cell.[17,23–28] The latter type of cell was originally described as a separate islet cell type by Bloom[29] and Thomas,[30] but it was later classified as either a precursor of the B cell[31] or a stage in the life cycle of the A cell.[32,33] Further doubts as to the existence of either the D cell or the A_1 and A_2 cells as distinct cell entities have been expressed in some quarters.[34–36] The localization of somatostatin to a separate islet cell type identified as the A_1 type has, however, presumably solved this controversy.[1–3] Electron-microscopic studies have also supported the view that in mammals the A_1 cells and the D cells are closely related,[37–39] and today these two designations can be regarded as interchangeable.

The A_2 or A Cell

The A_2 cell or the A cell is the source of pancreatic glucagon,[12,40–45] and these cells comprise 10 to 30% of the mammalian endocrine pancreas. The A_2 cells remain nonargyrophil with the Hellerström–Hellman[19] procedure, whereas in man and in several other species they are distinctly silver impregnated with the Grimelius technique.[46] In some species there is also a positive reaction for tryptophan in the A_2 cell,[20,47] possibly reflecting the presence of this amino acid in the glucagon molecule. In the rat, mouse, and hamster the A_2 cells are typically located in the islet periphery, whereas in the horse they are often found in the central core of the islets.[20] In man they occur both in the islet periphery and dispersed among the other islet cell types[16,46] (Fig. 3). Hereafter, the designation A_2 cell will be used synonymously with A cell.

The B Cell

The B cell has long been known to manufacture insulin and is by far the most well defined of the islet cell types. In the light microscope it produces characteristic tinctorial reactions with chrome-alum hematoxyline,[48] aldehyde fuchsin,[49] Victoria blue,[50] or pseudoisocyanine[51] (Fig. 4). B cells constitute 60 to 80% of the normal mammalian pancreas but may account for over 90% in some conditions (see below). For this reason the growth pattern of the pancreatic islets is to a large extent determined by the proliferation and loss of B cells.

The PP Cell

The PP cell has recently been characterized by light- and electron-microscopic immunocytochemistry in a number of species including man, mouse, rat, hamster, guinea pig, rabbit, opossum, chinchilla, cat, and dog[52–54] (Figs. 5 and

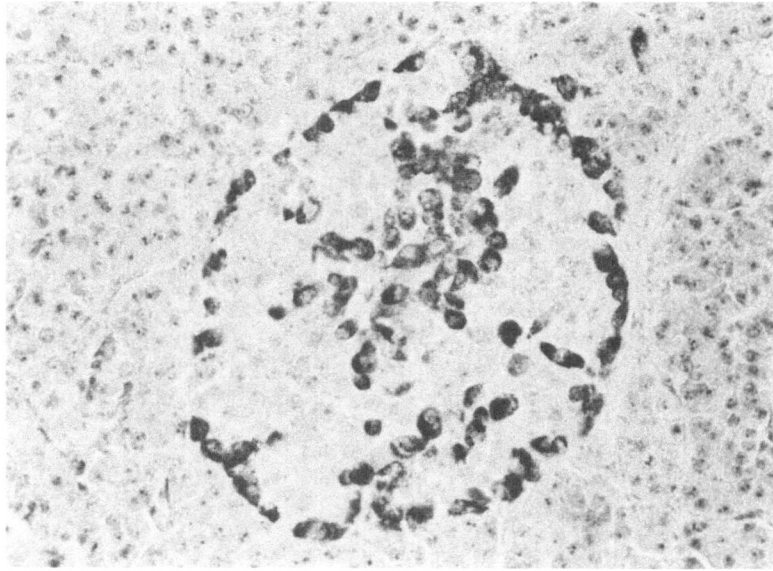

Figure 3. Human pancreatic section fixed in Bouin's solution and stained with the Grimelius[46] silver impregnation technique. Argyrophil A_1 cells are located both at the islet periphery and along capillaries within the islet. ×300.

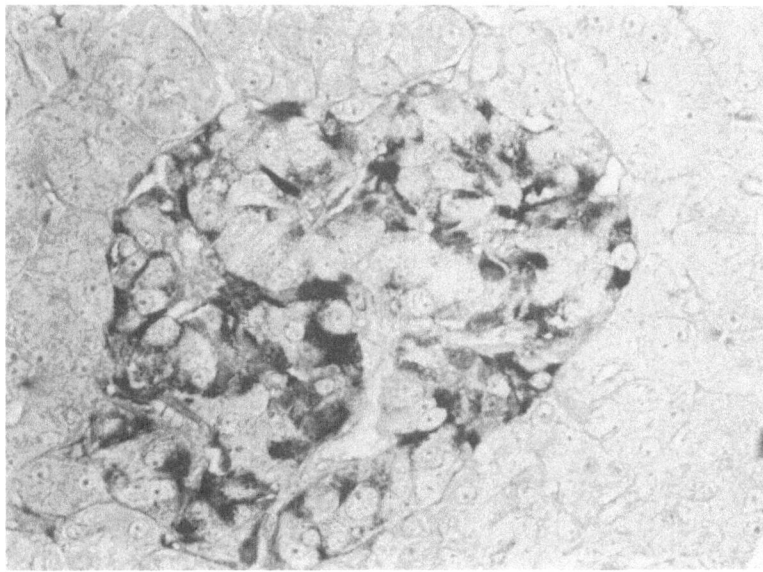

Figure 4. A Bouin-fixed section of a human pancreas stained with aldehyde-fuchsin trichrome. Dark (blue-violet) B cells are scattered all over the islet. ×400.

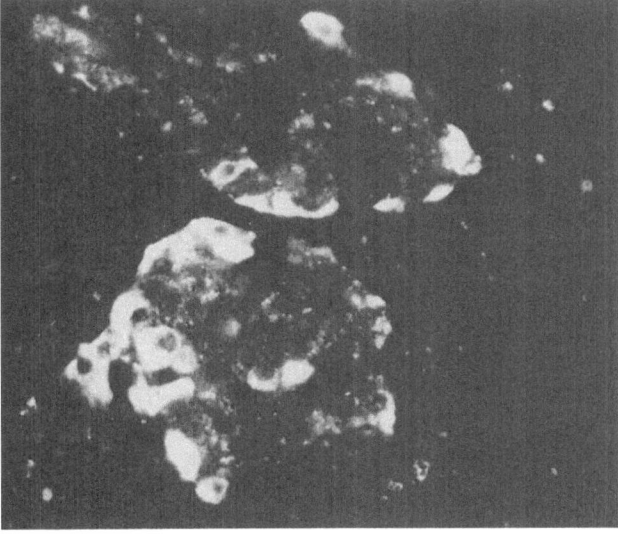

Figure 5. Immunofluorescent PP cells located at the periphery of two islets in a section of a human pancreas. The antiserum was directed toward human pancreatic polypeptide. ×560. The original micrograph was generously placed at the author's disposal by Dr. L.-I. Larsson, University of Aarhus, Denmark.

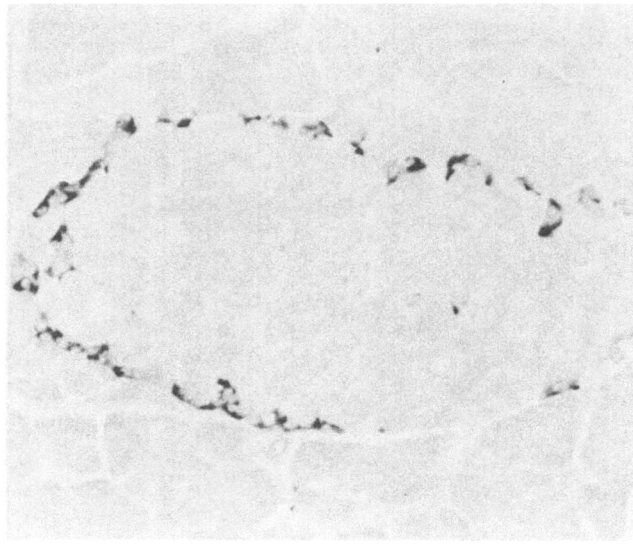

Figure 6. Immunoperoxidase staining of PP cells in the rat pancreas. The cells are located at the extreme periphery of the islet. ×370. Courtesy of Dr. L.-I. Larsson.

6). As the (tentative) name implies this cell is the source of pancreatic polypeptide,[55] a protein composed of 36 amino acid residues in a straight chain and chemically distinct from all known polypeptide hormones.[56] In the islets the PP cells are relatively rare but they occur also in the acinar parenchyma. They exhibit negative staining reactions to both aldehyde fuchsin[49] and the silver techiques of Hellerström–Hellman[19] and Grimelius,[46] but they have a relatively characteristic ultrastructural appearance.[54] Although their precise biological significance remains to be clarified, there is much evidence to suggest that they are true hormone-producing cells. They may be identical with the previously described F cells or X cells in cat and dog.[57–59] (See also Chapters 2, 5, and 15.)

The Agranular Cell

The agranular cell is rare in the adult mammalian islet but may be recognized in some islet cell tumors[60] and in the endocrine pancreas of lower vertebrates.[61] Since agranular cells occur in higher frequency during islet cell regeneration they have been regarded as precursors of granulated islet cells rather than true endocrine elements.[61,62]

Quantitation of the Number and Total Volume of the Islets: Methodological Considerations

Any detailed study of the growth pattern of the islets requires a thorough quantitation of their number and total volume. However, the dispersion of the islets throughout the pancreas and the overwhelming predominance of acinar tissue create great difficulties in quantitative measurements of the islet mass. Notwithstanding this, the regular spherical or ellipsoidal shape of the individual islet and the well-defined boundary between islets and exocrine parenchyma facilitate in most mammals the application of quantitative methods to the study of the islet organ. Some of the most reliable and widely used of these techniques will be reviewed below.

Number of Islets

Enumeration of the pancreatic islets has been used extensively in the past as a means of estimating changes in the total mass of the islet organ. Early techniques were based on the direct counting of islets visualized by intravital or supravital staining with neutral red or Janus green according to Bensley.[63] This technique was initially used to study the distribution and number of islets in the guinea pig[63] and in man.[64] Corresponding investigations were subsequently performed in the rat,[65-67] in the rabbit,[68] and in the mouse.[69] More recently Brunfeldt *et al.*[70] showed that mouse islets can be stained intravitally with diphenylthiocarbazone, a chelating agent which combines with zinc in the islets to form a visible red complex. Bunnag *et al.*[71] used this method to study changes in the islet number in mice which had been treated with tolbutamide.

Both techniques referred to above for counting islets in fresh pancreatic specimens involve the perfusion of the intact animal or dissected pancreas with a vital dye to visualize the islets. However, insufficient differentiation between islets and acini sometimes occurs, and many islets may be overlooked. In an attempt to overcome this source of error Mount[72] described a method for the direct counting of unstained islets in the mouse pancreas. By placing the whole organ between glass plates and illuminating the preparation with direct light the islets were claimed to become sufficiently visible to be counted. In our laboratory we have been unable to confirm this observation. The contrast between islet and acinar tissue could, however, be considerably improved simply by freezing and thawing the pancreas either before or after it was subdivided into small pieces which were placed between two glass plates (Nordin, Andersson, and Hellerström, unpublished observations). By this means detailed studies of the distribution of islets can be performed with a minimum of technical efforts in several small laboratory animals including the rat, mouse, and guinea pig.

Although the techniques for enumeration of whole islets described above are relatively simple, they have been criticized for being inaccurate.[73,74] In addition, they are unsuited for a size classification of the islets counted which is a prerequisite for the computation of the total islet volume (see below). If such information is also desired, fixed and adequately stained pancreatic sections should be employed, although preparation of these is much more tedious. However, the number of islet section surfaces counted in pancreatic sections (i.e., the apparent number of islets) is also widely different from the actual number of islets, which must be computed mathematically. The principles for this were first worked out by Tejning[73] who used the formulas derived by

Wiksell[75,76] to calculate both the actual number of islets and their distribution in different size classes in the rat. Tejning's[73] method was further extended in the careful work of Hellman[77-79] who pointed out the importance of defining precisely a lower size limit for the islet section surfaces to be counted. Since the size distribution of the islets is highly asymmetric with a marked predominance of smaller islets[73] and since a great number of these small cell conglomerations must inadvertently be overlooked in the microscope, any estimate of the actual islet number is meaningless unless the diameter of the smallest islet included has been defined.

Islet Volume or Weight

A number of techniques for estimating the total islet volume or weight have been suggested, but some have come under serious criticism and will not be referred to here. Among those regarded as reasonably accurate at least three principles have been employed, and all are based on the use of fixed and stained pancreatic sections. In the first, pancreatic sections are projected onto paper and scanned systematically for islet section surfaces, the outlines of which are then drawn on the paper. Islets exceeding a lower size limit are subsequently classified according to surface area by comparison with standard circles or ellipses,[74] and the islet volume (V) is calculated according to the formula

$$V = A \cdot T/M^2$$

where A is the total surface area of all recorded islet section surfaces; T is the thickness of the section unit (i.e., the distance between two representative sections taken at regular intervals from the serially sectioned pancreas); and M is the linear magnification of the microscope. The accuracy of the technique naturally is influenced by the width of the section unit, but this may be as large as 200 to 300 μm with a coefficient of variation of less than 10%.[74]

The second principle is based upon Tejning's application of the equations derived by Wiksell[75,76] and involves calculations of the actual islet number and size distribution. On the assumption that the islets are spherical or ellipsoidal and randomly distributed in the pancreas, the relationship between their apparent and actual distributions can be expressed by an Abelian integral equation, which after approximation into a linear equation system can be used for calculating the actual distribution from that observed in the sections. The total islet volume can then be computed from the number of islets in each size class. A comparison between this technique and the previous one showed a discrepancy of only 1% between estimates of the islet volume performed in the same rats.[74]

Other techniques for volume quantitation of islets are based on direct stereological analyses of pancreatic sections in the microscope. Of these, the point sampling method described by Chalkley[80] has been widely used in islet research. By fixing one or several points in the field of vision, for example, a hair cross in the ocular, and counting the components under the point(s) as they appear with a random step movement of the microscope stage, the relative volume (F) of different tissue components can be calculated according to the formula

$$F = h/n$$

in which h is the number of "hits" on the tissue component, e.g., islets, and n is the total number of points counted on the section. If the volume of the whole organ is known, the volume of the tissue component can then be calculated. Since it is much easier to measure accurately the weight than the volume of an organ, the results of point sampling are often transformed into the weights of the tissue components. This presupposes that the densities of the different components approximately equal the average density of the whole organ. In the pancreas the endocrine part seems to fulfill this criterion, provided fatty infiltration of the exocrine parenchyma is negligible.

Analyses of the islet volume using various light-microscopic line-sampling techniques have been applied in several studies.[81-88] Methods of this kind are particularly suited for automatic recording devices provided the tissue components can be differentially stained with sufficient contrast for photoelectric discrimination. An automatic scanning microscope adapted for measurements of the islet volume has been described by Tove *et al.*[81] During the scanning movements of the microscope stage blackened islets are projected onto a photocell close behind a diaphragm with a small aperture. The dark periods correspond to islet intercepts, which are measured and sorted electronically. A satisfactory staining of the islets against a light exocrine parenchyma was achieved in the mouse by the use of the sulfide–silver method for zinc,[89] which gives an intense blackening of the mouse islet cells. Because of the regular arrangement of the islet tissue (see below), the total islet volume can be computed directly from the number of longer islet intercepts counted in sections taken at regular intervals.[90]

Differential Counts of the Islet Cells

Separate quantitation of each islet cell type requires in the first place a satisfactory differential staining of the islet cells. Examples of such staining techniques have been given in the section on cell types of the pancreatic islets. Volume quantitation can then be performed with point sampling[15,91,92] or line scanning.[84] Alternatively, the relative frequency of each of the different islet cell types can be estimated by direct counting in representative sections. In this case the number of islets counted must be corrected with regard to the size of the cell or the cell nucleus as described by Floderus[93] and Hellman.[94]

Rates of Islet Cell Proliferation

The proliferative activity of individual islet cells can be estimated by measurements of the [^{3}H]thymidine incorporation into islet cells that duplicate their DNA in preparation for mitosis. The incorporation of thymidine can be quantitated either by direct counting in extracts of isolated islets or by radioautography. The proportion of labeled B cells ([³H]thymidine index) obtained by radioautography is a reasonably sensitive estimate of B cell replication. This approach can also be used to calculate, for example, the length of the S phase or the postsynthetic phase in the life cycle of the B cell.[95,96] Although measurements of thymidine incorporation into islet cells have so far been mostly carried out *in vivo,*[71,97–104] recent developments of methods for tissue culture of isolated islets[105] or monolayer culture of islet and acinar cells[106–108] make it now possible to study islet cell replication also in well-controlled *in vitro* conditions.[107,109] Such methods should become powerful tools for elucidating in detail the mitotic response of the B cell to various stimuli (Fig. 7).

Differentiation and Growth of the Islet Organ

Morphological and Functional Differentiation of the Islet Cells

The mammalian pancreas develops from two diverticula (dorsal and ventral) which appear as buds on the primitive gut.[32,110] Formation of endocrine cells has been demonstrated in the epithelium of these buds, and the endocrine cells gradually accumulate into clusters which represent primitive islets. This implies that the islet organ arises directly from the pancreatic endoderm and that exocrine and endocrine cells originate from common predifferentiated stem cells. Pearse and his colleagues[111,112] have, nevertheless, suggested that the islet cells may come from the ectoderm (neural crest) and migrate into the primitive pancreas very early in development. This concept was based on the fact that the islet cells, like several other endocrine cells, are able to accumulate and decarboxylate precursors of biogenic amines,[113,114] a property which they share with certain cells derived from the neuroectoderm. In testing this hypothesis Pictet *et al.*[115] followed the development of the B cells in organ cultures of rat embryos, which had been deprived of their ectoderm before formation of the neural crest. The occurrence of an apparently normal number of B cells in these preparations suggested that the B cells are not derived from the neural crest and that the common property of accumulating and decarboxylating amine precursors does not necessarily indicate an origin from the neural crest. It must, however, be noted that these observations do not clarify the origin of the other islet cell types. For example, the simultaneous occurrence of somatostatin in the islet A_1 cells[1–3] and in neurons of both the central and peripheral nervous systems[2] leaves the question open as to whether these islet cells are derived from the neuroectoderm.

Contrary to previous belief, there is now evidence to indicate that reversible transformation between differentiated acinar and islet cells does not occur during intrauterine development.[110] Instead, acinar and endocrine cells develop independently and in an asynchronous manner from a morphologically undifferentiated precursor cell, which may be common to all pancreatic cells.[110,116] In this sequence of events the first differentiated islet cell to be

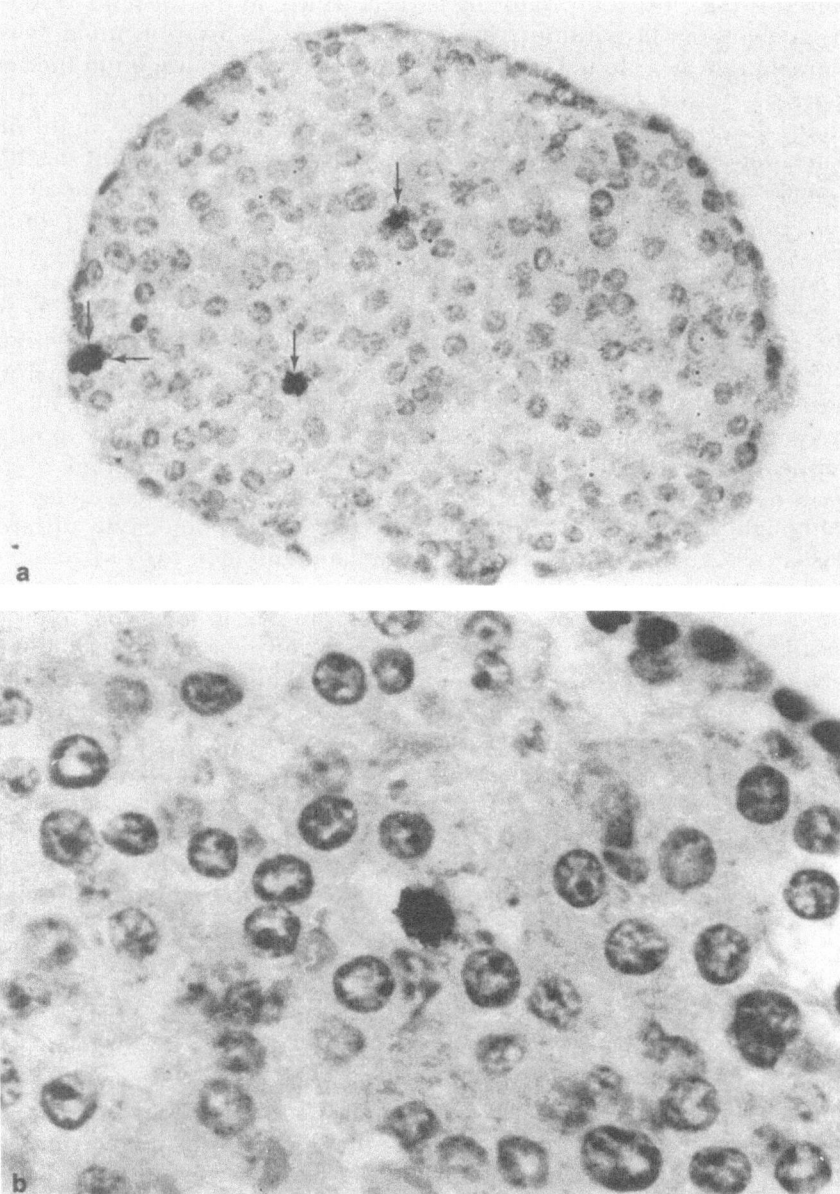

Figure 7. (a) Autoradiograph of an isolated mouse islet maintained in tissue culture[105] for 5 days in the presence of 16.7 mM glucose. During the last 24 hr [³H]thymidine was added to the culture medium at a concentration of 1 μCi/ml. Three distinctly labeled nuclei can be seen (arrows). ×400. (b) Detail of a mouse islet cultured and prepared for autoradiography as in Fig. 7a. Note a heavily labeled nucleus in the center of the picture. ×1000. The original micrographs were generously placed at the author's disposal by Dr. A. Andersson, University of Uppsala, Sweden.

recognized is the glucagon-producing A_2 cell, which, in the rat fetus, appears already at about the 11th intrauterine day.[110] These cells probably multiply at a considerable rate as reflected in a rapid accumulation of glucagon in the fetal rat pancreas.[110] The next cell to follow is the D cell (A_1 cell) on the 15th gestational day, whereas B cells cannot be recognized with certainty until 1 or 2 days later. Since insulin is extractable from the pancreas already on the 12th gestational day, the B cell may become functionally active before it attains its structurally recognizable characteristics. So far, information is lacking on the occurrence of either PP cells or of pancreatic polypeptide in the rat fetus.

The sequential order in which the islet cell types appear in the rat fetus seems to be the same also in other species. Thus, in the guinea pig fetus A_1 and A_2 cells can be recognized considerably earlier than the B cells.[92] In the human fetus, A_2 cells can be identified in the pancreas at 9 weeks gestational age followed by D cells and occasional B cells at 10.5 weeks of age[117] (Fig. 8). PP cells have recently been identified in the human fetus, but the precise time at which they appear has yet to be determined.[53] An extensive description of the embryogenesis of the islets in man is given in Chapter 6 of this volume.

Although the fetal endocrine pancreas contains morphologically differentiated islet cells, able to synthesize both insulin and glucagon early in gestation, there are a number of reports which indicate that the secretion of these hormones is regulated in a manner different from that in the adult. Thus, *in vivo* studies in premature babies and in fetuses and newborns of subhuman primates suggested that glucose is a poor stimulus of insulin secretion,[118,119] and this was later confirmed *in vitro*.[120–122] Similarly, the rat and the lamb have a low and sluggish insulin response to an acute glucose challenge during late and early neonatal life.[123–125] With regard to the release of glucagon, a relative lack of glucose sensitivity has been recorded in the fetal and neonatal rat and mouse, although the A_2 cells respond well to stimulation by arginine or to inhibition by fatty acids.[126–129] The transition to a mature regulation of insulin release takes place in the immediate neonatal period,[124] whereas for glucagon it occurs about 10 days postnatally.[126]

Islet Volume and Number at Different Ages

Quantitative studies of islet growth as a function of age have been restricted to postnatal life except for a relatively brief period toward the end of intrauterine development. In earlier embryonic life difficulties in specific staining of the different islet cell types have so far hampered a detailed quantitation of the islet mass. However, such studies in the perinatal period have demonstrated an extremely dynamic development of the islet organ. Thus, during the last 4 intrauterine days of the rat, the total islet number increases exponentially by doubling each day up to birth, followed by a declining rate during the immediate postnatal period.[130] In the same period the total islet volume increases by more than 100%.[131] The relative number of islets at birth is two to three times higher than in the adult rat, and the percentage contribution of islet cells to the total pancreatic mass is about three times higher.[130] In accordance

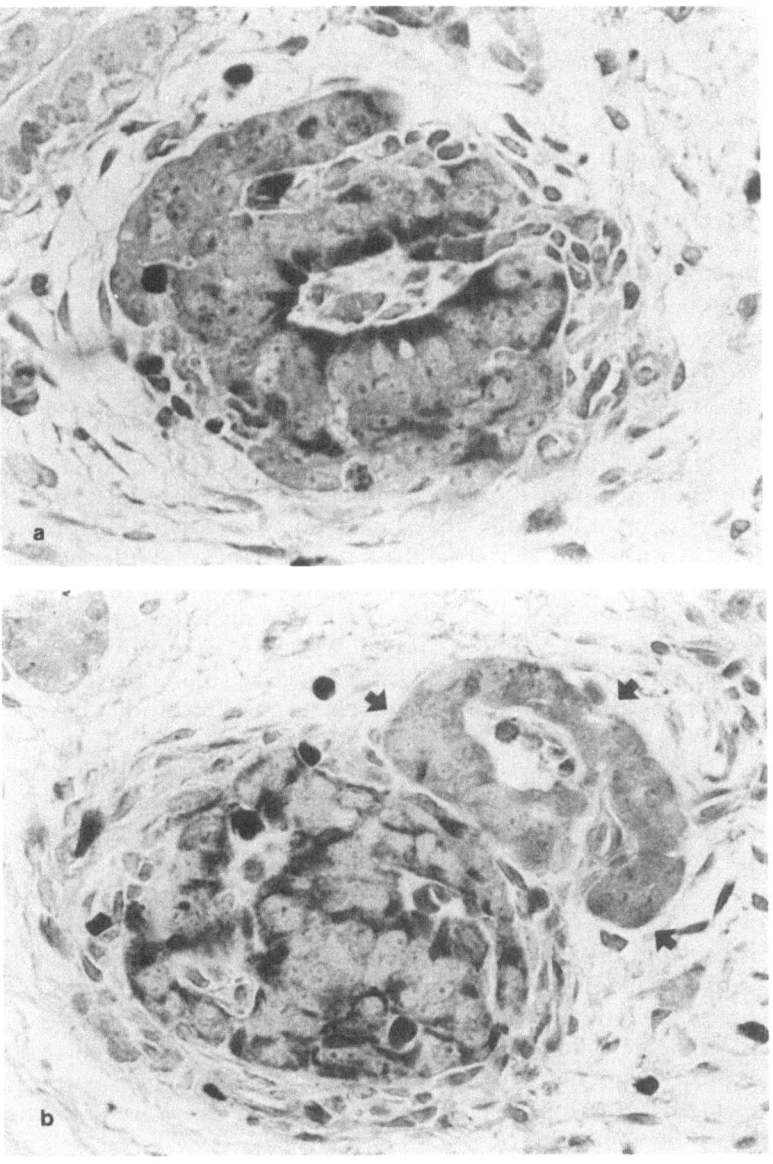

Figure 8. (a) Aldehyde-fuchsin trichrome stained islet in a pancreatic section from an 18 cm long human fetus. The wide central islet capillary is surrounded by B cells with their secretion granules polarized toward the capillary lumen. ×650. (b) Another aldehyde-fuchsin trichrome stained islet from an 18 cm long human fetus showing segregation between B and A₂ cells. The latter (brick red) cells are grouped around a capillary in the upper right part of the picture (arrows), whereas sparsely granulated (blue-violet) B cells form the main bulk of the islet. ×500.

with these observations the pancreatic insulin concentration of the rat shows an almost exponential rise during the last 4 to 6 days of intrauterine life and the total pancreatic insulin content shows a trebling during each of the last 4 days before birth.[130-133] Although insulin has biological effects on some fetal tissues,[134,135] it is of limited significance for the blood sugar homeostasis of the fetus,[136,137] and much of the explosive development of the islets may, therefore, occur in preparation for the increased demands of extrauterine life.

As soon as independent extrauterine life begins, the function of the islet organ becomes of decisive importance for the regulation of the carbohydrate metabolism of the newborn. A steep rise in the circulating glucagon concentration and a marked decrease of insulin in the immediate neonatal period probably serve to protect from hypoglycemia before commencement of feeding.[138-140] In the further postnatal development the number of islet cells adapts to the functional demands of the organism and a precisely regulated blood sugar homeostasis becomes manifest. The realization that the total islet mass might closely reflect its functional capacity has greatly stimulated studies on the postnatal development of the islet number and volume. Much of the earlier effort in this context was directed toward mere enumeration of islets after staining them with neutral red according to Bensley.[63] With the aid of this technique Overholser[65] counted the islets in rats between 1 and 364 days old. He concluded that the number of islets rose markedly in the first 20 days of life, reached a maximum at 50 days, and subsequently declined to a steady-state level in animals 90 to 150 days old. Using the same technique for visualization of the islets, Hess and Root[66] carried out corresponding studies in rats varying from 1 to 256 days of age. These authors found, however, an increasing number of islets during the whole observation period; at the beginning rapidly and later more slowly, approaching a constant maximum value. The latter observations were confirmed and extended by Haist and Pugh,[67] who studied rats in the weight range of 50 to 300 g. Also these authors noted a continuous increase of the islet number up to a body weight of about 200 g followed by a tendency to a steady-state level before the animals reached a weight of about 300 g. In the work of Hess and Root[66] the total number of islets counted was in the range of 700 at 1 day of age and 4500 at 256 days of age when the rats had a body weight of about 245 g. By contrast, Haist and Pugh[67] reported 4000 to 10,000 islets in the pancreas of rats weighing 50 g as compared to 15,000 to 24,000 in those weighing 300 g. It therefore seems either that the two strains of rats had widely different numbers of islets or that there were great discrepancies between the counting efficiencies of the islets.

Except for the rat, there are few other species in which the islets have been enumerated in relation to age. Using Bensley's method[63] Clark[64] determined the number of islets in adult man to be between 208,000 and 1,800,000. In a half-year-old baby the corresponding figure was 250,000. The mean number of islets per gram of adult pancreas was 14,800. Ogilvie[141] made an extensive study of the islet number in histologically stained sections of 100 human pancreatic glands obtained from subjects varying in age between newborn infants and 64-year-old adults. The average number of islets in five stillborn infants was

284,000. The number of islets subsequently increased up to 3 years of age, when it reached a steady state at 960,000 islets per pancreas. However, the procedure used by Ogilvie[141] to calculate the islet number has been seriously criticized[73] and the absolute values therefore cannot be accepted without reservation. It seems nevertheless reasonable to conclude from Ogilvie's[141] observations that there is a postnatal increase in the islet number in man. Similar observations have been made also in the mouse. Thus, Bunnag,[142] using intravital staining of islets with diphenylthiocarbazone counted 421 ± 30 islets in 1-month-old mice and 751 ± 47 in 14-month-old mice. The number of islets remained approximately constant after the age of 6-months in these animals. In a corresponding study with Bensley's[63] technique in mice aged between 10 days and 1 year, Parakkal and Ali[69] found a mean total islet number of 325 ± 51 in the youngest age group and 551 ± 140 in the oldest. In this study there was no apparent increase in the islet number between 28 days and 1 year of age, although no attempts were made to elucidate the possible occurrence of a peak value in this interval. When recalculated per dry pancreatic weight the number of islets in the 10-day-old mouse was not less than 224/mg pancreas followed by a marked drop to only 8 islets/mg in the 1-year-old group.

For a correct interpretation of the observations referred to above it is of crucial importance to know not only the method errors, but also the relation between the number of islets and the total islet mass. This problem was elucidated in the pioneering work of Tejning,[73] who showed for the first time the existence of a definite relationship between the total volume of the islet organ and the numerical or volumetric distributions of islets among various size classes. Thus, the numerical distribution of islets according to their size is excessively asymmetric with a progressive increase in the islet number with decreasing size (Fig. 9). On the other hand, the volume distribution shows a remarkable symmetry with average-sized islets comprising the largest volume of the islet organ (Fig. 10). It thus follows that the total volume of the relatively few islets in the largest size classes is of about the same magnitude as the total volume of the very numerous islets in the smallest size classes. Tejning[73] also showed that when the volume of the islet organ expands, the curve describing the volumetric distribution of the islet tissue moves to the right. This is demonstrated in Fig. 10, in which there is a gradual displacement to the right of the maxima as the total islet volume increases. Thus, as pointed out by Tejning,[73] the mere observation of an increased number of large islet section surfaces signifies an increased islet mass.

Tejning's[73] observations were further extended by Hellman[74,77,78] in his analyses of the islet organ at different ages in the rat. These studies showed conclusively that both the number and volume of the islets increased in the rat throughout the period of observation, i.e., between 1 and 480 days of age, and that the regular arrangement of the islet organ was retained at all ages.[74,77] During this time period the islet volume increased from 0.14 ± 0.02 mm³ in newborn rats to 3.39 ± 0.02 mm³ in the 480-day-old rats, a 24-fold increase. During the same period the actual number of islets exceeding a diameter of 47 μm increased from 243 ± 22 in the newborn to 3320 ± 48 in the oldest animal

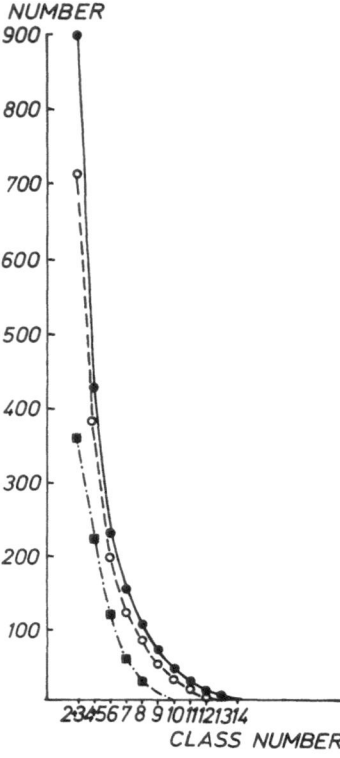

NUMBER

CLASS NUMBER

Figure 9. Numerical distribution on different size classes of the islets of three rats with total islet volumes comprising 2.85 mm³ (●——●), 1.75 mm³ (○----○), and 0.65 mm³ (■----■), respectively. The average islet diameter is 54 μm in class 2 and 375 μm in class 14. Redrawn from Tejning[73] with permission from the author.

group. Since the main contribution to the increase in the total islet volume between 100 and 480 days of age came from the B cells the observations were taken as suggesting that a growing influence of diabetogenic factors with age may be compensated in the rat by an increase of the B cell mass.

A regular arrangement of the islets, corresponding to that in the rat, has been found also in other species including man[21,143] and mouse.[14,144,145] Although in the human pancreas these techniques have not so far been applied for a detailed quantitation of the total islet volume and number, it is evident that the balance between the volume contribution of small and large islets is retained during the postnatal increase of the islet mass.[143] The islet growth is reflected as a broadening of the volume distribution curve and in a shift of the peak to the right, according to the same pattern as found in the rat (Fig. 11). The only deviation from the symmetrical arrangement of the islets was noted in a patient with islet fibrosis and hyalinization in whom there was an excess of larger islets. On the other hand, symmetrical curves have been recorded in several endocrine disorders associated with islet changes such as diabetes, insulinoma, and acromegaly.[146] The frequency of islets was calculated in the human as being between 12 and 30 per mm³ of pancreas without any marked variations between different regions of the gland.[143] The mean contribution of the islet volume to the total pancreatic volume was in the range of 0.9 to 1.9% in the human pancreas.

There have been few studies so far on the growth of the individual islet cell types during postnatal life. In the islet organ of the rat Hellman[147] found the relative volume contribution of the A cells to increase with age. Due to a lack of suitable differential staining techniques at that time, the contribution of A_1 and A_2 cells could not be evaluated separately. In the guinea pig the postnatal growth rates of the A_1, A_2, and B cells were, however, analyzed separately more recently by Petersson.[92] In this species the percentage contribution of the islet cells to the total pancreatic parenchyma was highest in the newborn at almost 12%, while in the 9-month-old guinea pig the value had decreased to about 6%.

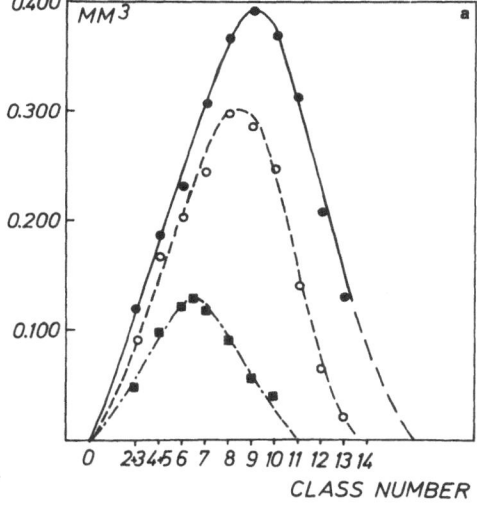

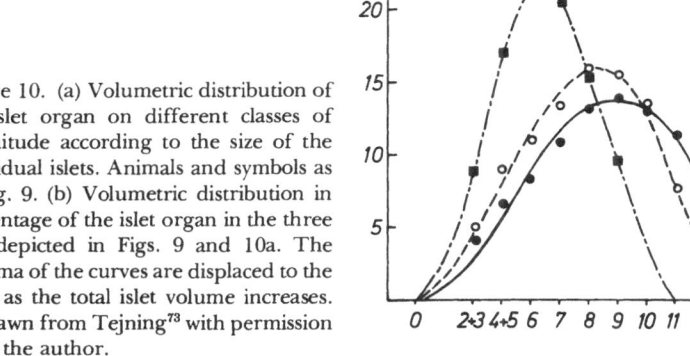

Figure 10. (a) Volumetric distribution of the islet organ on different classes of magnitude according to the size of the individual islets. Animals and symbols as in Fig. 9. (b) Volumetric distribution in percentage of the islet organ in the three rats depicted in Figs. 9 and 10a. The maxima of the curves are displaced to the right as the total islet volume increases. Redrawn from Tejning[73] with permission from the author.

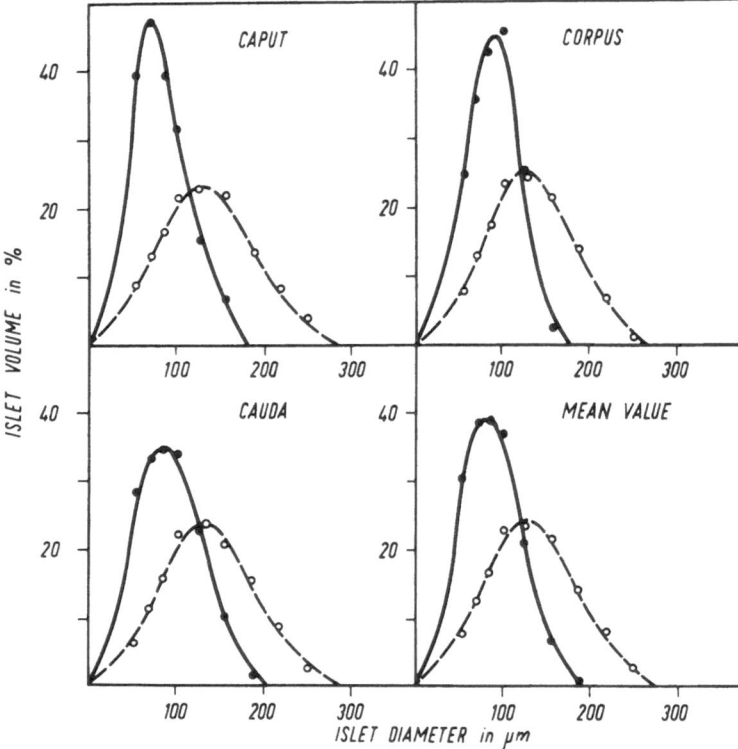

Figure 11. The percentage volume contribution of differently sized islets within the head, body, and tail of the human pancreas in a newborn infant (●——●) and an adult (○----○). In each age the volume curves in the three pancreatic regions are symmetrical. With the postnatal growth of the islet organ these curves become broader and their peaks are displaced to the right. Reproduced from Hellman and Hellerström[21] with permission from the publisher.

The percentual contributions of the different islet cell types to the islet parenchyma were, however, rather constant in the two age groups. Thus, the A_1 cell fraction comprised about 10%, the A_2 cells between 26 and 30%, and the B cells between 58 and 64%. The weight increases of the different types of islet cells in the age interval from 1 day before birth up to 9 months of age were for the A_1 cells from 1 to 10 mg, for the A_2 cells from 3 to 26 mg, and for the B cells from 5 to 65 mg. The observation of a linear relationship between the logarithm of the body weight at different ages and the weight of each of the different islet cell types indicated a growth rate of the islet cells proportional to that of the body weight. Another noteworthy finding was that the postnatal growth of the A_1 cells proceeded at the same rate as that of the two other islet cell types. This suggests that the production of somatostatin, or a somatostatin-like substance, which has been localized to the A_1 cell, is of biological significance throughout postnatal life.

Replication and Neogenesis of Islet Cells

It follows from the observations referred to above that during a substantial part of postnatal life there is a considerable expansion of the total islet mass. Such an increase may either occur through increase in size of the individual cells or through formation of new cells. Since the former process can account for only a small part of the observed changes, the occurrence of new islet cells must be of major significance. Early observations of a low frequency of mitotic figures among the B cells both in the fetal and postnatal islets led to the suggestion that proliferation of these cells occurred mainly by transformation of other cell types.[32,142,148,149] In the fetus, more recent studies have confirmed that although the rate of replication of differentiated islet cells is considerable, it is not as high as in the surrounding parenchyma.[110] There is, however, much evidence to suggest that in this period new islet cells arise from protodifferentiated cells comprising the epithelial matrix of the developing pancreas rather than from already differentiated cells.[110] In postnatal life, application of autoradiography to detect incorporation of [^{3}H]thymidine into islet cell DNA revealed that at least the B cells are able to duplicate, a finding which was further substantiated by the subsequent ultrastructural identification of mitotic B cells.[95,150-152] These observations were nevertheless insufficient to solve the controversy regarding the main source of new B cells, particularly in situations with a rapidly expanding B cell mass. Thus, Pictet and Gonet[153] and Orci *et al.*[154] reported the occurrence of mixed endocrine and exocrine cells in the islets of hyperglycemic spiny mice and suggested that these cells might represent exocrine cells undergoing endocrine transformation. Similar observations were reported by Leduc and Jones[155] in islets of C$_3$Hf mice. Furthermore, Sétáló,[156] Sétáló *et al.*,[157,158] Shorr and Bloom,[159] and Melmed *et al.*[160-162] presented evidence for mixed cells in the pancreas of the normal rat. The latter authors claimed the existence of intermediate forms between both A, B, and acinar cells, and after injections of alloxan or streptozotocin they observed a selective destruction in such cells of intracellular organelles morphologically similar to B granules.[162] Although the morphologic evidence presented so far no doubt favors the occurrence of pleomorphic cells in islet specimens prepared for electron microscopy, criticism has been directed toward the interpretation of these observations. It has thus been suggested that mixed cells are artifacts due to poor delineation of cell membranes or fusion and rupture of plasma membranes resulting in cytoplasmic confluence.[96] Cell fusion *in vitro* has actually been induced by increasing the cytoplasmic calcium concentration.[163] A mechanism of this kind might be operating in the intensely secreting B cells of hyperglycemic animals, since glucose-stimulated insulin release may be associated with accumulation of cytoplasmic calcium.[164] There is, furthermore, little to suggest that the mixed cells, if they exist *in vivo*, are transformed from exocrine to endocrine cells, and their significance for the expansion of the islet cell mass, therefore, cannot be evaluated. Further studies are obviously needed to solve this intricate problem.

The growth of the islet organ, as reflected in the replication of individual islet cells, has been evaluated in the mouse and rat. Denffer[95] studied the autoradiographic labeling of B cells with [³H]thymidine in mouse fetuses of various ages. Labeled B cells were positively identified by staining with dichlorpseudoisocyanine, which reacts metachromatically with insulin.[51] A maximal labeling frequency of the B cells amounting to not less than 21% was found on the 17th intrauterine day with a subsequent decline up to birth. This observation well accords with the rapid expansion of the islet volume and number in this period. By the use of double labeling the mean duration of DNA synthesis (S phase) in the B cell cycle was estimated as 5.6 hr and the whole generation time as 39 hr. The value for the S phase compares well with corresponding values of 5.6 hr and 4.5 to 5 hr calculated by Bunnag[142] and Logothetopoulos[96] respectively, in adult mice. Relatively little is known of the postnatal rate of B cell replication in relation to age. Blum *et al.*[150] observed a decrease in the labeling frequency of the rat B cells from 3.2% immediately before birth to 0.5% at 48 days of age. Corresponding observations have been made in the normal and obese hyperglycemic mouse.[103] In following the decline in the frequency of labeled islet cells after administration of [³H]thymidine to newborn rats, Hellman *et al.*[97] observed the retention of many labeled cells for as long as 5 months. After an initial rapid fall the curve expressing the percentage of labeled islet cells in various ages tended to reach a steady state, suggesting that some mature B cells remain in interphase for prolonged periods of time or indefinitely. Generally, it may be said that the rate of B cell renewal in the adult animal is low. Thus, Logothetopoulos,[96] using reported [³H]thymidine and mitotic indices, calculated that of 1000 B cells, only 5 to 20 divided during 24 hr in the adult mouse and rat. Nevertheless, this apparently low rate of islet cell replication is sufficient to gradually expand the islet mass indicating an even lower rate of degeneration and loss of islet cells.

Regulation of Growth of the Islet Organ

It has been known for a long time that an increased demand for insulin is met with a compensatory volume increase of the islet organ. Although all the different islet cell types may be involved in this process, except for the B cell, little is known about the magnitude of their responses. Since the capacity of the islets to synthesize and secrete insulin depends on the number of properly functioning B cells, their total number will also be of crucial significance for the development and outcome of diabetes. Recent observations suggesting a deficient regenerative capacity of the B cells in certain animals with hereditary diabetes[165] is of considerable interest in this context (see below). The following section will discuss the regulation of islet growth with particular reference to factors known to affect the B cell mass of normal animals.

Food Intake and Diet Composition

The positive correlation between a high food intake, obesity, and diabetes is well known, and much interest has been devoted to quantitative changes of the islet organ in relation to diet. The results of such studies have shown that the amount and composition of ingested food greatly affects the islet organ (Fig. 12). An insufficient food intake has been shown to retard the growth of the islets in both rats and mice.[91,166,167] For example, in obese hyperglycemic mice (genotype *ob,ob*) which are allowed free access to food, the total islet volume exceeds that of the lean littermates by five to ten times, whereas food restriction just sufficient to maintain a normal body weight decreased this ratio to only 1.5.[91] The presence of over 90% B cells in the islets of well-fed *ob,ob* mice indicates that a dietary restriction preferentially inhibits the proliferation of this cell type. Conversely, Tejning[73] showed that the islet organ of rats given free access to a carbohydrate-rich diet grows much faster than that of rats reared on a diet containing high amounts of either protein or fat. Hellman[147] subsequently reported that a carbohydrate-rich diet leads to a selective enlargement of the B cell mass in the rat, indicating a mitogenic effect of the dietary loading on the B cells. These studies are in accord with the earlier observations of Wissler *et al.,*[168] who showed that force feeding of rats with a carbohydrate-rich diet caused a considerable expansion of the islet organ. Despite the presence of glucosuria and degranulation of the B cells no evidence of degeneration of the islet cells or permanent diabetes was noted in this study. A number of recent reports, furthermore, indicate that chronic excessive carbohydrate intake, besides causing islet hyperplasia, also has a stimulating influence on

Figure 12. Effects of variations in the food intake on the total volume of the islet organ of mice and rats. (A) The left part of the picture shows that obese hyperglycemic mice (gene symbol *ob*) have an islet volume (left bar) which is about five times larger than that of their lean litter mates (right bar). When the body weight of the obese hyperglycemic animals was maintained at the same level as that of their lean litter mates by a reduced food intake, this ratio decreased to about 1.5 times (middle bar). Data from Petersson and Hellman.[91] (B) The right part of the picture shows the islet volume of 21-day-old rats which had been segregated into small litters (five animals per litter) or large litters (13 to 14 animals per litter) on the day after birth. The islet volume of the animals belonging to the small litters (left bar) was three times larger than that of the large litters (right bar). Data from Petersson *et al.*[167]

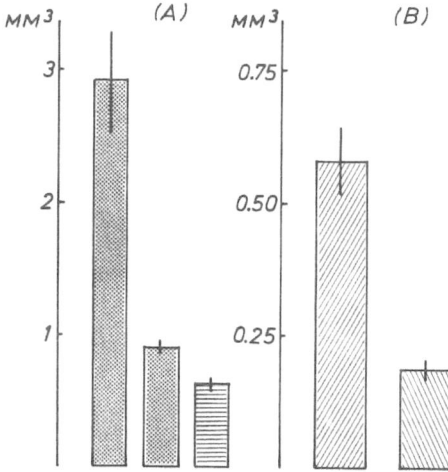

insulin release.[169] Conversely, starvation has been shown to induce a marked impairment of the insulinogenic response to glucose.[170] The marked correlation between these observations and the rate of islet growth again emphasizes that the functional demand on the islet cells is of great regulatory significance for the islet growth.

Hormones

The effect of hormones on B cell regeneration has been studied ever since the discovery by Hausberger and Ramsay[171] that cortisone induces morphological signs of both hyperplasia and an increased functional state of the B cells. This observation was confirmed and extended in a number of subsequent reports using different animal species and various steroid preparations. Thus, increases of both the frequency and the size of the islets in the pancreas of cortisone-treated guinea pigs have been confirmed by Abelove and Paschkis,[172] Fabbrini,[173,174] and Weinges and Maske.[175] Moreover, corresponding effects of cortisone administration in the islet tissue have been described in rabbits,[172,176−179] rats,[180−182] mice,[183] and monkeys.[184] In steroid-diabetic cats the functional load on the islets seems to cause severe hydropic degeneration of the B cells, but only little, if any, hyperplastic changes.[185] In a more detailed volume quantitation of the islet organ, Hellerström[13] demonstrated that guinea pigs treated with cortisone acetate for 40 days expanded their islet volume at least fourfold. Although most of the islet growth was due to B cell proliferation, evidence was presented also for hyperplasia of the A_1 cells. More recently, autoradiographic and ultrastructural studies of the islets of guinea pigs maintained hyperglycemic and glucosuric for up to 5 months by daily injections of prednisolone have been presented by Kern and Logothetopoulos.[186] Besides morphological signs of pronounced hyperfunction and glycogen infiltration of the B cells, there was a marked increase of the [^{3}H]thymidine-labeling index of these cells during the first 2 months of treatment. In guinea pigs killed after 3 to 4 months of steroid treatment, the labeling index had, however, returned to levels found in the untreated guinea pigs despite persistent hyperglycemia. Similar observations have been made in subhuman primates in which mild hyperglycemia was induced by daily injections of prednisolone for up to 3 weeks.[101] An increased number of labeled islet cells and of B cells undergoing mitotic division was directly correlated with the magnitude of serum insulin elevation. These observations are noteworthy, since they confirm that primates also respond to a diabetogenic stimulus by increasing their B cell mass.

A role of growth hormone as a mitogenic stimulus for the B cells was foreshadowed by the studies of Richardson and Young,[187] in which islet cell hyperplasia in dogs was induced by injection of an anterior pituitary extract. This treatment was found to result not only in increased mitotic activity, but there were also marked degenerative changes of the islet cells leading to permanent diabetes. Although the pituitary extracts used by the early workers in this field[187−190] consisted of crude preparations, both the diabetogenic and

insulotropic effects were subsequently confirmed in several studies using purified growth hormone and performed in various species.[179,191-194] The chronic
effects on the islets of very high circulating levels of growth hormone have been
particularly well documented in studies of rats bearing a growth-hormone-
producing, transplantable tumor (MtT-W15).[195,196] It was reported in these
studies that 7 weeks after tumor implantation the islet mass had increased by
more than four times and the pancreatic insulin content almost doubled. In
agreement with the observed volume expansion of the islet organ, there was a
significantly increased insulin biosynthesis and insulin release in response to
glucose in isolated islets from the tumor-bearing rats. Despite a 20-fold elevation of the fasting values of serum growth hormone, none of the animals
developed overt diabetes. The glucose tolerance was actually better and the
circulating insulin values were higher than in the controls. All in all, this study
amply demonstrates the efficiency with which the B cells of the rat respond to a
diabetogenic stimulus. Instead of degenerating, they are able to compensate for
a heavy functional load by multiplication to the extent that the glucose homeostasis is maintained within the normal range. As will be further discussed below,
this ability may be regarded as one of the crucial factors which determines
whether a given diabetogenic stimulus will induce the manifest disease.

In addition to cortisone and growth hormone the effects on the islet organ
of a large number of other endocrine influences have been evaluated, but so far
none has been found to exert a mitogenic response comparable to that of these
two hormones. For a more comprehensive review of these studies reference
should be made to Lazarus and Volk.[179] Some attention should, nevertheless, be
paid in this context to the effects of the islet hormones themselves on the
growth of the endocrine pancreas. Prolonged administration of glucagon has
been shown to cause involution of the A_2 cells, an effect that was interpreted as
indicating that this cell type is the source of glucagon.[12,40,41,43] The regressive
changes of the A_2 cells are particularly pronounced in the guinea pig in which
glucagon injections for 1 month were found to reduce the islet proportion of A_2
cells from about 25% to less than 4%.[12] Some hyperplasia of the B cells was also
suggested in this study by the finding of an unchanged islet volume and an
increased percentage of B cells (Fig. 13). Similar observations were made in
rabbits which, in addition, developed severe hydropic degeneration of the B
cells.[40] In support of a direct "feedback" effect of glucagon on the A_2 cell only
minimal retardation of body growth was found in these animals. Corresponding studies of the action of insulin on the islet organ are often complicated by
the development of antibodies towards this hormone. In addition to a marked
diabetogenic action by neutralizing insulin in the circulation, such antibodies
may exert adverse effects on the islets in several respects.[197,198] However, the rat
seems to have a relatively weak tendency for insulin antibody formation which
makes this species suited for studies of insulin effects on the islet organ. Haist[190]
reported that daily insulin injections into growing rats for 20 to 160 days
significantly inhibited the islet growth. In agreement with these observations,
regressive changes in individual B cells have been demonstrated when adequate

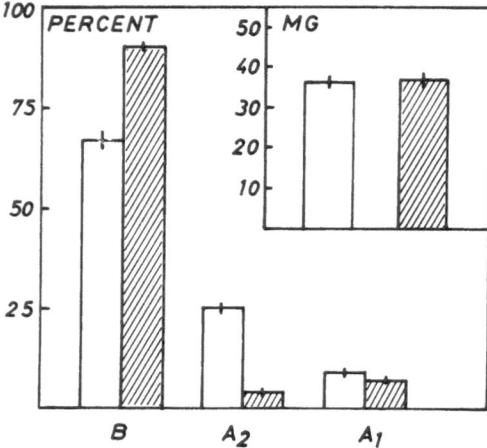

Figure 13. Percentage cellular composition of the pancreatic islets of guinea pigs, which had been injected every 8 hr for 30 days either with 0.4 mg/kg body wt. of crystalline glucagon (▨) or with the corresponding volume of the solvent for glucagon (☐). An increased contribution of B cells and a markedly decreased contribution of A$_2$ cells are evident. The insert shows that the glucagon treatment did not affect the total islet volume. Data from Hellman and Petersson.[11]

amounts of insulin were injected into rats over prolonged periods of time.[199-201] In the careful study of Logothetopoulos *et al.*[201] insulin injections for 2 months caused a marked diminution in the number of B cells, with degranulation and depletion of zinc. These changes occurred despite a 30% increase in the food intake and a rapidly growing body weight. The blood sugar concentration was subnormal until cessation of the insulin injections, when a transient diabetes appeared. It is thus conceivable that insulin administration induces regressive changes of the islets which may lead to a deficient blood sugar homeostasis when the exogenous insulin supply is withdrawn. To what extent these alterations are secondary to a decreased glycemic stimulus of the B cells remains to be clarified.

Pregnancy has for a long time been regarded as a stimulus to B cell replication,[202,203] which in this particular condition may reflect the action of both dietary and hormonal mechanisms. In studies of full-term pregnant mice, Hellerström[14] recorded a 25% increase of the total islet volume, and in the islets of gravid rats Hellman[204] found a pronounced increase in the proportion of B cells. These observations were recently confirmed by van Assche[205] who also demonstrated ultrastructural evidence of a raised insulin production by the individual B cells.[206] Marked functional alterations of the B cells were reported in pregnant rats by Green and Taylor,[207] who found a greatly increased *in vitro* sensitivity of the islet insulin release in response to both glucose, arginine, and theophylline. At least in part these changes could be attributed to the raised food intake during pregnancy, since pair feeding of pregnant and control rats reversed the functional changes toward normal.[208] It therefore appears that endocrine factors may be of minor significance for the islet growth in pregnancy.

Hypoglycemic Sulfonylureas

The reactions of the islet organ to the administration of sulfonylureas is of both theoretical and clinical interest. A stimulant action on the regeneration of the B cells by these compounds would signify that functional stimulations, in general, initiate mitotic activity of these cells irrespective of the blood glucose concentration. Conversely, the prolonged use of these drugs in maturity-onset diabetes leads, in a small number of cases, to "secondary failure," which raises the question of whether the islet cells become gradually damaged or exhausted by the treatment. Numerous studies have been conducted to solve these questions, but there is so far considerable disagreement in the literature as to the effects of sulfonylureas on the islet growth. Loubatières[209] concluded from a study in chlorpropamide-treated dogs that prolonged administration of these drugs induced hyperplasia of the B cells and protected them from degeneration or exhaustion. These observations, however, were not in agreement with those of Lazarow *et al.*,[210] who did not find any expansion of the islet organ or B cell volume in rats made subdiabetic by alloxan injections and subsequently treated with tolbutamide for up to 1 year. Treatment with sulfonylurea actually produced further deterioration of the glucose tolerance of the subdiabetic animals. On the other hand, Gepts *et al.*[144] noted an increased islet number and enlargement of individual islets in carbutamide-treated normal mice. However, no effects of this treatment were seen in mice with the obese–hyperglycemic syndrome. Also, Ashworth and Haist,[211] Davidson and Haist,[212] Bloodworth,[213] and Bunnag *et al.*[71] presented evidence suggesting neoformation of islets in both rat, mouse, and man after prolonged treatment with sulfonylurea. The weight of evidence, therefore, favors a modest enhancement of B cell regeneration by sulfonylureas, although the mechanism of this is entirely unknown.

Replication of the B Cell in Vitro

Although the studies referred to above clearly indicate that a number of stimuli are able to induce proliferation of the B cells *in vitro,* such studies do not elucidate the precise pathways which trigger the mitotic process. Various techniques for long-term incubations of islet cells *in vitro* have, therefore, been utilized in order to analyze the B cell replication in more rigidly controlled conditions. By using autoradiographic labeling with [^{3}H]thymidine of B cells in monolayer cultures of newborn rat pancreas, Chick[107] and Chick *et al.*[214] demonstrated a three- to fourfold increase in labeled B cells, when the glucose concentration of the medium was elevated from 1 to 3 mg/ml. A similar effect was observed with tolbutamide (100 μg/ml), whereas growth hormone (10 μg/ml) and glucagon (10 μg/ml) had no effect in this system. By contrast, dexamethazone (10 μg/ml) inhibited significantly the incorporation of thymidine. In other studies, Andersson[109] and Hellerström *et al.*[215] measured the specific incorporation of [³H]thymidine into DNA in intact isolated mouse islets maintained in culture for 5 days according to the technique of Andersson and Hellerström.[105] Exposure of these islets to 16.7 mM glucose markedly stimulated the DNA synthesis, while neither tolbutamide nor L-leucine were active in this respect. Again, cortisone was found to be a strong inhibitor of the DNA synthesis.

The most noteworthy result of these studies seems to be the unequivocal finding that glucose by itself is able to stimulate the replication of the B cells. Although the intimate mechanism of this action is so far obscure it further emphasizes the exceptional dependence of the B cell on this hexose. This observation also suggests that the growth-promoting effects of cortisone on the islets *in vivo,* as opposed to its inhibitory action on the DNA synthesis *in vitro,* is mediated through the ensuing hyperglycemia. The previously reported enlargement of islets after growth hormone or glucagon may reflect a similar mechanism. It is, on the other hand, difficult to explain the disparity as to the effects of tolbutamide except that differences in culture techniques or species or age may have been of significance. For instance, Chick[107] used islet cells from newborn mice, while Andersson[109] used adult islets. The lack of effect of L-leucine is, furthermore, worthy of note, since this amino acid, like glucose, stimulates both insulin biosynthesis and release and serves as a metabolic substrate for the B cells.[216,217] Thus, the intracellular signals which initiate the replication of the B cell genome may be dissociated from those regulating insulin production.

Islet Growth in Experimental and Spontaneous Diabetes

The capacity of the islet organ to respond to a diabetogenic stimulus by B cell renewal may be one of the key factors that determines the development, course, and outcome of diabetes mellitus. In a broad sense, diabetogenic influences are continuously active in the organism and are normally balanced precisely by adjustments of the B cell function. Irrespective of the nature of the diabetogenic agent, a deficient ability of the B cell to respond to the demand for insulin will lead to metabolic derangements eventually resulting in overt diabetes. It is conceivable that two mechanisms are operative in this context, namely, a minute-to-minute regulation of the insulin release from the individual B cell and a more long-term adaptation involving changes in the total B cell mass. Furthermore, it seems plausible that disturbances in either of these two mechanisms may be of etiologic significance for the manifestation of diabetes. It is the purpose of this section to discuss the adaptive responses of the islet cell mass in diabetes with particular attention to the kinetics of B cell proliferation and to factors of genetic or environmental nature which may interfere with this process.

Experimental Diabetes

A number of data referred to in previous sections of this chapter clearly show that hyperglycemia represents a powerful stimulus to B cell proliferation. Detailed studies of the [^{3}H]thymidine index of the islet B cells have disclosed a distinct pattern of DNA synthesis, when these cells are exposed to sustained hyperglycemia. Thus, when high blood sugar concentrations were maintained in mice by daily injections of insulin antibodies, incorporation of [^{3}H]thymidine into B cell DNA remained within the control range on the 1st day, reached a peak on the 3rd day, and subsequently declined in spite of sustained hyperglycemia.[198,218] Peak values were about four times higher than the control values, and a normal frequency of labeled cells was again observed by the 15th day. When the circulating antibody was neutralized by an excess of exogenous insulin, high [^{3}H]thymidine indices were still recorded on two subsequent days despite normal blood sugar concentrations.[96] The mitotic response was blocked by actinomycin D, suggesting that DNA replication in the B cell is in some way related to the synthesis of RNA. It was also found that the mitotic rate was decreased by 30 to 40% when mice were subjected to antibody stimulation for a second time. A similar pattern of response was found also after injection of alloxan or streptozotocin in that surviving B cells exhibited an initial wave of mitotic activity during the first week, followed by a gradual decline despite persistent hyperglycemia.[103] Further studies indicated that obese hyperglycemic mice (gene symbol *ob*), which have a high rate of B cell renewal early in life, were unable to respond to a hyperglycemic stimulus with increased B cell replication when reverted to a normoglycemic state.[103]

Altogether, these studies suggest that a high rate of mitotic activity of the B cells cannot be maintained continuously, but there is a gradual decline despite persisting hyperglycemia. On the basis of these observations Logothetopoulos *et al.*[103] and Logothetopoulos[96] suggested that the B cell genome is programmed for a finite number of mitotic cycles, which might be exhausted in situations with sustained mitogenic stimulation. The rate of B cell loss then becomes the important factor in maintaining or reducing the population of B cells in the islet organ.

An observation of so far unknown biological significance is the proliferative response of the A$_1$ cells in experimental diabetes. This was first demonstrated by Hellman and Petersson[11] in alloxan diabetic rats, which showed a significant increase in the total weight of the A$_1$ cell system 3 months after induction of diabetes. Morphological signs of a raised functional state of the A$_1$ cells have subsequently been reported in both steroid-diabetic and streptozotocin-diabetic guinea pigs[6,219,220] and in the newborn offspring of alloxan-diabetic rats.[221] More recently Orci *et al.*[15] showed a marked increase of immunofluorescent, somatostatin-containing islet cells in rats which had been made diabetic with streptozotocin. In support of these observations radioimmunoassay of the somatostatin content in extracts of islets isolated from streptozotocin-diabetic rats showed a striking increase of this peptide.[10] Although the islet glucagon content was also raised in the diabetic rats, there seems to be no corresponding increase of the total A_2 cell volume in diabetes.[11,15] Since the biological role of the somatostatin-like islet material is so far unknown, it is too early to suggest a precise interpretation of these results. The apparently similar reactions of the A_1 cells in alloxan- and streptozotocin-induced diabetes (with a diminished number of B cells) and in steroid diabetes (with proliferation of the B cells) may signify that the A_1 cells react with proliferation independent of the islet insulin content.

Spontaneous Diabetes

Further insight into the regulation of islet growth in diabetes has been gained in studies of various animal strains with hereditary diabetes. One of these, the diabetic Chinese hamster, exhibits a syndrome which develops from a prediabetic phase into a fulminant diabetes characterized by a diminished concentration of insulin in the blood, ketosis, and severe B cell degeneration.[85,222] Autoradiographic studies of [³H]thymidine-labeled islet cells of these animals have consistently shown an increased islet labeling in the early diabetic phase which is in accord with the simultaneous finding of some hyperglycemia and hyperinsulinemia.[223] With progression of the diabetes the number of B cells declined and islet labeling became infrequent. Furthermore, administration of glucocorticoids to these animals was without effect on the incidence of labeled B cells in the diabetic animals, whereas a similar treatment greatly enhanced the labeling of the B cells in normal control hamsters.[223] Thus, these observations support the notion that exhaustion of mitotic events might contribute to the development also of spontaneous diabetes in animals.[224]

One important question raised by the observations referred to above is to what extent the total capacity for B cell regeneration is determined by individual variations in the genetic background. Again, studies of spontaneously diabetic animals, and in particular certain mouse strains, have contributed to the elucidation of this problem. In several of these mouse strains there is a recessively inherited trait for diabetes characterized by gross obesity, hyperglycemia, and extreme insulin resistance.[225] Early in the development of the syndromes there is marked hyperplasia of the B cells, which may comprise over 90% of the enlarged islets, and high levels of circulating insulin. However, in some of the syndromes the well-compensated phase of the disease is followed by a ketoacidotic fulminant diabetes with a lack of circulating insulin and loss of the B cells. This development is, for example, characteristic of the diabetic mutant mouse (C57BL/KsJ-*db*).[99,226] In contrast, several other mouse strains with hereditary diabetic syndromes, for example, the yellow obese mouse (gene symbol *A^y*), the C57BL/6J-*ob* mouse, and the NZO mouse, remain hyperglycemic and hyperinsulinemic for most of their life span without any signs of decompensation.[225] The islets of these animals are greatly enlarged but lack degenerative changes, although the individual B cells show morphological signs of increased functional demand such as degranulation and nuclear hypertrophy.

It might be inferred from these observations that the phenotypic expression of the diabetic syndrome is determined entirely by the intensity of the diabetogenic stimulus which, of course, could vary in different animal strains. However, recent comparisons between two of these mouse strains, the obese-hyperglycemic mouse (gene symbol *ob*) and the diabetic mutant mouse (gene symbol *db*), have shown that each of the two genetic determinants (the *ob* gene or the *db* gene) attains a quite different phenotypic expression depending upon the genetic background upon which it has been introduced.[165,225,227] Thus, when the *db* gene was introduced on the C57BL/KsJ background, the diabetes became manifest as a severe, ketoacidotic disease with marked islet atrophy and insulin lack. However, when the same gene was introduced on the C57BL/6J background, the disease was much milder with marked B cell hyperplasia and no tendency for ketoacidosis.[227,229] Similar observations were reported by Coleman and Hummel[165,228] when the obese *(ob)* gene rather than the diabetic *(db)* gene was introduced on the same genetic background. A third variety, obtained by outcrossing C57BL/Ks-*db* mice with C57BL/6-*m* mice (gene symbol *m* stands for misty) followed by backcrossing for four generations to the Ks background has given rise to an intermediate form of diabetes with islet atrophy only at a relatively advanced age of the animal[230] (Fig. 14). Coleman and Hummel[165] have recently presented evidence that the observed modifications of the diabetic syndromes are under multigenic control and that modifiers that determine the milder diabetic syndrome associated with islet hypertrophy are dominant over those which cause the more severe condition with islet atrophy.

On the basis of the above observations it was suggested that the primary action of the modifying genes is to regulate the proliferation of the B cells in periods of hyperglycemic stress.[165] This may, indeed, be the inherited factor which determines the number of mitotic cycles through which the B cell genome is able to pass. That a mechanism of this kind could be operative in the C57BL/KsJ-*db* mice is suggested by the findings of Like and Chick[99] and Chick and Like[231] showing a marked decline in the number of [³H]thymidine-labeled B cells in these mice when they approached the terminal phase of the syndrome. Although so far inconclusive, these data serve to emphasize the possible significance of the background genome for the manifestations of the diabetic syndrome and also underline the complexity involved in the inheritance of the disease.

Diabetes in Man

The observations on spontaneously diabetic animals raise the question of whether an inherited restriction on the maximum number of mitoses which a B cell can undergo represents a significant pathogenetic factor also in the development of human diabetes. As in laboratory animals, mitotic figures are extremely rare in normal human islets, but they may increase considerably in

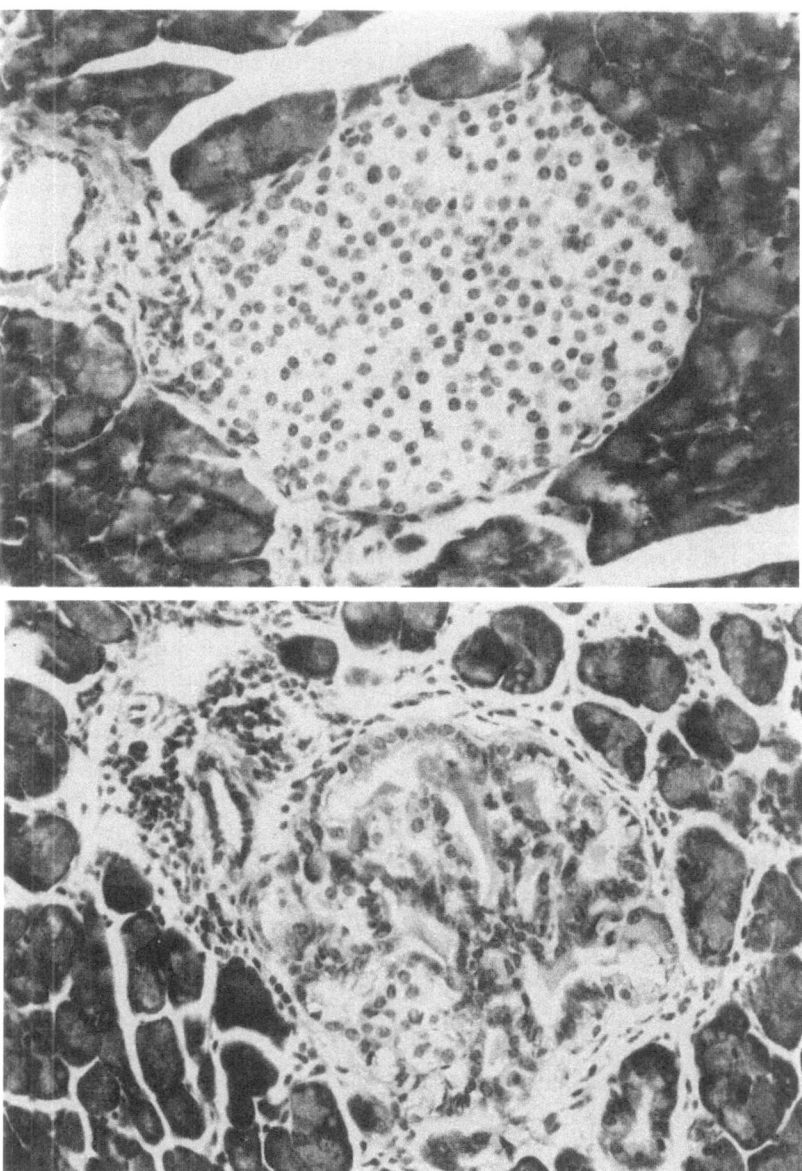

Figure 14. (top) Pancreatic islet from a 50-week-old nondiabetic mouse originating from the C57BL/KsJ strain. Chrome-hematoxylin ponceau fuchsin stain. ×250. (bottom) Pancreatic islet from a 50-week-old C57BL/KsJ-*dbm* mouse exhibiting marked obesity and diabetes.[230] There is a pronounced atrophy of endocrine cells, which have been replaced by proliferating ductlike structures. Chrome-hematoxylin ponceau fuchsin stain. ×250.

patients with acute liver disease.[232,233] Although these mitotic cells have not been classified according to type, the observations indicate a potential for regeneration of islet cells also in adult man. That this regenerative capacity may be present in the B cells is indicated by the observation of B cell hyperplasia in obese persons[234,235] and in prediabetic individuals.[236] On the other hand, the extensive studies by Gepts[237-240] have shown conclusively an almost complete disappearance of the B cells in chronic juvenile diabetes with few, if any, signs of regenerative activity. While an accelerated loss of human B cells may be caused by a number of factors such as viruses and/or autoimmune reactions[241-243] the only way to compensate for this loss is by formation of new B cells. It could be that in both animals and man the key factor which determines whether diabetes will become manifest in a given individual is the genetic potential for B cell divisions. It is of considerable interest in this context that a finite number of mitotic events is a characteristic of normal human fibroblasts[244] and that such cells derived from diabetic or prediabetic patients show a diminished capacity for replication[245-247]. If this is shown to be a general property of somatic cells in diabetics, it would explain not only their (so far hypothetical) deficient capacity for B cell regeneration, but it would also serve as a future genetic marker for individuals with an increased risk of developing diabetes.

Acknowledgment

The work by the author included in this review was supported by the Swedish Medical Research Council, the Swedish Diabetes Association, the Nordic Insulin Fund, Expressens Prenatalforskningsfond, and the United States Public Health Service.

References*

1. Polak, J. M., Pearse, A. G. E., Grimelius, L., and Bloom, S. R.: *Lancet,* **1**:1220, 1975.
2. Hökfeldt, T., Efendic, S., Hellerström, C., Johansson, O., Luft, R., and Arimura, A.: *Acta Endocrinol., Suppl. 200,* **80**:1, 1975.
3. Orci, L., Baetens, D., Dubois, M. P., and Rufener, C.: *Horm. Metab. Res.,* **7**:400, 1975.
4. Lomsky, R., Lange, F., and Vortel, V.: *Nature (London),* **223**:618, 1969.
5. Greider, M. H., and McGuigan, J. E.: *Amer. J. Pathol.* **59**:76A, 1970.
6. Erlandsen, S. L., Hegre, O. D., Parsons, J. A., McEvoy, R. C., and Elde, R. P.: *J. Histochem. Cytochem.* **24**:883, 1976.
7. Larsson, L.-I., Rehfeld, J. F., Sundler, F., and Håkansson, R.: *Nature (London),* **262**:609, 1976.
8. Lostra, F., van der Loo, W., and Gepts, W.: *Diabetologia,* **10**:291, 1974.
9. Dubois, M. P.: *Proc. Nat. Acad. Sci., U.S.A.,* **72**:1340, 1975.
10. Patel, Y. C., and Weir, G. C.: *Clin. Endocrinol.,* **5**:191, 1976.
11. Hellman, B., and Petersson, B.: *Endocrinology,* **72**:238, 1963.
12. Petersson, B., and Hellman, B.: *Acta Endocrinol.,* **44**:139, 1963.

*The survey of the literature was concluded in May, 1976.

13. Hellerström, C.: *Acta Soc. Med. Upsal.*, **68**:1, 1963.

14. Hellerström, C.: *Acta Soc. Med. Upsal.*, **68**:17, 1963.

15. Orci, L., Baetens, D., Rufener, C., Amherdt, M., Ravazzola, M., Studener, P., Malaisse-Lagae, F., and Unger, R. H.: *C. R. Acad. Sci., Paris*, **281**:1884, 1975.

16. Hellman, B., and Hellerström, C.: *Acta Endocrinol.*, **36**:22, 1961.

17. Fujita, T.: *Z. Zellforsch.*, **69**:363, 1966.

18. Van Assche, F. A.: Thesis. Louvain, 1970.

19. Hellerström, C., and Hellman, B.: *Acta Endocrinol.*, **35**:518, 1960.

20. Hellerström, C., Hellman, B., Petersson, B., and Alm, G.: In: *The Structure and Metabolism of the Pancreatic Islets.* Edited by S. E. Brolin, B. Hellman, and H. Knutsson. Pergamon Press, Oxford, 1964, p. 117.

21. Hellman, B., and Hellerström, C.: In: *Handbuch des Diabetes Mellitus.* Edited by E. F. Pfeiffer, J. F. Lehmanns Verlag, München, 1969, p. 89.

22. Hellerström, C., and Asplund, K.: *Z. Zellforsch.* **70**:68, 1966.

23. Fujita, T.: In: *The Structure and Metabolism of the Pancreatic Islets.* Edited by S. E. Brolin, B. Hellman, and H. Knutsson. Pergamon Press, Oxford, 1964, p. 11.

24. Fujita, T.: *Arch. Histol. Jap.*, **29**:1, 1968.

25. Solcia, E., and Sampietro, R.: *Z. Zellforsch.*, **65**:131, 1965.

26. Solcia, E., and Sampietro, R.: *Z. Zellforsch.*, **68**:689, 1965.

27. Epple, A.: *Endocrinol. Jap.*, **15**:107, 1968.

28. Titlbach, M.: *Folia Morphol.*, **17**:1, 1969.

29. Bloom, W.: *Anat. Rec.*, **49**:363, 1931.

30. Thomas, T. B.: *Amer. J. Anat.*, **62**:31, 1937.

31. Conklin, J. L.: *Amer. J. Anat.*, **111**:181, 1962.

32. Ferner, H.: *Das Inselsystem des Pankreas.* Georg Thieme, Stuttgart, 1952, p. 62.

33. Like, A. A.: *Lab Invest.*, **16**:937, 1967.

34. Bencosme, S., and Lechago, J.: *Lab Invest.*, **18**:715, 1968.

35. Kern, H. F., and Kern, D.: *Symposium der Deutschen Gesellschaft für Endokrinologie*, **14**:186, 1968.

36. Faller, A.: *Z. Zellforsch.*, **97**:226, 1969.

37. Sato, T., Herman, L., and Fitzgerald, P. I.: *Gen. Comp. Endocrinol.*, **7**:132, 1966.

38. Titlbach, M.: *Folia Morphol.*, **17**:17, 1969.

39. Wellmann, K. F., Volk, B. W., and Brancato, P.: *Lab. Invest.*, **25**:97, 1971.

40. Logothetopoulos, J., Sharma, B. B., Salter, J. M., and Best, C. H.: *Diabetes*, **9**:278, 1960.

41. Volk, B. W., and Lazarus, S. S.: *Diabetes*, **9**:53, 1960.

42. Unger, R. H., and Lefèbvre, P. J.: In: *Glucagon.* Edited by P. J. Lefèbvre and R. H. Unger. Pergamon Press, Oxford, 1972, p. 213.

43. Hellerström, C., and Hellman, B.: *Acta Endocrinol.*, **41**:116, 1962.

44. Baum, J., Simons, Jr., B. E., Unger, R. H., and Madison, L. L.: *Diabetes*, **11**:371, 1962.

45. Lundquist, G., Brolin, S. E., Unger, R. H., and Eisentraut, A. M.: In: *The Structure and Metabolism of the Pancreatic Islets.* Edited by S. Falkmer, B. Hellman, and I.-B. Täljedal. Pergamon Press, Oxford, 1970, p. 115.

46. Grimelius, L.: *Acta Soc. Med. Upsal.*, **73**:243, 1968.

47. Lange, H.: In: *Handbuch der Histochemie.* Edited by W. Graumann and K. Neumann. G. F. Verlag, Stuttgart, 1973, Vol. 8, p. 1.

48. Gomori, G.: *Amer. J. Pathol.*, **17**:395, 1941.

49. Gomori, G.: *Amer. J. Clin. Pathol.*, **20**:665, 1950.

50. Ivic, M.: *Anat. Anz.*, **107**:347, 1959.

51. Schiebler, T. H., and Schiessler, S.: *Histochemie*, **1**:445, 1959.

52. Larsson, L.-I., Sundler, F., Håkansson, R., Pollock, H. G., and Kimmel, J. R.: *Histochemistry*, **42**:377, 1974.

53. Larsson, L.-I., Sundler, F., and Håkansson, R.: *Cell Tiss. Res.*, **156**:167, 1975.

54. Larsson, L.-I., Sundler, F., and Håkansson, R.: *Diabetologia*, **12**:211, 1976.

55. Kimmel, J. R., Pollock, H. G., and Hazelwood, R. L.: *Endocrinology*, **83**:1323, 1968.

56. Kimmel, J. R., Pollock, H. G., and Hazelwood, R. L.: *Fed. Proc.*, **30**:1318, (Abst.), 1971.

57. Lazarus, S. S., and Shapiro, S. H.: *Anat. Rec.,* **169**:487, 1971.
58. Munger, B. L., Caramia, P. E., and Lacy, P. E.: *Z. Zellforsch.,* **67**:776, 1965.
59. Lacy, P. E., and Greider, M. H.: In: *Handbook of Physiology.* Sect. 7, Vol. 1. Edited by D. F. Steiner and N. Freinkel. American Physiological Society, Washington, D.C., 1972, p. 77.
60. Boquist, L., and Falkmer, S.: In: *The Structure and Metabolism of the Pancreatic Islets.* Edited by S. Falkmer, B. Hellman, and I.-B. Täljedal, Pergamon Press, Oxford, 1970, p. 25.
61. Falkmer, S., and Patent, G. J.: In: *Handbook of Physiology;* Sect. 7, Vol. 1. Edited by D. F. Steiner and N. Freinkel. American Physiological Society, Washington, D.C., 1972, p. 1.
62. Edström, C.: *Umeå Univ. Med. Diss.,* **10**:1, 1972.
63. Bensley, R. R.: *Amer. J. Anat.,* **12**:297, 1911.
64. Clark, E.: *Anat. Anz.,* **43**:81, 1913.
65. Overholser, M. D.: *Endocrinology,* **9**:439, 1925.
66. Hess, W. N., and Root, C. W.: *Amer. J. Anat.,* **63**:489, 1938.
67. Haist, R. E., and Pugh, E. J.: *Amer. J. Physiol.,* **152**:36, 1948.
68. Jaffé, F. A.: *Anat. Rec.,* **11**:109, 1951.
69. Parakkal, R. F., and Ali, M. A.: *Rev. Can. Biol.,* **20**:781, 1961.
70. Brunfeldt, K., Hunhammar, K., and Skouby, A. D.: *Acta Endocrinol.,* **29**:473, 1958.
71. Bunnag, S. C., Warner, N. E., and Bunnag, S.: *Diabetes,* **15**:597, 1966.
72. Mount, L. E.: *J. Endocrinol.,* **5**:243, 1948.
73. Tejning, S.: *Acta Med. Scand.,* Suppl. 198, **128**:1, 1947.
74. Hellman, B.: *Acta Pathol. Microbiol. Scand.,* **47**:35, 1959.
75. Wiksell, S. D.: *Biometrika,* **17**:84, 1925.
76. Wiksell, S. D.: *Biometrika,* **18**:151, 1926.
77. Hellman, B.: *Acta Endocrinol.,* **32**:78, 1959.
78. Hellman, B.: *Acta Endocrinol.,* **31**:91, 1959.
79. Hellman, B.: *Acta Pathol. Microbiol. Scand.,* **47**:21, 1959.
80. Chalkley, H. W.: *J. Nat. Cancer Inst.,* **4**:47, 1943.
81. Tove, P. A., Brolin, S., and Hellman, B.: *Rev. Sci. Instr.,* **32**:1343, 1961.
82. Lazarow, A., and Carpenter, A. M.: *J. Histochem. Cytochem.,* **10**:324, 1962.
83. Carpenter, A. M., and Lazarow, A.: *J. Histochem. Cytochem.,* **10**:329, 1962.
84. Carpenter, A. M.: *J. Histochem. Cytochem.,* **11**:834, 1966.
85. Carpenter, A. M., Gerritsen, G. C., Dulin, W. E., and Lazarow, A.: *Diabetologia,* **6**:168, 1970.
86. Hegre, O. D., McEvoy, R. C. Bachelder, V., and Lazarow, A.: *In Vitro,* **7**:366, 1972.
87. McEvoy, R. C., Lazarow, A., and Hegre, O. D.: *Differentiation,* **3**:69, 1975.
88. McEvoy, R. C., and Hegre, O. D.: *Differentiation.* 1976 (in press).
89. Voigt, G. E.: *Virchows Arch. Pathol. Anat.,* **332**:295, 1959.
90. Brolin, S. E., and Hellman, B.: *Diabetes,* **12**:62, 1963.
91. Petersson, B., and Hellman, B.: *Metabolism,* **11**:342, 1962.
92. Petersson, B.: *Z. Zellforsch.,* **75**:371, 1966.
93. Floderus, S.: *Acta Pathol. Microbiol. Scand., (Suppl. 53)*:1, 1944.
94. Hellman, B.: *Acta Pathol. Microbiol. Scand.,* **45**:336, 1959.
95. Denffer, H. V.: *Histochemie,* **21**:338, 1970.
96. Logothetopoulos, J.: In: *Handbook of Physiology.* Sect. 7, Vol. 1. Edited by D. F. Steiner and N. Freinkel. American Physiological Society, Washington, D.C., 1972, p. 67.
97. Hellman, B., Hellerström, C., and Petersson, B.: *Diabetes,* **10**:470, 1961.
98. Crane, W. A. J., and Dutta, L. P.: *J. Endocrinol.,* **28**:341, 1964.
99. Like, A. A., and Chick, W. L.: *Diabetologia,* **6**:207, 1970.
100. Like, A. A., and Chick, W. L.: *Diabetologia,* **6**:216, 1970.
101. Like, A. A., and Chick, W. L.: *Amer. J. Pathol.,* **75**:329, 1974.
102. Logothetopoulos, J., and Bell, E. G.: *Diabetes,* **15**:205, 1966.
103. Logothetopoulos, J., Brosky, G., and Kern, H. F.: In: *The Structure and Metabolism of the Pancreatic Islets.* Edited by S. Falkmer, B. Hellman, and I.-B. Täljedal, Pergamon Press, Oxford, 1970, p. 15.
104. Chick, W. L., and Like, A. A.: *Amer. J. Physiol.* **221**:202, 1971.

105. Andersson, A., and Hellerström, C.: *Diabetes, Suppl. 2,* **21**:546, 1972.
106. Lambert, A. E., Blondel, B., Kanazawa, Y., Orci, L., and Renold, A. E.: *Endocrinology,* **90**:239, 1972.
107. Chick, W. L.: *Diabetes,* **22**:687, 1973.
108. Braaten, T., Järlfors, O., Smith, D. S., and Mintz, D. H.: *Tiss. Cell,* **4**:747, 1975.
109. Andersson, A.: *Endocrinology,* **96**:1051, 1975.
110. Pictet, R., and Rutter, W. J.: In: *Endocrine Pancreas. Handbook of Physiology.* Sect. 7, Vol. 1. Edited by D. F. Steiner and N. Freinkel. Williams & Wilkins, Baltimore, 1972, p. 25.
111. Pearse, A. G. E., and Polak, J. M.: *Gut,* **12**:173, 1971.
112. Welbourn, M. A., Pearse, A. G. E., Polak, J. M., Bloom, S. R., and Joffe, S. N.: *Med. Clin. North. Amer.,* **58**:1359, 1974.
113. Falck, B., and Hellman, B.: *Experientia,* **19**:139, 1963.
114. Cegrell, L., and Falck, B.: *Acta Physiol. Scand. Suppl.* **314**:35, 1968.
115. Pictet, R. L., Rall, L. B., Phelps, P., and Rutter, W. J.: *Science,* **191**:191, 1976.
116. Pictet, R. L., Rall, L., Gasparo, M., and Rutter, W. J.: In: *Early Diabetes in Early Life.* Edited by R. A. Camerini-Davalos and H. S. Cole. Academic Press, New York, 1975, p. 25.
117. Like, A. A., and Orci, L.: *Diabetes, Suppl. 2,* **21**:511, 1972.
118. Grasso, S., Saporito, N., Messina, A., and Reitano, G.: *Lancet,* **2**:755, 1968.
119. Chez, R. A., Mintz, D. H., and Hutchinson, D. L.: *Metabolism,* **20**:805, 1971.
120. Espinosa de los Monteros Mend, A. M., Driscoll, S. G., and Steinke, J.: *Science,* **168**:1111, 1970.
121. Milner, R. D. G., Ashworth, M. A., and Barson, A. J.: *J. Endocrinol.* **52**:497, 1972.
122. Milner, R. D. G., Leach, F. N., and Jack, P. M. B.: In: *Carbohydrate Metabolism in Pregnancy and the Newborn.* Edited by H. W. Sutherland, and J. M. Stowers. Churchill Livingstone, Edinburgh, 1975, p. 83.
123. Asplund, K., Westman, S., and Hellerström, C.: *Diabetologia,* **5**: 260, 1969.
124. Asplund, K.: *Eur. J. Clin. Invest.,* **3**:338, 1973.
125. Shelley, H. J., Bassett, J. M., and Milner, R. D. G.: *Brit. Med. Bull.,* **31**:37, 1975.
126. Edwards, J. C., Asplund, K., and Lundquist, G.: *J. Endocrinol.,* **54**:493, 1972.
127. Lernmark, A., and Wenngren, B. I.: *J. Embryol. Exp. Morphol.* **28**:607, 1972.
128. Jarrouse, C., Rancon, F., Rosselin, G., and Freychet, P.: *C. R. Acad. Sci., Paris,* **276**:797, 1973.
129. Jarrousse, C., and Rosselin, G.: *Endocrinology,* **96**:168, 1975.
130. Freie, H. M. P., Pasma, A., and Bouman, P. R.: *Acta Endocrinol.* **80**:657, 1975.
131. Murata, J., Eguchi, Y., Morikawa, Y., and Hashimoto, Y.: *Endocrinol. Jap.,* **19**:163, 1972.
132. Lambert, A. E.: Thesis, Louvain, 1970.
133. Hegre, O., McEvoy, R. C., Bachelder, V., and Lazarow, A.: *Diabetes,* **22**:577, 1973.
134. Fricke, R., and Clark, Jr., C. M.: *Amer. J. Physiol.,* **224**:117, 1973.
135. Asplund, K.: *Horm. Res.,* **6**:12, 1975.
136. Picon, L., and Montané, M.: *C. R. Acad. Sci., Paris, Ser. D,* **267**:860, 1968.
137. Britton, H. G., and Blade, M.: *Biol. Neonat.,* **16**:370, 1970.
138. Felix, J. M., Sutter, M. T., Sutter, B. C., and Jacquot, R.: *Horm. Metab. Res.,* **3**:71, 1971.
139. Girard, J. R., Cunendet, G. S., Marliss, E. B., Kervran, A., Rientort, M., and Assan, R.: *J. Clin. Invest.,* **52**:3190, 1973.
140. Blázquez, E., Montoya, E., and Lopez Quijada, C.: *J. Endocrinol.* **48**:553, 1970.
141. Ogilvie, R. F.: *Quart. J. Med.,* **6**:287, 1937.
142. Bunnag, S.: *Diabetes,* **15**:480, 1966.
143. Hellman, B.: *Acta Soc. Med. Upsal.,* **64**:432, 1959.
144. Gepts, W., Christophe, J., and Mayer, J.: *Diabetes,* **9**:63, 1960.
145. Hellman, B., Brolin, S., Hellerström, C., and Hellman, K.: *Acta Endocrinol.* **36**:609, 1961.
146. Hellman, B., and Angervall, L.: *Acta Pathol. Microbiol. Scand.,* **53**:230, 1961.
147. Hellman, B.: *Acta Soc. Med. Upsal.,* **64**:393, 1959.
148. Patent, G. J., and Alfert, M.: *Acta Anat.,* **66**:504, 1967.
149. Falin, L. I.: *Acta Anat.,* **68**:147, 1967.

150. Blum, B., Heggestad, C., and Lazarow, A.: *Anat. Rec.,* **145**:309, 1963.
151. Like, A. A., and Chick, W. L.: *Science,* **163**:941, 1969.
152. Westman, J., Andersson, A., Petersson, B., and Hellerström, C.: *Acta Diabet. Lat.,* **7**:557, 1970.
153. Pictet, R., and Gonet, A.: *C. R. Acad. Sci., Paris,* **262**:1123, 1966.
154. Orci, L., Rufener, C., Pictet, R., Renold, A. E., and Rouiller, C.: In: *The Structure and Metabolism of the Pancreatic Islets.* Edited by S. Falkmer, B. Hellman, and I.-B. Täljedal. Pergamon Press, Oxford, 1970, p. 37.
155. Leduc, E. H., and Jones, E. E.: *J. Ultrastr. Res.,* **24**:165, 1968.
156. Sétáló, G.: *Acta Biol. Hung.,* **18**:323, 1967.
157. Sétáló, G., Blatniczky, L., and Vigh, S.: *Acta Biol. Sci. Hung.,* **22**:361, 1971.
158. Sétáló, G., Blatniczky, L., and Vigh, S.: *Excerpta Med.,* **280**:5, 1973.
159. Shorr, S. S., and Bloom, F. E.: *Yale J. Biol. Med.,* **43**:47, 1970.
160. Melmed, R. N., Benitez, C. J., and Holt, S. J.: *J. Cell Sci.,* **11**:449, 1972.
161. Melmed, R. N., Turner, R. C., and Holt, S. J.: *J. Cell Sci.,* **13**:279, 1973.
162. Melmed, R. N., Benitez, C. J., and Holt, S. J.: *J. Cell Sci.,* **13**:297, 1973.
163. Ahkong, Q. F., Tampion, W., and Lucy, J. A.: *Nature (London),* **256**:208, 1975.
164. Howell, S. L., and Montague, W.: *FEBS Lett.,* **52**:48, 1975.
165. Coleman, D. L., and Hummel, K. P.: *Israel J. Med. Sci.,* **11**:708, 1975.
166. Ashworth, M. A., Kerbel, N. C., and Haist, R. E.: *J. Physiol. (London),* **171**:25, 1952.
167. Petersson, B., Hellerström, C., and Hellman, B.: *Acta Endocrinol.* **35**:533, 1960.
168. Wissler, R. N., Findley, J. W., and Frazier, L. E.: *Proc. Soc. Exp. Biol. Med.,* **71**:308, 1949.
169. Blazquez, E., and Lopez-Quijada, C.: *J. Endocrinol.,* **44**:107, 1969.
170. Malaisse, W. J.: In: *Handbook of Physiology,* Sect. 7, Vol. 1. Edited by D. F. Steiner and N. Freinkel. American Physiological Society, Washington, D.C., 1972, p. 237.
171. Hausberger, F. X., and Ramsay, A. J.: *Endocrinology,* **53**:423, 1953.
172. Abelove, W. A., and Paschkis, K. E.: *Endocrinology,* **55**:637, 1954.
173. Fabbrini, A.: *Z. Zellforsch.,* **43**:307, 1955.
174. Fabbrini, A.: *Folia Endocrinol.* **9**:95, 1956.
175. Weinges, K., and Maske, H.: *Arch. Exp. Pathol. Pharmakol.,* **231**:440, 1957.
176. Lazarus, S. S., and Bencosme, S. A.: *Amer. J. Clin. Path.,* **26**:1146, 1956.
177. Creutzfeldt, W.: *Verh. Deutsch. Ges. Pathol.* **42**:85, 1959.
178. Volk, B. W., and Lazarus, S. S.: *Diabetes,* **9**:264, 1960.
179. Lazarus, S. S., and Volk, B. W.: *The Pancreas in Human and Experimental Diabetes.* Grune & Stratton, New York, 1962, p. 102.
180. Franckson, J. R. M., Gepts, W., Bastenie, P. A., Conrad, V., Cordier, N., and Kovacs, L.: *Acta Endocrinol.,* **14**:153, 1953.
181. Houssay, B. A., Rodriguez, R. R., and Cardeza, A. F.: *Endocrinology,* **54**:550, 1954.
182. Yoshinaga, T., Katayama, T., Nakajima, I., and Nishikawa, M.: *Endokrinologie,* **51**:211, 1967.
183. Hausberger, F. X.: *Fed. Proc.,* **17**:67, 1958.
184. Rivière, M., and Combescat, C.: *C. R. Soc. Biol., Paris,* **148**:93, 1954.
185. Lukens, F. D. W., Cohen, S. N., and Goto, Y.: *Diabetes,* **10**:182, 1961.
186. Kern, H., and Logothetopoulos, J.: *Diabetes,* **19**:145, 1970.
187. Richardson, K. C., and Young, F. G.: *Lancet,* **116**:1098, 1938.
188. Ham, A. W., and Haist, R. E.: *Amer. J. Pathol.,* **17**:787, 1941.
189. Dohan, F. C., and Lukens, F. D. W.: *Amer. J. Physiol.,* **125**:188, 1939.
190. Haist, R. E.: *Proc. Amer. Diab. Assoc.,* **9**:53, 1949.
191. Mosca, L.: *Folia Endocrinol., Pisa,* **4**:335, 1951.
192. Ogilvie, R. F., and Maclean, F.: *Diabetes,* **9**:38, 1960.
193. Volk, B. W., and Lazarus, S. S.: *Diabetes,* **11**:426, 1962.
194. Cicchitti, L. F.: *Acta Physiol. Lat. Amer.,* **14**:324, 1964.
195. Martin, J. M., Akerblom, H. K., and Garay, G.: *Diabetes,* **17**:661, 1968.
196. Bencosme, S. A., Tsutsumi, V., Martin, J. M., and Akerblom, H. K.: *Diabetes,* **20**:15, 1971.
197. Toreson, W. E., Lee, J. C., and Grodsky, G. M.: *Amer. J. Pathol.,* **52**:1099, 1968.

198. Freytag, G.: *Beitr. Path. Anat.*, **137**:121, 1968.
199. Bell, E. T.: *Diabetes*, **2**:125, 1953.
200. Latta, J. S., and Harvey, H. T.: *Anat. Rec.*, **82**:281, 1942.
201. Logothotepoulos, J., Kraicer, J., and Best, C. H.: *Diabetes*, **10**:367, 1961.
202. Akehi, T.: *Jap. J. Obstet. Gynecol.*, **13**:427, 1930.
203. Florentine, P., and Picard, D.: *Rév. Franc. Endocrinol.*, **14**:1, 1936.
204. Hellman, B.: *Acta Obstet. Gynecol. Scand.*, **39**:331, 1959.
205. Van Assche, F. A.: *Amer. J. Obstet. Gynecol.* **118**:39, 1974.
206. Aerts, L., and Van Assche, F. A.: *Diabetologia*, **11**:285, 1975.
207. Green, I. C., and Taylor, K. W.: *J. Endocrinol.*, **62**:137, 1974.
208. Green, I. C., and Taylor, K. W.: *J. Endocrinol.*, **54**:317, 1972.
209. Loubatières, A.: In: *The Structure and Metabolism of the Pancreatic Islets*. Edited by S. E. Brolin, B. Hellman, and H. Knutsson. Pergamon Press, London, 1964, p. 437.
210. Lazarow, A., Carpenter, A. M., Morgan, C., and Wright, D.: *Diabetes*, **11**:103, 1962.
211. Ashworth, M. A., and Haist, R. E.: *Can. Med. Assoc. J.*, **74**:975, 1956.
212. Davidson, J. K., and Haist, R. E.: *Diabetes*, **11**:115, 1962.
213. Bloodworth, Jr., J. M. B.: *Metabolism*, **12**:287, 1963.
214. Chick, W. L., Lauris, V., Flewelling, J. H., Andrews, K. A., and Woodruff, J. M.: *Endocrinology*, **92**:212, 1973.
215. Hellerström, C., Andersson, A., and Gunnarsson, R.: *Acta Endocrinol. Suppl.*, **205**:145, 1976.
216. Andersson, A.: *Biochim. Biophys. Acta*, **437**:345, 1976.
217. Andersson, A.: *Diabetologia*, **13**:59, 1977.
218. Logothetopoulos, J., and Bell, E. G.: *Diabetes*, **15**:205, 1966.
219. Howell, S. L., Edwards, J. C., and Whitfield, M.: *Horm. Metab. Res.*, **3**:37, 1971.
220. Petersson, B., Hellerström, C., and Gunnarsson, R.: *Horm. Metab. Res.*, **2**:313, 1970.
221. Angervall, L., Hellerström, C., and Hellman, B.: *Pathol. Microbiol.*, **25**:389, 1962.
222. Gerritsen, G. C., and Dulin, W. E.: *Diabetologia*, **3**:74, 1967.
223. Like, A. A., Gerritsen, G. C., Dulin, W. E., and Gaudreau, P.: *Diabetologia*, **10**:509, 1974.
224. Boquist, L.: Thesis. University of Umeå., Umeå, 1969.
225. Cameron, D., Stauffacher, W., and Renold, A. E.: In: *Endocrine Pancreas. Handbook of Physiology*, Sect. 7, Vol. 1. Edited by D. F. Steiner and N. Freinkel. William & Wilkins, Baltimore, 1972, p. 611.
226. Coleman, D. L., and Hummel, K. P.: *Diabetologia*, **3**:238, 1967.
227. Hummel, K. P., and Coleman, D. L.: *Biochem. Genet.*, **7**:1, 1972.
228. Coleman, D. L., and Hummel, K. P.: *Diabetologia*, **9**:287, 1973.
229. Boquist, L., Hellman, B., Lernmark, A., and Täljedal, I.-B.: *J. Cell Biol.*, **62**:77, 1974.
230. Gunnarsson, R.: *Diabetologia*, **11**:431, 1975.
231. Chick, W. L., and Like, A. A.: *Diabetologia*, **6**:243, 1970.
232. LeCompte, P. M., and Merriam, J. C.: *Diabetes*, **11**:35, 1962.
233. Potvliege, P., Gepts, W., and Carpent, G.: *Beitr. Pathol. Anat.*, **128**:335, 1963.
234. Ogilvie, R. F.: In: *The Structure and Metabolism of the Pancreatic Islets*. Edited by S. E. Brolin, B. Hellman, and H. Knutsson. Pergamon Press, London, 1964, p. 499.
235. Warren, S., LeCompte, P. M., and Legg, M. A.: *The Pathology of Diabetes Mellitus*. Lea & Febiger, Philadelphia, 1966.
236. Scully, R. E.: *N. Engl. J. Med.*, **273**:41, 1965.
237. Gepts, W.: Contribution à l'étude morphologique des îlots de Langerhans au cours du diabète. Les Editions Acta Medica Belgica. Bruxelles, 1957.
238. Gepts, W.: In: *The Structure and Metabolism of the Pancreatic Islets*. Edited by S. E. Brolin, B. Hellman, and H. Knutsson. Pergamon Press, London, 1964, p. 513.
239. Gepts, W.: *Diabetes*, **14**:619, 1965.
240. Gepts, W.: In: *Endocrine Pancreas. Handbook of Physiology*. Sect. 7, Vol. 1. Edited by D. F. Steiner and N. Freinkel. Williams & Wilkins, Baltimore, 1972, p. 289.
241. Gamble, D. R., Kinsley, M. L., Fitzgerald, M. G., Bolton, R., and Taylor, K. W.: *Brit. Med. J.*, **3**:627, 1969.

242. Craighead, J. E.: In: *Endocrine Pancreas. Handbook of Physiology.* Sect. 7, Vol. 1. Edited by D. S. Steiner and N. Freinkel. Williams & Wilkins, Baltimore, 1972, p. 289.
243. Nerup, J., Andersen, O. O., Bendixen, G., Egeberg, J., Gunnarsson, R., and Poulsen, J. E.: *Proc. Royal Soc. Med.,* **6**:506, 1974.
244. Hayflick, L.: *J. Amer. Geriatr. Soc.,* **22**:1, 1974.
245. Goldstein, S., Littlefield, J. W., and Soeldner, J. S.: *Proc. Nat. Acad. Sci. USA* **64**:155, 1969.
246. Vracko, R., and Benditt, E. P.: *Fed. Proc.,* **33**:607, 1974.
247. Goldstein, S., Niewiarowski, S., and Singal, D. P.: *Fed. Proc.,* **34**:56, 1975.

Chapter 4

Histology, Cell Types, and Functional Correlation of Islets of Langerhans

Klaus F. Wellmann and Bruno W. Volk

Histology

The pancreatic islets, first described in 1869 by Langerhans,[1] are compact round, ovoid, or less regular groups of polygonal epithelial cells irregularly distributed within the lobules of the exocrine portion of the organ (Fig. 1). The question whether or not the islets are surrounded by a connective tissue capsule has received a good deal of attention, mainly because of its presumed importance for theories of transitions between exocrine and endocrine cells. The most extensive review of this problem is that of Kraus,[2] who lists many of the earlier authors in the field as supposing the existence of a true capsule, but also quotes a nearly equal number of writers as being opposed to that supposition. The present consensus, already intimated by Kraus and reflected in more recent reviews[3,15,4,44]* appears to be that the islands are surrounded by a more or less complete "pseudocapsule" formed by connective tissue fibers which are continuous with those of the interstitial septa of the exocrine part of the pancreas. While there is a gradual increase in the amount of intra- and extrainsular connective tissue with advancing age,[5] the formation of a true capsule around the islets does not occur in the healthy organ.

The islets of Langerhans have an unusually rich blood supply characterized by the presence of wide, thin-walled, anastomosing sinusoids that form glomerulus-like networks.[6,7,96,8] In general, only one afferent arteriole feeds the sinusoidal net through which the blood flows rapidly.[9] Several efferent capillaries connect the islet circulation with that of the surrounding tissue. The architectural arrangement of the capillary net mirrors the architecture of the islet itself.[7,101] While Kracht[10,11] interpreted hyperemia in the blood vessels of

*Reference and page number therein.

Klaus F. Wellmann and Bruno W. Volk • Isaac Albert Research Institute of the Kingsbrook Jewish Medical Center, and Downstate Medical Center, State University of New York, Brooklyn, New York. Present address of K.F.W.: Beekman Downtown Hospital, New York, New York. Present address of B. W. V.: University of California, Irvine, California.

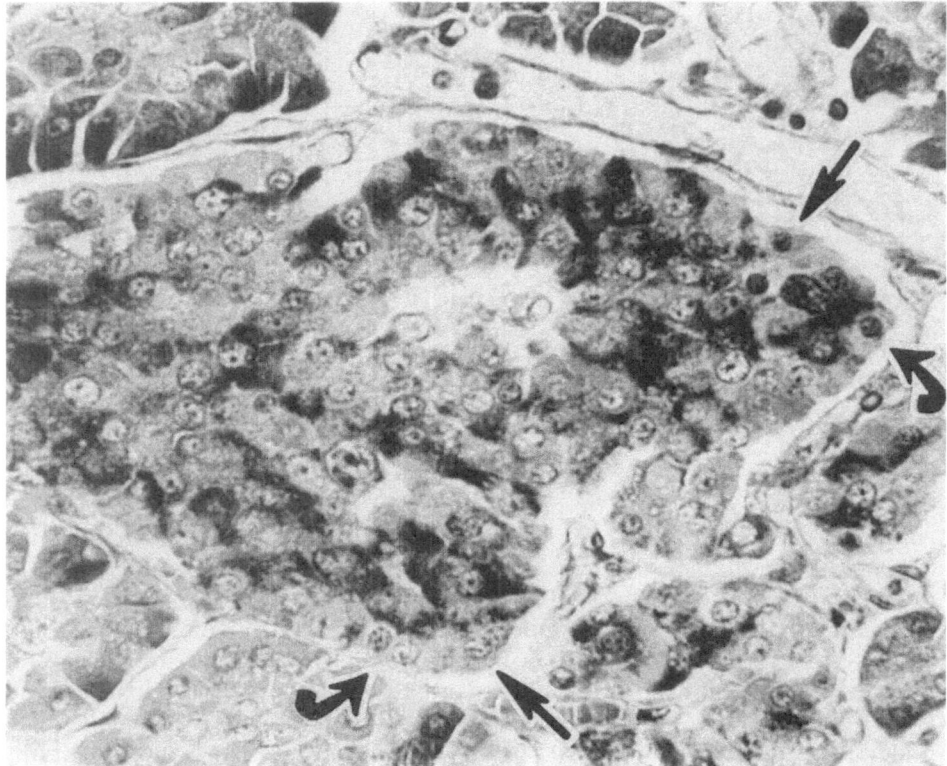

Figure 1. Pancreatic islet of nondiabetic patient. B cells black, A cells gray (straight arrows), D cells light gray (curved arrows). Aldehyde fuchsin trichrome stain. ×650. Reproduced at 110%.

the islet as an indicator for enhanced insulin synthesis, Hellerström *et al.*[12] found an increased erythrocyte content in the islets of starved rats associated with a decreased B cell function, as determined by karyometry, and these authors concluded that the red cell content of an islet cannot be used as a reliable index of the functional state of the B cell.

That there are "certain connections" between the islets and the nervous system was already recognized by Langerhans[1] who detected nerve fibers and ganglion cells in close proximity to groups of islet cells. Pensa[13] observed nerve fibers entering the islets with the blood vessels and following their ramifications. A more intimate, organoid association between neural and epithelial elements has been recorded by van Campenhout,[14,15] who spoke of "complexes sympathico-insulaires," and especially by Simard,[16] who preferred the term "complexes neuro-insulaires" as he was not certain about the sympathetic nature of these structures. They contain A and B cells, are located in the inter- and intralobular septa of the pancreas, have been found in several mammalian species,[17] and were regarded by Simard[16] as metasympathetic paraganglia having a neurocrine function. Ferner,[7,104] however, did not recognize the functional independence of these structures which he considered rare, fortuitous associations between neural and insular elements. More recently, Munger[18] has reaffirmed the existence of neuroinsular complexes, at least for the mouse, the raccoon, and the puppy; his electron-microscopic study in the latter shows ganglion and A cells side by side, without separating basal lamina.

The presence of autonomic terminals in islets has been observed ultrastructurally in several animals,[19-23] but there is as yet no consensus on their exact nature and distribution.[18] Proceeding from the premise that sympathetic stimulation will result in glycogenolysis, while parasympathetic stimuli are followed by glycogenogenesis, a premise supported by experimental evidence in the cat[24,25] Ferner[7.104] concluded that the A cells are innervated by sympathetic nerve fibers while the B cells receive parasympathetic ones. Also in the cat, however, newer enzyme histochemical and autoradiographic methods provided evidence for adrenergic and cholinergic innervation of both A and B cells.[26] In this species, sympathetic stimulation apparently sets in motion the secretory cycle of the A cell.[27] In the rat, Shorr and Bloom[28] found nerve endings on both A and B cells; most of them were of the cholinergic type. Fluorescence microscopy has also been helpful in demonstrating the presence of adrenergic nerve fibers in the islets of several species including cat, dog, guinea pig, and golden hamster.[22,29-31]

In freeze-fracture replicas of pancreatic islets of the rat, Orci *et al.*[32] recently found typical tight and gap junctions between A and B cells. These cells may thus be interconnected by a functional syncytium through which chemical information can be transmitted from cell to cell. Since only a small fraction of the total number of islet cells—estimated at less than 10% by Woods and Porte[33]—receive axon terminals, this system may also function to disperse neural signals throughout the islets. The complex problem of neural–pancreatic interactions has been the subject of a recent interdisciplinary conference, the results of which have been published in summary form.[33]

Cell Types

Diamare,[34] in 1899, and Schulze,[35] one year later, were the first to suggest that the islets of Langerhans contain more than one cell type. The latter, working with the guinea pig, observed small cells with chromatin-rich nuclei and larger cells with darker cytoplasm and centralized chromatin clumps. In 1902, Mankowski[36] confirmed the presence of two cell types in this species. In the same year, Ssobolew[37] expanded on these earlier studies. In the guinea pig and in the rabbit, he found that most of the islet cells (those later called B cells) were characterized by a pale, finely granular cytoplasm and ovoid nuclei with a well-developed chromatin network. The cells of the second type (subsequently known as A cells), of which he never encountered more than five or ten in any one section, were located in the periphery of the islets; they were larger and more nearly rounded, and they contained a coarsely granular cytoplasm stained deeply red by safranin. Their nuclei possessed distinct nucleoli, while their chromatin network was only poorly visible.

In 1906, Tschassownikow[38] devised a method that for the first time permitted a tinctorial differentiation between the two cell types then known. In rabbit pancreas fixed with Hermann's fluid (platinum chloride and osmic acid) and stained with safranin and methyl green, the majority of the islet cells (the B cells) appeared green, while some cells located in the periphery (the A cells) distinguished themselves by a red cytoplasm. Tschassownikow[38] and some other early observers[37,39] also noted the presence of granules in the cytoplasm of islet cells that were not identical with the zymogen granules of the exocrine acinar cell. Lane,[40] in 1907, found that after fixation of the guinea pig pancreas in 50–70% alcohol the granules of the A cells stained violet with Bensley's neutral gentian, while the B cell granules remained unstained. After fixation in aqueous chrome sublimate fluid, however, the B cell granules assumed a violet color following staining with gentian. Lane was the first to actually employ the term "A cells" (derived probably from his conviction that these cells were fixed by alcohol), but inexplicably he called the second cell type "β cells" and not "B cells." Four years later, however, his teacher Bensley[41] changed "β" to "B," but the confusion between the Greek and Roman letters as designations for these elements has persisted to this date. Lane also deserves credit for clearly recognizing the nature of these cells; he stated that the "islets of Langerhans are structures which in all probability have the function of producing a twofold substance which, poured into the blood stream, has an important effect upon metabolism." He added that these substances are "different from zymogen."

Bensley,[41] in 1911, published results of several fixation and staining experiments conducted on the pancreas of the guinea pig. With Lane's chrome sublimate fixative and a neutral gentian and acid fuchsin stain, the A cells appeared red and the B cells blue. After fixation in acetic osmic bichromate and staining with anilin fuchsin and methyl green, the A cells were deeply red while the B cells displayed a green color. In similarly fixed sections stained with safranin acid violet, the A cells showed a violet and the B cells a red cytoplasm. Bensley also identified a few agranular or "clear" cells in the pancreas of the guinea pig; he believed that these elements represented a "stage in the physiological activity" of the cells of one of the two known types, or perhaps that they were the source of the A cells. The term "C cell," attached to this cell by later observers,[3,42] does not appear in Bensley's original article.[41] Thomas,[12] investigating the pancreatic islets of 41 mammalian species, found C cells only in the guinea pig.

Working with a teleost fish, the gray snapper *(Neomaenis griseus)*, Bowie,[43] in 1924, used Zenker's fluid with acetic acid as fixative and neutral ethyl violet plus Biebrich's scarlet for staining. He identified A and B cells as well as a third cell type characterized by a lightly stained, faintly granular cytoplasm and an oval, pale nucleus; these "γ cells" were believed by him to be precursors of A and B cells. Ukai,[44] in 1926, utilized neutral formol and Zenker's fixative with a modified Mallory aniline blue method; in pancreatic islets of the cat and of the guinea pig, the A cells stained red and the B cells stained blue. Five years later, Bloom[45] combined the same fixative with Mallory's azan stain in an investigation of human pancreases derived from autopsies. In addition to A cells, which were red, and B cells staining orange, he was able to identify a third cell type displaying a pale blue cytoplasm with or without darker blue granules. He called it "D cell" and wondered whether it was a transitional element, intermediate between A and B cell, or whether it might be related to Bowie's γ cell (which he thought possible) or to Bensley's C cell (which he deemed unlikely).

Some additional cell types have been found in the pancreatic islets of certain species. The most nebulous of these is the "Mankowski cell" of the guinea pig. Mankowski's original article[36] does not contain a usable definition for this cell; it is not mentioned at all in Ferner's[7,111] careful analysis of the constituents of the guinea pig islet. In the opossum, Thomas[42] identified the "E cell" which is characterized by magenta-colored granules in tissue fixed with Helly's fluid and stained with Heidenhain's azan. Baumann,[46] Wolter,[47] and Ferner[7,126] found groups of polygonal cells with brown cytoplasmic pigmentation in the central portions of the pancreatic islets of the horse. This pigment disappears after alcohol fixation, in xylene, and under the influence of light but is enhanced by formalin. The cells are silver-negative and react similar to A cells in granule stains. They were called "X cells" by Ferner.[7,126] To confuse matters, Bencosme and Liepa,[48] who were unaware of Ferner's earlier assignation, applied the same term to a cell found in the islets, acini, and ducts of the dog and cat pancreas. The granules of this "X cell" stained brown with Gomori's chrome hematoxylin, pale green with Gomori's aldehyde fuchsin, and red with both the Masson trichrome method and with Mallory–Heidenhain's azan stain. Bencosme and Liepa thought that the cell might correspond to the Mankowski cell[36] of the guinea pig, to the "granular cells of the acini" observed by Bayley[49] in the same species, and to certain cells described in the pancreases of snakes.[50] It is silver-negative[51] and has certain ultrastructural features including secretory granules varying in electron density depending on what fixative has been used.[51,52] The X cell of Bencosme and Liepa was called "F cell" by Munger *et al.*[52]

In ultrastructural studies, two additional cell types have been described in the human pancreas by Deconinck *et al.*[53] These authors distinguished between A cells, B cells, D cells (called "type IV" by them), and cells of types III and V. Type III cells, termed "G cells" by Kubes and Jirásek,[54] resemble the gastrin-secreting cells of the gastric and duodenal mucosa[55-58]; the suggestion that they have a similar function receives support from the immunofluorescent demonstration of gastrin in some human islet cells.[59] Type V cells were found to be similar to the serotonin-producing cells of the gastrointestinal tract of rats[55] and of man.[58]

Gomori[60-62] summarized the application of various fixatives (Bouin's solution, Bayley's modified Zenker-formaldehyde, and Stieve's fluid) and of specific staining methods (Mallory–Heidenhain's azan stain, Mallory's PTAH method, and Gomori's chromium hematoxylin–phloxin stain) to the pancreases of man and animals. His aldehyde fuchsin trichrome stain[63] as modified by Lazarus and Volk[3,261] is one of the most frequently employed differential stains for the pancreatic islets; with it, the B cell granules are purple, those of the A cells are red, and the D cells display a homogeneous translucent green cytoplasm.

Summaries of special staining techniques for islet cells can be found in the monographs of Lazarus and Volk[3.257] and of Warren, LeCompte, and Legg.[4.499] Among recent discussions of islet cell types differentiated by light- and electron-microscopic techniques are those of Hellman and Hellerström,[64] Greider *et al.*,[65] and Lacy and Greider.[66] Various methods for the demonstration of B cell granules have been described by von Denffer and Mertz[67] and by Klessen.[68]

Silver impregnation methods have added another dimension to the study of pancreatic islet cells every since Piazza,[69] in 1911, first demonstrated that silver-impregnable cells occur in this organ. All such cells are argyrophilic rather than argentaffin as they will reduce silver not spontaneously (as truly argentaffin cells do) but only after the addition of a reducing substance. Most of the earlier workers[7.13,70−78] employed the Gros–Schultze method of silver impregnation, or a modification of it, usually on frozen sections. This technique apparently stains the A cells but is noted for its capriciousness as it will often not stain all potentially argyrophilic cells, especially when the reaction time is cut short, and it may also stain some of the B cells.[78] More islet cells are argyrophilic with the Gros–Schultze method than with Bodian's technique, but the latter also stains A cells[65,79,80] as do the procedures of Grimelius[81] and of Sevier and Munger.[82] On the other hand, modifications of the Davenport silver impregnation technique such as the ones devised by Volk *et al.*[83] and by Hellerström and Hellman[84−86] will stain D cells rather than A cells.[65,66,87−92]

Nevertheless, none of the silver impregnation methods appears to be absolutely specific. Thus, a comparison between the Hellerström–Hellman and the Sevier–Munger techniques, studied by staining adjacent sections, indicated that a small population of islet cells may at times be stained by both methods.[65] In ultrastructural investigations employing a modification of the Davenport silver nitrate procedure, it was shown that small silver particles concentrate over the internal structures of the secretory granules of the D cells; but a few silver particles were also observed in the A and B cells.[91] Similar overlaps were recorded in light-microscopic studies by others, too.[81,84,87]

In 1960, Hellerström and Hellman[84] classified the cells stained by their modification of the Davenport technique with the A cells, calling them A_1 cells and distinguishing them from the A_2 cells which remained silver-negative (see Chapter 3). Whereas the Swedish authors[64,81,84−87,91,92] have continued to employ these terms, most other observers equate the A_2 cell with the A cell and consider the A_1 cell to be identical with the D cell.[65,66,89,90]

The B Cell and Insulin

In all species, the B cells are the most numerous constituents of the pancreatic islets, and their function was elucidated earlier than that of any of the other cell types. The extraction of a blood-sugar-lowering substance from the pancreas by Banting and Best[93] in 1922 verified older conjectures assigning a role to the islets in carbohydrate metabolism.[34,40,94] In 1938, Richardson and

Young[95] observed degranulation, hydropic degeneration, and destruction of B cells in dogs made permanently diabetic by the injection of anterior pituitary extracts; these histological changes, interpreted to represent functional exhaustion induced by the diabetic state, suggested that the B cells were the source of insulin. Conclusive evidence for this supposition was, however, not available until 1943 when Dunn *et al.*[96] showed that the selective destruction of the pancreatic B cells by alloxan monohydrate induces severe diabetes in experimental animals. The cytotoxicity of alloxan for B cells of several species has been confirmed in subsequent histological studies.[97-103] Other B cell cytotoxins including, in particular, streptozotocin[104-109] have been employed with similar results. These investigations, summarized by Frerichs and Creutzfeldt[110] and by Rerup,[111] have gone far in providing evidence for the origination of the blood-sugar-lowering principle, insulin, from the pancreatic B cells.

Data obtained through several different experimental techniques corroborate and expand the observations related to the actions of the B cell cytotoxins. In one group of experiments, it has been shown that the infusion of glucose solutions into the living animal is promptly followed by a degranulation of the pancreatic B cells[112-114]; the granules reappear when the blood sugar levels regain normal values.[113] In dogs given large doses of glucose continuously for up to 9 days, a latent period of normoglycemia lasting for 3 to 7 days develops after an initial, transitory rise in blood sugar and before sustained hyperglycemia is seen[114]; this may be taken to indicate the eventual exhaustion of the capability of the B cell to produce sufficient insulin under conditions of long-continued demand. These experiments also helped verify the view that it is hyperglycemia, per se, and not hypoinsulinemia that is the appropriate stimulus for B cell degranulation.

Direct perfusion of the pancreas of an experimental animal with glucose also results in degranulation of the B cells,[115] while the venous effluent contains greatly increased amounts of insulin.[116,117] Under such conditions it has been found that the rate of insulin secretion is a continuous function of the blood sugar level.[117]

There is good correlation between the amount of insulin extractable from the pancreas and the number of B cell granules visualized in microscopic studies. This has been shown for both animals with experimentally induced diabetes[118,119] and adult human diabetics[118,120,121] as well as for metabolically intact control patients.[120,121] Good general agreement between the two parameters was also found in a similar investigation on 40 infants and fetuses of diabetic and control mothers.[122]

The administration of exogenous insulin is followed by a number of functional and structural changes, all of which indicate that there occurs a diminution in both production and liberation of insulin by the pancreatic B cells. In rats, the B cell granules disappear more or less completely,[123-125] even though there may be an initial, transitory increase in their numbers.[123] After the cessation of insulin treatment, regranulation occurs[123] which may require 6 to 10 days in order to become complete.[125] Other authors have described B cell atrophy[126] or an inhibition of islet cell growth and proliferation[127,128] following the injection of insulin. Insulin administration also leads to a decrease of the insulin content in the pancreas, as determined in rats[129-131] and in the pancreatic vein, as observed in dogs.[132] Again, there is close correlation between the diminished pancreatic insulin concentrations and the decreased numbers of the B cell granules as seen in histologic sections.[129,131]

Hormones other than insulin have an effect on the pancreatic B cell, too. The injection of anterior pituitary extracts in experimental animals causes B cell degranulation[95,126,133,134] and often further changes such as hydropic degeneration and even necrosis of B cells.[95,134] The insulin content in the pancreas of such animals is diminished.[131] Gradual disappearance of secretory granules associated with a distinctive type of vacuolar change, "ballooning degeneration," has been described by Volk and Lazarus[147,148] in dogs subjected to growth hormone treatment for several weeks. The administration of adrenal steroids in rabbits is followed by a loss of B cell granules observable after 24 to 48 hr; complete regranulation occurs within 7 days after the cessation of treatment.[135] Since in such cases insulin output increases much earlier than B cell degranulation becomes evident in light-microscopic sections, it has been suggested that aldehyde fuchsin and pseudoisocyanin stain the membranous sacs of the B cell granules, rather than the secretory substance (insulin) contained within them,[3,136-138] or that both of these components are stained.[139]

Dietary factors also influence B cell granulation and insulin content of the pancreas, even though the observed effects are not the same in all species. While starvation does not diminish the granules in rabbits,[135] degranulation has been described in the rat[124,125]; in starved Carneau pigeons, B cell "inactivity" has been recorded.[126] Once normal feeding is resumed after a period of starvation, rats recover their B cell granules within 3 to 8 days.[125] The pancreases of starved rats show reduced insulin stores,[131,140] even if the calorically insufficient diet is nutritionally balanced.[141] The lack of certain amino acids may also adversely affect insulin synthesis; thus, a considerably diminished pancreatic insulin content has been encountered in rabbits fed a diet deficient in methionine and cysteine.[142] On the other hand, it was only after very prolonged exposure to a diet high in carbohydrates and low in fat and protein that adult rabbits displayed some visible loss of B cell granules,[143] while no degranulation at all was encountered in the offspring of such animals.[144] Lastly, a diet very rich in fat, or restricted to fat, also induces degranulation of B cells[124] and a concomitant reduction in the assayable pancreatic insulin stores.[131,140,145]

While histochemical methods for the indirect demonstration of insulin, such as the one devised by Barnett *et al.*[146] which depends on the presence of disulfide groups in the cytoplasmic proteins, lack specificity, direct evidence for the presence of insulin in the pancreatic B cell has been obtained by fluorescent antibody techniques for both insulin[149-152] and proinsulin.[153] Microdissection of B cells from freeze-dried pancreatic sections of the rabbit[154] and the rat[155] and subsequent bioassay of their insulin content provided further proof that it is the B cells that contain the insulin.

Although other modes of insulin release from the B cell into the blood stream have been discussed from time to time,[156,157] the data obtained thus far from ultrastructural studies and from subcellular fractionation techniques support the concept first clearly enunciated by Lacy, that emiocytosis is the major and probably the only mechanism of insulin secretion.[157–160] Emiocytosis, also called "exocytosis" by some,[161] involves the fusion of the membranous sac of the secretory granule with the plasma membrane of the cell, the rupture of the cell membrane at this point, and the release of the granule into the extracellular space where it dissolves. Microtubules and microfilaments have been implicated in the secretory process; possibly, the translocation of the B cell granules to the cell surface occurs along a calcium-dependent microtubular–microfilamentous system[153,161–164] (see Chapter 8).

The A Cells and Glucagon

Whereas the existence of the pancreatic A cell[34–37] and its tinctorial difference from the B cell[38,40,41] had been established shortly after the turn of the century, it proved much more difficult to clarify its functional status. One role attributed to the A cells was that of secreting a lipotropic factor in the form of a hypothetical hormone termed "lipo-caic".[165,166] However, subsequent investigations negated the possibility that the A cells were in any way responsible for the observed lipotropic activity of pancreatic preparations.[167,168]

Soon after pancreatic extracts and insulin preparations began to be used for the purpose of treating diabetic patients it became apparent that these substances induced unexpected, transient initial hyperglycemia, both in humans and in experimental animals, before lowering the blood sugar.[169–174] While some authors attributed this effect to impurities in the preparations and applied terms such as "toxic fraction"[170] or "antiinsulin," Murlin and his associates[172–174] first suggested that the observed hyperglycemic factor was an additional pancreatic hormone for which they coined the name "glucagon." Bürger[175–177] further investigated the action of glucagon which he described as a substance preformed in the pancreas and causing hyperglycemia by mobilizing hepatic glycogen stores. He was able to inactivate insulin by weak alkali solutions without abolishing the hyperglycemic activity of pancreatic extracts. The chemical characterization of glucagon, begun by Bürger and Brandt[178] in 1935, culminated in the preparation and crystallinization of this protein by Staub *et al.*[179] 18 years later.

While it had thus been shown that glucagon behaved like a hormone derived from the pancreas, its exact site of elaboration within that organ remained to be established. To this end, several lines of investigation were followed. Gaede *et al.*[180] ligated the pancreatic ducts in dogs causing fibrosis and obliteration of the exocrine acini and subsequently administered alloxan which destroyed the B cells of the islets of Langerhans; as extracts prepared from these pancreases still induce an unequivocal hyperglycemic reaction in experimental animals, the undamaged A cells were suspected of being the source of glucagon. The discovery that the uncinate process of the canine pancreas is virtually devoid of A cells provided a means of conducting a negative test; and since extracts from this portion of the organ did fail to elicit hyperglycemia when injected, the hypothesis that the A cells were, in fact, responsible for the secretion of glucagon received further support.[181]

The availability of agents which selectively damage or destroy the pancreatic A cells in experimental animals opened new avenues of research in this field. One of the most widely employed A cell cytotoxins has been cobaltous chloride ($CoCl_2$) first utilized for this purpose by van Campenhout and Cornelis[182] in 1951. These authors concluded that the hyperglycemia observed by them in the guinea pig after the injection of this substance was caused by the release of glucagon from the damaged A cells. One year later, Goldner *et al.*[183] recorded hyperglycemia in rabbits given cobaltous chloride, and while the blood sugar levels returned to normal within 4 or 5 hr after the injections, severe selective damage was demonstrable histologically in the A cells, most of which had disappeared by the end of the second day. Six days after the administration of the same substance in guinea pigs, Vuylsteke *et al.*[184] found an average diminution of the pancreatic glucagon content by 60%. Although A cell regeneration became obvious on the sixth day following cobalt treatment in rabbits, the injurious effects were seen by Volk and co-workers[185] to persist for as long as 10 days after the injections. In the same species, Kadota and Kurita[186] observed transient hyperglycemia and destruction of A cells also after the administration of nickelous chloride.

Damage after cobaltous chloride injection is rarely complete in the sense that all A cells are demonstrably afflicted. Fodden,[187] for instance, noted degenerative morphologic changes in the A cells of rabbits so treated, but the induced alterations apparently were not sufficient in either extent or severity to cause any disturbance of the carbohydrate metabolism. In radioautographic studies in normal and alloxan-diabetic rats, Ulrich and Copp[188] failed to obtain any evidence that ^{60}Co in this organ might be concentrated in the islets. In a review article, Creutzfeldt[189] even suggested that the effects of certain A cell cytotoxins, including $CoCl_2$, can be explained by extrapancreatic mechanisms and may not be the direct result of the histologically demonstrable A cell lesions. Nevertheless, Bencosme and Frei[190] successfully utilized the incompleteness of the A cell cytotoxicity of cobaltous chloride in order to obtain additional evidence for the origination of glucagon from A cells. They found that pancreatic extracts of cobalt-treated guinea pigs with severe lesions failed to induce significant hyperglycemia when assayed in cats; however, if well-granulated A cells remained in amounts roughly estimated above 25% of normal, the extracts from these pancreases invariably elicited hyperglycemia indistinguishable from that of the normal organ. While Kern[191] noted that cobaltous chloride in single or multiple injections acts primarily on the exocrine pancreatic tissue leading to degranulation and ultimately to destruction of acinar cells, he did reaffirm, in ultrastructural studies conducted on the pancreas of the guinea pig, that this substance also damages the A cells of the islets of Langerhans whereas B cells remain unaffected.

In 1951, Kadota and Midorikawa[192] tested 24 different reagents in rabbits and found that two of them, sodium diethyldithiocarbamate (NaDDC) and potassium ethylxanthate (KEX), produced hyperglycemia and caused A cell damage; the latter was more pronounced with NaDDC and involved degeneration and eventual disappearance of such cells. In a later experiment in rabbits and rats, however, Galin *et al.*[193] were unable to detect consistent histological changes in the pancreas and concluded that the hyperglycemia following the injection of NaDDC was essentially extrapancreatic in nature and required the integrity of the adrenal glands.

Davis,[194] in 1952, noted certain histological changes in the islets of rabbits treated with NaDDC, but these did not include selective A cell necrosis. This author introduced another A cell cytotoxin, Synthalin A, a guanidine derivative (decamethylenediguanidine hydrochloride) originally recommended and tested as a blood-sugar-lowering agent in diabetic patients[195] but soon abandoned for this purpose because of severe side effects on liver and kidneys.[196,197] Both Davis[194] and Fodden[187] recorded degranulation and gross hydropic degeneration of the A cells of the rabbit pancreas as well as distinct and at times severe hypoglycemia following a rather prolonged initial hyperglycemic response. Other authors[198-200] confirmed these observations on the action of Synthalin A in rabbits, rats, and guinea pigs, even though the severity of the obtained alterations was not the same in each species. While most investigators[194,198-200] considered the histologic and physiologic changes induced by this compound to be the direct result of A cell damage, Creutzfeldt and his coworkers[189,201-203] surmised that Synthalin A primarily afflicts the liver and that all other alterations, including those in the pancreatic islets, are only secondary effects. Creutzfeldt and Moench[202] also recorded vacuolization and degranulation of the pancreatic A cells of guinea pigs following the administration of a related substance, Synthalin B (dodecamethylenediguanidine), while in the rabbit Davis[194] had seen no such alterations, even though there were blood sugar changes after the injection of this agent. Synthalin has been used by Munger[204] in his electron-microscopic studies on the secretory cycle of the pancreatic A cell in the rabbit. He made the interesting observation that cytoplasmic vacuolization following Synthalin administration is seen only in cells with at least a few secretory granules present and most certainly does not occur in completely degranulated cells. Hence, Synthalin may affect some particular phase of the secretory cycle of these cells.

Another guanidine derivative, phenylethyldiguanide (DBI), also induces A cell degranulation but not in all of the cases tested and rarely completely so.[202] Initially, the hypoglycemic effect of *p*-aminobenzenesulfonamidoisopropylthiodiazole (IPTD) had also been ascribed to its supposed A cell toxicity,[200] but in later investigations[205-207] no evidence was found to maintain the view that this substance, and other hypoglycemic agents including tolbutamide and carbutamide,[207] affect the pancreatic A cells in a deleterious manner.

Common to all A cell cytotoxins examined thus far is the fact that it is usually not possible to achieve a complete and permanent destruction of the A cells in this manner.[189,208,209] The isolation and crystallinization of porcine pancreatic glucagon by Staub and co-workers[179,210] and its subsequent availability, after 1953, opened another line of research into the role of the A cell and its involvement in glucagon production. Applying the well-known principle that the exogenous administration of a hormone tends to suppress its endogenous elaboration, Kracht[211,212] was able to demonstrate atrophy and degranulation of A cells in rats and rabbits as well as concomitant B cell hypertrophy after the injection of glucagon for up to 38 days. Lazarus and Volk[213–215] confirmed and extended these observations in studies on rabbits and guinea pigs. They noted a partial degranulation of the A cells and an apparent reduction in their numbers and concluded that glucagon is a hormone derived from the A cells. A progressive involution of A cells in glucagon-treated rabbits was also recorded by Logothetopoulos and Salter.[216] In other experiments, glucagon administration failed to induce A cell changes in dogs[215] and rats[217]; this was attributed to species differences or to the possibility that glucagon could have been given in suboptimal doses or for an insufficient length of time.

Attempts to demonstrate the presence of glucagon directly in the pancreatic A cells began with the development of a technique for the intracellular staining of protein-bound indole derivatives including tryptophane by Glenner and Lillie[218] in 1957; the tryptophane-containing protein noted in rabbit A cells was surmised to be glucagon.[219] In 1962, Baum *et al.*[220] provided the first direct evidence for the production of glucagon in the A cells of the bovine pancreas by applying immunofluorescent techniques. Later, Lundquist and co-workers[221] were able to demonstrate this hormone by radioimmunochemical microassay in isolated guinea pig A cells.

Not many investigators have concerned themselves with the mechanism of secretion in pancreatic A cells. Munger[18,204] proposed that the A cells degranulate by a disintegration of their granules; the resulting secretory particles were thought to pass through the plasma membrane of the A cell into the capillary endothelial cell. Other authors[27,222–224] have suggested that margination and emiocytosis (exocytosis) of the intact granule are involved.

Biochemical and immunochemical studies[225–228] as well as ultrastructural investigations[55,56,229] have established in the gastrointestinal tract of several species the presence of endocrine cells that are morphologically and functionally indistinguishable from pancreatic A cells. The secretion of glucagon by these extrapancreatic cells, reaffirmed in recent immunochemical studies,[230,231] explains the findings of continued glucagon immunoreactivity in plasma even after pancreatectomy.[230] Glucagon derived from this source, as well as pancreatic glucagon, may also play an important role in the pathophysiology of diabetes[232–235] (see Chapter 10). The suppression of glucagon secretion by somatostatin, the newly identified secretory product of the pancreatic D cell (see following section), reduces or abolishes hyperglycemia in insulin-deficient dogs[234] as well as in human diabetics[232]; in the latter, the results indicate that excessive glucagon secretion accounts for about 25% of the fasting plasma glucose levels. Diabetes has, therefore, been looked upon as representing a bihormonal abnormality[233,235]; in this view, the major consequence of absolute or relative insulin lack is glucose underutilization, whereas absolute or relative glucagon excess is the principal factor in the overproduction of glucose in the diabetic patient.

The D Cell and Somatostatin

Until recently, the functional role of the pancreatic D cells remained a complete mystery. Ferner[75] dismissed them as degenerating cells of no particular significance, a view reiterated in 1961 by Robb.[236] Gomori[61] surmised that D cells were aged A cells, while other investigators[237,238] considered them to be precursors of either the A or the B cells, or of both. The possibility that the D cell produces gastrin has also been entertained.[66]

The answer to the question of what the D cell does derived from studies in a field not primarily related to pancreatic islet cell physiology at all. In a series of experiments initiated late in 1971, Vale and his co-workers[239] had noted that some ovine hypothalamic extracts consistently and dramatically inhibited the secretion of growth hormone. The substance responsible for this effect, first known as somatotropin (or growth hormone)-release-inhibiting factor (SRIF or GHRIF), could soon be isolated, purified, and characterized; it is a polypeptide with 14 amino acids now called "somatostatin," and its synthetic replicate proved biologically active.[240] Then, in 1973, Alberti *et al.*[241] discovered that somatostatin injected into healthy human subjects lowers the basal plasma insulin levels; in intravenous glucose tolerance tests in five normal persons, glucose-induced insulin release was markedly suppressed, and the glucose disappearance rate was lowered. In perfusion experiments on the isolated canine pancreas, these authors showed that somatostatin appears to act directly on the B cells, causing suppression of the initial and the late sustained release phase.

Other investigators soon confirmed and extended these initial observations. Koerker *et al.*[242] observed that somatostatin inhibits the basal insulin secretion in fasted cats and rats; in fasted baboons, both the basal and the arginine-stimulated secretion of insulin and of glucagon are suppressed. Somatostatin appeared to act directly on the endocrine pancreas; its action was dose-related, rapid in onset, and readily reversed. In infusion studies on human diabetic patients, Gerich *et al.*[232] found that after the administration of somatostatin (1 mg over 2 hr) plasma glucose fell from a mean of 260 ± 20 to 191 ± 21 mg/100 ml, whereas the fasting plasma glucagon level decreased from 150 ± 15 to 77 ± 10 pg/ml. Similar responses occurred in a hypophysectomized diabetic patient, indicating that these effects were independent of somatostatin-induced suppression of growth hormone secretion. In additional studies, somatostatin infusion combined with insulin completely abolished postprandial hyperglycemia in four diabetic patients and was more effective than insulin alone.

Fujimoto and co-workers[243] showed that dihydrosomatostatin, in concentrations between 0.001 and 1.0 μg/ml, inhibited both insulin and glucose secretion in monolayer cell cultures of newborn rat pancreas. When cultures were incubated with somatostatin and then rinsed, the effect of the hormone appeared to last longer on the A than on the B cells as indicated by a more prolonged inhibition of glucagon secretion than of insulin release. Submaximal inhibition of glucose-stimulated insulin release by somatostatin was partially reversed by increasing the concentration of glucose. These experiments suggest that the effect of somatostatin is mediated directly on the pancreatic endocrine cells. In subsequent work with monolayer cultures of rat endocrine pancreas, Fujimoto[244] demonstrated that somatostatin inhibits not only the basal insulin release but also insulin secretion induced by glucose, tolbutamide, theophylline, cytochalasin B, and calcium. Since net calcium uptake by the B cell, or intracellular translocation of calcium within the B cell from an organelle-bound pool to a cytoplasmic pool, may trigger secretion through interaction of calcium with the microtubular–microfilamentous system, this author proposed that somatostatin may act by supressing calcium influx. The inhibition of insulin secretion by somatostatin in cell cultures was confirmed by Vale *et al.*[239] who found that 1 nmol of the hormone lowered the insulin output of hamster insulinoma cells from 91 ± 6.5 to 56 ± 3.8 ng/dish/4 hr.

From the data reviewed thus far it should have become obvious that somatostatin exerts a powerful effect upon the function of both the A and the B cell of the mammalian pancreas. Most recently, however, it has been discovered that the connections between this polypeptide hormone and the pancreatic islets are even closer than had been suspected. Thus, Vale *et al.*[239] found evidence for bioassayable somatostatin-like activity in crude extracts of fetal rat pancreas while Arimura and co-workers[245] identified somatostatin by radioimmunoassay in the rat stomach and pancreas in a concentration similar to that in the hypothalamus; the hormone was also encountered in the duodenum and jejunum, albeit in lesser concentrations. At the same time, several investigators succeeded in demonstrating directly within the pancreatic islets the presence of somatostatin, employing immunohistochemical[246] or immunofluorescent[92,247–249] techniques at the light-microscopic level. Pelletier *et al.*[246] encountered a positive reaction for somatostatin in only a few cells of the rat islet; these cells had an irregular shape and were more commonly located at the periphery of the islet. Hökfelt and co-workers,[92] also working with the rat, noted the same topographical relationship and found in parallel studies with glucagon antibodies that the somatostatin-positive cells and the glucagon-positive cells were not identical even though they were localized extremely close to each other. Furthermore, with the Hellman–Hellerström silver-staining technique it could be shown that virtually all somatostatin-positive cells were argyrophilic, and vice versa. The authors concluded that it was the D cell that produced somatostatin. Orci *et al.,*[248] investigating the pancreas of the pigeon, also suggested that the distribution of the somatostatin immunofluorescent cells corresponded to that of the D cells which are particularly numerous in this species. This view is being shared by Polak *et al.*[249] and by Dubois[247] who found that the somatostatin-reactive cells differed from those containing glucagon or insulin. In view of the intensity of the immunofluorescence reaction, and because of the selectivity of these cells, the last-mentioned author deemed it unlikely that the observed fluorescence was due to nonspecific absorption of circulating somatostatin; instead, the D cells themselves appeared to synthesize and store the hormone. The presumed derivation of pancreatic endocrine cells from the neural crest anlage[251] could explain how pancreatic cells would secrete a peptide observed originally in cellular elements of the central nervous system.[247]

Both Goldsmith *et al.*[251] and Pelletier and co-workers[246] were able to confirm and extend these light-microscopic observations at the ultrastructural level. Again, the immunostaining was found to be restricted to a few cells located in the periphery of the rat islet. The positive reaction demonstrated by the accumulation of PAP (peroxidase–antiperoxidase complex) molecules was mainly observed over the secretory granules, although there was some degree of diffusion into the surrounding cytoplasm. The positive secretory granules measured about 170–210 nm. The A and the B cells remained negative.

It has thus been established beyond doubt that the pancreatic D cells produce and store somatostatin. Still to be investigated is the effect that the exogenous administration of this hormone would exert upon its endogenous elaboration. It is also not yet known in what manner the D cell discharges its secretory product. Limited observations by Gomez-Acebo *et al.*[223] in the rabbit pancreas suggest that secretion in the D cell occurs by emiocytosis of the entire granule.

In 1960, Hellerström and co-workers[252] alleged that the topographic location of any given B cell within the confines of an islet may be of importance for its function. More recently, Orci and Unger[253] have pointed out that insulin-producing B cells, glucagon-producing A cells, and somatostatin-producing D cells are not randomly arranged within the islets. Wherever A cells are found in the islet, they are accompanied by D cells; most B cells, on the other hand, are in contact only with other B cells. In view of the inhibitory effect of somatostatin on both insulin and glucagon secretion, the arrangement of A, B, and D cells would seem important to the normal and pathological functioning of the islets. The suggestion that somatostatin modulates the specific secretion of neighboring A and B cells, a process perhaps facilitated by the presence of gap junctions between cells of different types,[32] is shared by other authors[245–247]; thus, glucose homeostasis can be maintained within tightly constricted boundaries.

Other Cell Types

Additional cell types recently identified in the mammalian pancreatic islet include the PP cells and agranular cells. These have been discussed in Chapters 2, 3, 5, and 15.

References

1. Langerhans, P.: Beiträge zur mikroskopischen Anatomie der Bauchspeicheldrüse. Inaugural-Dissertation, G. Lange, Berlin, 1869.
2. Kraus, E. J.: In: *Handbuch der speziellen pathologischen Anatomie und Histologie,* Vol. V, part 2. Edited by F. Henke and O. Lubarsch. Springer, Berlin, 1929, p. 631.
3. Lazarus, S. S., and Volk, B. W.: *The Pancreas in Human and Experimental Diabetes.* Grune & Stratton, New York, 1962.
4. Warren, S., LeCompte, P. M., and Legg, M. A.: *The Pathology of Diabetes Mellitus.* 4th Ed. Lea & Febiger, Philadelphia, 1966.
5. Schultrich, S.: *Z. Mikrosk. Anat. Forsch.,* **73**:506, 1965.
6. Neubert, K.: *Anat. Anz.,* **61**:243, 1926.
7. Ferner, H.: *Das Inselsystem des Pankreas.* G. Thieme, Stuttgart, 1952.
8. Beck, J. S. P., and Berg, B. N.: *Amer. J. Pathol.,* **7**:31, 1931.
9. Beck, J. S. P., and Peterson, P.: *Amer. J. Pathol.,* **8**:573, 1932.
10. Kracht, J.: *Endokrinologie,* **36**:146, 1958.
11. Kracht, J.: *Verh. Dtsch. Ges. Pathol.* **42**:116, 1959.
12. Hellerström, C., Westman, S., Zachrisson, U., and Hellman, B.: *Acta Endocrinol.,* **34**:611, 1960.
13. Pensa, A.: *Int. Mschr. Anat. Physiol.,* **22**:90, 1905.
14. Van Campenhout, E.: *Arch. Biol. Liège,* **35**:45, 1925.
15. Van Campenhout, E.: *Arch. Biol. Liège,* **37**:121, 1927.
16. Simard, L. C.: *Arch. Anat. Micr.,* **33**:49, 1937.
17. Feyrter, F.: *Erg. Allg. Path. Path. Anat.* **36**:3, 1943.
18. Munger, R. L.: In: *Glucagon: Molecular Physiology, Clinical and Thereapeutic Implications.* Edited by P. J. Lefebvre and R. H. Unger. Pergamon Press, Oxford, 1972, p. 7.
19. Stahl, M.: *Z. Mikrosk. Anat. Forsch.,* **70**:62, 1963.
20. Lange, R.: *Z. Zellforsch.,* **65**:176, 1965.
21. Legg, P. G.: *Z. Zellforsch.,* **80**:307, 1967.
22. Legg, P. G.: *Z. Zellforsch.,* **88**:487, 1968.
23. Watari, N.: *Z. Zellforsch.,* **85**:291, 1968.
24. Sergeyeva, M. A.: *Anat. Rec.,* **77**:297, 1940.
25. Sergeyeva, M. A.: *Rev. Can. Biol.,* **2**:495, 1943.
26. Esterhuizen, A. C., Spriggs, T. L. B., and Lever, J. D.: *Diabetes,* **17**:33, 1968.
27. Esterhuizen, A. C., and Howell, S. L.: *J. Cell Biol.,* **46**:593, 1970.
28. Shorr, S. S., and Bloom, F. E.: *Z. Zellforsch.,* **103**:12, 1970.
29. Falk, B., and Hellman, B.: *Experientia,* **19**:139, 1963.
30. Falk, B., and Hellman, B.: *Acta Endocrinol.,* **45**:133, 1964.
31. Cegrell, L.: *Acta Physiol. Scand., Suppl.,* **314**:17, 1967.
32. Orci, L., Malaisse-Lagae, F., Ravazzola, M., Rouiller, D., Renold, A. E., Perrelet, A., and Unger, R.: *J. Clin. Invest.,* **56**:1066, 1975.
33. Woods, S. C., and Porte, D., Jr.: *Fed. Proc.,* **35**:1117, 1976.
34. Diamare, V.: *Int. Mschr. Anat. Physiol.,* **16**:155, 1899.
35. Schulze, W.: *Arch. Mikr. Anat.,* **56**:491, 1900.
36. Mankowski, A.: *Arch. Mikr. Anat.,* **59**:286, 1902.
37. Ssobolew, L. W.: *Virchows Arch. Pathol. Anat.,* **168**:91, 1902.
38. Tschassownikow, S.: *Arch. Mikr. Anat.,* **67**:758, 1906.
39. DeWitt, L. M.: *J. Exp. Med.,* **8**:193, 1906.
40. Lane, M. A.: *Amer. J. Anat.,* **7**:409, 1907.
41. Bensley, R. R.: *Amer. J. Anat.,* **12**:297, 1911.
42. Thomas, T. B.: *Amer. J. Anat.,* **62**:31, 1937/38.
43. Bowie, J. D.: *Anat. Rec.,* **29**:57, 1924.
44. Ukai, S.: *Mitt. Allg. Path. Path. Anat.,* **3**:1, 1926.
45. Bloom, W.: *Anat. Rec.,* **49**:363, 1931.
46. Baumann, A.: *Z. Mikrosk. Anat. Forsch.,* **46**:223, 1939.

47. Wolter, J.: *Z. Zellforsch.*, **35**:229, 1950.
48. Bencosme, S. A., and Liepa, E.: *Endocrinology*, **57**:588, 1955.
49. Bayley, J. M.: *J. Pathol. Bacteriol.*, **44**:272, 1937.
50. Thomas, T. B.: *Anat. Rec.*, **82**:327, 1942.
51. Lazarus, S. S., and Shapiro, S. H.: *Anat. Rec.*, **169**:487, 1971.
52. Munger, B. L., Caramia, F., and Lacy, P. E.: *Z. Zellforsch.*, **67**:776, 1965.
53. Deconinck, J. F., Potvliege, P. R., and Gepts, W.: *Diabetologia*, **7**:266, 1971.
54. Kubeš, L., and Jirásek, K.: *Sbornik vědeckých praci Lék. fak. KU Hradci Králove*, **14**:481, 1971.
55. Orci, L., Pictet, R., Forssmann, W. G., Renold, A. E., and Rouiller, C.: *Diabetologia*, **4**:56, 1968.
56. Forssmann, W. G., Orci, L., Pictet, R., Renold, A. E., and Rouiller, C.: *J. Cell Biol.*, **40**:692, 1969.
57. Lechago, J., and Bencosme, S. A.: *Lab. Invest.*, **22**:504, 1970.
58. Pearse, A. G. E., Coulling, I., Weavers, B., and Friesen, S.: *Gut*, **11**:649, 1970.
59. Lomský, R., Langr, F., and Vortel, V.: *Nature (London)*, **223**:618, 1969.
60. Gomori, G.: *Anat. Rec.*, **74**:439, 1939.
61. Gomori, G.: *Amer. J. Pathol.*, **17**:395, 1941.
62. Gomori, G.: *Arch. Pathol.*, **36**:217, 1943.
63. Gomori, G.: *Amer. J. Clin. Pathol.*, **20**:665, 1950.
64. Hellman, B., and Hellerström, C.: In: *Handbuch des Diabetes mellitus*, Vol. 1. Edited by E. F. Pfeiffer. Lehmann, Munich, 1969, p. 89.
65. Greider, M. H., Bencosme, S. A., and Lechago, J.: *Lab. Invest.*, **22**:344, 1970.
66. Lacy, P. E., and Greider, M. H.: In: *Handbook of Physiology*, Sect. 7, Vol. I. Edited by R. O. Greep, and E. B. Astwood. American Physiological Society, Washington, D.C., 1972, p. 77.
67. Von Denffer, H., and Mertz, M.: *Histochemie*, **29**:54, 1972.
68. Klessen, C.: *Histochemistry*, **45**:203, 1975.
69. Piazza, C.: *Anat. Anz.*, **38**:127 & 167, 1911.
70. Takahashi, K.: *Trans. Jap. Pathol. Soc.*, **17**:65, 1927.
71. Van Campenhout, E.: *Proc. Soc. Exp. Biol. Med.*, **30**:617, 1933.
72. Nagelschmidt, L.: *Z. Mikrosk. Anat. Forsch.*, **45**:200, 1939.
73. Lasowsky, J. M.: *Frankf. Z. Pathol.*, **41**:1, 1931.
74. Ferner, H.: *Z. Mikrosk. Anat. Forsch.* **44**:451, 1938.
75. Ferner, H.: *Virchows Arch. Pathol. Anat.*, **309**:87, 1942.
76. Ferner, H.: *Virchows Arch. Pathol. Anat.*, **319**:390, 1951.
77. Hultquist, G. T., Dahlen, M., and Helander, C.: *Schweiz. Z. Pathol. Bacteriol.*, **11**:570, 1948.
78. Creutzfeldt, W.: *Beitr. Pathol. Anat.*, **113**:133, 1953.
79. Hamperl, H.: *Virchows Arch. Pathol. Anat.*, **321**:482, 1952.
80. Hellweg, G.: *Virchows Arch. Pathol. Anat.*, **327**:502, 1955.
81. Grimelius, L.: *Acta Soc. Med. Upsal.*, **73**:243 & 271, 1968.
82. Sevier, A. C., and Munger, B. L.: *J. Neuropathol. Exp. Neurol.*, **24**:130, 1965.
83. Volk, B. W., Goldner, M. G., and Crowley, H. F.: *Metabolism*, **4**:491, 1955.
84. Hellerström, C., and Hellman, B.: *Acta Endocrinol.*, **35**:518, 1960.
85. Hellman, B., and Hellerström, C.: *Z. Zellforsch.*, **52**:278, 1960.
86. Hellman, B., and Hellerström, C.: *Acta Endocrinol.*, **36**:72, 1961.
87. Björkman, N., Hellerström, C., Hellman, B., and Petersson, B.: *Z. Zellforsch.*, **72**:425, 1966.
88. Epple, A.: *Stain Technol.*, **42**:53, 1967.
89. Fujita, T.: *Arch. Histol. Jap.*, **29**:1, 1968.
90. Wellmann, K. F., Volk, B. W., and Brancato, P.: *Lab. Invest.*, **25**:97, 1971.
91. Grimelius, L., and Strand, A.: *Virchows Arch. Abt. A*, **364**:129, 1974.
92. Hökfelt, T., Efendic, S., Hellerström, C., Johansson, O., Luft, R., and Arimura, A.: *Acta Endocrinol. Suppl.*, **200**:5, 1975.
93. Banting, F. G., and Best, C. H.: *J. Lab. Clin. Med.*, **7**:251, 1922.
94. Schäfer, E. A.: *Lancet*, **2**:321, 1895.
95. Richardson, K. C., and Young, F. G.: *Lancet*, **1**:1098, 1938.
96. Dunn, J. S., Sheehan, H. L., and McLetchie, N. G. B.: *Lancet*, **1**:484, 1943.
97. Bailey, O. T., Bailey, C. C., and Hagen, W. H.: *Amer. J. Med. Sci.*, **208**:450, 1944.

98. Duff, G. L.: *Amer. J. Med. Sci.*, **210**:381, 1945.
99. Lukens, F. D.: *Physiol. Rev.*, **28**:304, 1948.
100. Burton, P. R., and Vensel, W. H.: *J. Morphol.*, **118**:91, 1966.
101. Wellmann, K. F., Volk, B. W., and Lazarus, S. S.: *Diabetes*, **16**:242, 1967.
102. Boquist, L.: *Virchows Arch. Abt. B*, **1**:157, 1968.
103. Hinkley, R. E., and Burton, P. R.: *Anat. Rec.*, **166**:67, 1970.
104. Rakieten, N., Rakieten, M. L., and Nadkarni, M. V.: *Cancer Chemother. Rep.*, **29**:91, 1963.
105. Arison, R. N., Ciaccio, E. I., Glitzer, M. S., Cassaro, J. A., and Pruss, M. P.: *Diabetes*, **16**:51, 1967.
106. Junod, A., Lambert, A. E., Orci, L., Pictet, R., Gonet, A. E., and Renold, A. E.: *Proc. Soc. Exp. Biol. Med.*, **126**:201, 1967.
107. Brosky, G., and Logothetopoulos, J.: *Diabetes*, **18**:606, 1969.
108. Pitkin, R. M., and Reynolds, W. A.: *Diabetes*, **19**:85, 1970.
109. Lazarus, S. S., and Shapiro, S. H.: *Diabetes*, **21**:129, 1972.
110. Frerichs, H., and Creutzfeldt, W.: Diabetes durch Beta-Zytotoxine. In: *Handbuch des Diabetes Mellitus*. Vol. 1. Edited by E. F. Pfeiffer. J. F. Lehmann, Munich, 1969, p. 811.
111. Rerup, C. C.: *Pharmacol. Rev.*, **22**:485, 1970.
112. Woerner, C. A.: *Anat. Rec.*, **71**:33, 1938.
113. Gomori, G., Friedman, N. B., and Caldwell, D. W.: *Proc. Soc. Exp. Biol. Med.*, **41**:567, 1939.
114. Barron, S. S., and State, D.: *Arch. Pathol.*, **48**:297, 1949.
115. Brown, E. M., Jr., Dohan, F. C., Freedman, L. R., DeMoor, P., and Lukens, F. D. W.: *Endocrinology*, **50**:644, 1952.
116. Anderson, E., and Long, J. A.: *Endocrinology*, **40**:92, 1947.
117. Metz, R.: *Diabetes*, **9**:89, 1960.
118. Bell, E. T.: *Diabetes*, **2**:125, 1953.
119. Wrenshall, G. A., Hartroft, W. S., and Best, C. H.: *Diabetes*, **3**:444, 1954.
120. Wrenshall, G. A., Bogoch, A., and Ritchie, R. C.: *Diabetes*, **1**:87, 1952.
121. Hartroft, W. S., and Wrenshall, G. A.: *Diabetes* **4**:1, 1955.
122. Steinke, J., and Driscoll, S. G.: *Diabetes*, **14**:573, 1965.
123. Latta, J. S., and Harvey, H. T.: *Anat. Rec.*, **82**:281, 1942.
124. Barron, S. S.: *Arch. Pathol.*, **46**:159, 1948.
125. Nerenberg, S. T.: *Amer. J. Clin. Pathol.*, **23**:340, 1953.
126. Miller, R. A.: *Endocrinology*, **31**:535, 1942.
127. McJunkin, F. A., and Roberts, B. D.: *Proc. Soc. Exp. Biol. Med.*, **29**:893, 1932.
128. Evans, M. A., and Haist, R. E.: *Amer. J. Physiol.*, **167**:176, 1951.
129. Best, C. H., Haist, R. E., and Ridout, J. H.: *J. Physiol.*, **97**:107, 1939.
130. Best, C. H., and Haist, R. E.: *J. Physiol.*, **100**:142, 1941.
131. Haist, R. E.: *Physiol. Rev.*, **24**:409, 1944.
132. Zunz, E., and La Barre, J.: *C. R. Soc. Biol.*, **96**:1045, 1927.
133. Ham, A. W., and Haist, R. E.: *Nature (London)*, **144**:835, 1939.
134. Ham, A. W., and Haist, R. E.: *Amer. J. Pathol.*, **17**:787, 1941.
135. Lazarus, S. S., and Bencosme, S. A.: *Amer. J. Clin. Pathol.*, **26**:1146, 1956.
136. Lazarus, S. S., and Barden, H.: *J. Histochem. Cytochem.* **9**:628, 1961.
137. Lazarus, S. S., and Volk, B. W.: *Diabetes 11, Suppl.*, p. 2, 1962.
138. Fujita, T., Hasegawa, N., Koga, Y., Kameda, Y., and Takaya, K.: *Arch. Histo. Jap.*, **29**:313, 1968.
139. Volk, B. W., Wellmann, K. F., and Lazarus, S. S.: *Lab. Invest.*, **14**:1375, 1965.
140. Haist, R. E., and Best, C. H.: *Science*, **91**:410, 1940.
141. Haist, R. E., and Best, C. H.: *Proc. Amer. Diab. Assoc.*, **1**:29, 1941.
142. Griffiths, M.: *J. Biol. Chem.*, **184**:289, 1950.
143. Volk, B. W., and Lazarus, S. S.: *Amer. J. Pathol.*, **37**:121, 1960.
144. Wellmann, K. F., Adachi, M., and Volk, B. W.: *Virchows Arch. Abt. A*, **360**:327, 1973.
145. Haist, R. E., Ridout, J. H., and Best, C. H.: *Amer. J. Physiol.*, **126**:518, 1939.
146. Barnett, R. F., Marshall, R. B., and Seligman, A. M.: *Endocrinology*, **57**:419, 1955.
147. Volk, B. W., and Lazarus, S. S.: *Diabetes*, **11**:426, 1962.

148. Lazarus, S. S., and Volk, B. W.: *Arch. Pathol.*, **67**:456, 1959.
149. Lacy, P. E., and Davies, J.: *Diabetes*, **6**:354, 1957.
150. Lacy, P. E., and Davies, J.: *Stain Technol.*, **34**:85, 1959.
151. Lacy, P. E.: *Amer. J. Med.*, **31**:851, 1961.
152. Lazarus, S. S., and Volk, B. W.: In: *The Structure and Metabolism of the Pancreatic Islets.* Wenner-Gren Series, Vol. 16. Edited by S. Falkmer, B. Hellman, and I. B. Täljedal. Pergamon Press, Oxford, 1970, p. 159.
153. Logothetopoulos, J., Yip, C., and Coburn, M. E.: In: *The Structure and Metabolism of the Pancreatic Islets.* Wenner-Gren Series, Vol. 16. Edited by S. Falkmer, B. Hellman, and I. B. Täljedal. Pergamon Press, Oxford, 1970, p. 381.
154. Lacy, P. E., and Williamson, J. R.: *Diabetes*, **11**:101, 1962.
155. Dixit, P. K., Lowe, I., and Lazarow, A.: *Nature (London)*, **195**:388, 1962.
156. Creutzfeldt, W., Creutzfeldt, C., and Frerichs, H.: In: *The Structure and Metabolism of the Pancreatic Islets.* Wenner-Gren Series, Vol. 16. Edited by S. Falkmer, B. Hellman, and I. B. Täljedal. Pergamon Press, Oxford, 1970, p. 181.
157. Lacy, P. E., and Howell, S. L.: In: *The Structure and Metabolism of the Pancreatic Islets.* Wenner-Gren Series, Vol. 16. Edited by S. Falkmer, B. Hellman, and I. B. Täljedal. Pergamon Press, Oxford, 1970, p. 171.
158. Lacy, P. E.: *Diabetes*, **19**:895, 1970.
159. Lacy, P. E.: *Amer. J. Pathol.*, **79**:170, 1975.
160. Orci, L., Amherdt, M., Malaisse-Lagae, F., and Renold, A. E.: *Science*, **179**:82, 1973.
161. Pipeleers, D. G., Pipeleers-Marichal, M. A., and Kipnis, D. M.: *Science*, **191**:88, 1976.
162. Van Obberghen, E., Somers, G., Devis, G., Vaughan, G. D., Malaisse-Lagae, F., Orci, L., and Malaisse, W. J.: *J. Clin. Invest.*, **52**:1041, 1973.
163. Van Obberghen, E., Somers, G., Devis, G., Ravazzola, M., Malaisse-Lagae, F., Orci, L., and Malaisse, W. J.: *Endocrinology*, **95**:1518, 1974.
164. Devis, G., van Obberghen, E., Somers, G., Malaisse-Lagae, F., Orci, L., and Malaisse, W. J.: *Diabetologia*, **10**:53, 1974.
165. Dragstedt, L. R., von Prohaska, J., and Harms, H. P.: *Amer. J. Physiol.*, **117**:175, 1936.
166. Dragstedt, L. R.: *J. Amer. Med. Assoc.*, **114**:29, 1940.
167. Ralli, E. P., Rubin, S. H., and Present, C. H.: *Amer. J. Physiol.*, **122**:43, 1938.
168. Montgomery, M. L., Entenman, C., Chaikoff, I. L., and Nelson, C.: *J. Biol. Chem.*, **137**:693, 1941.
169. Collip, J. B.: *Amer. J. Physiol.*, **63**:391, 1923.
170. Fisher, N. F.: *Amer. J. Physiol.*, **67**:57, 1924.
171. De Jongh, S. E.: *Biochem. J.*, **18**:833, 1924.
172. Murlin, J. R., Clough, H. G., Gibbs, C. B. F., and Stokes, A. M.: *J. Biol. Chem.*, **56**:253, 1923.
173. Kimball, C. P., and Murlin, J. R.: *J. Biol. Chem.*, **58**:337, 1923.
174. Collens, W. S., and Murlin, J. R.: *Proc. Soc. Exp. Biol. Med.*, **26**:485, 1929.
175. Bürger, M.: *Amer. J. Physiol.*, **90**:302, 1929.
176. Bürger, M.: *Klin. Wochenschr.*, **10**:351, 1931.
177. Bürger, M.: *Klin. Wochenschr.*, **16**:361, 1937.
178. Bürger, M., and Brandt, W.: *Z. Gesamte Exp. Med.*, **96**:375, 1935.
179. Staub, A., Sinn, L., and Behrens, O. K.: *Science*, **117**:628, 1953.
180. Gaede, K., Ferner, H., and Kastrup, H.: *Klin. Wochenschr.*, **28**:388, 1950.
181. Bencosme, S. A., Liepa, E., and Lazarus, S. S.: *Proc. Soc. Exp. Biol. Med.*, **90**:387, 1955.
182. Van Campenhout, E., and Cornelis, G.: *C. R. Soc. Biol.*, **145**:933, 1951.
183. Goldner, M. G., Volk, B. W., and Lazarus, S. S.: *Metabolism*, **1**:544, 1952.
184. Vuylsteke, C. A., Cornelis, G., and de Duve, C.: *Arch. Int. Physiol.*, **60**:128, 1952.
185. Volk, B. W., Lazarus, S. S., and Goldner, M. G.: *Proc. Soc. Exp. Biol. Med.*, **82**:406, 1954.
186. Kadota, I., and Kurita, M.: *Metabolism*, **4**:337, 1955.
187. Fodden, J. H.: *Amer. J. Clin. Pathol.*, **23**:1002, 1953.
188. Ulrich, F., and Copp, D. H.: *Arch. Biochem. Biophys.*, **31**:148, 1951.
189. Creutzfeldt, W.: *Diabetes*, **6**:135, 1957.
190. Bencosme, S. A., and Frei, J.: *Proc. Soc. Exp. Biol. Med.*, **91**:589, 1956.

191. Kern, H. F.: In: *The Structure and Metabolism of the Pancreatic Islets.* Wenner-Gren Series, Vol. 16. Edited by S. Falkmer, B. Hellman, and I. B. Täljedal. Pergamon Press, Oxford, 1970, p. 99.
192. Kadota, I., and Midorikawa, O.: *J. Lab. Clin. Med.,* **38**:671, 1951.
193. Galin, M. A., Reisman, M., Rudolph, I., and Fink, H.: *Diabetes,* **6**:154, 1957.
194. Davis, J. C.: *J. Pathol. Bacteriol.,* **64**:575, 1952.
195. Frank, E., Nothmann, M., and Wagner, A.: *Klin. Wochenschr.* **5**:2100, 1926.
196. Hornung, S.: *Klin. Wochenschr.,* **7**:69, 1928.
197. Varela, B., Collazo, J. A., and Rubino, P.: *C. R. Soc. Biol.,* **99**:1441, 1928.
198. Runge, W.: *Klin. Wochenschr.,* **32**:748, 1954.
199. Von Holt, C., Von Holt, L., Kröner, B., and Kühnau, J.: *Naturwissenschaften,* **41**:166, 1954.
200. Von Holt, C., Von Holt, L., Kröner, B., and Kühnau, J.: *Arch. Exp. Pathol. Pharmacol.* **224**:66, 1955.
201. Creutzfeldt, W., and Tecklenborg, E.: *Arch. Exp. Pathol. Pharmacol.,* **227**:23, 1955.
202. Creutzfeldt, W., and Moench, A.: *Endokrinologie,* **36**:167, 1958.
203. Creutzfeldt, W., and Tecklenborg, E.: *Klin. Wochenschr.,* **33**:43, 1955.
204. Munger, B. L.: *Lab. Invest.,* **11**:885, 1962.
205. Gepts, W., Christophe, J., and Bellens, R.: *Ann. Endocrinol.,* **16**:946, 1956.
206. De Bastiani, G., and Granata, L.: *Arch. Ital. Scienze Farm.,* **7**:3, 1957.
207. Lundbaek, K., and Nielsen, K.: *Acta Endocrinol.,* **27**:325, 1958.
208. Korp, W., and LeCompte, P. M.: *Diabetes,* **4**:347, 1955.
209. Creutzfeldt, W.: In *Diabetes.* Edited by R. H. Williams. Paul B. Hoeber, New York, 1960, p. 52.
210. Staub, A., Sinn, L., and Behrens, O. K.: *J. Biol. Chem.,* **214**:619, 1955.
211. Kracht, J.: *Naturwissenschaften,* **41**:336, 1954.
212. Kracht, J.: *Naturwissenschaften,* **42**:50, 1955.
213. Lazarus, S. S., and Volk, B. W.: *Endocrinology,* **63**:359, 1958.
214. Lazarus, S. S., and Volk, B. W.: *Diabetes,* **8**:294, 1959.
215. Volk, B. W., and Lazarus, S. S.: *Diabetes,* **9**:53, 1960.
216. Logothetopoulos, J., and Salter, J. M.: *Diabetes,* **9**:31, 1960.
217. Lacy, P. E., Cardeza, A. F., and Wilson, W. D.: *Diabetes,* **8**:36, 1959.
218. Glenner, G. G., and Lillie, R. D.: *J. Histochem. Cytochem.,* **5**:279, 1957.
219. Levine, H. J., and Glenner, G. G.: *J. Nat. Cancer Inst.,* **20**:63, 1958.
220. Baum, J., Simon, B. E., Jr., Unger, R. H., and Madison, L. L.: *Diabetes,* **11**:371, 1962.
221. Lundquist, G., Brolin, S. E., Unger, R. H., and Eisentraut, A. M.: In: *The Structure and Metabolism of the Pancreatic Islets.* Wenner-Gren Series, Vol. 16. Edited by S. Falkmer, B. Hellman, and I. B. Täljedal. Pergamon Press, Oxford, 1970, p. 115.
222. Machino, M., Onoe, T., and Sakuma, H.: *J. Electron Microsc.,* **15**:249, 1966.
223. Gomez-Acebo, J., Parrilla, R., and R-Candela, J. L.: *J. Cell Biol.,* **36**:33, 1968.
224. Lazarus, S. S., Shapiro, S., and Volk, B. W.: *Diabetes,* **17**:152, 1968.
225. Sutherland, E. W., and de Duve, C.: *J. Biol. Chem.,* **175**:663, 1948.
226. Unger, R. H., Eisentraut, A., Sims, K., McCall, M. S., and Madison, L. L.: *Clin. Res.,* **9**:53, 1961.
227. Unger, R. H., Ketterer, H., and Eisentraut, A. M.: *Metabolism,* **15**:865, 1966.
228. Samols, E., Tyler, J., Megyesi, C., and Marks, V.: *Lancet,* **2**:727, 1966.
229. Forssmann, W. G., Orci, L., Pictet, R., and Rouiller, C.: *Acta Anat.,* **68**:605, 1967.
230. Sasaki, H., Rubalcava, B., Baetens, D., Blazquez, E., Srikant, C. B., Orci, L., and Unger, R. H.: *J. Clin. Invest.,* **56**:135, 1975.
231. Baetens, D., Rufener, C., Srikant, C. B., Dobbs, R., Unger, R., and Orci, L.: *J. Cell Biol.,* **69**:455, 1976.
232. Gerich, J. E., Lorenzi, M., Schneider, V., Karam, J. H., Rivier, J., Guillemin, R., and Forsham, P. H.: *N. Engl. J. Med.,* **291**:544, 1974.
233. Unger, R. H., and Orci, L.: *Lancet,* **1**:14, 1975.
234. Dobbs, L., Sakurai, H., Sasaki, H., Faloona, G., Valverde, I., Baetens, D., Orci, L., and Unger, R.: *Science,* **187**:544, 1975.
235. Unger, R. H.: *Diabetes,* **25**:136, 1976.

236. Robb, P.: *Quart. J. Exp. Physiol.,* **46**:335, 1961.
237. Ito, T., Takahashi, Y., Aoki, H., and Yamamoti, T.: *Arch. Histol. Jap.,* **21**:415, 1961.
238. Liu, H. M., and Potter, E. L.: *Arch. Pathol.* **74**:439, 1962.
239. Vale, W., Brazeau, P., Rivier, C., Brown, M., Boss, B., Rivier, J., Burgus, R., Ling, N., and Guillemin, R.: *Rec. Progr. Horm. Res.,* **31**:365, 1975.
240. Brazeau, P., Vale, W., Burgus, R., Ling, N., Butcher, M., Rivier, J., and Guillemin, R.: *Science,* 179:77, 1973.
241. Alberti, K. G. M. M., Christensen, N. J., Christensen, S. E., Hansen, A. P., Iversen, J., Lundbaek, K., Seyer-Hansen, K., and Ørskov, H.: *Lancet,* **2**:1299, 1973.
242. Koerker, D. J., Ruch, W., Chideckel, E., Palmer, J., Goodner, C. J., Ensinck, J., and Gale, C. C.: *Science,* **184**:482, 1974.
243. Fujimoto, W. Y., Ensinck, J. W., and Williams, R. H.: *Life Sci.,* **15**:1999, 1974.
244. Fujimoto, W. Y.: *Endocrinology,* **97**:1494, 1975.
245. Arimura, A., Sato, H., Dupont, A., Nishi, N., and Schally, A. V.: *Science,* **189**:1007, 1975.
246. Pelletier, G., Leclerc, R., Arimura, A., and Schally, A. V.: *J. Histochem. Cytochem.,* **23**:699, 1975.
247. Dubois, M.: *Proc. Nat. Acad. Sci., USA* **72**:1340, 1975.
248. Orci, L., Baetens, D., Dubois, M. P., and Rufener, C.: *Horm. Metab. Res.,* **7**:400, 1975.
249. Polak, J., Pearse, A. G. E., Grimelius, L., Bloom, S. R., and Arimura, A.: *Lancet,* **1**:1220, 1975.
250. Weichert, R. F.: *Amer. J. Med.,* **49**:232, 1970.
251. Goldsmith, P. C., Rose, J. C., Arimura, A., and Ganong, W. F.: *Endocrinology,* **97**:1061, 1975.
252. Hellerström, C., Petersson, B., and Hellman, B.: *Acta Endocrinol.,* **34**:449, 1960.
253. Orci, L., and Unger, R. H.: *Lancet,* **2**:1243, 1975.

Chapter 5

Quantitative Studies of the Islets of Nondiabetic Patients

Bruno W. Volk and Klaus F. Wellmann

In view of the fact that the islets of Langerhans are dispersed into numerous different-sized bodies within the pancreas, the various methods used to determine the number of islets, their volume, and A:B ratio has led to divergent results. Some investigators counted the islets in representative sections. Laguesse,[1] by reconstructing a single pancreatic lobule, observed that the actual number of islets was considerably in excess of that obtained by counting them in representative sections. Bensley,[2] using his staining procedure, emphasized that when such pancreatic fragments are carefully selected they are to the same extent representative of the part of the organ from which they are taken. He also postulated that a large number of pancreases must be examined in order to ensure a reasonable range of individual variations. Gepts[3] warned that the estimation of weight or volume of islets presents a difficult problem and that the estimate should be considered as very rough. He further stated that as a result of errors in the methodology of sampling, quantitative methods are without value for the determination of the proportion of insular tissue in any given pancreas.

It is generally agreed that the islets of the adult human pancreas are more numerous in the tail than in the head or the body.[4-13] Opie[5] observed that the head of the pancreas contains 36.66, the body 36, and the tail 68 islets/cm². This is in general agreement with the findings of other investigators,[7-9] although some of them reported moderately higher values.

Various authors studied the total volume or weight of the pancreatic islets. Thus, Laguesse[10] noted that the islets occupy 1% of the total pancreatic mass. De Witt[14] observed that they comprise approximately 2% of the organ and Heiberg[15] estimated that a pancreas weighing 80 g contains 2.4 g of insular tissue. Gündisch[16] observed that the islet tissue in a person weighing 75 kg amounts approximately to 0.4 g for the entire organ. Clark,[4] on the other hand,

Bruno W. Volk and Klaus F. Wellmann • Isaac Albert Research Institute of the Kingsbrook Jewish Medical Center, and Downstate Medical Center, State University of New York, Brooklyn, New York. Present address of B. W. V.: University of California, Irvine, California. Present address of K. F. W.: Beekman Downtown Hospital, New York, New York.

determined that 1 g of human pancreatic tissue contains between 3 and 27 islets, while Weichselbaum[17] calculated that 4.3% of the pancreas is occupied by islet tissue. In similar studies Gündisch[16] estimated that 0.6 to 2.11% of the pancreas, and according to Susman[18] 0.9 to 3.5% of this organ, is occupied by the islets.

Other investigators also made extensive quantitative studies of the islets. Ogilvie[19] observed that the average weight of the pancreas increased from 2.6 g at birth to 66 g for patients over 21 years of age. However, he found that the weight of the islets varied through a wider range than that of the total pancreas. For the first 2 years, the rate of increase of the islets and that of the total pancreas runs parallel and is greater than the rate of body growth. From the ages of 4 to 12 years, the rate of increase of insular tissue is about one-half that of the total pancreas and of the body as a whole. At the time of adolescence the rates are equal again. Ogilvie,[19] in agreement with other authors,[20–22] calculated that the number of islets remains constant from the 3rd year on and estimated that the weight of the average islet increases from 0.350 μg at birth to 1.469 μg in adult life. However, the weights fluctuate over a wide range, even in the adult with a mean varying from 0.478 to 2.738 μg. During fetal life and in the newborn the islets seem to be more numerous than after birth, particularly in comparison with the adult. It has been shown by various authors[20–22] that during the period from the 26th to 32nd week of gestation the fetal pancreas contains the largest number of islets, the tail from 600 to 700 islets/50 mm^2. From then on the number of islets declines until after birth when the number of islets averages 550/mm^2. From this time on, there is a gradual and persistent decrease of the total number until the fifth year, at which time a total of 130 islets/mm^2 have been counted.

Other authors who also attempted to count the islets observed wide variations. Laguesse[10] counted 0.8 to 1.5 islets/mm^2 and Dubs[23] observed 1.0 to 1.02 islets/mm^2. Gellé[24] examined the pancreases of four executed criminals and estimated that the human adult pancreas contains 1.0 to 1.5 islets/mm^2. In a study of the total islets of six nondiabetic executed criminals Clark[4] observed a wide variation in the number of islets ranging from 250,000 to 1,750,000. Ogilvie's counts[19] varied greatly from 117,000 to 226,000 in a 1-year-old female and 2,325,123 islets in an 8-month-old male. He estimated that the number of islets of adults amounted to approximately 1,000,000 and that the range was as wide as that seen in infants. Heiberg[7] estimated that the islets made up approximately 3% of the total pancreas, and Bargmann[25] gave counts in five adults which varied from 208,369 to 1,760,000. He also estimated that the pancreas of a 6-month-old child contains approximately 120,323 islets.

Hellman[26] observed, on the basis of a study of 14 nondiabetic pancreases ranging from newborn to 84 years of age, that at all ages and regions of the pancreas, the number of islets increased progressively as the diameter decreased. He[26–28] also noted that the bulk of insular volume was composed of medium-sized islets and observed that the endocrine pancreas was arranged in a regular way, independent of age. When the number of islets was plotted in relation to the islet diameter, highly asymmetric curves were obtained. He concluded that the main part of the endocrine pancreas is composed of medium-sized islets, while the many small islets contribute approximately equally to the volume of the endocrine pancreas as do the substantially fewer large islets.

Because the estimation of the total number of islets in the pancreas varied considerably, several authors attempted to determine the size of the islets and to compare their volume in relation to that of the pancreas. Thus, Laguesse[10] observed that distinct differences in islet diameter occur within one and the same organ. However, he noted no differences in islet size in different areas of the pancreas. He observed that the largest diameter was 460 μm, although such dimensions were very rare. Heiberg[7] measured the longest diameter of the islets and observed that 71% of them averaged 100 to 225 μm. The largest islet in his study measured 360 × 560 μm in diameter. Burkhardt[29] suggested that those islets in which the diameter exceeded 500 to 600 μm should be considered as giant size.

Differential Count of Normal Pancreatic Islets

Schulze[30] and Diamare[31] for the first time suggested the existence of more than one cell type in the mammalian islets of Langerhans. Lane,[32] who devised a method for distinguishing the two types of granules in the islets, demonstrated that some of the islet cells (A cells) stained after fixation in 70% alcohol, the other islet cells (B cells) stained after fixation in chrome sublimate. He concluded that the islets of Langerhans contained two types of cells exhibiting a characteristic difference with regard to the alcohol solubility of the secretory granules. Moreover, the stain permitted a distinction between islet cell granules and those of the exocrine cells of the pancreas. Bloom[33] in 1931, in combining Zenker-formol fixation with the Heidenhain–Mallory azan stain, observed the presence of D cells within the islets which contained closely packed blue granules. While some authors have regarded these latter cells as precursors[34] or aged varieties[35,36] of the A cells, others[37,38] have concluded that they are related to the B cells. In more recent years it was thought that the D cells secrete gastrin.[39,40] However, since then it was shown, with the use of immunocytochemical techniques, that the D cells are responsible for the storage or synthesis[41,42] of somatostatin, a somatotropin-release-inhibiting factor, which also inhibits the release of both glucagon and insulin.[43–47] Gomori in 1939[35,48,49] introduced the chrome alum hematoxylin phloxine technique for differential stains of the islet cells. With this method the A cells stain various shades of red, while the B cells stain purple, depending on the counterstain. When combined with a modified Masson trichrome counterstain the islet cells are particularly well demonstrated.[50]

Kon[51] in 1933, showed that silver impregnation demonstrates the A cells seemingly specifically. Subsequently, Ferner[52] introduced the Gros–Schultze method for silver impregnation of formalin-fixed frozen sections of the pancreas. In his monograph in 1952[36] he felt that the silver impregnation method was preferable to granule stains in the differentiation of the islet cells, particularly in human postmortem material, since it permitted the distinction between A and B cells quite clearly. However, other investigators[53-55] considered this procedure to be unreliable for the identification of A cells. Creutzfeldt[54] emphasized that the Gros–Schultze method is capable of staining the B cells as well as the A cells. Bencosme[55] has shown that when the chrome alum hematoxylin method with a phloxine counterstain is used all cells staining red have to be considered A cells, despite the fact that the phloxine also stains D cells. Another shortcoming of the silver-impregnation method is the fact that thick frozen sections make cell counting difficult.

In order to eliminate the frozen sections Hamperl,[56] Hellweg,[48] and Grimelius[58] used the Bodian method and Volk *et al.*[59] utilized a modification of the Davenport method for silver impregnation in paraffin-embedded section material for the demonstration of A cells. A modification of the Davenport method in paraffin-embedded sections, in which the islet cells were first impregnated with silver and then after removal of the silver by oxidation with permanganate were stained differentially with one of the usual granule stains, was used extensively by Hellerström and Hellman.[60,61] These authors concluded that there are two types of A cells which they called A_1 and A_2, depending on the presence or absence of cytoplasmic argyrophilia. They[62] found differences as to their position in the islets, nuclear size, cell size, cytoplasmic granulation, and cytochemical properties. Using various staining histochemical reactions they concluded that the A_2 cells are probably the source of glucagon, while the function of the argyrophil A_1 cells at that time remained unknown. They further believed that the agranular C cells described by Thomas[63] in the guinea pig are probably identical with the A_1 cells in that species, and that the D cells described by Bloom[33] in man probably correspond to the relatively scarce A_1 cells in this species, also that the D cells in the dog most likely are the equivalent to the A_1 cells. (See also Chapter 3.)

These conclusions derived at by Hellman and Hellerström[60,61] have not been generally accepted, particularly in view of the fact that in electron-microscopic examinations of various species a multiplicity of morphologic cell types of doubtful or unknown functions have been observed, some of which were previously recognized by light microscopy. Thus, Caramia *et al.*[64] reported in the guinea pig three subtypes of A cell which they called A_a, A_b, and A_c. Munger *et al.*[65] observed the C cells in the guinea pig as having no granules and the E cells in the opossum, which was previously described by Thomas,[63] as having large granules as well as an F cell in the uncinate process of the dog pancreas which was previously called "X" cell by Bencosme *et al.*[66] and Lazarus and Shapiro.[67] These authors conjectured that these morphologically distinct cell types possibly serve different functions. They, as well as Fujita[68] and Petersson *et al.*,[69] believed that the silver-positive A_1 cells are identical with the D cells.

In 1974 Deconinck *et al.*[70,71] identified in ultramicroscopic studies four main cell types. Type I was identified with the B cells and type II with the A cells. Two other cell types were temporarily called types III and IV, and a fifth cell type, type V, was not observed in the islets but was present among the acinar cells. The authors conjectured that they had a certain resemblance to the serotonin secreting cells which are found in the digestive tract. Deconinck *et al.*[71] found these cells in the islets of neonates, with the exception of type V, which was absent. Compared with the islets of the adults, type III cells were more numerous in the newborn. In 1973, Solcia *et al.*[72] concluded that there are four islet cell types: A, B, and D, corresponding to type III of Deconinck *et al.*[70,71]; and D_1, corresponding to type IV of the same authors. (See also Chapter 2.)

Like and Orci[73] studied the developing pancreases of 20 human embryos and fetuses 8 to 23 weeks gestational age. They identified A cells at 9 weeks, followed by D cells, and subsequently B cells at 10.5 weeks. They recognized also other endocrine cells tentatively in the developing human pancreas (serotonin-, gastrin-, epinephrine-, and norepinephrine-producing cells).

In 1968, Kimmel *et al.*[74,75] isolated from chicken pancreas a polypeptide with physical characteristics similar to those of insulin, but which could be separated from it by displacement chromatography on DEAE cellulose. Later on, Linn and Chance[76-78] isolated a similar factor from bovine and porcine pancreases.

In 1975 Larsson *et al.*,[79] in histochemical studies, observed a small population of pancreatic islet cells which showed strong immunofluorescence after staining with anti-human pancreatic polypeptide (HPP) serum. HPP cells were mainly localized at the periphery of the islets, and sometimes they were scattered in the exocrine pancreas, as well as within the epithelium of small to medium-sized ducts. While they are rare in the pancreas of adult man, HPP cells were found in relatively large numbers in some parts of the pancreas of 18- to 20-week-old fetuses. Subsequently, Larsson *et al.*[80] observed PP cells in the islets of several mammals, and in the opossum and dog they were also seen in the gastric mucosa. Their staining properties showed them to be distinct from the A, B, and D cells of the pancreatic islets. Electron microscopically, in the rat, guinea pig, and chinchilla the PP cell granules are small and have an electron-lucent halo between the dense core and the surrounding membrane.[80] The human PP cells contain small dense granules with the membrane closely applied to the dense core. Larsson *et al.*[80] believed that the islet cells described by Deconinck *et al.*[70,71] as type V correspond to the PP cells. The physiologic function of this polypeptide is not known as yet, but there is evidence that it acts as a hormone.[76-78,81,82] (See also Chapters 3 and 12.)

Discovered by Vale *et al.*,[83] somatostatin, which inhibits the release of growth hormone as well as of glucagon and insulin, was shown by immunocytochemical techniques to be either synthesized or stored in cells of the islets of Langerhans.[84,85] Moreover, the cells, believed to be D cells, are arranged in a way which suggests an inhibitory action of these cells on the A cells.[86]

Several workers have utilized a modification of the silver impregnation method of Gros–Schultze for calculating the number of A cells and differential staining of the islet cells in the human pancreas. Thus, Ferner,[87] using the Gros–Schultze technique, found that 10 of 11 human pancreases showed 20%

A cells in the islets, while in one case the A cells included 33% of the total cells. Despite this last figure, which he considered to be the result of inanition of the patient, he believed that the number of A cells was consistent and amounted to 20% of the total islet cells. He claimed that the cellular proportions are the same and are equally distributed in the head, body, and tail of the pancreas. Hess[88] confirmed Ferner's observation and Terbrüggen[89] similarly reported in a group of nondiabetic individuals that the silver cells varied from 14 to 33%.

Other investigators, however, were unable to confirm the consistency of the proportion of A:B cells that was claimed by Ferner[87] and Hess.[88] Thus, Creutzfeldt[54] found 9 to 58% of A cells in 52 nondiabetic pancreases and Hultquist *et al.*[90] observed in 13 cases a range from 27 to 47% A cells. Ferner[36,87] believed that the variations of results observed by different investigators were due to subjective factors in counting the cells and that the material used by them did not represent appropriate controls. He also proposed that various disturbances, such as cachexia, could have modified or influenced the proportion of the cell types. Creutzfeldt[54] failed to concur with this interpretation and believed that the considerable variability of the figures observed by a number of investigators was the result in part of individual variations, and also in part due to the capriciousness of the silver-staining techniques for A cells. With other techniques of silver impregnation which could be applied to paraffin sections Gepts[91,92] found 16 to 55% in 35 nondiabetic pancreases and Creutzfeldt and Theodossiou[93] reported 24 to 65% in 48 cases.

There are only a few reports concerning the ratio of cell types in the islets of Langerhans using the chrome alum hematoxylin phloxine technique. Gomori[94] first observed the A:B cell ratio in 55 cases to vary from 8 to 45%. However, in two-thirds of the cases these values ranged from 11 to 25%. Using the same technique in a series of 30 nondiabetic pancreases Maclean and Ogilvie[95] found figures which varied from 18 to 33%.

By combining the results of different cell counts with estimations of the total islet volume Maclean and Ogilvie[95] have calculated the total weight of A and B cells in the islets of nondiabetics. They found that the mean total weight of the islets was 1.06 g (0.51 to 2.89 g); that of the B cells was 0.64 g (0.36 to 1.07 g), and that of the A cells was 0.22 g (0.10 to 0.43 g). Gepts[96] observed a total mean weight of the islets of 1.36 g (0.44 to 2.48 g), for the B cells 0.75 g (0.24 to 1.51 g) and for the A cells 0.34 g (0.08 to 0.78 g).

References

1. Laguesse, E.: *Rev. Gen. Histol.* **2**:1, 1906.
2. Bensley, R. R.: *Amer. J. Anat.*, **12**:297, 1911.
3. Gepts, W.: *Ann. Soc. R. Sci. Méd. Nat. Brux.*, **10**:34, 1957.
4. Clark, E.: *Anat. Anz.*, **43**:81, 1913.
5. Opie, E. L.: *Bull. Johns Hopkins Hosp.*, **11**:205, 1900.
6. Flint, J. M.: *Arch. Anat. Entwcklngsgesch.*, **27**:61, 1903.
7. Heiberg, K. A.: *Anat. Anz.*, **29**:49, 1906.
8. Heiberg, K. A.: *Anat. Anz.*, **37**:545, 1910.

9. Sauerbeck, E.: *Ergeb. allg. Pathol. Anat.*, **8**:539, 1902.
10. Laguesse, E.: *C. R. Soc. Biol.*, **58**:504, 1905.
11. Pochon: *Arch. Wissensch. Prakt. Tierh.*, **34**:581, 1908.
12. Maximow, A., and Bloom, W.: *A Textbook of Histology.* 5th ed. W. B. Saunders, Philadelphia, 1948, p. 443.
13. Schaffer, J.: *Lehrbuch der Histologie und Histogenese.* 3rd ed. Wilhelm Engelmann, Leipzig, 1933.
14. De Witt, L. M.: *J. Exp. Med.*, **8**:193, 1906.
15. Heiberg, K. A.: *Ergeb. Anat. Entwickl.-Gesch.*, **19**:948, 1909.
16. Gündisch, M.: *Cluj. Med.*, **15**:406, 1934.
17. Weichselbaum, A.: *Sitzungsb. Akad. Math.-Naturw. K.*, **119**:73, 1910.
18. Susman, W.: *J. Clin. Endocrinol.*, **2**:97, 1942.
19. Ogilvie, R. R.: *Quart. J. Med.*, **6**:287, 1937.
20. Seyfarth, C.: *Klin. Wochenschr.*, **3**:1085, 1924.
21. Nakamura, N.: *Virchows Arch.*, **253**:286, 1924.
22. Wilms, C.: In: *von Möllendorff's Handbuch der Mikroskopischen Anatomie des Menschen.* J. Springer, Berlin, 1939, p. 209.
23. Dubs: Quoted in *von Möllendorff's Handbuch der Mikroskopischen Anatomie des Menschen.* J. Springer, Berlin, 1939, p. 209.
24. Gellé: *Ergeb. Anat. Entwickl.-Gesch.*, **20**:1042, 1911.
25. Bargmann, W.: *von Möllendorff's Handbuch der Mikroskopischen Anatomie des Menschen.* J. Springer, Berlin, 1939, p. 209.
26. Hellman, B.: *Acta Soc. Med. Upsal.*, **64**:432, 1959.
27. Hellman, B.: *Nature (London)* **184**:1498, 1959.
28. Hellman, B.: *Acta Soc. Med. Upsal.*, **64**:461, 1959.
29. Burkhardt, L. W.: *Virchows Arch.*, **296**:655, 1936.
30. Schulze, W.: *Arch. Mikr. Anat.*, **56**:491, 1900.
31. Diamare, V.: *Int. Mschr. Anat. Physiol.*, **16**:155, 1899.
32. Lane, M. A.: *Amer. J. Anat.*, **7**:409, 1907.
33. Bloom, W.: *Anat. Rec.*, **49**:363, 1931.
34. Miller, R. A.: *Endocrinology*, **31**:535, 1942.
35. Gomori, G.: *Amer. J. Pathol.* **17**:395, 1939.
36. Ferner, H.: *Das Inselsystem des Pankreas.* Georg Thieme Verlag, Stuttgart, 1952, p. 17.
37. Ito, T., Takahashi, Y., Aoki, H., and Yamamoto, T.: *Arch. Histol. Jap.* **21**:415, 1961.
38. Conklin, J. L.: *Amer. J. Anat.*, **111**:181, 1962.
39. Lomsky, R. F., Langer, F., and Vortel, V.: *Nature (London)*, **223**:618, 1969.
40. Greider, M. H., and McGuigan, J. E.: *Diabetes*, **20**:387, 1971.
41. Pelletier, G., LeClerc, R., Arimara, A., and Schally, A. V.: *J. Histochem. Cytochem.*, **23**:699, 1975.
42. Orci, L., Baetens, D., Dubois, M. P., and Rufener, C.: *Horm. Metab. Res.*, **7**:400, 1975.
43. Mortimer, C. H., Turnbridge, W. M. G., Carr, D., Yeomans, L., Lind, T., Coy, D. H., Bloom, S. R., Kastin, A., Mallinson, C. N., Besser, G. M., Schally, A. V., and Hall, R.: *Lancet*, **1**:697, 1974.
44. Koerker, D. J., Ruch, W., Chideckel, E., Palmer, J., Goodner, C. J., Ensinck, J., and Gale, C. C.: *Science*, **184**:482, 1974.
45. Johnson, D. G., Ensinck, J. W., Koerker, D. J., Palmer, J., and Goodner, C. J.: *Diabetes, Suppl. 1*, **23**:374, 1974.
46. Iverson, J.: *Scand. J. Clin. Lab. Invest.*, **33**:125, 1974.
47. Efendic, S., Luft, R., and Grill, V.: *FEBS Lett.*, **42**:169, 1974.
48. Gomori, G.: *Amer. J. Pathol.*, **15**:497, 1939.
49. Gomori, G.: *Amer. J. Clin. Pathol.*, **20**:665, 1950.
50. Lazarus, S. S., and Volk, B. W.: *The Pancreas in Human and Experimental Diabetes.* Grune & Stratton, New York, 1962, p. 262.
51. Kon, A.: *Über die Silberreaktion der Zellen.* G. Fischer Verlag, Jena, 1933, p. 47.
52. Ferner, H.: *Z. Mikr.-Anat. Forsch.*, **44**:451, 1938.
53. Creutzfeldt, W.: *Z. Zellforsch.*, **34**:280, 1949.
54. Creutzfeldt, W.: *Beitr. Path. Anat.*, **133**:113, 1953.
55. Bencosme, S. A.: *Arch. Pathol.*, **53**:87, 1952.

56. Hamperl, H.: *Virchows Arch.*, **321**:482, 1952.
57. Hellweg, G.: *Virchows Arch.*, **327**:502, 1955.
58. Grimelius, L.: In: *The Structure and Metabolism of the Pancreatic Islets.* Edited by S. E. Brolin, B. Hellman, and H. Knutson. Macmillan, New York, 1964, p. 99.
59. Volk, B. W., Goldner, M. G., and Crowley, H. F.: *Metabolism*, **4**:491, 1955.
60. Hellman, B., and Hellerström, C.: *Z. Zellforsch. Mikrosk. Anat. Abt. Histochem.*, **52**:278, 1960.
61. Hellman, B., and Hellerström, C.: In: *Handbuch des Diabetes Mellitus.* Edited by E. F. Pfeiffer. J. F. Lehmanns Verlag, München, 1969, p. 89.
62. Hellerström, C., Hellman, B., Petersson, B., and Alm, G.: In: *The Structure and Metabolism of the Pancreatic Islets.* Edited by S. E. Brolin, B. Hellman, and H. Knutson. Macmillan, New York, 1964, p. 117.
63. Thomas, T. B.: *Amer. J. Anat.*, **62**:31, 1937.
64. Caramia, F., Munger, B. L., and Lacy, P. E.: *Z. Zellforsch.*, **67**:533, 1965.
65. Munger, B. L., Caramia, F., and Lacy, P. E.: *Z. Zellforsch.*, **67**:776, 1965.
66. Bencosme, S. A., Lazarus, S. S., and Liepa, E.: *Proc. Soc. Exp. Biol. Med.*, **90**:387, 1955.
67. Lazarus, S. S., and Shapiro, S. H.: *Anat. Rec.*, **169**:487, 1971.
68. Fujita, T.: *Arch. Histol. Jap.*, **25**:189, 1964.
69. Petersson, B., Hellerström, C., and Hellman, B.: *Z. Zellforsch.*, **57**:559, 1962.
70. Deconinck, J., Potvliege, P. R., and Gepts, W.: *Diabetologia*, **7**:266, 1971.
71. Deconinck, J., van Assche, F., Potvliege, P. R., and Gepts, W.: *Diabetologia*, **8**:326, 1972.
72. Solcia, E., Pearse, A. G. E., Grube, D., Kobayashi, S., Bussolati, G., Creutzfeldt, W., and Gepts, W.: *Rend. Gastroenterol.*, **5**:13, 1973.
73. Like, A. A., and Orci, L.: *Diabetes, Supp. 2*, **21**:511, 1972.
74. Kimmel, J. R., Pollock, H. G., and Hazelwood, R. L.: *Endocrinology*, **83**:1323, 1968.
75. Kimmel, J. R., Pollock, H. G., and Hazelwood, R. L.: *Fed. Proc.*, **30**:1318, (Abst.), 1971.
76. Lin, T. M., and Chance, R. E.: *Gastroenterology*, **82**:852 (Abst.), 1972.
77. Lin, T. M., Chance, R. E., and Evans, D.: *Gastroenterology*, **64**:865, 1973.
78. Lin, T. M., Evans, D. C., and Chance, R. E.: *Gastroenterology*, **6**:852, 1974.
79. Larsson, L.-I., Sundler, F., and Hakanson, R.: *Cell. Tiss. Res.*, **156**:167, 1975.
80. Larsson, L.-I., Sundler, F., and Hakanson, R.: *Diabetologia*, **12**:211, 1976.
81. Hazelwood, R. E., Turner, S. D., Kimmel, J. R., and Pollock, H. G.: *Gen. Comp. Endocrinol.* **21**:485, 1973.
82. Schwartz, T. W., Rehfeld, J. F., Stadil, F., Larsson, L. J., Chance, R. E., and Moon, N.: *Lancet*, **1**:1102, 1976.
83. Vale, W., Brazeau, G., Grant, A., Nussey, R., Burgus, J., Rivier, N., Ling, N., and Guillemin, C. R.: *C. R. Acad. Sci.*, **275**:2913, 1972.
84. Liljenquist, J. E., Bomboy, J. D., Lewis, S. B., Sinclair-Smith, B. C., Felts, P. W., Lacy, W. W., Crofford, O. B., and Liddle, W.: *J. Clin. Invest.*, **53**:190, 1974.
85. Pelletier, G., Leclerc, G., Arimura, A., and Schally, A. V.: *J. Histochem. Cytochem.*, **23**:699, 1975.
86. Orci, L., and Unger, R. H.: *Lancet*, **2**:1243, 1975.
87. Ferner, H.: *Virchows Arch.*, **309**:87, 1942.
88. Hess, W.: *Schweiz. Z. Pathol. Bakteriol.*, **9**:46, 1946.
89. Terbrüggen, A.: *Virchows Arch.*, **315**:407, 1948.
90. Hultquist, G. T., Dahlen, M., and Helander, C. G.: *Schweiz. Z. Pathol. Bakteriol.* **11**:570, 1948.
91. Gepts, W.: *Ann. Soc. R. Sci. Med. Nat. Brux.*, **10**:5, 1957.
92. Gepts, W.: *Endocrinologie*, **36**:185, 1958.
93. Creutzfeldt, W., and Theodossiou, A.: *Beitr. Pathol. Anat.*, **117**:235, 1957.
94. Gomori, G.: *Arch. Pathol.*, **36**:217, 1943.
95. Maclean, N., and Ogilvie, R. R.: *Diabetes*, **4**:367, 1955.
96. Gepts, W.: In: *Handbuch of Diabetes Mellitus.* Edited by E. F. Pfeiffer, J. F. Lehmann, Munich, Vol. II, 1971, p. 3.

Chapter 6

Histochemistry and Electron Microscopy of Islets

Lennart Boquist

General Ultrastructural Appearance

Cellular Composition of the Islets

The islets of highly different species are composed of parenchymal cells, blood vessels, nervous elements, and connective tissue. The parenchymal cells are either diffusely intermingled with each other, or, more often, the B (β) cells are localized to the central portion of the islets, and the A (α_2) and D (α_1) cells* are localized to the periphery, sometimes with a tendency toward interposition of the D cells between the central B cells and the peripheral A cells (Fig. 1). The differentiation of the parenchymal cell types is based mainly upon the structural appearance of their secretory granules. In most species B, A, and D cells are found, which usually can be easily distinguished by ultrastructural techniques.

In addition, other cell types or subtypes of one or more of the generally accepted cell types have been reported with more or less convincing evidence in some species under normal and/or pathological conditions. The A cells have thus been subclassified into light and dark variants in the rat[1] and into A_a, A_b, and A_c types in the guinea pig[2] and mouse.[3] However, obviously there is only one population of A cells in most species.[4] The difference in the size of the α granules of the guinea pig appears to represent stages in the life cycle of the same cells, rather than different cells concerned with the production of different secretory products.[5]

---

*Opinions differ as to whether or not there is an identity between D cells and α_1 cells which has led to some confusion in the literature. In order not to make the nomenclature of the parenchymal cells too complicated, the D and α_1 cells will be regarded as identical. Where possible, the revised Wiesbaden classification will be followed. Hence, the islet parenchymal cells will be called A, B, or D cells. Their secretory granules will be called α, β, and δ granules, respectively.

Lennart Boquist • University of Umea, Umea, Sweden.

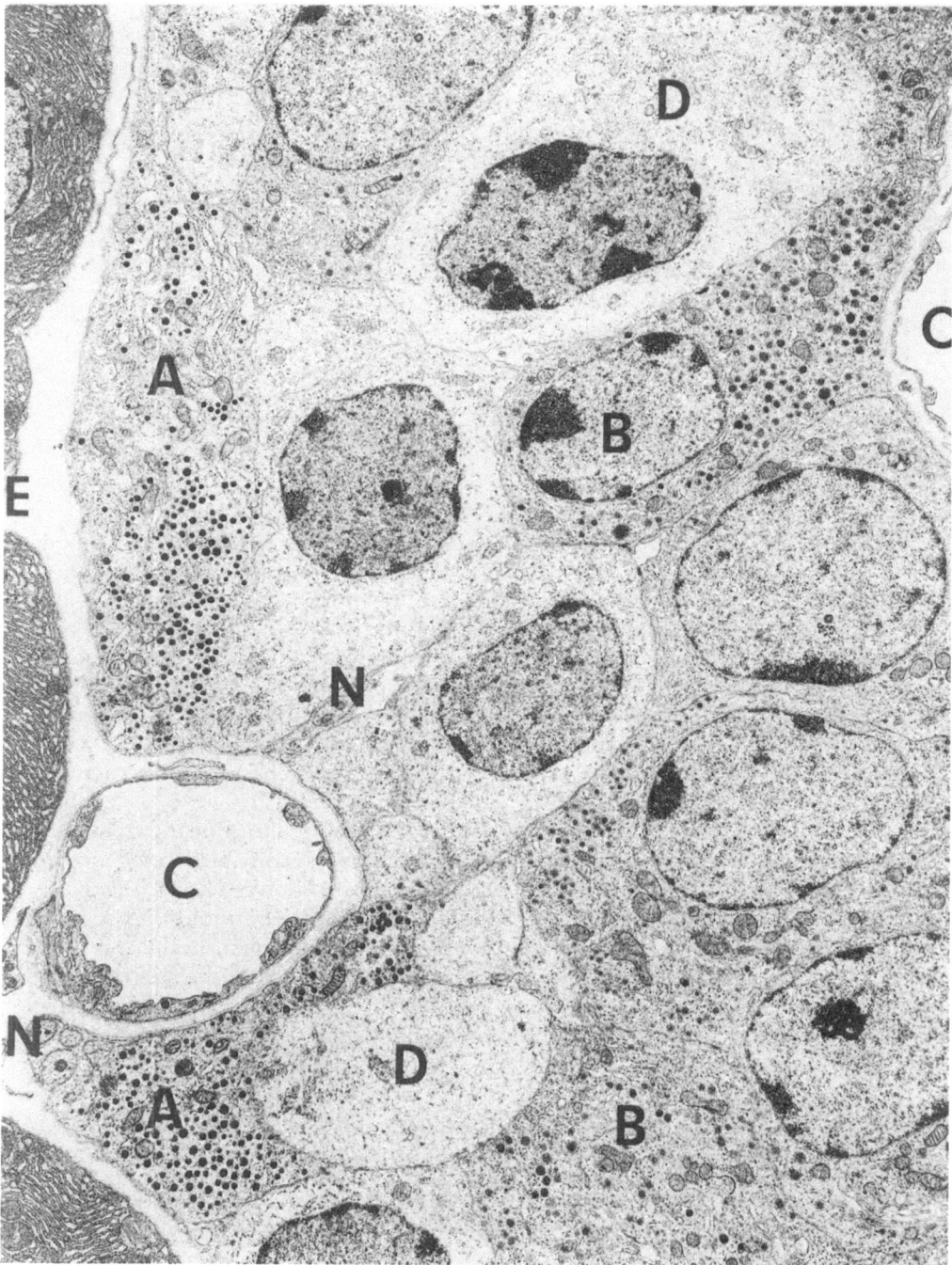

Figure 1. Survey of peripheral portion of pancreatic islet of normal Mongolian gerbil showing peripheral A cells (A), central B cells (B), and D cells (D) with an intermediate position and only faintly visible granules. Capillaries (C), nervous elements (N), and exocrine parenchyma (E) are also seen. ×3000. Reproduced at 90%.

The D cells have been suggested to represent resting B cells,[6] morphologically altered but viable A cells,[7] or stages in the secretory cycle of B and A cells.[8] After a review of the subject, Fujita[9] concluded that the D cell is a separate cell type and a normal constituent of the endocrine pancreas of vertebrates from elasmobranchs to mammals.

Mixed or intermediate cells have frequently been described in the endocrine pancreas of different species, e.g., transitional forms between A and D cells and between B and D cells.[6] Exocrine–endocrine and ductular–endocrine cells have also been reported, e.g., in the pancreas of genetically obese rats with hypertrophic islets.[10] Melmed *et al.*[11] suggested a widespread occurrence of cells intermediate between those of exocrine and endocrine type, serving as a source of insulin additional or alternative to that provided by the genuine endocrine cells.

A C cell, devoid of secretory granules, was recorded in the early electron microscopic studies of the guinea pig pancreas,[2,12,13] whereas no such cells could be disclosed in this species in later ultrastructural investigations.[5] The C cells in the endocrine pancreas of the guinea pig reported by earlier investigators obviously represent D cells.[9]

Cells lacking secretory granules have been identified in some species also in later ultrastructural investigations. Thus, so-called agranular cells, presumed to represent precursors to the granulated cells,[14] occur at a high frequency in lower vertebrates and in the human fetus[15] and at a lower frequency in rodents[16] (Fig. 2). In addition to agranular cells, there are sparsely granulated parenchymal cells, which may represent a stage in the development from agranular to granulated parenchymal cell types. In the Chinese hamster, agranular (clear) cells and/or sparsely granulated cells have been recorded both among nondiabetic animals[17] and among animals with experimental[18] or spontaneous[19,20] diabetes. Similar cells also occur in neonatal rabbits.[21]

Other cells with sparse granulation may represent cells which have been degranulated as a result of excessive hormone release and/or partial or total inhibition of hormone storage. Such seemingly degranulated cells of B type are often encountered in animals with experimental or spontaneous diabetes (Fig. 3). In contrast to the agranular cells, the degranulated cells often exhibit a prominent endoplasmic reticulum and Golgi complex, suggesting a high functional activity.

Furthermore, there are occasional reports of other cell types without any clarified functional role. An E cell possessing large (400 to 500 μm) secretory granules is described in the opossum.[22] F cells, showing kidney-shaped, U-shaped, triangular, rectangular, or rounded secretory granules, occur in the uncinate portion of the dog pancreas.[22] G cells, showing granules of different shape and electron density without any halo, and S cells (small granule cells) are present in the horse.[23] Type II enterochromaffin cells, identical to those of the rat intestine, are observed in the endocrine pancreas of the rabbit,[24] and endocrine cells of types III, IV, and V are present in the toad pancreas.[25] In rodent species there are occasional reports of up to eight different islet parenchymal cell types[3] which, however, have not been verified in other studies of those species. Still other cell types have also been reported.

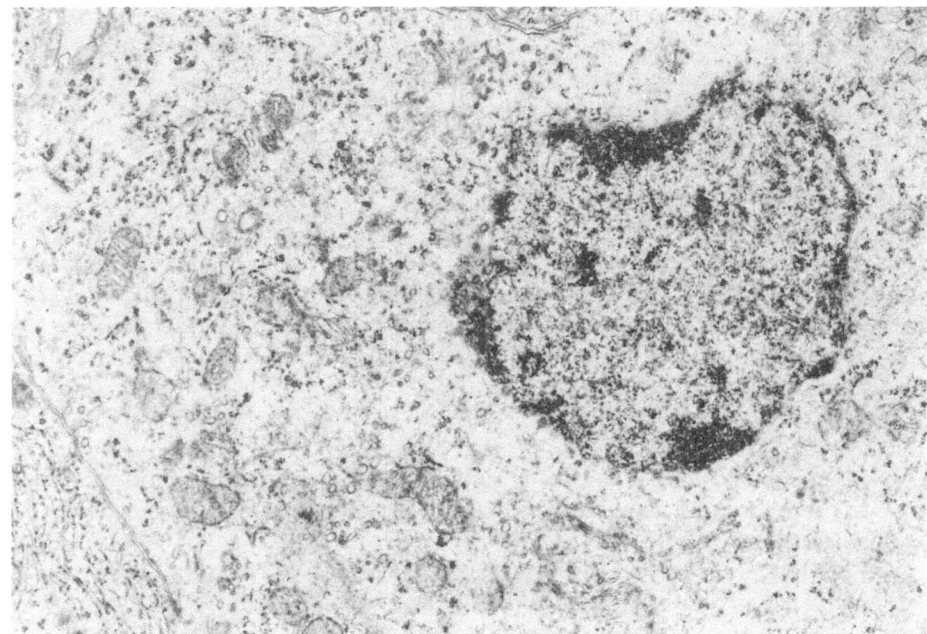

Figure 2. Portion of agranular cell in pancreatic islet of normal Chinese hamster exhibiting rather low cytoplasmic electron density, a small Golgi complex, mitochondria, and free ribosomes. ×7000. Reproduced at 85%.

Islet cell differentiation begins already during the fetal period in rabbits,[21] mice,[26,27] rat,[28-30] and man.[31,32] Pictet and Rutter[33] maintain that the A cells appear about 3 days earlier than the B cells in mouse and rat fetuses, and that the former cells may be precursors to the latter.

Vascular Supply and Innervation of the Islets; Some Ultrastructural and Histochemical Characteristics

The islets possess a great number of capillaries (Fig. 1) composed of fenestrated endothelial cells. Between the endothelium and the parenchymal cells there are two basement membranes, one associated with the endothelial cells and the other associated with the vascular surface of the endocrine cells. Ultrastructural investigation using horseradish peroxidase shows that the fenestrated endothelium has a high permeability.[34]

Whereas histochemical and ultrastructural studies have disclosed neural elements in the endocrine pancreas of most species, opinions differ as to the presence of an innervation of the pancreatic islets of birds. A close correlation exists in various species between peripheral nerve fibers and A, B, and D cells (Fig. 1). The nerves are usually ensheathed by nonmyelinating Schwann cells, and the nerve terminals lack synaptic specializations.[35] In dog islets there are structurally modified Schwann cells which contain cytoplasmic processes encompassing large portions of endocrine parenchyma, and which may play a role in the neural control of islet function.[36] Neural elements in juxtaposition to islet cells are sometimes designated "neuroinsular complexes" (complexe neuro-insulaire).

The neural elements can be differentiated into cholinergic, mainly containing electron-lucent (agranular) vesicles, and adrenergic, mainly exhibiting electron-lucent vesicles with dense cores. A distribution of the adrenergic innervation to smooth muscles of arteries and a mixed cholinergic–adrenergic distribution to the parenchymal cells are found in the cat.[37]

The functional role of the innervation of the pancreatic islets is not elucidated. However, stimulation of the parasympathetic nerve system causes insulin secretion, and stimulation of the sympathetic system inhibits insulin secretion, whereas the opposite responses are found for glucagon.[38,39]

Structures believed to represent dystrophic nerve terminals have been recorded in alloxan-treated rats, indicating that alloxan may induce autonomic nerve ending changes in the endocrine pancreas of this species.[40] An absence of nerve fibers characterizes the islets of spiny mice, which may be related to the insulin secretory defect of those animals.[41]

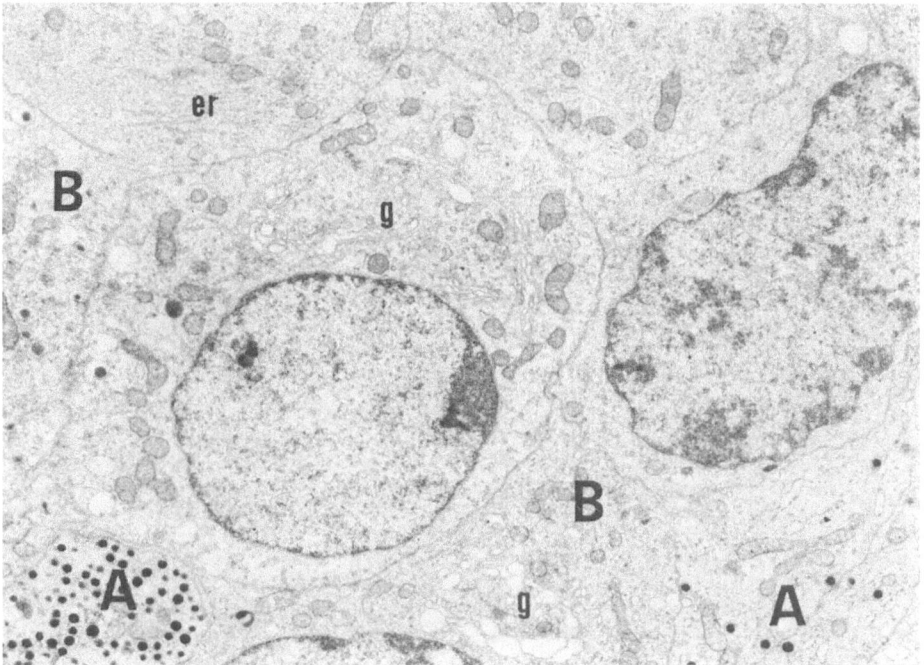

Figure 3. Pancreatic islet of diabetic Chinese hamster showing A cells (A) with dense secretory granules, and degranulated B cells (B) with prominent Golgi complexes (g), lamellar endoplasmic reticulum (er), and few or no secretory granules. ×5000. Reproduced at 85%.

B Cells

Ultrastructural Characteristics of the B Cells

The fine structural appearance of the B cells varies somewhat in different species, and there are structural variations depending upon the technique used for fixation, tissue preparation, and staining. Since it is not the aim of this chapter to give a presentation of all these variations, the description below will mainly, although not exclusively, be concerned with structural features common to the B cells of most species when applying current techniques for electron microscopy.

Generally, the B cells possess rounded or oval nuclei with a moderately distinct nucleolus. The chromatin is finely dispersed and the nuclear membranes and pores are easily discerned. The electron density of the cytoplasm varies; most often it is moderately dense (Fig. 4). Occasionally, B cells with a low and those with a high density can be seen in one and the same islet. The cause of this difference in cytoplasmic density is not clearly known, but it may be of functional significance.

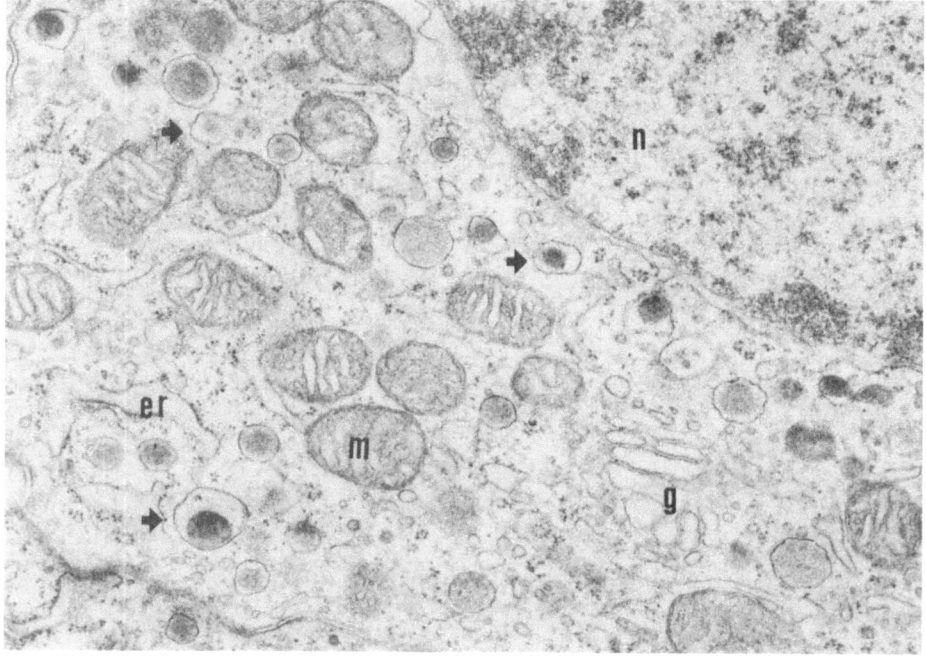

Figure 4. Portion of B cell of normal mouse (C57BL-KsJ-+/+) showing a moderate cytoplasmic density, Golgi complex (g), mitochondria (m), endoplasmic reticulum (er), nucleus (n), and secretory granules (arrows) of varying size and density. ×15,000. Reproduced at 85%.

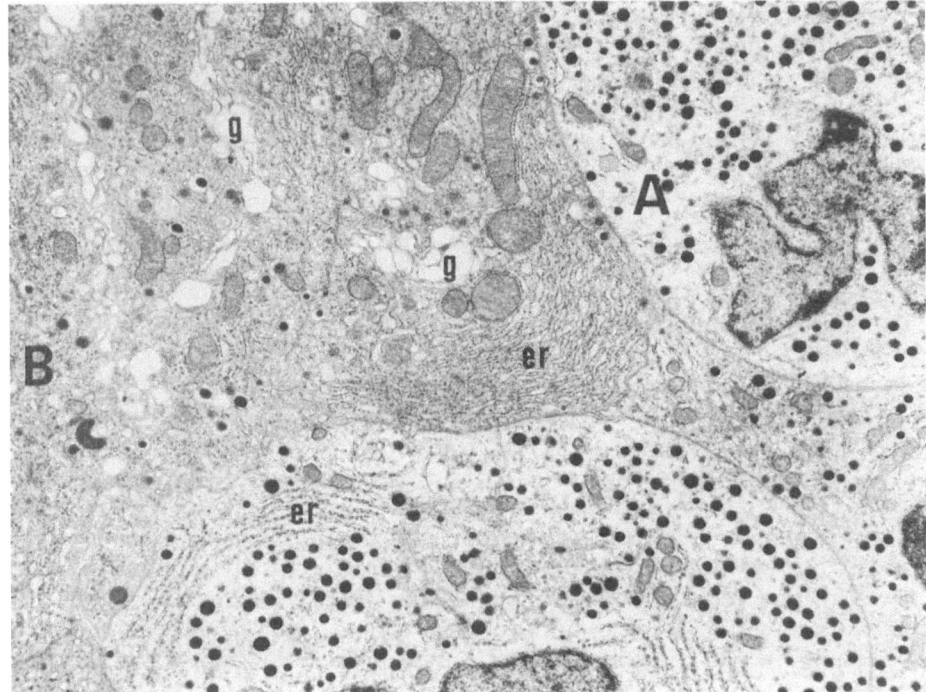

Figure 5. Islet of diabetic mouse (C57BL-6J-*db/db*) showing B cells (B) and A cells (A) with typical secretory granules, and prominent Golgi complexes (g) and endoplasmic reticulum (er). ×6000. Reproduced at 85%.

The endoplasmic reticulum is of rough type and exhibits a vesicular or lamellar appearance. At high synthetic activity the endoplasmic reticulum is prominent, lamellar (Fig. 5), and occasionally whorled, whereas it is less conspicuous at low synthetic activity. Free ribosomes occur in the cytoplasm. The Golgi complex is composed of cisterns, vesicles, and vacuoles and is expanded at high functional activity and small at low activity.

The mitochondria are usually medium-sized, rounded, oval, or elongated and possess a moderate number of mainly transverse cristae. The inner mitochondrial compartment exhibits a moderate electron density. The number of mitochondria varies in different cells, probably reflecting differences in functional activity; usually a moderate number of mitochondria are encountered. Small intramitochondrial granules of high density are seldom observed.

Lipoid bodies occur in the cytoplasm. They are usually rounded and moderately electron dense. Lysosomal bodies of varying appearance are also present. Microtubules can be identified in the cytoplasm; only rather seldom are they seen in obvious contact with secretory granules. In the B cells of rats, microtubules have been reported to extend in all directions from the outer nuclear membrane to the plasma membrane.[42]

A cell web is present in the B cells, consisting of a layer of short interconnected filaments, 40 to 70 Å in diameter, situated close to the plasma membrane.[43] By a combination of immunofluorescent and electron-microscopic techniques, actin is demonstrated in the cytoplasm of isolated, cultivated islet cells, suggesting that this protein is a component of the cytoplasmic web.[44] The area which the cell web occupies is virtually free from cytoplasmic structures with the exception of granules undergoing extrusion, pinocytotic vesicles, and ribosomes.[43]

The cell membranes are easily distinguished, and the cellular outline is rather smooth with occasional indentations, bulbous projections, and microvilli. Time-lapse cinematography of monolayer cultures shows that the addition of the ionophore A 23187 causes active membrane ruffling and surface expansion, as well as cytoplasmic vacuolization of the islet cells.[45]

Desmosomes occur on opposed cell membranes, but tight junctions (zonulae occludentes) are not observed at routine electron microscopy, which has been suggested to be consistent with the rapid access of the reaction product after administration of horseradish peroxidase to sand rats, and to explain the almost immediate response of the B cells to metabolic and pharmacologic agents.[34] However, tight junctions can be ultrastructurally demonstrated on freeze-fracture replicas of B cells.[46] These junctions are normally only sparsely occurring, but they are highly developed after exposure of the islet cells to proteolysis by low concentrations of either pronase or pancreatic protease, suggesting the induction of a drifting of preexisting particles to specific regions on the cell membrane or a new formation of particles at specific sites.[46,47]

Freeze-fracture technique splits the B cell membrane, like other membranes, and exposes its inner structure and reveals the gap junctions (nexuses).[48] In studies of other tissues, the gap junctions are ascribed a role as low-resistance pathways in the cell-to-cell transfer of ions, metabolites, and other possible types of signal molecules, and the same may hold true for the gap junctions occurring in the islets.[48]

A surface coat, presumably representing a polysaccharide–protein complex, is revealed on the B cells of islets stained with ruthenium red or Alcian blue; it may play a role in the control of the interaction between the cell and its external environment.[46]

The main distinguishing structural feature of the B cells is represented by the secretory granules, which show considerable species variation in morphological appearance. Variation may also be recorded among the secretory granules of single B cells of the same islet. The structural variations may be due to differences in the chemical or physical form of insulin.[7,13] In rodent species, the secretory granules are characteristically rounded, whereas they are rectangular, square, hexagonal, and irregular or rounded in humans.[7]

Generally, the β granules are composed of a central core, usually of moderate, homogeneous, or slightly heterogeneous electron density, and an external single-layered membrane with a rather large space between the core and the membrane (Fig. 4). Compared with the α granules, the β granules possess less electron-dense and more heterogeneous cores and a larger clear space between the core and the membrane. In comparison with the δ granules, the β granules exhibit more electron-dense and more heterogeneous cores and a larger clear space. The β granules are usually diffusely distributed in the cytoplasm. Signs of formation of secretory granules are occasionally observed in the Golgi region.

Both in the fetal[32] and adult human pancreas, the β granules are either dark or pale; presumably the latter predominate in conditions with a rapid turnover of insulin.[4] Dark and pale granules are also present in the rabbit,[49] even in the fetal and neonatal periods.[21,50] In this species an increased number of pale granules is found after experimental B cell stimulation.[50-52] An increase in the volume and number of light granules is also found in pregnant rats.[53] It has been proposed that the light granules are responsible for the immediate release of insulin, while the dark ones represent the insulin reserve.[54]

In many species the β granules possess a periodical substructure, suggesting a crystalloid nature. Possibly such periodicity is present in the β granules of all species and represents a crystalline storage form of insulin[7,55,56] or precursor or breakdown forms of dark β granules,[57] or perhaps it depends in some way on the process of tissue preparation.[58]

Apart from β granules with a crystalline substructure, there are reports of those with a fibrillar appearance. Thus, fibrillar subunits, often in parallel arrangement, are found among the β granules of the teleost fish *Scorpaena scropha*[59] (Fig. 6). Fibrils associated with the granule core are suggested to originate from the surrounding membrane and to be subsequently packed to form granules,[8] or to interact in the development of immature granules into mature ones.[60]

In addition to the well-known and more or less generally appearing organelles described above, other structures are occasionally encountered in the B cells, some with a completely unknown significance. Thus, annulate lamellae are recorded in the B cell cytoplasm of chick embryos[61] and in the endocrine cells of the islet organ of the hagfish *(Myxine glutinosa)*[62] (Fig. 7) which in many respects represents the most primitive of all vertebrate species. Annulate lamellae have, so far, not been reported in the endocrine pancreas of other species. The occurrence of these organelles in the chick embryo is consistent with the view that they are of transitory nature and are common to many different kinds of cells during the early embryonic differentiation,[61] and their presence in the islet organ of the hagfish is probably related to the high phylogenetic age of this species.[62]

The islet organ of the hagfish also exhibits crystalline inclusions in cisterns of rough endoplasmic reticulum[62] (Fig. 7). They are probably of proteinaceous nature and show a close association to the annulate lamellae, which may denote a functional relationship. Some cisterns of rough endoplasmic reticulum with such inclusions are in contact with the perinuclear space, suggesting a possible role of the nucleus in the development or possible function of the crystalline inclusions, similar to that believed to exist between nuclei and annulate lamellae in many tissues.

So-called multiple rough endoplasmic reticulum cisterns have been recorded in the different islet cells of the adult rat, believed to be normal constituents, and play a role in the secretory activity.[63] These cisterns possess

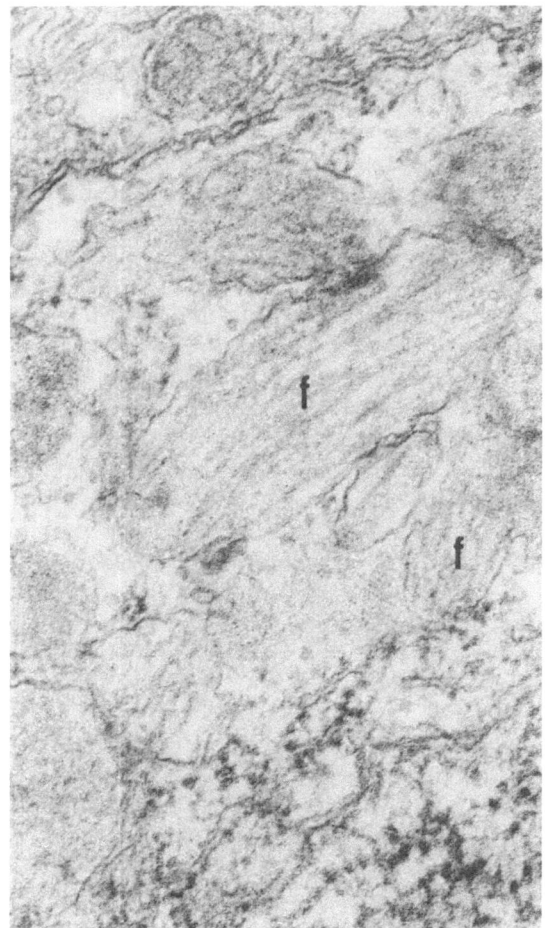

Figure 6. Portion of two B cells of teleost fish *Scorpaena scropha* showing secretory granules composed of fibrillar subunits (f). ×21,000.

ribosomes on the outermost, but not on the inner membranes, and are separated by narrow electron-lucent spaces of uniform width.

Bodies with a periodical substructure, without any direct association to secretory granules, occur in the cytoplasm and nuclei of the islet parenchymal cells of rodent species. Thus, tubular bodies are present in the B cell cytoplasm of rabbits,[64] Chinese hamsters,[65] and mice and are possibly derived from mitochondria.[66] Similar bodies are present in the B cells of mice treated with vinblastine *in vivo*, believed to be associated with the binding of vinblastine to microtubular protein.[67]

Rod-shaped structures composed of parallel fibrillar or tubular elements occur also in the nuclei of B cells of Mongolian gerbils[65] and obese-hyperglycemic mice and their lean litter mates[68] and in the A and B cells of the normal rabbit, rat, hedgehog, pig,[69] and ground squirrel.[70]

Signs of centriole replication are seen in the ductule cells of newborn rodents,[71] and cilia, usually of 9 + 2 or 9 + 0 type, are present in the islets of different species. In the Mongolian gerbil, the cilia are often swollen and contain heterogeneous vesicular particles (Fig. 8), possibly representing secretory material.[72] Cilia in endocrine cells may be chemo-receptors, have sensory of motile abilities, be nonfunctioning rudimentary structures, or play some role in cell division.

Histochemistry of the B Cells: Demonstration of Insulin

The B cells are characteristically stained by aldehyde fuchsin[73–75] (Fig. 9), probably due to interaction with sulfonic acid groups formed by the splitting of the disulfide bonds of the insulin molecule produced at preliminary oxidation with permanganate.[76] A correlation has been reported between the aldehyde

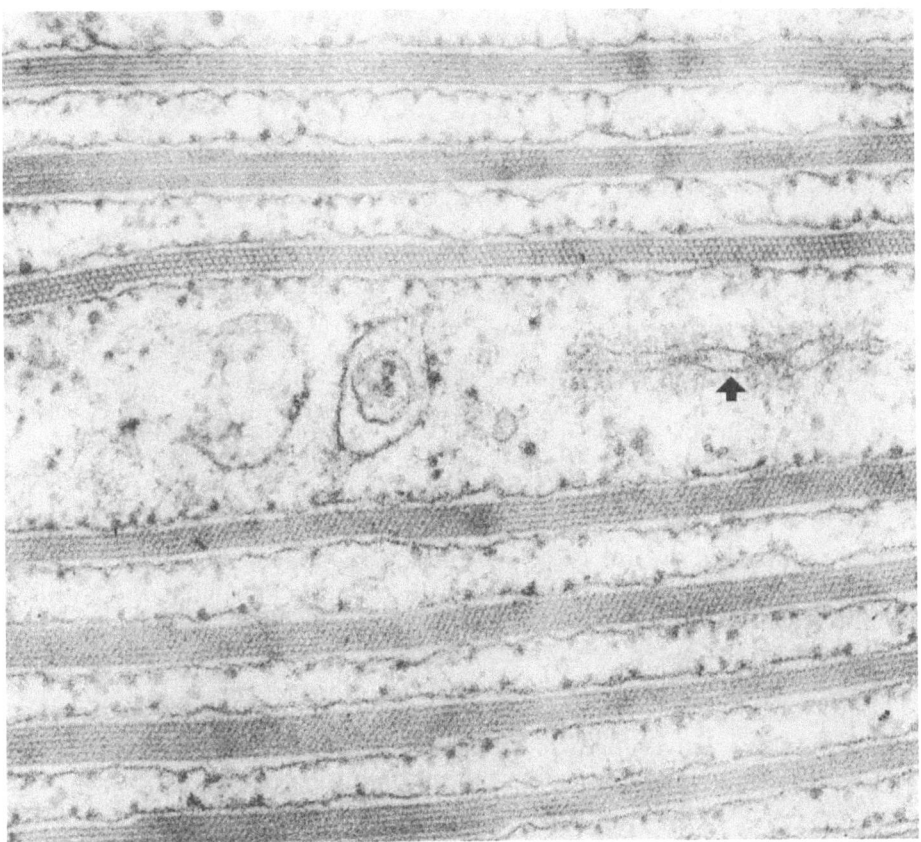

Figure 7. Cytoplasm of B cell from hagfish *Myxine glutinosa* showing lamellar cisterns of rough endoplasmic reticulum with crystalline inclusions, and annulate lamellae (arrow). ×40,000.

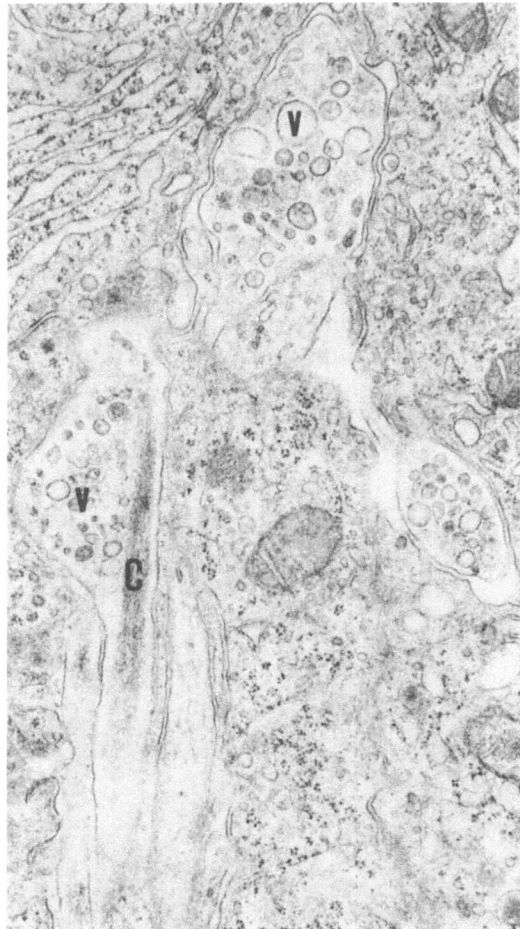

Figure 8. Intercellular area in B cell region of normal Mongolian gerbil showing swollen cilia (C) containing vesicular particles (v) of varying size and configuration. ×8000.

fuchsin staining and the number of β granules, and the intensity of this staining has been used as a histochemical index of the content of insulin in the B cells.[77] Pseudoisocyanin also visualizes insulin in oxidized pancreatic sections. It gives a metachromasia attributed to sulfonic acid groups in the oxidized A chain of the insulin molecule.[78]

Opinions differ about the specificity of aldehyde fuchsin and pseudoisocyanin staining. A positive aldehyde fuchsin reaction is suggested to be given only by proteins with few closely neighboring sulfonic acid groups, as in the A chain of insulin.[79] However, Lange[80] proposed that aldehyde fuchsin binds to other groups in addition to sulfonic acid residues and that it is not entirely specific for B cells. Several reports indicate that aldehyde fuchsin binds to the β granule membrane rather than to the supposedly hormone-containing granule

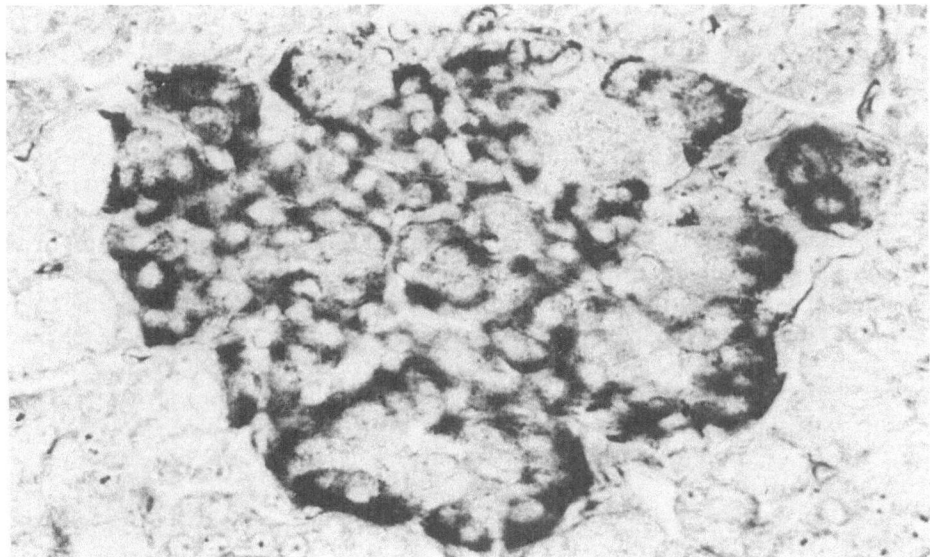

Figure 9. Aldehyde fuchsin staining of pancreatic islet from normal guinea pig showing positive reaction in the B cells which are seen both centrally and peripherally. ×400. Reproduced at 110%.

core.[81–84] On the other hand, experimental studies show that insulin has an affinity for both aldehyde fuchsin[85] and pseudoisocyanin,[78,86] and aldehyde fuchsin has been stated to be specific for insulin fixed in polyacrylamide gel by disc electrophoresis, although it is not sufficiently sensitive to detect normal serum levels of the hormone.[87] Blocking of the aldehyde fuchsin staining is possible by methylation, by acetylation, and by treating the sections with alcohols at high temperature in the presence of hydrochloric acid.[81]

A strong metachromatic reaction, believed to be due to interaction with sulfonic acid groups, is obtained in pancreatic sections treated with potassium permanganate.[88] Furthermore, the B cells can be demonstrated by a performic acid–colloidal iron reaction dependent upon oxidation of the insulin molecule with performic acid and the formation of sulfonic acid groups, thereby forming the basis for the reaction with colloidal iron.[89] It is also possible to detect disulfide groups of insulin by a histochemical method for demonstration of protein-bound sulfhydryl and disulfide groups in tissue sections.[90] The specificity of this method is somewhat limited since other sulfur-containing polypeptides are also demonstrated.[91]

In addition, the B cells are demonstrated more or less specifically by chrome hematoxylin, toluidine blue O,[88] Victoria Blue,[92] and crotonaldehyde diaminobenzophenone.[93] B cells treated with trypsin exhibit a strong basophilia, which is attributed to the formation of carboxylic end groups in the hydrolyzed insulin molecule.[94] Insulin[52,95] and proinsulin[96] can be detected in the B cells also by immunofluorescent techniques.

Insulin can be identified in rodent[97−99] and human[100] fetuses already during the fetal period by histochemical, biochemical, and immunofluorescent techniques.

Correlation of Morphology, Histochemistry, and Function of the B Cells

The first step in the production of insulin is represented by the synthesis of (preproinsulin? and) proinsulin in the rough endoplasmic reticulum, from which the proinsulin is transported to the Golgi complex, either through direct intracisternal communications or through vesicles pinched off from the endoplasmic reticulum. The conversion of proinsulin to insulin probably takes place in the Golgi complex by removal of the C peptide through interaction of a proteolytic enzyme which seems to be present in the membranes of the Golgi complex.[101,102] Coated vesicles, present in the Golgi area, may transfer enzyme(s) to immature secretory granules for conversion of proinsulin to insulin.[45]

After the conversion to insulin, the hormone is stored in the secretory granules which apparently originate from the Golgi complex. However, a direct formation of secretory granules from the endoplasmic reticulum has also been suggested.[103,104] The sequence of insulin synthesis and storage described above has been verified by electron-microscopic autoradiography showing that radioactively labeled amino acids at 5 to 10 min are localized to the endoplasmic reticulum, at 20 to 45 min mainly to the Golgi complex, and at 60 min to the secretory granules.[105] By correlation of the degree of B cell granulation with the content of insulin in the pancreas, evidence has been obtained that insulin is stored in the granules,[106] and localization of insulin to the β granules has been demonstrated by electron-microscopic immunohistochemistry.[107]

In addition to insulin, the secretory granules contain zinc, and apparently insulin is stored as a zinc–insulin complex in the granules.[108] 5-Hydroxytryptamine has been demonstrated in the β granules of guinea pigs by electron microscopy,[109] and the extramitochondrial SH-dependent ATPase of the B cells is probably associated with the secretory granules.[110] The contents of the clear space between the core and the membrane of the β granules are not clearly known.

The B cells secrete insulin in response to adequate stimuli. The release of stored hormone occurs through emiocytosis (Fig. 10), which means a fusion of the granule membrane with the plasma membrane after which the contents of the granule are delivered extracellularly and dissolved. Pentalaminar fusions have been observed to connect the plasma and granule membranes, and the solubilization and release of insulin have been proposed to be preceded by the formation of permeable membrane junctions.[111]

Signs of emiocytosis are rather seldom encountered in standard transmission electron micrographs of the B cells from most species but are reported to be frequent in genetically obese rats,[10] and the recognition of the process of emiocytosis may be facilitated with the aid of horseradish peroxidase.[112] Scan-

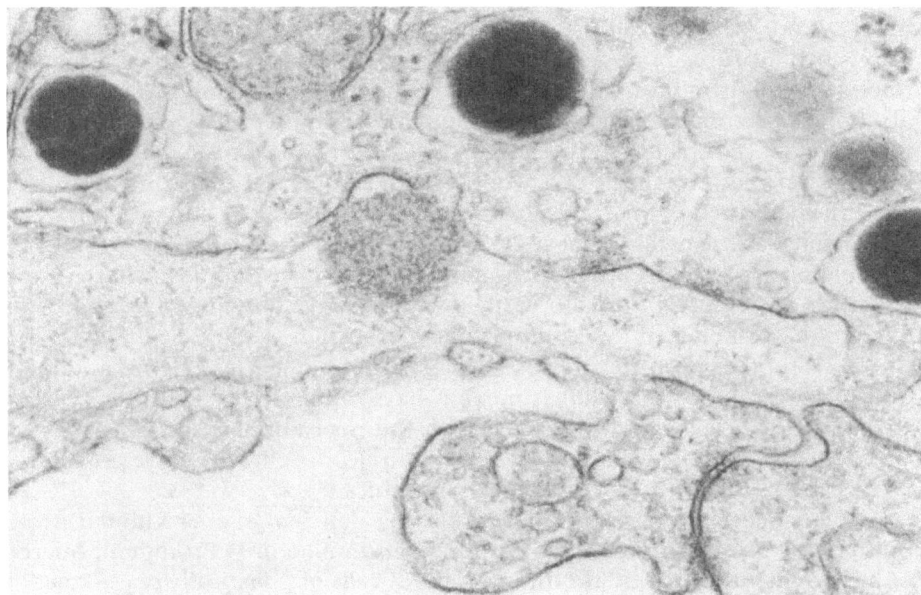

Figure 10. Emiocytosis in B cell from a newborn rodent (from Boquist, L.: *Diabetes,* **21**:1051, 1972). ×42,000. Reproduced at 110%.

ning electron microscopy of isolated islets shows cytoplasmic projections on the surface of the B cells, believed to be associated with emiocytosis,[113] and surface blebs and irregularities increase in number on the B cells during glucose stimulation with associated elevation of the serum insulin level.[114]

The view of a role of emiocytosis in insulin secretion does not eliminate the possibility that the hormone may be released by other means under certain conditions. Thus, newly formed insulin may be directly released without any storage stage, possibly representing basal insulin secretion,[115] and in the presence of sustained hyperglycemia.[116] Occasionally, discontinuities are found in the membranes of the β granules, through which intracytoplasmic release of hormone has been suggested to take place.[117] Moreover, there may be an intracytoplasmic dissolution of preformed secretory granules followed by an efflux of dissolved insulin.[118,119] Such dissolution may be an active process, since it can be blocked by diazoxide.[120] Isolated β granules exposed to glucose or other insulin secretagogues, or subjected to pH 4.0 and 6.0, are not disintegrated, whereas those subjected to sodium deoxycholate or pH 4.0 and 8.5 are solubilized, which has been interpreted to indicate that intracellular solubilization of the granules with subsequent diffusion of insulin into the extracellular space is not a likely mode of insulin secretion *in vivo*.[121]

Before emiocytosis occurs, the secretory granules must be transported to the cell membrane, possibly through interaction of the microtubular–microfilament system of the B cells,[122,123] which seems to represent a single, synergistically working functional system.[124] Agents which destroy (colchicine, vinblastine, and vincristine) or stabilize (deuterium oxide, hexylene glycol, and ethyl alcohol) microtubules inhibit glucose- or tolbutamide-induced release of insulin,[122,125] and colchicine induces structural alterations and a reduction of the number of microtubules.[126] Lacy and Greider[127] believe that some β granules are attached to the microtubular–microfilament system and are ready for immediate release after a transport to the cell surface elicited by a contraction or a change in the physical conformation of the microtubules, whereas other granules are free in the cytoplasm and attached subsequently. This would explain the presence of two compartments of insulin in the B cells. The role of the microtubules in insulin release has been questioned by Ericson and Lundquist[67] who advocate that vinblastine may have other effects on insulin secretion than those which may be associated with the microtubular system. Moreover, the secretory response evoked by sulfonylureas does not require an oriented intracellular transport of the secretory granules.[128]

Spiny mice with spontaneous diabetes are deficient in microtubular protein and release insulin only slowly after glucose stimulation.[46] Prominent microtubules, on the other hand, are found in the B cells of genetically obese rats.[10]

The contraction or the change in the physical conformation of the microtubular–microfilament system is suggested to be triggered by calcium,[124] since this cation is required for insulin release.

Cytochalasin B, which in other tissues causes disruption of the microfilamentous cell web beneath the plasma membrane,[129] potentiates glucose- and tolbutamide-induced insulin secretion,[43,130] suggesting that the cell web may represent a barrier to the rate of insulin release; under the influence of cytochalasin B this barrier would be destroyed, resulting in an increased rapidity of insulin release.[43] Van Obberghen *et al.*[131] believe that cytochalasin B-sensitive microfilamentous structures provide an exocytotic release of β granules.

Since the concept of emiocytosis involves a continuous addition of membranous substances to the plasma membrane of the B cells, continued release of insulin by this process would lead to an increase in the volume of the plasma membrane and possibly to a depletion of membranous substances in the cytoplasm. This could be counteracted either by recycling or degradation of the membranes of the secretory granules after completed emiocytosis.[46] Recycling would mean that membranous substances are pinched off after emiocytosis and returned as microvesicles to the cytoplasm. Evidence for the existence of such recycling in the B cells is obtained using horseradish peroxidase as an extracellular marker.[132]

Those granules which are not released from the B cells may undergo intracellular lysosomal digestion.[45,55] This is evident in rats in which the release of insulin has been blocked by diazoxide.[120] A similar process with an increased occurrence of lysosomes is observed in the A cells of Chinese hamsters[133] and spiny mice with spontaneous diabetes, as well as in rats with streptozotocin-induced diabetes.[134]

Some Ultrastructural and Histochemical B Cell Changes in Experimental and Spontaneous Diabetes

It is not the purpose of this chapter to give detailed information about electron microscopic and histochemical alterations in the B cells under pathological conditions. However, a few examples of such alterations will be given. The selective damaging action of alloxan upon the B cells of most species is very well known. It is also well known that streptozotocin has a damaging effect upon the B cells of most species, which is less selective than that of alloxan, in that A cell damage occasionally appears in addition to B cell necrosis.[135] Freeze-etching technique demonstrates that both alloxan and streptozotocin produce a reduction in the number of particles in the plasma membrane and a rearrangement of the individual particles already at a time when no structural change can be detected in the B cells by conventional electron microscopy,[136] suggesting an effect of these compounds upon the plasma membrane.

Cortisone also causes structural changes among the B cells; degranulation occurs in rabbits after administration of subsequent small doses of cortisone,[49,137] but regranulation follows within a few days after cessation of the cortisone treatment.[49,138] Cortisone treatment may induce B cell hyperplasia and hyperglycemia in rabbits[79] and Chinese hamsters[139,140] and an increase in the islet activity of isocitric dehydrogenase in both diabetic and nondiabetic patients, whereas the activity of this enzyme is decreased in the islets of nontreated diabetics.[141]

In spontaneous diabetes various structural changes have been reported in the islets of different species. Mice with mutation diabetes[142-147] exhibit necrosis of the B cells and a decline of the serum insulin level; the severely diabetic phase is associated with inhibited growth or loss of body weight, and B cell atrophy. Chinese hamsters with spontaneous diabetes show degranulation, glycogen infiltration, degeneration, necrosis, and atrophy of the B cells, and in early stages occasionally lymphocytic infiltration (Fig. 11). An increased number of nuclear pores in the A cells of diabetic Chinese hamsters points to alterations in the membrane systems associated with diabetes.[148]

Enlarged mitochondria (Fig. 12), occasionally of giant size, are present in the B cells of diabetic Wellesley hybrid, Swiss-Hauschka,[149,150] and diabetic mutant mice.[142] Increased mitochondrial volume and an associated enhanced activity of the mitochondrial marker enzyme L-3-hydroxyacyl-CoA-dehydrogenase are found in isolated mouse islets cultured at low glucose concentration compared with islets cultured at high glucose.[151]

The course and outcome of many diabetic syndromes may depend upon the ability of the organism to produce new B cells. New formation of endocrine cells from pancreatic ducts takes place in fetuses, and also in rodent species neonatally.[71] A similar process may be encountered in adult animals.[18] The intraislet ducts observed in mice with mutation diabetes[142,146] (Fig. 13) have been reported to form the basis for a new formation of endocrine cells,[144] although Like and Chick[147] find no evidence for an association between these ducts and neoformation of islet cells. Central cavitation of unknown signifi-

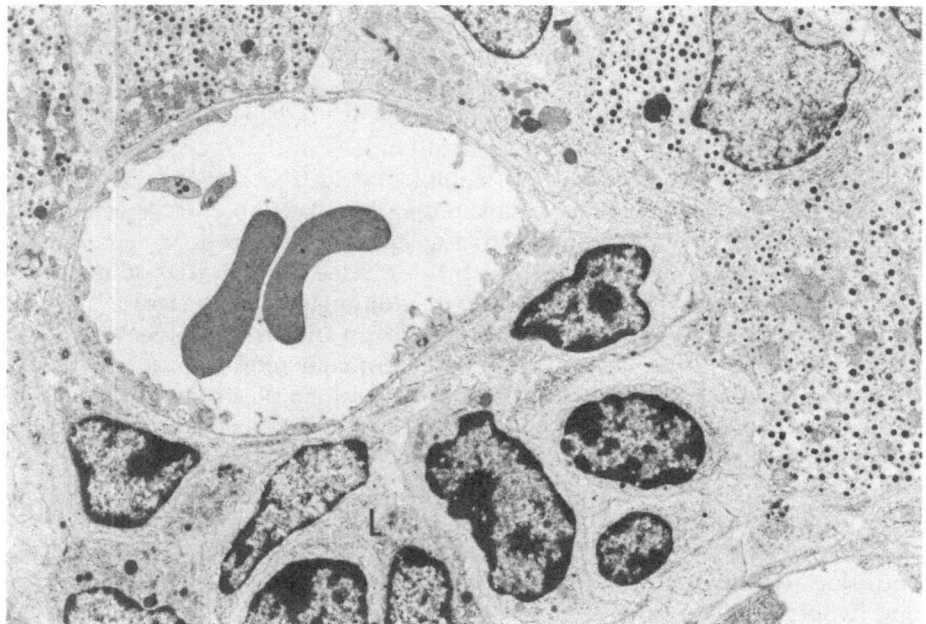

Figure 11. Area of pancreatic islet of Chinese hamster with spontaneous diabetes of short duration showing lymphocytic infiltration (L) close to a capillary. ×2500. Reproduced at 85%.

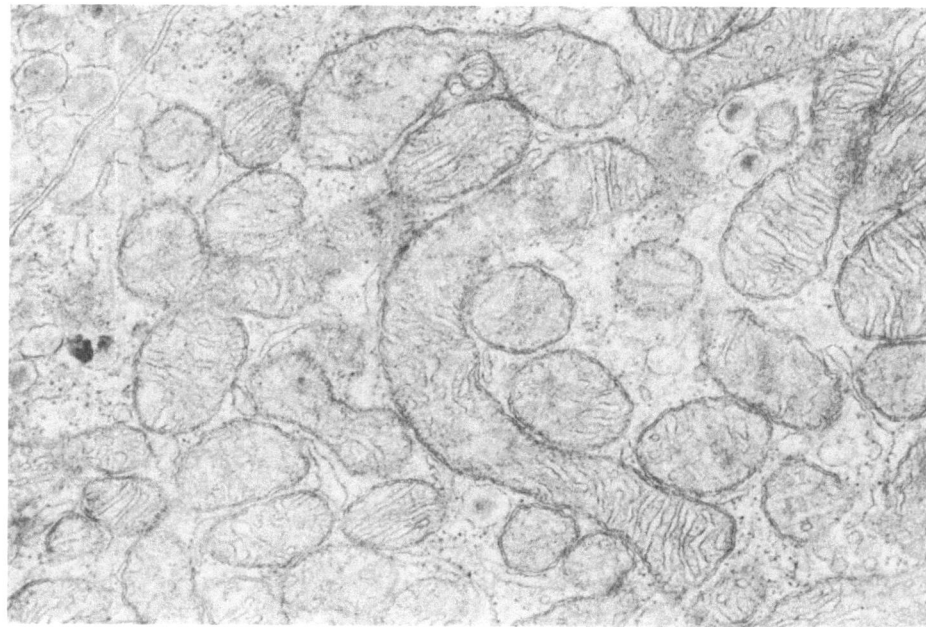

Figure 12. Portion of B cell from diabetic mouse (C57BL-KsJ-*db/db*) showing a great number of rather large mitochondria and some secretory granules. ×12,000. Reproduced at 85%.

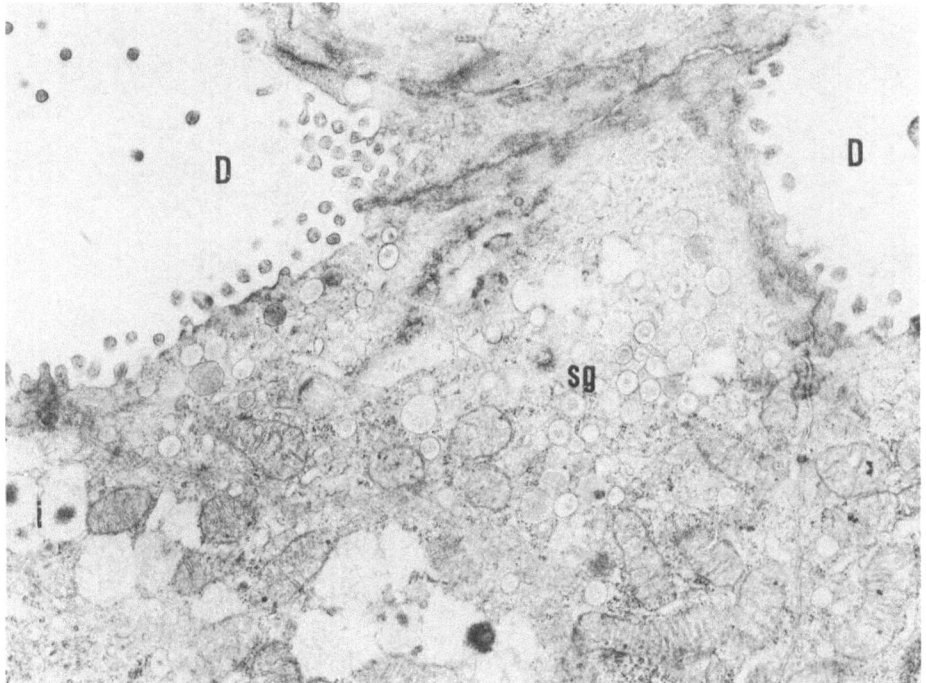

Figure 13. Pancreatic islet of diabetic mouse (C57BL-KsJ-*db/db*) demonstrating intraislet ducts (D) lined by epithelial cells possessing microvilli and secretory granules of varying size and configuration; some are endocrine-like (sg), others resemble those of intestinal epithelium (i). ×8500. Reproduced at 85%.

cance, somewhat similar to the intraislet ducts, is present in hyperplastic islets of obese-hyperglycemic mice,[152] diabetic Toronto-KK mice,[153] and in the islet organ of *Myxine glutinosa*.[154]

New formation of islet cells by mitotic division occurs in embryos and neonates[71] whereas the mitotic activity is low under normal conditions in most species, even after a 12-hr mitotic block with colchicine.[33] However, mitotic activity may be readily observed among the islet parenchymal cells in the adult period under pathological and experimental conditions, e.g., in genetically diabetic mice,[155] Mongolian gerbils with obesity and islet hyperplasia[156] (Fig. 14), rats with experimental diabetes,[157] and in association with hepatic injury in man.[158,159] A considerable proliferative capacity, leading to B cell hyperplasia, may be induced in some rodent species by continuous glucose stimulation. This is the case in *ob/ob* mice,[152] KK mice,[160] C57BL-6J-*db/db* mice,[142] genetically obese rats (Zucker-"fatty"),[10] and obese Mongolian gerbils.[156] B cell hyperplasia is also induced in rats treated with trypsin inhibitor, cholecystokinin–pancreozymin, or raw soybeans.[161] The maintenance of the animals under laboratory conditions with free access to laboratory diet and limited possibility for motion probably plays a prominent role in the development of islet hyperplasia and

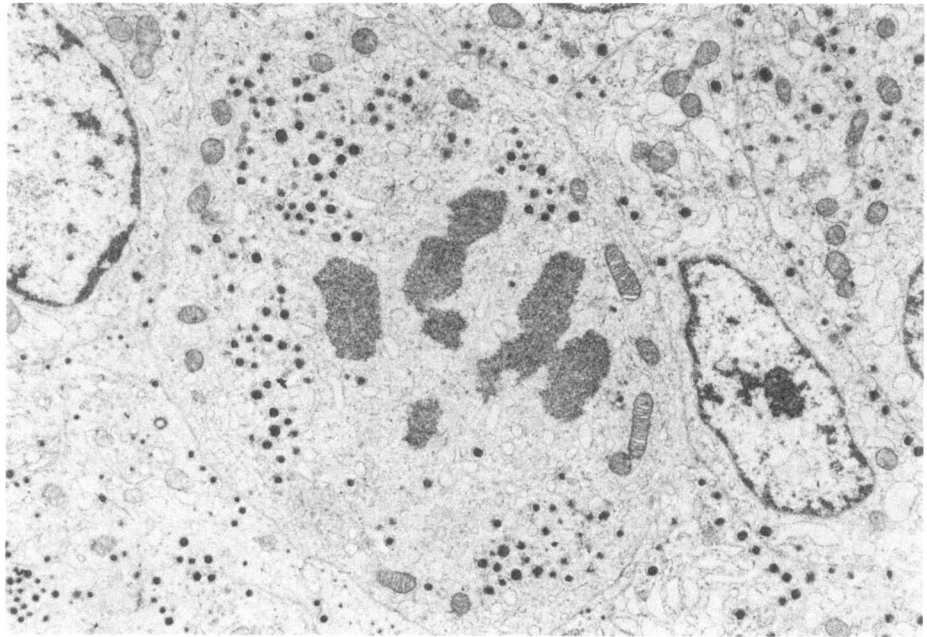

Figure 14. Hyperplastic pancreatic islet from obese Mongolian gerbil exhibiting mitosis in one B cell. ×6000. Reproduced at 85%.

obesity; the hyperplasia may reflect a compensatory adaptation to an increased demand of insulin associated with the obesity.

Occasionally, the regenerative capacity is high enough to cause development of tumor-like (adenomatous) islets.[156,162,163] Congenital hyperplasia of the endocrine pancreas is found in spiny mice *(Acomys cahirinus),*[164] whereas absence of neoformation of B cells may play a role in the development of spontaneous diabetes in the Chinese hamster,[165] in which the disease may be a manifestation of a genetically defined defect of B cell replication.[166] An exhaustion of a primarily existing capacity for new formation of islet cells is recorded in rats developing diabetes 40 to 60 days after subtotal pancreatectomy.[167]

A Cells

Ultrastructural Characteristics of the A (α₂) Cells

The glucagon-producing A cells are in most species situated peripherally in the islets (Fig. 1). However, in some species, e.g., man and guinea pig, they are diffusely distributed in the islet parenchyma, and in the horse they are localized to the central portion.[23,168] In the duct there are separate (dark) islets composed of A and D cells, and other (light) islets containing B and some D cells.[169,170] The main distinguishing feature of the A cells is represented by their secretory granules, which possess a rounded core of high density and a closely applied membrane with only a small clear space between the core and the membrane (Figs. 3 and 5). The number of secretory granules in the A cells is usually high, and the granules are diffusely distributed in the cytoplasm. The details of the other organelles and the nucleus are essentially similar to those of the B cells and, therefore, no further description will be given of these cellular components. The cytoplasm usually exhibits a moderate or low electron density.

The release of hormone from the A cells is suggested to occur by emiocytosis.[171,172] An intracytoplasmic dissolution of α granules with subsequent discharge of the hormonal product without any emiocytosis has also been ascribed a role in the process of glucagon release.[173] An A cell microtubular–microfilamentous system may be involved in glucagon secretion.[174]

Histochemistry of the A (α₂) Cells

Glucagon is demonstrated by fluorescent antibody technique in the beef pancreas,[175] and study of separate samples of A cells on one hand and of D cells on the other, microdissected from freeze-dried sections of guinea pig and horse pancreas, disclosed that only the A cells contain immunoreactive glucagon.[176] Indirect evidence for the production of glucagon by the A cells is obtained by the finding that these cells are virtually absent from the uncinate portion of the dog pancreas[177] which contains little or no glucagon-like activity.[178] Furthermore, glucagon administration to rats and guinea pigs causes an involution of the A cells, which exhibit a reduction in number[179] and nuclear size.[180,181]

Since glucagon, but not insulin, possesses a high content of tryptophan,[182] the postcoupled benzylidene reaction[183] has been used for detection of proteins rich in tryptophan, notably glucagon; the reaction is positive among the A cells of rodent species.[177,181,184] The xanthydrol and *o*-phthalaldehyde methods have been stated to be specific histochemical tests for glucagon.[185]

The A cells are impregnated with silver when applying Grimelius'[186] method (Fig. 15). Ultrastructural modification of this method discloses silver grains localized to the halo of the granules (Fig. 16),[187–189] which does not react with antiglucagon antibodies or phosphotungstic acid, in contrast to the core which shows no silver grains but a positive reaction to antiglucagon antibodies and phosphotungstic acid and which seems to represent glucagon.[185]

D Cells

Ultrastructural Characteristics of the D (α₁) Cells

The D cells are either diffusely distributed or in most species localized to the periphery of the islets, occasionally interposed between the peripheral A cells and the central B cells (Fig. 1). They possess rather large secretory granules with a rounded core of low or moderate density and a closely applied membrane (Fig. 17), usually occurring in great number, diffusely distributed in

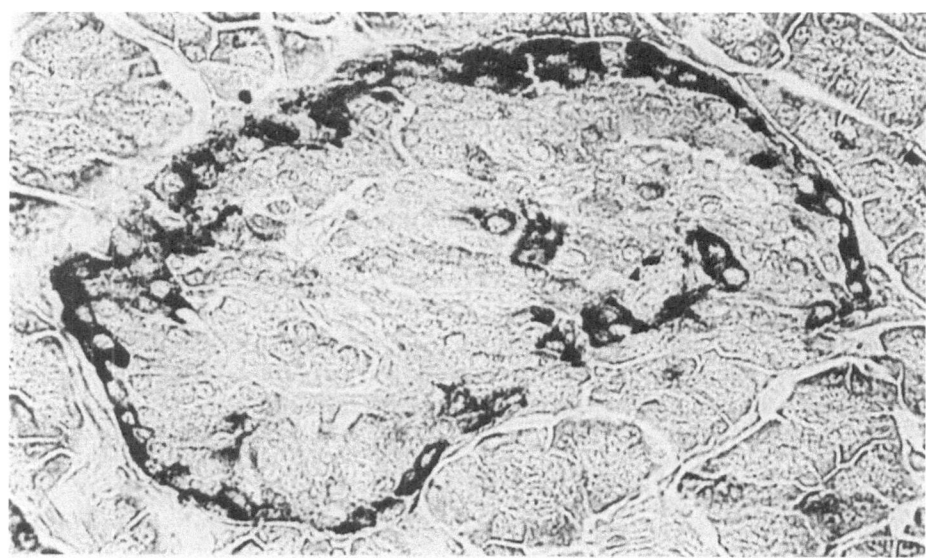

Figure 15. Silver impregnation according to Grimelius showing positive reaction in the peripheral A cells of a normal Chinese hamster islet. ×350. Reproduced at 110%.

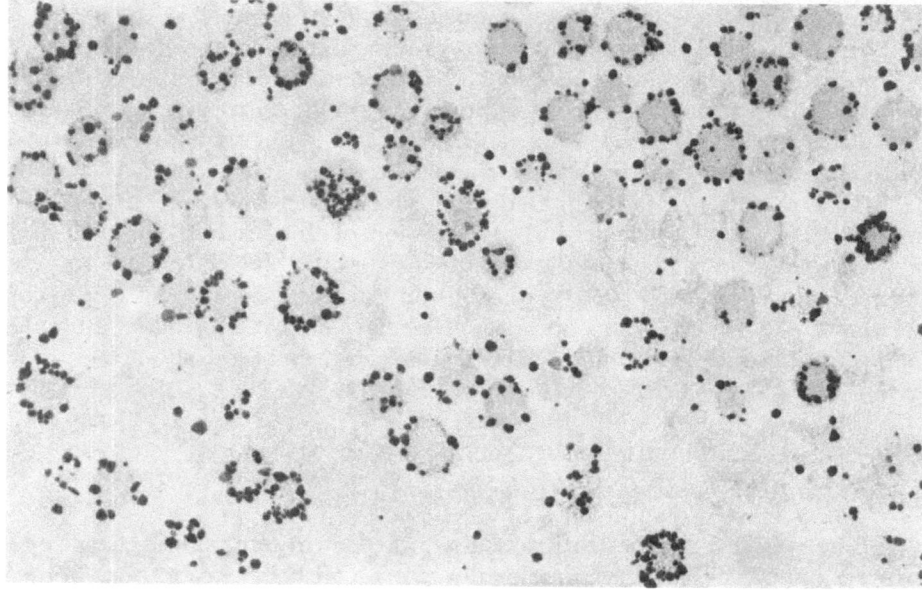

Figure 16. Ultrastructural modification of Grimelius' silver impregnation showing dense precipitates, mainly localized to the halo and the periphery of the core of the secretory granules in an A cell of a normal Chinese hamster. ×12,000. Reproduced at 110%.

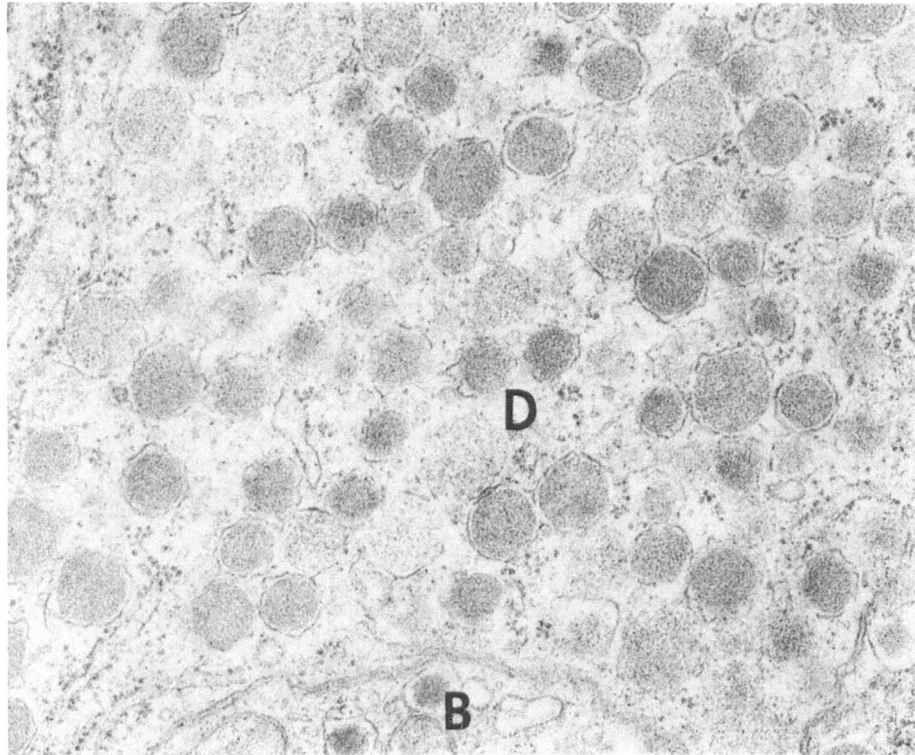

Figure 17. Portion of one B cell (B) and one D cell (D) of Mongolian gerbil. The secretory granules of the D cell are rather large and possess finely granular cores of low to moderate density and rather closely applied membranes. ×15,000. Reproduced at 85%.

the cytoplasm. The other organelles and the nucleus are structurally essentially similar to those of the B and A cells, and, therefore, no further description of them will be given. The cytoplasmic ground substance exhibits a low or moderate density.

Stimulated D cell function is reported after treatment with compounds which damage the B cells and induce experimental diabetes, e.g., alloxan,[85,190] streptozotocin,[191] and steroids.[192] Islets rich in D and A cells, with a predominance of the latter type, have been isolated from guinea pigs treated with streptozotocin.[193]

Histochemistry of the D (α_1) Cells

The D cells stain metachromatically with toluidine blue at pH 5 in tissue fixed with Bouin's fluid.[194,195] No such staining is obtained after methylation, or below pH 4.5, but alkaline demethylation restores the metachromatic reaction.[196] The D (α_1) cells differ from other islet cells in being impregnated with the modified Davenport silver.[197] Ultrastructural modifications of this technique disclose small silver grains associated with the secretory granules of the D (α_1) cells, localized to the interior portion or covering the whole granule.[188,198] The D cells of the duck show strong staining reactions for acid phosphatase and leucyl β-naphthylamide-splitting enzymes.[170]

With the aid of fluorescent antibodies against gastrin, a positive reaction is obtained in some species in peripheral cells believed to represent D cells,[199,200] and the D cells of the human pancreas also show immunochemical and radioimmunological signs of gastrin content, allegedly indicating that these cells would synthesize and store gastrin.[201] In guinea pigs injected with gastrin, no gastrin reaction could be found in any of the parenchymal cells.[202] The human D cells (and also other non-B cells) have been suggested to be the cell of origin of ulcerogenic tumors of the pancreas (Zollinger–Ellison syndrome). These tumors seem to originate from islet cells, but their light-microscopic staining characteristics[201] and ultrastructural appearance[203] are different from those of the D, B, and A cells, and the cellular origin of the neoplasms has not yet been clarified.

Using immunofluorescent techniques, somatostatin has been disclosed in the D cells of various species.[204–208] Somatostatin has also been localized to cells believed to represent D cells of rats by electron-microscopic immunocytochemistry.[209] This tetradecapeptide exerts an inhibitory effect on glucagon and insulin secretion, so far investigated in rat,[210–213] dog,[214,215] baboon,[216] and man.[212,214]

General Histochemistry of the Islets

The presentation given below, including that dealing with enzyme histochemistry, represents no complete review of the histochemistry of the pancreatic islets. More information and further references are given in other works.[79,80,217–223] Attention will be paid to zinc, calcium, glycogen, and biogenic amines which play an essential, although not completely clarified, role in the physiology and/or pathology of the islets.

Zinc

Heavy metals, including zinc, have repeatedly been demonstrated in the islets of many species, using histochemical techniques on the light-microscopic level. A histochemical method for demonstration of heavy metals was described by Okamoto,[224] based upon a complex binding of zinc ions with diphenylthiocarbazone (dithizone) modified by the utilization of a complex-forming buffer solution masking the reaction with metals other than zinc.[225] The sulfide silver method for histochemical demonstration of heavy metals is also employed for the detection of zinc in the islets[226] (Fig. 18). Control experiments should be used since the specificity of the sulfide silver technique is limited.[227] Ultrastructural modifications exist both of the dithizone[228] and the sulfide silver

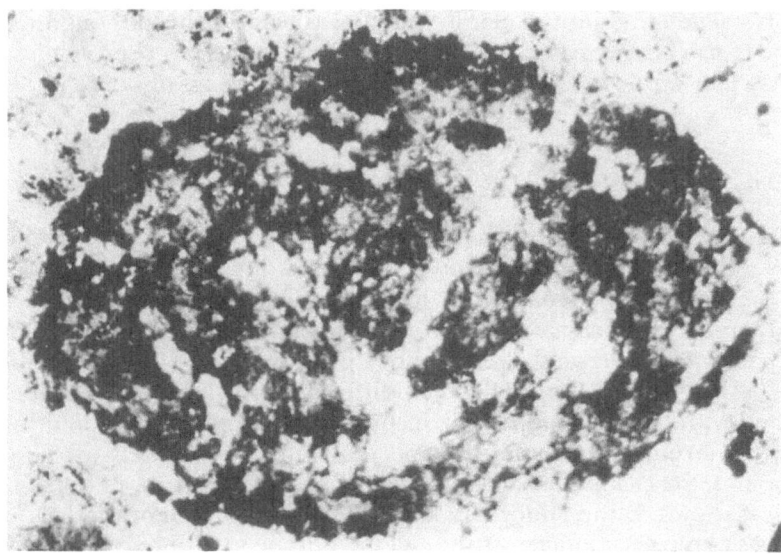

Figure 18. Pancreatic islet treated with sulfide silver for localization of heavy metals showing positive reaction both in the central B cells and in the peripheral D and A cells of a normal Mongolian gerbil. ×400.

method.[229] A fluorescent technique using 2-methyl-8-hydroxyquinoline is also used for identification of zinc.[230]

Histochemically detectable zinc occurs in the islets of most species, including man. However, in a few species, e.g., the guinea pig, only traces of zinc, or no zinc at all, can be recorded. The cellular distribution of zinc shows considerable species variations.[231–234] Electron microscopy demonstrates zinc localized to the β granules of the Chinese hamster,[17] rabbit,[235] dog, cat, and rat.[236] The granules close to the Golgi complex have been reported to contain less zinc than those situated at some distance from the Golgi area.[237]

Functionally, there is a close relationship between zinc and insulin. Zinc is believed to play a role in the storage of insulin.[60,124,231,238,240] Crystalline insulin contains zinc which is chemically bound to the insulin,[241] and X-ray analysis shows that rhombohedral zinc–insulin crystals are composed of two zinc ions and six insulin molecules.[242] It is, however, not known whether this holds true also for the zinc–insulin complexes presumed to exist in the β granules.

The content of zinc in the B cells seems to be related to their functional state; zinc is mobilized in association with insulin secretion,[234] and is almost lacking in degranulated B cells.[239] The islet content of zinc is also decreased and the glucose tolerance is impaired in Chinese hamsters fed a zinc-deficient diet.[238] The content of zinc decreases in the islets after alloxan administration.[243,244] Findings in genetically diabetic yellow KK mice indicate that zinc may play a role in the conversion of pale granules into dark ones.[54] An experimental diabetes can be induced in rabbits by injection of dithizone, which binds zinc.[245]

Crystalline glucagon generally contains traces of zinc, although this metal does not form an integral part of the crystals,[182] and it has been suggested that zinc may play a role in the synthesis, storage, and release of both glucagon and insulin.[246]

Calcium

Calcium can be demonstrated in the islets by light microscopy using the GBHA [glyoxal bis(2-hydroxyanyl)] reaction, and electron microscopically using the potassium pyroantimonate technique and X-ray elemental analysis (Figs. 19 and 20). Herman *et al.*[247] found pyroantimonate precipitates localized to the cell membrane and the secretory granules of the B cells in mice and rabbits. Schäfer and Klöppel[248] noted differences in calcium distribution demonstrated with the pyroantimonate technique in normo-, hypo-, and hyperglycemia; in normoglycemia the deposits were mainly localized to the granule membranes, the cell membranes, and the cytoplasmic matrix; in hyperglycemia there was a shift to the endoplasmic reticulum and the mitochondria, whereas there was a translocation across the cell membrane to its inner surface and into

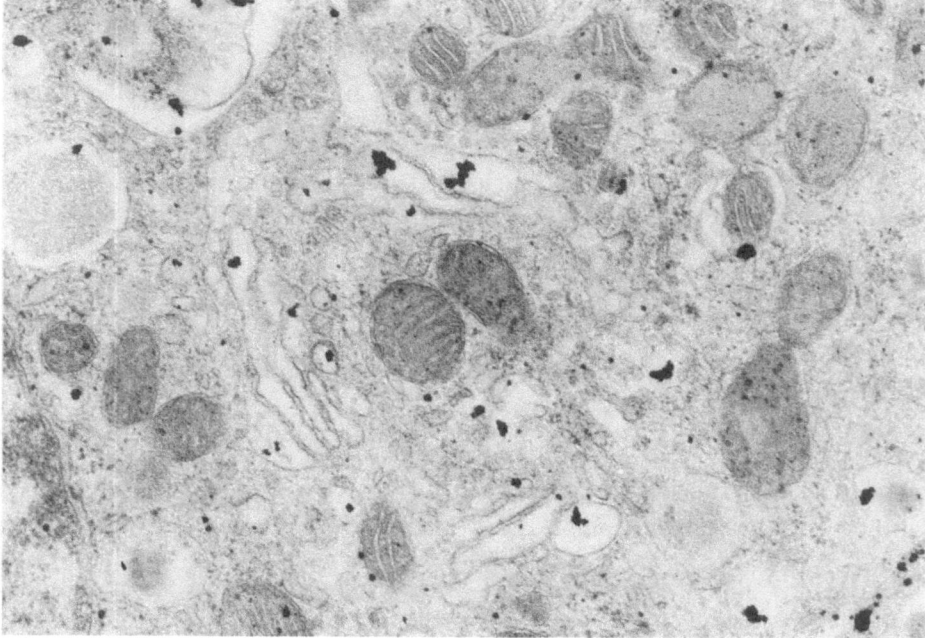

Figure 19. B cell from normal mouse (C57BL-KsJ-+/+) subjected to pyroantimonate fixation for ultrastructural demonstration of cations showing electron-dense precipitates in Golgi cisterns, halos of secretory granules, and mitochondria. X-ray elemental analysis has shown that this precipitation contained calcium. ×19,000. Reproduced at 85%.

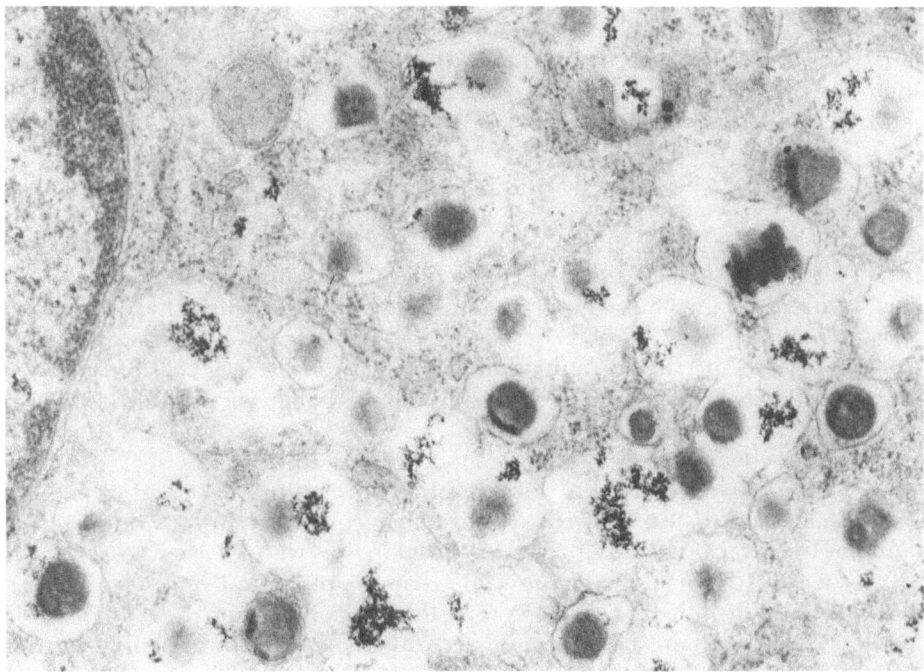

Figure 20. Another B cell from normal mouse (C57BL-KsJ-+/+) subjected to pyroantimonate fixation demonstrating electron-dense precipitate, mainly localized to the halo of the secretory granules. X-ray elemental analysis has shown that this precipitation contained calcium. ×20,000. Reproduced at 85%.

the halos of the secretory granules in hyperglycemia. X-ray microanalysis of areas in frozen sections of unfixed rat islets discloses the highest concentrations of calcium in the secretory granules and mitochondria of the B cells; accumulation of $^{45}Ca^{2+}$ by isolated organelles studied in homogenates and isolated subcellular fractions indicates that the B cells contain readily exchangeable pools of calcium mainly in the mitochondria but also in the endoplasmic reticulum.[249]

Calcium is well known to be essential for the secretion of insulin, and this cation is thought to be involved in the contraction or the change in the physical conformation of the microtubular–microfilament system of the B cells.[124] Study of isolated secretory vesicles by freeze-cleavage technique shows that calcium causes an aggregation of membrane-associated particles and a fusion of vesicles, suggesting that this cation may act as a final intracellular trigger in stimulus–secretion coupling.[250]

The ionophore A 23187 facilitates the movement of Ca^{2+} across the cell membrane and in the direction of the diffusion gradient for the ion. Experiments with this ionophore disclose that calcium, in the absence of stimulators of insulin release, can induce high rates of sustained insulin secretion from the B cells.[45] Using the potassium pyroantimonate technique and X-ray elemental analysis, differences in the intracellular distribution of calcium have been demonstrated in the presence and absence of the ionophore A 23187 (Boquist and Hellman, unpublished).

Glycogen

Glycogen is normally present in the B cells, although the stores are small[251-253] and usually not detected by light-microscopic techniques, and the islet content of enzymes for glycogen metabolism is richer than that of the exocrine pancreas.[254] A good correlation is reported between the activity of the phosphorylase and the accumulation of glycogen in the islet cells of the guinea pig,[255] and between the degree of degranulation and glycogen infiltration in the B cells of the cat.[256]

Increased amounts of glycogen occur in diabetic states.[252,257-259] Toreson[260] found glycogen in the B cells both of human diabetics and rabbits with experimental diabetes induced by alloxan or cortisone administration; in the animals the glycogen was regularly observed in cells with light-microscopic signs of so-called hydropic degeneration. Electron-microscopically, glycogen infiltration may be a prominent feature in the islets of diabetic animals,[116,261,262] and in diabetic Chinese hamsters glycogen accumulation is found not only in the B cells,[19,20,148,263,264] but also reportedly in the A and D cells of a few animals which have been diabetic for almost 1 year before development of ketonuria.[265]

Opinions differ about the physiological role of glycogen in the B cells. Hellman and Idahl[252] believe that glycogen is essential for the action of agents which have an effect upon the concentration of cyclic 3':5' AMP. Glycogenolysis represents one way in which glucose-6-phosphate can be formed in the islets, and there is a good correlation between the glycogen content of the B cells and the glucose concentration to which they are exposed.[251,252]

The significance of glycogen infiltration in experimental and spontaneous diabetes is not clearly known, but it is obviously associated with an abnormal glucose and glycogen metabolism. The glycogen deposited in diabetes may be secondary to hypoinsulinism[257] or hyperglycemia,[256,266] or it may be the result of an increased insulin production associated with beginning insufficiency.[267] Gepts[268] maintains that glycogen infiltration in diabetic states always is a secondary alteration, and Warren[269] reports that significant amounts of glycogen were found in the islets of diabetics mainly before the era of insulin treatment.

Biogenic Amines

The fluorescence obtained at exposure of freeze-dried sections to formaldehyde vapors indicates that the B cells contain a tryptamine derivative, apparently 5-hydroxytryptamine (5-HT).[270] These cells also contain dopamine (DA) and monoamine oxidase (MAO),[271] and the precursors of 5-HT and DA are taken up by the B cells and are decarboxylated.[271-273]

Species differences exist in the type of cell possessing the monoamines and in the type of monoamine. In the guinea pig all islet cells are fluorescent after intraperitoneal injection of the biogenic amine precursor L-dopa.[271] A positive reaction for MAO is obtained in the B cells, and a negative reaction is observed in the A cells of rat, guinea pig, cat, rabbit, and man.[274]

Ultrastructurally, the monoamines are localized to the secretory granules.[109,275] Electron-microscopic autoradiography discloses that 5-HT, formed from injected precursors, is localized to the secretory granules of the A and B cells, whereas no autoradiographic reaction is obtained over the D cells; the absence of a reaction product in the D cells may indicate that monoamines are not formed in these cells, or that they possess a storage mechanism for mono-amines different from that of the A and B cells.[276]

The role of the biogenic amines in the islets is not known, but they have been suggested to play a role in the synthesis, storage, or release of insu-lin.[39,275,277-279] A correlation has been reported between MAO and zinc in the islets,[274] and MAO inhibitors have been found to alter insulin secretion by decreasing the monoamine degradation in the B cells.[280]

Enzyme Histochemistry of the Islets

Enzymes Active in Glucose Metabolism

The metabolism of glucose in the B cells is of great importance since it is known that the ambient glucose concentration regulates the synthesis and release of insulin. However, so far it is not known whether this regulation is achieved by the glucose molecule itself or by some of its metabolites. After its entrance into the cell, the glucose molecule is phosphorylated to glucose-6-phosphate by adenosine triphosphate (ATP) in the presence of hexokinase and magnesium. The islets possess a higher capacity for phosphorylation of glucose than either the exocrine pancreas or the liver.[281] In the B cells of normal[282] and obese-hyperglycemic[258] mice two varieties of hexokinase have been identified; one with a low and another with a high Michaelis–Menten constant (K_m) value for glucose. In the rat some authors have found only a low K_m islet hexoki-nase,[253] whereas others have identified also a high K_m hexokinase.[283]

Different fates are available for the glucose-6-phosphate produced in the B cells. The islets are well equipped with enzymes for glucose degradation. The enzymes of the glycolytic pathway, which predominates in the glucose utiliza-tion of the B cells, have been studied in different species using staining histochemistry[221,285-288] and quantitative microtechniques.[141,254,289-293] These enzymes exhibit higher activity in the islets than in the exocrine pancreas, with the exception of lactate dehydrogenase, in rat, obese and hyperglycemic New Zealand mice, rabbit, and man.[281,290,291,294,295] As to lactate dehydrogenase, the islets of obese-hyperglycemic mice possess a high percentage of M subunits, suggesting that their B cells are well equipped for anaerobic glucose metabolism.[222] The activity of glucose-6-phosphatase in the B cells is inhibited by glucose[282,296] and is increased in association with cellular hyperfunction.[296] The islets are well equipped for a glycolytic formation of ATP; the associated enzymes are more richly represented in the islets than in the acinar parenchyma in mice[297] and man.[219]

The high activity of glucose-6-phosphate dehydrogenase (G-6-PD) observed in the B cells suggests an active role of the phosphogluconate pathway (pentose phosphate shunt).[79] This enzyme is demonstrated in the B cells by staining histochemistry[221,284,287,298-300] and by direct measurements on islets.[290-291,301] The kinetics of islet G-6-PD have been studied in cryostat sections[302] and islet homogenates.[303] The G-6-PD activity is markedly decreased in spontaneous diabetes[304] and after alloxan administration.[110,305]

Assays of 6-phosphogluconate carried out on isolated islets[301,306] lend further support to the existence of an active phosphogluconate pathway in the B cells. The supply of triosephosphates from the phosphogluconate pathway to the glycolytic pathway may be limited since transketolase and transaldolase activities are low.[297]

Hydrolysis of glucose-6-phosphate which is achieved by glucose-6-phosphatase (G-6-Pase), has been demonstrated in the islets of several species by staining histochemistry.[284-286,288,300] The G-5-Pase of the islets possesses properties similar to those of the specific G-6-Pase of liver.[293,307] The activity of islet G-6-Pase is inhibited by glucose.[296] Ultrastructural investigations in rabbits show that the G-6-Pase activity is limited to the inner surface of the lamellar endoplasmic reticulum and the nuclear membranes, indicating a role of the enzyme in insulin synthesis.[308] The amount of G-6-Pase available for cell metabolism may be a limiting factor controlling the rate of insulin release.[79] An increased activity of G-6-Pase has been recorded in hyperfunctioning B cells[296] and in the B cells of diabetic KK mice.[309]

Enzymes Active in the Utilization of Amino Acids, Nucleotides, and Lipids

The free amino acid pool in the B cells is suggested to be partly regulated by protein catabolism[222] because of rather high activities of peptidase observed in mouse islets.[310,311] A prominent role of transamination processes is also proposed since there are high activities of glutamate–oxaloacetate transaminase and glutamate–pyruvate transaminase in the islets of different species.[222] Hellerström and Brolin,[297] however, have reported a rather low activity of glutamate–pyruvate transaminase.

Histochemical staining shows extramitochondrial ATP-splitting activity in the B cell cytoplasm of rabbits, disappearing during degranulation.[83,110]

ATP-splitting enzyme activity is also present in mouse islet homogenates,[312,313] and the B cells of rats show a strong staining reaction for AMP-splitting enzyme activity.[284] Histochemical staining[284] and determination on islet homogenates[314] disclose that this activity is enhanced by cortisone.

Light and electron microscopy have revealed inosine diphosphate- and pyrophosphate-splitting enzymes in the Golgi area of the B cells.[315] Three different enzymes acting on inosine diphosphate have been demonstrated, tentatively identified as alkaline phosphatase, thiamine pyrophosphatase, and Golgi-associated nucleoside diphosphatase.[316] Glutathione reductase is high in the islets, which may be of significance for the NADP$^+$/NADPH turnover.[297] The NADP$^+$/NADPH-converting enzymes in the islets of New Zealand obese mice exhibit activities suggesting a rapid turnover of the islet NADP$^+$/NADPH pool.[317]

Lipids have been reported to be more numerous in the A than in the B cells of the guinea pig.[318] The nonspecific esterase activity is low in the islets compared with that of the exocrine parenchyma.[319] In the rat the nonspecific esterase activity is mainly localized to the A cells.[79] Mouse islets possess a high activity for β-hydroxyacyl-CoA dehydrogenase,[320] which conforms to a high rate of octanoate oxidation.[321] Furthermore, adenosine triphosphate citrate lyase is particularly active in these islets, thereby providing an essential enzymatic prerequisite for the synthesis of fatty acids and cholesterol in the cytosol.[317]

Enzymes Active in the Citric Acid Cycle and Respiratory Chain

The enzymatic activity of the citric acid cycle in the islets is incompletely known, so far. Some of the associated enzymes have been studied by staining histochemistry. Isocitrate dehydrogenase shows a strong activity in the B cells,[300,322] whereas the activity of succinate dehydrogenase is rather low.[168,170,221,298,322] Quantitative histochemistry of the B cells shows high activities of malate dehydrogenase[290-292,317] and NADP$^+$-linked isocitrate dehydrogenase.[303,317,323] The activity of the latter enzyme is lower in diabetics than in nondiabetics.[141] The staining intensity for cytochrome oxidase is approximately similar in the endocrine and exocrine pancreas.[110]

Among the intermediates of the citric acid cycle, the islet concentrations of citrate and α-ketoglutarate have been determined and have been found to be rather unaffected by variations in the functional activity of the B cells.[253,324] The respiration of microdissected islets is markedly stimulated by glucose and succinate, less stimulated by citrate and oxaloacetate, and not affected at all by pyruvate, isocitrate, α-ketoglutarate, fumarate, and malate.[325]

Alkaline Phosphatase Activity

A varying degree and distribution of alkaline phosphatase activity (Fig. 21) occurs in the islets of different species. In the rat, mouse, and hamster this activity is mainly localized to the A cells,[218,221,318] whereas it is found in the B cells of the duck,[170,221] and in both A and B cells of cat, sheep, and cattle.[300] The reactions for alkaline phosphatase are negative in the islets of the pig and guinea pig.[223] In the rabbit the pancreatic ducts, but not the islets, show alkaline phosphatase activity.[286] A strong activity for alkaline phosphatase is in many species present in the capillary walls, and in some species, e.g., man, it is restricted to the vessels.[298]

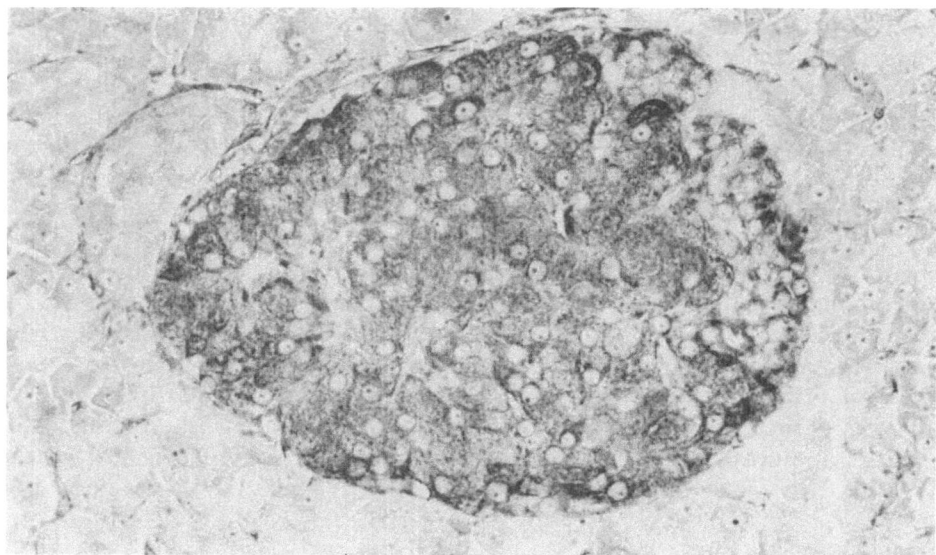

Figure 21. Pancreatic islet of normal Mongolian gerbil showing positive reaction to alkaline phosphatase both in the central B cells and in the peripheral D and A cells. ×350. Reproduced at 110%.

The role of alkaline phosphatase in the islets is not known. The high activities of different kinds of phosphatases recorded in fetal and neonatal rats[326] may indicate a role in the growth of the islets.[168] A decrease or a complete loss of the islet alkaline phosphatase activity is reported after insulin injection[327] or insulin injection combined with adrenalectomy,[328] whereas increased activity appears after fasting or administration of glucose[327] or gluca-gon.[329] The islet capillaries of normal mice exhibit a high alkaline phosphatase activity, whereas those of obese-hyperglycemic mice lack such activity.[330] Reduced activity of alkaline phosphatase has also been observed in the islets of diabetic KK mice compared with findings in nondiabetic mice.[309]

Acid Phosphatase Activity

Great species differences exist in the histochemical staining for acid phos-phatase in the islets; the B cells of rat, rabbit, and adult man show strong reactions.[220,221] Acid phosphatase activity has been reported in the islets of human fetuses,[15,331] whereas Gössner[319] found no acid phosphatase activity in human B cells in the neonatal period, but an activity comparable to that of adults was found from the 7th postnatal month on. A positive staining reaction for acid phosphatase is present in the A cells of the rabbit[286] and in the D cells of the duck.[170]

The acid phosphatase activity in the B cells exhibits different activity optima (around pH 3.5 and 5.3),[312,332] and electrophoretically, two types of nonspecific acid phosphatase have been differentiated.[316]

The activity of acid phosphatase in the islet cells is ultrastructurally localized to lysosomal bodies (Fig. 22) as in other kinds of cells. In addition, acid phosphatase activity can be observed in the Golgi complex of the B cells.[70,333] The secretory granules are usually free from acid phosphatase, but signs of acid phosphatase activity have occasionally been recorded in association with the β granules of rat,[334] ground squirrel,[70] and Chinese hamster.

The significance of islet acid phosphatase is poorly known. It may play a role in insulin synthesis,[79,286] although Gössner[221] could not find any evidence for a direct participation of this enzyme. Orci *et al.*[334] believe that it is involved in the "preparation" of the secretory granules for insulin release in response to secretory stimulation.

The acid phosphatase activity is slightly reduced after repeated injections of guinea pig antiinsulin serum,[335] and a decreased activity has been reported in alloxan diabetes, usually at a time when the B cells already are necrotic.[110,221,305,336] The islet activity of acid phosphatase is also reduced in "experimental congenital diabetes,"[304] and in old diabetic KK mice[309] in which the reduction may be consistent with an impairment of insulin release.[160] In human diabetics the islet acid phosphatase activity is depressed[268] or absent.[319]

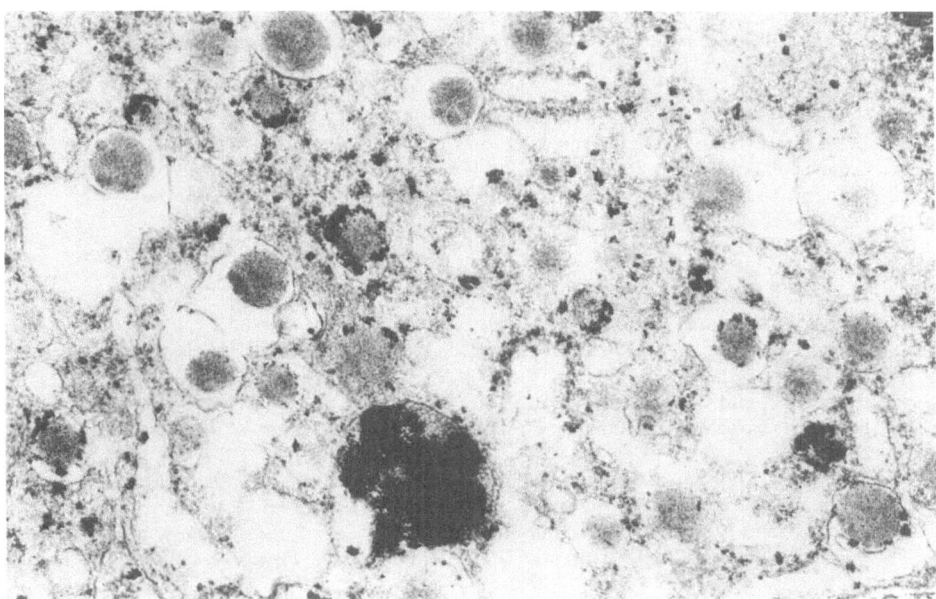

Figure 22. Cytoplasm of B cell of normal Chinese hamster showing positive reaction to acid phosphatase (modified Gomori technique) in a lysosomal body and in association with secretory granules. ×14,000. Reproduced at 110%.

Acknowledgment

Investigations of the author and his collaborators, providing part of the background for this review, were supported by grants from the Swedish Medical Research Council (Project No. 12X-718).

References

1. Caramia, F.: *Amer. J. Anat.*, **112**:53, 1963.
2. Caramia, F., Munger, B. L., and Lacy, P. E.: *Z. Zellforsch.*, **66**:533, 1965.
3. Hoyos-Guevara, E., de: *Z. Zellforsch.*, **101**:28, 1969.
4. Greider, M. H., Bencosme, S. A., and Lechago, J.: *Lab. Invest.*, **22**:344, 1970.
5. Bencosme, S. A., and Lechago, J.: *Lab. Invest.*, **18**:715, 1968.
6. Faller, A.: *Z. Zellforsch.*, **97**:226, 1969.
7. Like, A. A.: *Lab. Invest.*, **16**:937, 1967.
8. Sato, T., Herman, L., and Fitzgerald, P. J.: *Gen. Comp. Endocrinol.*, **7**:132, 1966.
9. Fujita, T.: *Arch. Histol. Jap.*, **29**:1, 1968.
10. Shino, A., Matsuo, T., Iwatsuka, H., and Suzuoki, Z.: *Diabetologia*, **9**:413, 1973.
11. Melmed, R. N., Benitez, C. J., and Holt, S. J.: *J. Cell Sci.*, **11**:449, 1972.
12. Lacy, P. E.: *Anat. Rec.*, **128**:255, 1957.
13. Lacy, P. E.: *Diabetes*, **6**:498, 1957.
14. Falkmer, S., Hellman, B., and Voigt, G. E.: *Acta Pathol. Microbiol. Scand.*, **60**:47, 1964.
15. Björkman, N., Hellerström, C., Hellman, B., and Petersson, B.: *Z. Zellforsch.*, **72**:425, 1966.
16. Boquist, L., and Falkmer, S.: In: *The Structure and Metabolism of the Pancreatic Islets*. Edited by S. Falkmer, B. Hellman, and I.-B. Täljedal. Pergamon Press, Oxford, 1970, p. 25.
17. Boquist, L.: *Acta Soc. Med. Upsal.*, **72**:345, 1967.
18. Boquist, L.: *Virchows Arch. Abt.´ Zellpath.*, **1**:169, 1968.
19. Boquist, L.: *Acta Pathol. Microbiol. Scand.*, **75**:399, 1969.
20. Luse, S. A., Caramia, G., Gerritsen, G., and Dulin, W. E.: *Diabetologia*, **3**:97, 1967.
21. Lazarus, S. S., Shapiro, S. H., and Volk, B. W.: *Lab. Invest.*, **16**:330, 1967.
22. Munger, B. L., Caramia, F., and Lacy, P. E.: *Z. Zellforsch.*, **67**:776, 1965.
23. Forssmann, A.: *Cell Tiss. Res.*, **167**:179, 1976.
24. Parrilla, R., Gomez-Acebo, J., and R-Candela, J. L.: *J. Ultrastruc. Res.*, **26**:1, 1969.
25. Kobayashi, K.: *Arch. Histol. Jap.*, **26**:439, 1966.
26. Munger, B. L.: *Amer. J. Anat.*, **103**:275, 1958.
27. Wessels, N. K., and Evans, J.: *Develop. Biol.*, **17**:413, 1968.
28. Orci, L., Lambert, A. E., Rouiller, C., Renold, A. E., and Samols, E.: *Horm. Metab. Res.*, **1**:108, 1969.
29. Perrier, H., and Billat, C.: *Diabetologia*, **6**:605, 1970.
30. Pictet, R., Clark, W. R., Renold, A. E., Williams, R. H., and Rutter, W. J.: *J. Cell Biol.*, **39**:105A, 1968.
31. Deconinck, J. F., Van Assche, F. A., Potvliege, P. R., and Gepts, W.: *Diabetologia*, **8**:326, 1972.
32. Wellmann, K. F., Volk, B. W., and Brancato, P.: *Lab. Invest.*, **25**:97, 1971.
33. Pictet, R., and Rutter, W. J.: In: *Handbook of Physiology*, Sect. 7, *Endocrinology*, Vol. 1, *Endocrine Pancreas*. Edited by R. O. Greep and E. B. Astwood. Amer. Physiol. Soc., Washington, 1972, p. 25.
34. Like, A. A.: *Amer. J. Pathol.*, **59**:225, 1970.
35. Woods, S. C., and Porte, Jr., D.: *Physiol. Rev.*, **54**:596, 1974.
36. Smith, P. H.: *Amer. J. Anat.*, **144**:513, 1975.
37. Lever, J. D.: In: *Subcellular Organization and Function in Endocrine Tissues*. Edited by H. Heller and K. Lederis. Cambridge University Press, Cambridge, 1971, p. 839.
38. Esterhuizen, A. C., and Howell, S. L.: *J. Cell Biol.*, **46**:593, 1970.

39. Malaisse, W., Malaisse-Lagae, F., Wright, P. H., and Ashmore, J.: *Endocrinology,* **80**:975, 1967.
40. Shorr, S. S., and Bloom, F. E.: *J. Biol. Med.,* **43**:47, 1970.
41. Orci, L., Lambert, A. E., Amherdt, M. L., Dameron, D., Kanazawa, Y., and Stauffacher, W.: *Acta Diab. Lat.,* **7**, *Suppl.* **1**:184, 1970.
42. Kern, H. F.: *Cell Tiss. Res.,* **164**:261, 1975.
43. Orci, L., Gabbay, K. H., and Malaisse, W. J.: *Science,* **175**:1128, 1972.
44. Gabbiani, G., Malaisse-Lagae, F., Blondel, B., and Orci, L.: *Endocrinology,* **95**;1630, 1974.
45. Sharp, G. W. G., Wollheim, C., Müller, W. A., Gutzeit, A., Trueheart, P. A., Blondel, B., Orci, L., and Renold, A. E.: *Fed. Proc.,* **34**:1537, 1975.
46. Orci, L.: *Diabetologia,* **10**:163, 1974.
47. Orci, L., Amherdt, M., Henquin, J. C., Lambert, A. E., Unger, R. H., and Renold, A. E.: *Science,* **180**:647, 1973.
48. Orci, L., Unger, R. H., and Renold, A. E.: *Experientia,* **29**:1015, 1973.
49. Wellmann, K. F., Brancato, P., Lazarus, S. S., and Volk, B. W.: *Arch. Pathol.,* **84**:251, 1967.
50. Wellmann, K. F., Volk, B. W., Lazarus, S. S., and Brancato, P.: *Diabetes,* **18**:138, 1969.
51. Bencosme, S. A., and Martinez-Palomo, A.: *Lab. Invest.,* **18**:746, 1968.
52. Lazarus, S. S., and Volk, B. W.: In: *The Structure and Metabolism of the Pancreatic Islets.* Edited by S. Falkmer, B. Hellman, and I.-B. Täljedal. Pergamon Press, Oxford, 1970, p. 159.
53. Aerts, L., and Van Assche, F. A.: *Diabetologia,* **11**:285, 1975.
54. Shino, A., and Iwatsuka, H.: *Acta Histochem. Cytochem.,* **6**:273, 1973.
55. Boquist, L.: *Horm. Metab. Res.,* **2**:166, 1970.
56. Greider, M. H., Howell, S. L., and Lacy, P. E.: *J. Cell Biol.,* **41**:162, 1969.
57. Bencosme, S. A., Wilson, M. D., Aleyassine, H., de Bold, A. J., and de Bold, M. L.: *Diabetologia,* **6**:399, 1970.
58. Grossner, D.: *Z. Zellforsch.,* **83**:82, 1967.
59. Boquist, L., and Patent, G.: *Z. Zellforsch.,* **115**:416, 1971.
60. Kawanishi, H.: *Endocrinol. Jap.,* **13**:384, 1966.
61. Benzo, C. A.: *Amer. J. Anat.,* **140**:139, 1974.
62. Boquist, L., and Östberg, Y.: *Cell Tiss. Res.,* **158**:78, 1975.
63. Wasserman, D.: *Cell Tiss. Res.,* **160**:539, 1975.
64. Martinez-Palomo, A., and Bencosme, S. A.: *J. Micros. (Paris),* **5**:259, 1966.
65. Boquist, L.: *Acta Diab. Lat.,* **7**:590, 1970.
66. Boquist, L.: *Z. Zellforsch.,* **106**:69, 1970.
67. Ericson, L. E., and Lundquist, I.: *Diabetologia,* **11**:467, 1975.
68. Boquist, L.: *J. Cell Biol.,* **43**:377, 1969.
69. Donev, A., and Petkov, P.: *Arch. Histol. Jap.,* **33**:351, 1971.
70. Petkov, P. E., and Ogneva, V.: *Acta Anat.,* **88**:348, 1974.
71. Boquist, L.: *Diabetes,* **21**:1051, 1972.
72. Boquist, L.: *J. Cell Biol.,* **45**:532, 1970.
73. Bangle, Jr., R.: *Amer. J. Pathol.,* **32**:349, 1956.
74. Gabe, M.: *Bull. Micr. Appl.,* **3**:153, 1953.
75. Gomori, G.: *Amer. J. Clin. Pathol.,* **20**:665, 1950.
76. Scott, H. R., and Clayton, B. P.: *J. Histochem. Cytochem.,* **1**:336, 1953.
77. Lever, J. D., and Findlay, J. A.: *J. Anat.,* **98**:55, 1964.
78. Schiebler, T. H., and Schiessler, S.: *Z. Zellforsch,* **1**:445, 1969.
79. Lazarus, S. S., and Volk, B. W.: *The Pancreas in Human and Experimental Diabetes.* Grune & Stratton, New York, 1962, p. 21.
80. Lange, R. H.: In: *Handbuch der Histochemie.* Edited by W. Graumann and K. Neumann. Gustav Fischer Verlag, Stuttgart, Vol. VIII/1, 1973, p. 1.
81. Denffer, v., H.: *Histochemie,* **36**:97, 1973.
82. Fujita, T., Nasegawa, N., Koga, Y., Kameda, Y., and Takaya, K.: *Arch. Histol. Jap.,* **29**:313, 1968.
83. Lazarus, S. S., and Barden, H.: *J. Histochem. Cytochem.,* **9**:628, 1961.
84. Lazarus, S. S., Shapiro, S., and Volk, B. W.: *J. Histochem. Cytochem.,* **17**:191, 1969.
85. Kvistberg, D. R., Lester, G., and Lazarow, A.: *J. Histochem. Cytochem.,* **14**:609, 1966.

86. Schirner, H.: *Z. Naturforsch.,* **14b**:690, 1959.

87. Rosenbloom, A. L., and Rennert, O. W.: *Stain. Technol.,* **45**:25, 1970.

88. Fujita, T., and Takaya, K.: *Stain. Technol.,* **43**:329, 1968.

89. Klessen, C.: *Histochemistry,* **45**:203, 1975.

90. Barnett, R. J., and Seligman, M.: *J. Histochem. Cytochem.,* **2**:462, 1954.

91. Denffer, v., H., and Mertz, M.: *Histochemie,* **29**:54, 1972.

92. Ivic, M.: *Anat. Anz.,* **107**:347, 1959.

93. Bock, R., and Ockenfels, H.: *Histochemie,* **21**:181, 1970.

94. Mansini, A. M., Frizzera, G., and Vecchi, A.: *Histochemie,* **6**:301, 1966.

95. Lacy, P. E.: *Exp. Cell. Res.,* **7**:296, 1959.

96. Logothetopoulos, J., Yip, C. C., and Coburn, M. E.: In: *The Structure and Metabolism of the Pancreatic Islets.* Edited by S. Falkmer, B. Hellman, and I.-B. Täljedal. Pergamon Press, Oxford, 1970, p. 381.

97. Grillo, T. A. I.: *J. Endocrinol.,* **31**:67, 1964.

98. Han v. Dorsche, H., Harfelt, E., Pehrmann, P., and Sulzmann, R.: *Acta Histochem.,* **43**:342, 1972.

99. Orci, L., Lambert, A. E., Kanazawa, Y., Amherdt, M., Rouiller, C., and Renold, A. E.: *J. Cell Biol.,* **50**:565, 1971.

100. Grillo, T. A. I., and Shima, K.: *J. Endocrinol.* **36**:151, 1966.

101. Grant, P. T., and Coombs, T. L.: *Biochemistry,* **6**:69, 1970.

102. Kemmler, W., and Steiner, D. F.: *Biochem. Biophys. Res. Commun.,* **41**:1223, 1970.

103. Lacy, P. E.: *Diabetes,* **11**:509, 1962.

104. Volk, B. W., and Lazarus, S. S.: *Diabetes,* **13**:60, 1964.

105. Howell, S. L., Kostianovsky, M., and Lacy, P. E.: *J. Cell Biol.,* **42**:695, 1969.

106. Hartroft, W. S., and Wrenshall, G. A.: *Diabetes,* **4**:1, 1955.

107. Misugi, K., Howell, S. L., Greider, M. H., Lacy, P. E., and Sørenson, G. D.: *Arch. Pathol.,* **89**:97, 1970.

108. Blundell, T. G., Dodson, G., Hodgkin, D., and Mercola, D.: *Adv. Protein Chem.,* **26**:279, 1972.

109. Jaim-Etcheverry, G., and Zieher, L. M.: *Endocrinology,* **83**:917, 1968.

110. Lazarus, S. S., Barden, H., and Bradshaw, M.: *Arch. Pathol.,* **73**:210, 1962.

111. Berger, W., Dahl, G., and Meissner, H.-P.: *Cytobiologie,* **12**:119, 1975.

112. Rhoten, W. B.: *Amer. J. Anat.,* **138**:481, 1973.

113. Lacy, P. E.: *Diabetes,* **19**:895, 1970.

114. Zimny, M. L., and Blackard, W. G.: *Cell Tiss. Res.,* **164**:467, 1975.

115. Creutzfeldt, W., Creutzfeldt, C., and Frerichs, H.: In: *The Structure and Metabolism of the Pancreatic Islets.* Edited by S. Falkmer, B. Hellman, and I.-B. Täljedal. Pergamon Press, Oxford, 1970, p. 181.

116. Like, A. A., and Miki, E.: *Diabetologia,* **3**:143, 1967.

117. Lever, J. D., and Findlay, J. A.: *Z. Zellforsch.,* **74**:317, 1966.

118. Findlay, J. A., Gill, J. R., Irvine, G., Lever, J. D., and Randle, P. J.: *Diabetologia,* **4**:150, 1968.

119. Haist, R. E.: In: *On the Nature and Treatment of Diabetes.* Edited by B. S. Leibel, and G. A. Wrenshall. Excerpta Medica, Amsterdam, 1965, p. 12.

120. Creutzfeldt, W., Creutzfeldt, C., Frerichs, H., Perings, E., and Sickinger, K.: *Horm. Metab. Res.,* **1**:53, 1969.

121. Howell, S. L., Young, D. A., and Lacy, P. E.: *J. Cell Biol.,* **41**:167, 1969.

122. Lacy, P. E., Howell, S. L., Young, D. A., and Fink, C. J.: *Nature (London)* **219**:1177, 1968.

123. Lacy, P. E., and Malaisse, W. J.: *Rec. Progr. Horm. Res.,* **29**:199, 1973.

124. Lacy, P. E.: *Amer. J. Pathol.,* **70**:170, 1975.

125. Lacy, P. E., Walker, M. M., and Fink, C. J.: *Diabetes,* **21**:987, 1972.

126. Somers, G., Van Obberghen, E., Devis, G., Ravazzola, M., Malaisse-Lagae, F., and Malaisse, W. J.: *Europ. J. Clin. Invest.,* **4**:299, 1974.

127. Lacy, P. E., and Greider, M. H.: In: *Handbook of Physiology,* Sect. 7, *Endocrinology,* Vol. 1, *Endocrine Pancreas.* Edited by R. O. Greep and E. B. Astwood. Amer. Physiol. Soc., Washington, 1972, p. 77.

128. Van Obberghen, E., Devis, G., Somers, G., Ravazzola, M., Malaisse-Lagae, F., and Malaisse, W. J.: *Eur. J. Clin. Invest.*, **4**:307, 1974.
129. Wessels, N. K., Spooner, B. S., Ash, J. F., Bradley, M. O., Luduena, M. A., Taylor, E. L., Wrenn, J. T., and Yamada, K. M.: *Science*, **17**:135, 1971.
130. Lacy, P. E., Klein, N. J., and Fink, C. J.: *Endocrinology*, **92**:1458, 1973.
131. Van Obberghen, E., Somers, G., Devis, G., Ravazzola, M., Malaisse-Lagae, F., Orci, L., and Malaisse, W. J.: *Diabetes*, **24**:892, 1975.
132. Orci, L., Malaisse-Lagae, F., Ravazolla, M., Amherdt, M., and Renold, A. E.: *Science*, **181**:561, 1973.
133. Orci, L., Stauffacher, W., Dulin, W. E., Renold, A. E., and Rouiller, C.: *Diabetologia*, **6**:199, 1970.
134. Orci, L., Junod, A., Pictet, R., Renold, A. E., and Rouiller, C.: *J. Cell Biol.*, **38**:462, 1968.
135. Wilander, E., and Boquist, L.: *Horm. Metab. Res.*, **4**:426, 1972.
136. Orci, L., Amherdt, M., Stauffacher, W., Like, A. A., Rouiller, C., and Renold, A. E.: *Diabetes, (Suppl. 1)* **21**:326, 1972.
137. Lazarus, S. S., and Volk, B. W.: *Diabetes*, **13**:54, 1964.
138. Lazarus, S. S., and Bencosme, S. A.: *Amer. J. Clin. Pathol.*, **26**:1145, 1956.
139. Campbell, J., Rastogi, K. S., and Hausler, H. K.: *Endocrinology*, **79**:749, 1966.
140. Frenkel, J. K.: *Progr. Exp. Tumor Res.*, **16**:300, 1972.
141. Gepts, W., Gregoire, F., Van Assche, A., and de-Gasparo, M.: In: *The Structure and Metabolism of the Pancreatic Islets.* Edited by S. Falkmer, B. Hellman, and I.-B. Täljedal. Pergamon Press, Oxford, 1970, p. 283.
142. Boquist, L., Hellman, B., Lernmark, A., and Täljedal, I.-B.: *J. Cell Biol.*, **62**:77, 1974.
143. Coleman, D. L., and Hummel, K. P.: *Diabetologia*, **3**:238, 1967.
144. Coleman, D. L., and Hummel, K. P.: In: *Diabetes, Proc. VI Congr. Int. Diab. Fed., Exc. Med. Int. Congr. Ser. No. 172.* Edited by J. Östman. 1967, p. 813.
145. Hummel, K. P., Coleman, D. L., and Lane, P. W.: *Biochem. Genet.*, **7**:1, 1972.
146. Like, A. A., and Chick, W. L.: *Diabetologia*, **6**:207, 1970.
147. Like, A. A., and Chick, W. L.: *Diabetologia*, **6**:216, 1970.
148. Orci, L., Amherdt, M., Malaisse-Lagae, F., Perrelet, A., Dulin, W. E., Gerritsen, G. C., Malaisse, W. J., and Renold, A. E.: *Diabetologia*, **10**:529, 1974.
149. Like, A. A., and Jones, E. E.: *Diabetologia*, **3**:179, 1967.
150. Like, A. A., Steinke, J., Jones, E. E., and Cahill, Jr., G. F.: *Amer. J. Pathol.*, **46**:621, 1965.
151. Borg, L. A. H., Andersson, A., Berne, C., and Westman, J.: *Cell Tiss. Res.*, **162**:313, 1975.
152. Westman, S.: *Acta Soc. Med. Upsal.*, **73**:81, 1968.
153. Appel, M. C., Chang, A. Y., and Dulin, W. E.: *Diabetologia*, **10**:625, 1974.
154. Östberg, Y., and Boquist, L.: *Acta Zool.*, **57**:41, 1976.
155. Like, A. A., and Chick, W. L.: *Science*, **163**:941, 1969.
156. Boquist, L.: *Diabetologia*, **8**:274, 1972.
157. Cavallero, C., and Mosca, L.: *J. Pathol.*, **66**:147, 1953.
158. LeCompte, P. M., and Merriam, Jr., J. C.: *Diabetes*, **11**:35, 1962.
159. Potvliege, P., Gepts, W., and Carpent, G.: *Beitr. Path. Anat.*, **128**:335, 1963.
160. Nakamura, H.: *Z. Zellforsch.*, **65**:340, 1965.
161. Yanatori, Y., and Fujita, T.: *Arch. Histol. Jap.*, **39**:67, 1976.
162. Boquist, L.: *Virchows Arch. Abt. B. Zellpath.*, **1**:157, 1968.
163. Steiner, H., Oelz, O., Zahnd, G., and Froesch, E. R.: *Diabetologia*, **6**:558, 1970.
164. Gonet, A. E., Stauffacher, W., Pictet, R., and Renold, A. E.: *Diabetologia*, **1**:162, 1965.
165. Boquist, L.: The Endocrine pancreas in the Chinese hamster. Studies on non-diabetic, alloxan-treated, zinc-deficient, and spontaneously diabetic animals. Thesis, University of Umeå, Umeå, Sweden, 1969.
166. Like, A. A., Gerritsen, G. C., Dulin, W. E., and Gaudreau, P.: *Diabetologia*, **10**:501, 1974.
167. Marx, M., Schmidt, W., and Goberna, R.: *Z. Zellforsch.*, **110**:569, 1970.
168. Björkman, N., Hellerström, C., Hellman, B., and Rothman, U.: *Z. Zellforsch.*, **59**:535, 1963.
169. Björkman, N., and Hellman, B.: *Acta Anat.*, **56**:348, 1964.

170. Hellerström, C.: *Z. Zellforsch.,* **60**:688, 1963.
171. Gomez-Acebo, J., Parilla, R., and R-Candela, J. L.: *J. Cell Biol.,* **36**:33, 1968.
172. Unger, R. H.: *Diabetes,* **25**:136, 1976.
173. Munger, B. L.: *Lab. Invest.,* **2**:855, 1962.
174. Leclercq-Meyer, V., Marchand, J., and Malaisse, W. J.: *Diabetologia,* **10**:215, 1974.
175. Baum, J., Simons, Jr., B. E., Unger, R. H., and Madison, L. L.: *Diabetes,* **11**:371, 1962.
176. Lundquist, G., Brolin, S. E., Unger, R. H., and Eisentraut, A. M.: In: *The Structure and Metabolism of the Pancreatic Islets.* Edited by S. Falkmer, B. Hellman, and I.-B. Täljedal. Pergamon Press, Oxford, 1970, p. 115.
177. Hellman, B., Wallgren, A., and Hellerström, C.: *Nature (London),* **194**:1201, 1962.
178. Bencosme, S. A., Liepa, E., and Lazarus, S. S.: *Proc. Soc. Exp. Biol. Med.,* **90**:387, 1955.
179. Petersson, B., and Hellman, B.: *Acta Endocrinol.,* **44**:139, 1963.
180. Hellerström, C., and Hellman, B.: *Acta Endocrinol.,* **41**:116, 1962.
181. Petersson, B., Hellerström, C., and Hellman, B.: *Z. Zellforsch.,* **57**:559, 1962.
182. Bromer, W. W., Sinn, L. G., Staub, A., and Behrens, O. K.: *J. Amer. Chem. Soc.,* **78**:3858, 1956.
183. Levine, H. J., and Glenner, G. G.: *J. Natl. Cancer Inst.,* **20**:63, 1958.
184. Boquist, L.: *Acta Soc. Med. Upsal.,* **72**:331, 1967.
185. Bussolati, G., Capella, C., Vassalo, C., and Solcia, E.: *Diabetologia,* **7**:181, 1971.
186. Grimelius, L.: *Acta Soc. Med. Upsal.,* **73**:243, 1968.
187. Grimelius, L.: *Acta Soc. Med. Upsal.,* **74**:28, 1969.
188. Suzuki, H.: *J. Electr. Microsc.,* **23**:33, 1974.
189. Vassalo, G., Capella, C., and Solcia, E.: *Stain Technol.,* **46**:7, 1971.
190. Hellman, B., and Petersson, B.: *Endocrinology,* **72**:238, 1963.
191. Petersson, B., Hellerström, C., and Gunnarsson, R.: *Horm. Metab. Res.,* **2**:313, 1970.
192. Hellerström, C.: *Acta Soc. Med. Upsal.,* **68**:1, 1963.
193. Petersson, B.: In: *The Structure and Metabolism of the Pancreatic Islets.* Edited by S. Falkmer, B. Hellman, and I.-B. Täljedal. Pergamon Press, Oxford, 1970, p. 123.
194. Lehy, T., and Zeitoun, P.: *Stain Technol.,* **45**:63, 1970.
195. Manocchio, I.: *Zbl. Allg. Pathol.,* **101**:1, 1960.
196. Solcia, E., and Sampietro, R.: *Z. Zellforsch.,* **65**:131, 1965.
197. Hellerström, C., and Hellman, B.: *Acta Endocrinol.,* **35**:518, 1960.
198. Grimelius, L., and Strand, A.: *Virchows Arch. Abt. A Pathol. Anat.,* **364**:129, 1974.
199. Greider, M. H., and McGulgan, J. E.: *Amer. J. Pathol.,* **59**:76, 1970.
200. Lomsky, R., Langr, F., and Vortel, V.: *Nature (London)* **223**:618, 1969.
201. Greider, M. H., and McGuigan, J. E.: *Diabetes,* **20**:389, 1971.
202. Petersson, B.: *Acta Pathol. Microbiol. Scand.,* **72**:553, 1968.
203. Greider, M. H., Rosai, J., and McGuigan, J. E.: *Cancer,* **33**:1423, 1974.
204. Dubois, M. P.: *Proc. Nat. Acad. Sci.,* **72**:1340, 1975.
205. Hökfelt, T., Efendić, S., Hellerström, C., Johansson, O., Luft, R., and Rimura, A.: *Acta Endocrinol. Suppl.* **200**:1, 1975.
206. Luft, R., Efendić, S., Hökfelt, T., Johansson, O., and Arimura, A.: *Med. Biol.,* **52**:428, 1974.
207. Orci, L., Baetens, D., Dubois, M. P., and Rufener, C.: *Horm. Metab. Res.,* **7**:400, 1975.
208. Polak, J. M., Pearse, A. G. E., Grimelius, L., Bloom, S. R., and Arimura, A.: *Lancet,* **1**:1220, 1975.
209. Goldsmith, P. C., Rose, J. C., Arimura, A., and Ganong, W. F.: *Endocrinology,* **97**:1061, 1975.
210. Curry, D. L., Bennett, L. L., and Li, C. H.: *Biochem. Biophys. Res. Commun.,* **58**:885, 1974.
211. Efendić, S., Luft, R., and Grill, V.: *FEBS Lett.,* **42**:169, 1974.
212. Gerich, J. E., Lorenzi, M., Schneider, V., Kwan, C. W., Karam, J. H., Guillemin, R., and Forsham. P. H.: *Diabetes,* **23**:876, 1975.
213. Weir, G. C., Knowlton, S. D., and Martin, D. B.: *Endocrinology,* **95**: 1744, 1974.
214. Alberti, K. G. M. M., Christensen, N. J., Christensen, S. E., Hansen, A. P., Iversen, J., Lundbaek, K., Seyer-Hansen, K., and Orskov, H.: *Lancet,* **2**:1299, 1973.
215. Iversen, J.: *Scand. J. Clin. Lab. Invest.,* **33**:125, 1974.
216. Koerker, D., Ruch, W., Chideckel, E., Palmer, J., Goodner, C., Ensinck, J., and Gale, C.: *Science,* **184**:482, 1974.

217. Arvy, L. (Ed.): *Histo-enzymologie des glandes endocrines.* Gauthier-Villars Éditeur, Paris, 1963, p. 105.
218. Arvy, L.: In: *Modern Trends in Physiological Sciences.* Edited by P. Alexander and Z. M. Bacq. Pergamon Press, Oxford, 1971, p. 249.
219. Gepts, W., and Gregoire, F.: In: *Recent Advances in Quantitative Histo- and Cytochemistry.* Edited by V. C. Dubach and V. Schmidt. Hans Huber, Bern, 1971, p. 284.
220. Gössner, W.: In: *Fortschritte der Diabetesforschung.* Edited by K. Oberdisse and K. Jahnke. Georg Thieme Verlag, Stuttgart, 1963, p. 140.
221. Gössner, W.: In: *Handbuch des Diabetes Mellitus,* Band 1. Edited by E. F. Pfeiffer. J. F. Lehmanns Verlag, München, 1969, p. 63.
222. Hellman, B., and Täljedal, I.-B.: In: *Handbook of Physiology,* Sect. 7, *Endocrinology,* Vol. 1, *Endocrine Pancreas.* Edited by R. O. Greep, and E. B. Astwood. Amer. Physiol. Soc., Washington, 1972, p. 91.
223. Schätzle, W.: *Acta Histochem.,* **6**:93, 1958.
224. Okamoto, K.: *Trans. Soc. Pathol. Jap.,* **32**:99, 1942.
225. McNary, Jr., W. F.: *J. Histochem. Cytochem.,* **2**:185, 1954.
226. Voigt, G. E.: *Arch. Pathol. Anat. Physiol.,* **332**:295, 1959.
227. Schmidt, R., Drosner, H.-P., and Schultka, R.: *Morphol. Jb.,* **115**:344, 1970.
228. Okamoto, K., and Kawanishi, K.: *Endocrinol. Jap.,* **13**:305, 1966.
229. Pihl, E.: *Histochemie,* **10**:126, 1967.
230. Hahn v. Dorsche, H., and Fiedler, H.: *Acta Histochem.,* **38**:359, 1970.
231. Petkov, P. E., and Galabova, R.: *Acta Histochem.,* **32**:93, 1969.
232. Petkov, P. E., Galabova, R., and Gospodinov, C.: *Histochemie,* **15**: 318, 1968.
233. Stampfl, B.: *Verh. Dtsch. Ges. Pathol.,* **42**:137, 1959.
234. Wolff, H., and Ringleb, D.: *Z. Ges. Exp. Med.,* **124**:326, 1954.
235. Yokoh, S., Aoji, O., Matsuno, Z., and Yoshida, H.: *Diabetologia,* **5**:137, 1969.
236. Pihl, E.: *Acta Pathol. Microbiol. Scand.,* **74**:145, 1968.
237. Falkmer, S., and Pihl, E.: *Diabetologia,* **4**:239, 1968.
238. Boquist, L., and Lernmark, Å.: *Acta Pathol. Microbiol. Scand.,* **76**:215, 1969.
239. Logothetopoulos, J., Kaneko, M., Wrenshall, G. A., and Best, C. H.: In: *The Structure and Metabolism of the Pancreatic Islets.* Edited by S. E. Brolin, B. Hellman, and H. Knutson. Pergamon Press, Oxford, 1964, p. 333.
240. Maske, H.: *Diabetes,* **6**:335, 1957.
241. Scott, D. A., and Fisher, A. M.: *Biochem. J.,* **29**:1048, 1935.
242. Adams, M. J., Blundell, T. L., Dodson, E. J., Dodson, G. G., Vijayan, M., Baker, E. N., Harding, M. M., Hodgkin, D. C., Rimmer, B., and Sheat, S.: *Nature (London),* **224**:491, 1969.
243. Maske, H.: *Z. Naturforsch.,* **8b**:96, 1953.
244. Schmidt, R., Schultka, R., Wiemann, B., and Straub, E.: *Acta Histochem.,* **50**:200, 1974.
245. Kadota, I.: *J. Lab. Clin. Med.,* **35**:568, 1950.
246. Schmidt, R.: In: *Handbuch der Allgemeinen Pathologie,* Vol. VI/4. Springer Verlag, Berlin/Heidelberg/New York, 1972, p. 582.
247. Herman, L., Sato, T., and Hales, C. N.: *J. Ultrastruct. Res.,* **42**:298, 1973.
248. Schäfter, H.-J., and Klöppel, G.: *Virchows Arch. Abt. A Pathol. Anat.,* **362**:231, 1974.
249. Howell, S. L., Montague, W., and Tyhurst, M.: *J. Cell Sci.,* **19**:395, 1975.
250. Dahl, G., and Gratzl, M.: *Cytobiologie,* **12**:344, 1976.
251. Hellman, B., and Idahl, L.-A.: *Endocrinology,* **84**:1, 1969.
252. Hellman, B., and Idahl, L.-A.: In: *The Structure and Metabolism of the Pancreatic Islets.* Edited by S. Falkmer, B. Hellman, and I.-B. Täljedal. Pergamon Press, Oxford. 1970, p. 253.
253. Matschinsky, F. M., Ellerman, J. E., Landgraf, R., Krzanowski, J., Kotler-Brajtburg, J., and Fertel, R.: In: *Recent Advances in Quantitative Histo- and Cytochemistry. Methods and Applications.* Edited by U. C. Dubach and U. Schmidt. Hans Huber, Bern, 1971, p. 143.
254. Brolin, S. E., and Berne, C.: In: *The Structure and Metabolism of the Pancreatic Islets.* Edited by S. Falkmer, B. Hellman, and I.-B. Täljedal. Pergamon Press, Oxford. 1970, p. 245.
255. Pagundes, L. A., and Cohen, R. B.: *Lab. Invest.,* **15**:312, 1966.
256. Williamson, J. R., and Lacy, P. E.: *Arch. Pathol.,* **72**:637, 1961.

257. Duff, G. L., and Toreson, W. E.: *Endocrinology*, **48**:298, 1951.
258. Matschinsky, F. M., and Ellerman, J. E.: *J. Biol. Chem.*, **243**:2730, 1968.
259. Volk, B. W., and Lazarus, S. S.: *Diabetes*, **12**:162, 1963.
260. Toreson, W. E.: *Amer. J. Anat.*, **62**:31, 1951.
261. Pictet, R., Orci, L., Gonet, A. E., Rouiller, C., and Renold, A. E.: *Diabetologia*, **3**:188, 1967.
262. Volk, B. W., Lazarus, S. S., and Wellmann, K. F.: *Diabetes*, **14**:792, 1965.
263. Carpenter, A. M., Gerritsen, G. C., Dulin, W. E., and Lazarow, A.: **3**:92, 1967.
264. Carpenter, A. M., Gerritsen, G. C., Dulin, W. E., and Lazarow, A.: *Diabetologia*, **6**:168, 1970.
265. Soret, M. G., Dulin, W. E., Mathews, J., and Gerritsen, G. C.: *Diabetologia*, **10**:567, 1974.
266. Lazarus, S. S., and Volk, B. W.: *Arch. Pathol.*, **66**:59, 1958.
267. Theodossiou, A.: *Klin. Wochenschr.*, **34**:1161, 1956.
268. Gepts, W.: In: *Handbuch des Diabetes Mellitus*. Edited by E. F. Pfeiffer. J. F. Lehmanns Verlag, München, 1971, p. 3.
269. Warren, S.: *Diabetes*, **2**:257, 1953.
270. Falck, B., and Hellman, B.: *Acta Endocrinol.*, **45**:133, 1964.
271. Cegrell, L.: *Acta Physiol. Scand., Suppl.*, **314**, 1968.
272. Gershon, M. D., and Ross, L. L.: *J. Physiol.*, **186**:477, 1966.
273. Ritzén, M., Hammarström, L., and Ullberg, S.: *Biochem. Pharmacol.*, **14**:313, 1965.
274. Petkov, P. E.: *Ann. Histochim.*, **10**:17, 1965.
275. Lundquist, I., Sundler, F., Håkanson, R., Larsson, L.-I., and Heding, L. G.: *Endocrinology*, **97**:937, 1975.
276. Ekholm, R., Ericson, L. E., and Lundquist, I.: *Diabetologia*, **7**:339, 1971.
277. Feldman, J. M., and Lebovitz, H. E.: *Endocrinology*, **86**:66, 1970.
278. Owman, C., Håkanson, R., and Sundler, F.: *Fed. Proc.*, **32**:1785, 1973.
279. Wong, K. K., Symchowicz, S., Staub, M. S., and Tabachnick, J. J. A.: *Life Sci.*, **6**:2285, 1967.
280. Feldman, J. M., and Chapman, B.: *Diabetologia*, **11**:487, 1975.
281. Brolin, S. E., Borglund, E., and Ohlsson, A.: *Acta Soc. Med. Upsal.*, **71**:334, 1966.
282. Ashcroft, S. J. H., and Randle, P. J.: In: *The Structure and Metabolism of the Pancreatic Islets*. Edited by S. Falkmer, B. Hellman, and I.-B. Täljedal. Pergamon Press, Oxford, 1970, p. 225.
283. Andersson, A., Grill, V., Asplund, K., Berne, C., Ågren, A., and Hellerström, C.: In: *Early Diabetes in Early Life*. Edited by R. A. Camerini-Davalos and H. S. Cole. Academic Press, New York, 1975, p. 49.
284. Gepts, W., and Toussaint, D.: In: *The Structure and Metabolism of the Pancreatic Islets*. Edited by S. E. Brolin and B. Hellman. Pergamon Press, Oxford, 1964, p. 357.
285. Hellman, B., and Hellerström, C.: *Acta Endocrinol.*, **39**:474, 1962.
286. Lazarus, S. S.: *Proc. Soc. Exp. Biol. Med.*, **101**:819, 1959.
287. Lazarus, S. S., and Bradshaw, M.: *Proc. Soc. Exp. Biol. Med.*, **102**:463, 1959.
288. Petersson, B.: *Histochemie*, **7**:116, 1966.
289. Brolin, S. E., Berne, C., Petersson, B., and Larsson, A.: *J. Histochem. Cytochem.*, **16**:654, 1968.
290. Kissane, J. M., Lacy, P. E., Brolin, S. E., and Smith, C. H.: In: *The Structure and Metabolism of the Pancreatic Islets*. Edited by S. E. Brolin, B. Hellman, and H. Knutson. Pergamon Press, Oxford, 1974, p. 281.
291. Lacy, P. E.: *Diabetes*, **11**:96, 1962.
292. Lazarow, A., Dixit, P. K., Lindall, A., Moran, J., Hostetler, K., and Cooperstein, S. J.: In: *The Structure and Metabolism of the Pancreatic Islets*. Edited by S. E. Brolin, B. Hellman, and H. Knutson. Pergamon Press, Oxford, 1964, p. 249.
293. Täljedal, I.-B.: *Biochem. J.*, **114**:387, 1969.
294. Dixit, P. K., and Lazarow, A.: *Metabolism*, **13**:285, 1964.
295. Dixit, P. K., and Lazarow, A.: *Diabetologia*, **18**:589, 1969.
296. Täljedal, I.-B.: In: *The Structure and Metabolism of the Pancreatic Islets*. Edited by S. Falkmer, B. Hellman, and I.-B. Täljedal. Pergamon Press, Oxford, 1970, p. 233.
297. Hellerström, C., and Brolin, S. E.: In: *Handbook of Experimental Pharmacology*. Edited by G. V. R. Born, O. Eichler, A. Farah, H. Herken, and A. D. Welch. Vol. 32/2 Insulin II. Edited by A. Hasselblatt and F. v. Bruchhausen. Springer Verlag, Berlin/Heidelberg, 1975, p. 57.
298. Hellerström, C., and Hellman, B.: *Acta Pathol. Microbiol. Scand.*, **55**:385, 1962.

299. Hellman, B., and Hellerström, C.: *Z. Zellforsch.*, **56**:97, 1962.
300. Petkov, P. E.: In: *The Structure and Metabolism of the Pancreatic Islets.* Edited by S. Falkmer, B. Hellman, and I.-B. Täljedal. Pergamon Press, Oxford, 1970, p. 213.
301. Matschinsky, F. M., Kauffman, F. C., and Ellerman, J. E.: *Diabetes*, **17**:475, 1968.
302. Täljedal, I.-B.: *Histochemie*, **21**:307, 1970.
303. Randle, P. J., and Aschcroft, S. J. H.: *Acta Diab. Lat. 7, Suppl.*, **1**:159, 1970.
304. Yoshikawa, O.: *Endocrinol. Jap.*, **16**:609, 1969.
305. Petkov, P. E., Verne, J., and Wegmann, R.: *Ann. Histochim.*, **10**:257, 1965.
306. Montague, W., and Taylor, K. W.: *Biochem. J.*, **115**:257, 1969.
307. Täljedal, I.-B.: *Histochemie*, **19**:355, 1969.
308. Lazarus, S. S., and Barden, H.: *Diabetes*, **14**:146, 1965.
309. Nakamura, M., and Yamada, K.: *Z. Zellforsch.*, **66**:396, 1965.
310. Hellerström, C. and Hellman, B.: *Acta Endocrinol.*, **42**:615, 1963.
311. Idahl, L.-A., and Täljedal, I.-B.: *Biochem. J.*, **106**:161, 1968.
312. Hellerström, C., Hellman, B., Täljedal, I.-B.: In: *The Structure and Metabolism of the Pancreatic Islets.* Edited by S. E. Brolin, B. Hellman, and H. Knutson. Pergamon Press, Oxford, 1964, p. 311.
313. Täljedal, I.-B., Hellman, B., and Hellerström, C.: *J. Histochem. Cytochem.*, **12**:491, 1964.
314. Hellerström, C., Täljedal, I.-B., and Hellman, B.: *Endocrinology*, **76**:315, 1965.
315. Lazarus, S. S., and Barden, H.: *J. Histochem. Cytochem.*, **10**:368, 1962.
316. Täljedal, I.-B.: *Acta Endocrinol.*, **55**:153, 1967.
317. Berne, C.: *J. Histochem. Cytochem.*, **23**:660, 1975.
318. Petkov, P. E., Gospodinov, C. Izmirov, I., and Donev, S.: *Acta Histochem.*, **39**:185, 1971.
319. Gössner, W.: *Verh. Dtsch. Ges. Pathol.*, **42**:125, 1959.
320. Hammar, H., and Berne, C.: *Diabetologia*, **6**:526, 1970.
321. Berne, C.: *Diabetologia*, **8**:364, 1972.
322. Wegmann, R., and Petkov, P.: *Ann. Histochim.*, **10**:93, 1965.
323. Hellman, B.: *Diabetologia*, **3**:222, 1966.
324. Danielsson, Å., Hellman, B., and Idahl, L.-A.: *Horm. Metab. Res.*, **2**:28, 1970.
325. Hellerström, C., Westman, S., Marsden, N., and Turner, D. S.: In: *The Structure and Metabolism of the Pancreatic Islets.* Edited by S. Falkmer, B. Hellman, and I.-B. Täljedal. Pergamon Press, Oxford, 1970, p. 315.
326. Hellerström, C., Brolin, S. E., Larsson, S., and Hellman, B.: *Acta Endocrinol.*, **40**:604, 1962.
327. Verne, J., and Petkov, P.: *Ann. Endocrinol.*, **22**:500, 1961.
328. Weiss, I., and Hildebrandt, H.-J.: *Anat. Anz.*, **125**:541, 1969.
329. Täljedal, I.-B., Hellman, B., Peterson, B., and Hellerström, C.: *Nature (London)*, **209**:409, 1966.
330. Hellman, B., Hellerström, C., Larsson, S., and Brolin, S.: *Z. Zellforsch.*, **55**:235, 1961.
331. Jirásek, J. E.: *Acta Histochem.*, **22**:62, 1965.
332. Hellerström, C., Täljedal, I.-B., and Hellman, B.: *Acta Endocrinol.*, **45**:476, 1964.
333. Lazarus, S. S., Volk, B. W., and Barden, H.: *J. Histochem. Cytochem.*, **14**:233, 1966.
334. Orci, L., Stauffacher, W., Rufener, C., Lambert, A. E., Rouiller, C., and Renold, A. E.: *Diabetes*, **20**:385, 1971.
335. Klöppel, G., Freytag, G., and Bommer, G.: *Diabetologia*, **8**:19, 1972.
336. Ihara, N.: *Endocrinol. Jap.*, **12**:215, 1965.

Chapter 7

Morphology of Membrane Systems in Pancreatic Islets

Lelio Orci and Alain Perrelet

In the last few years, membrane systems have been identified as key effectors in cell function. In parallel with this awareness of the importance of membranes, much effort has been spent to gain a detailed knowledge of their structure in a great variety of cells. It is the purpose of this chapter to review the evidence accumulated up to now concerning the ultrastructure of intracellular and plasma membranes in pancreatic islet cells. The normal architecture of the membrane will be reviewed first, followed by the alterations of this structure during normal or pathological functioning of the islet cells. An earlier review of the subject has been published.[1]

Normal Architecture

Membranes in islet cells fall in two categories: intracellular membranes and plasma membranes. Intracellular membranes bound a large number of specific cytoplasmic compartments such as the nucleus, the rough and smooth endoplasmic reticulum, and vesicles of various sizes, including transfer microvesicles, secretory granules, and the Golgi apparatus. Plasma membranes bound the cell cytoplasm and several cytoplasmic differentiations such as microvilli and endocytotic vesicles; moreover, they are involved in intercellular junctions (see below).

Thin Section

Plasma and intracellular membranes of islet cells show the classical trilaminar "unit"[2] structure (Fig. 1).

Intracellular Membranes. As in other cell types,[3] membranes limiting the rough endoplasmic reticulum, the transfer microvesicles, and the outer (convex) Golgi cisternae are thinner (~60 Å) than those limiting the inner (concave)

Lelio Orci and Alain Perrelet • Institute of Histology, Medical School, University of Geneva, Geneva, Switzerland.

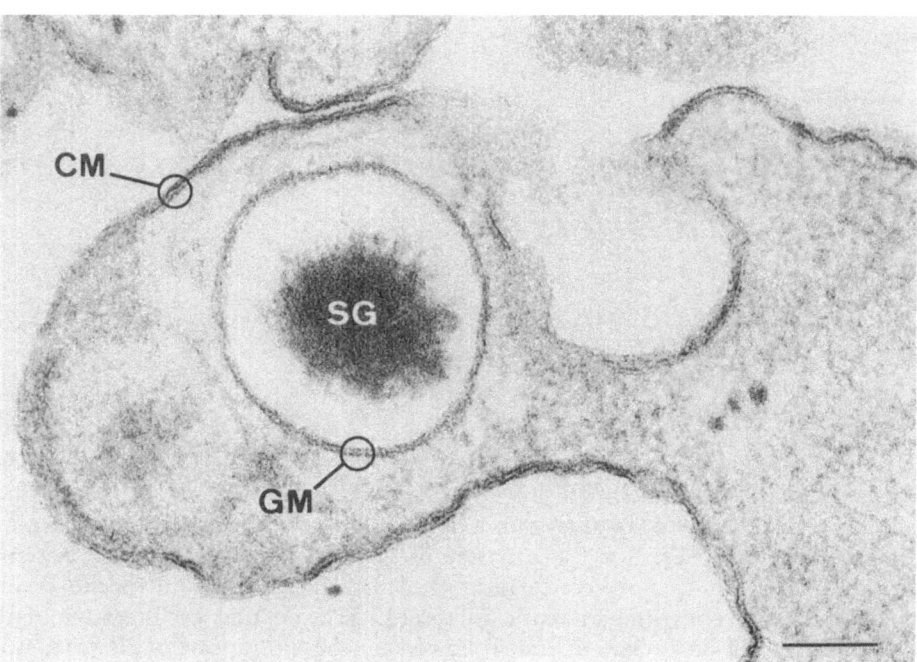

Figure 1. Portion of an islet cell in thin section revealing the trilaminar "unit" structure of the cell (plasma) membrane (CM) and of the limiting membrane (GM) of a secretory granule (SG). The trilaminar "unit" structure consists of two dense lines sandwiching a less dense intermediate layer. ×126,000. The horizontal bar represents 0.1 μm. Courtesy of Ciba Foundation, Symposium No. 41, Elsevier/Excerpta Medica.[40]

Golgi stacks and the secretory granules; these latter two have a thickness similar to that of the plasma membrane (~75 Å). The change in membrane thickness was originally believed to indicate a change in the composition of the membrane; this hypothesis recently found support in freeze-fracturing studies (see below).

Plasma Membrane.   Although it is generally recognized at present that the "unit" structure of the membrane as seen in thin-sectioned material cannot be interpreted in terms of macromolecular organization, thin sections of fixed, dehydrated, and embedded cells remain useful in identifying nonmembrane layers associated with the outer and inner leaflets of the plasma membrane.[4]

Cell Coat.   The layer attached to the outer leaflet is most evident after staining with cationic dyes such as ruthenium red or Alcian blue. This layer, the cell coat, is present at the periphery of all islet cells (Fig. 2a–c), and as in other cell types it probably represents extended glucidic residues attached to the membrane proteins and lipids (glycoproteins and glycolipids). The cell coat seems to be involved in cellular recognition and cellular adhesion,[5] and many receptors and binding sites are currently thought to be part of this specialized layer of the cell membrane[6] (see below).

Cell Web. The layer attached to the plasma membrane's inner leaflet is called the cell web (Fig. 3). Immunofluorescent staining,[7] special cytochemical reactions (heavy meromyosin binding),[8] as well as ultrastructural evidence[9] indicated that the cell web is made up principally of thin (40 to 60 Å) filaments (microfilaments) whose constitutive protein is chemically similar to muscle actin. Myosin has also been detected in the cell web.[10] Microfilaments of the cell web are thought to be responsible, at least in part, for the active movement of the plasma membrane (ruffling, endocytosis, exocytosis),[9] and recent evidence[11] indicates that they could also be involved, together with microtubules, in the control of the mobility of specific sites in the membrane (see below). Selected ultrastructural images indicate a close relationship between the extremity of microfilaments and the inner leaflet of the plasma membrane. Although it is

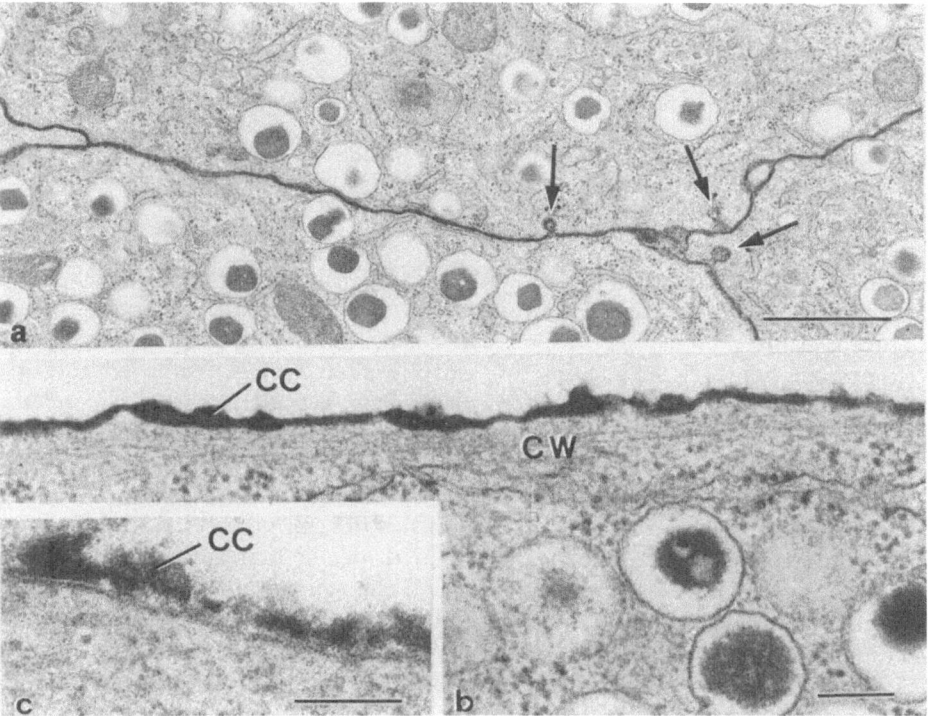

Figure 2. (a) B cell from isolated rat islet stained with ruthenium red. Ruthenium-red-stained material (in black) is visible in intercellular spaces and fills three micropinocytotic invaginations of the plasma membrane (arrows). (b) B cell from a monolayer culture of rat endocrine pancreas treated with Alcian blue. A dense, irregular coat (CC) is stained at the external surface of the cell; the association of the coat (CC) with the outer leaflet of the plasma membrane is seen in part c. A microfilamentous cell web (CW) underlines the plasma membrane in parts b and c. (a) ×17,000; (b) ×52,000; (c) ×143,000. The horizontal bar represents (a) 1 μm, (b) 0.2 μm, and (c) 0.1 μm. Courtesy of International Congress Series No. 132, *Diabetes*, Elsevier/Excerpta Medica.[4]

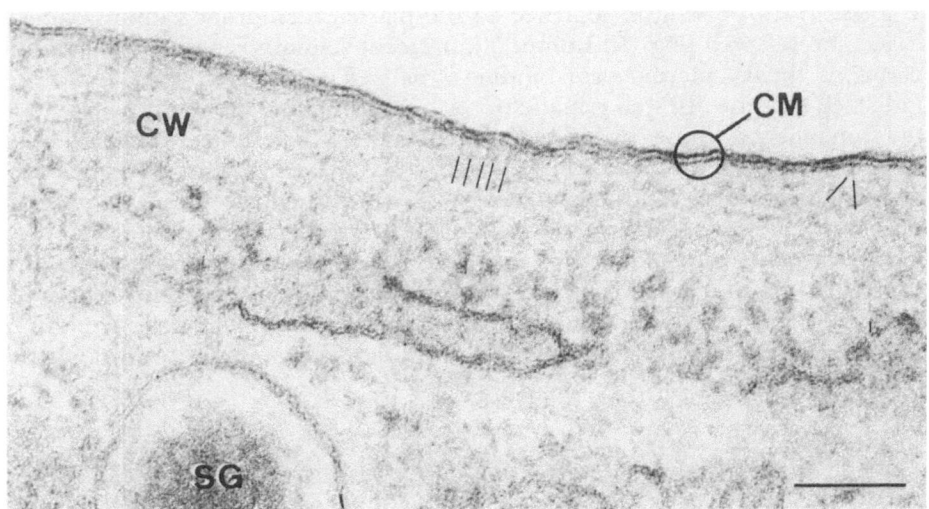

Figure 3. Thin section of the periphery of a B cell showing the association of a microfilamentous cell web (CW) with the cell membrane (CM). Individual microfilaments appear either in parallel or in polygonal arrays and the outermost (underlined by short black lines) can be seen in close relationship with the inner leaflet of the cell membrane. SG, secretory granule. ×147,000. The horizontal bar represents 0.1 µm.

certain that microfilaments (and microtubules) form a complex network webbing the entire cytoplasm, the relationships of these elements with intracellular membranes are not clear at present. The realization that the "unit" membrane is so intimately associated with its two peripheral layers has prompted authors to introduce descriptive terms to account for this fact: Names such as "greater membrane"[12] or "cell boundary"[4] have been used to describe the triple layer, cell coat–unit membrane–cell web, and it is widely thought that many of the plasma membrane functions may depend on this triple association.

Intercellular Junctions. At several points of the cell periphery, thin sections reveal that the plasma membrane takes part in specific morphological differentiations. These differentiations, called intercellular junctions, represent regions in which the plasma membranes of neighboring cells come into well-defined relationships with one another which may involve one of the following three features[13]: (1) fusion of the outer leaflets of the membranes (tight junction); (2) juxtaposition of the outer leaflets along a narrow (20 to 40 Å) gap of intercellular space (gap junction); or (3) focal condensation of extracellular material between the neighboring membranes (desmosomes). Each of these specializations may exist separately or in association with any of the other two in islet cells (Fig. 4a–c). Notably, junctions may be found not only between homologous cells (two or more B cells, for example), but also between heterologous cells (i.e., A and B cells). The possible functional role and detailed ultrastructure of tight and gap junctions is best understood by examination of freeze-fracture replicas

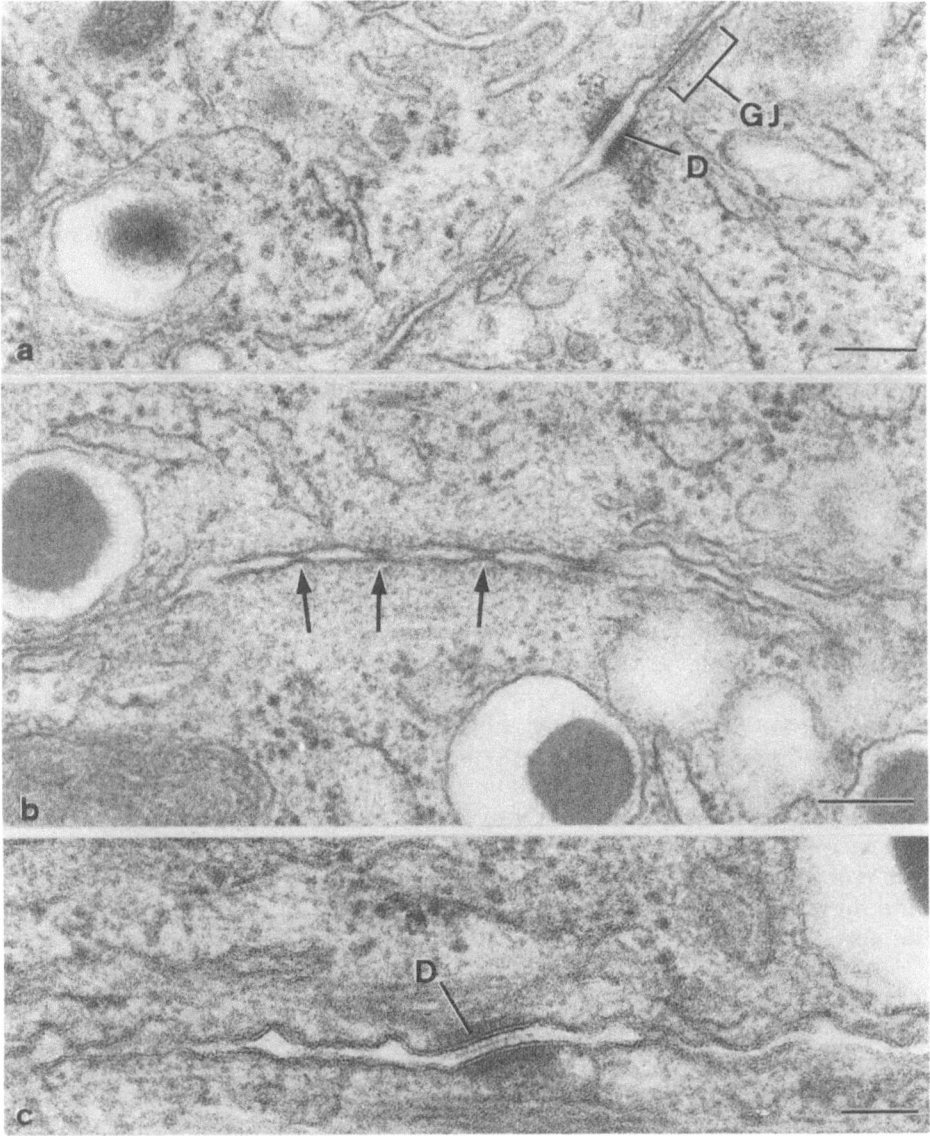

Figure 4. (a) Thin section of the periphery of two B cells showing a desmosome (D) and a probable gap junction (GJ) associated along the same stretch of intercellular space. (b) Periphery of two B cells showing several points of close relationships between the respective plasma membranes (arrows). Such points could correspond to tight junctions. (c) High magnification illustrating the fine structure of a desmosome (D). The desmosome consists of the accumulation of tonofilaments at the inner aspect of the plasma membrane and of a dense line in the middle of the intercellular space. See the freeze-fracture appearance of the desmosome in Fig. 12b. (a) ×56,000; (b) ×65,000; (c) ×102,000. The horizontal bar represents (a, b) 0.2 μm and (c) 0.1 μm.

of islet cells. These two junctions will be discussed accordingly in the relevant section. By contrast, the fine structure of the desmosome is well appreciated in thin sections of islets (cf. Fig. 4c). The admitted functional role of the desmosome is cell-to-cell adhesion.

This chapter on the morphology of membrane systems in pancreatic islets would have come to an abrupt end at this very point—except for a few details of minor importance—had the freeze-fracture technique not been discovered nearly 20 years ago[14] and applied to islet cells for a little more than 7 years.

Freeze-Fracture

It is not too strong to say that freeze-fracture has literally revolutionized the field of membrane ultrastructure and given a new insight into structure–function relationships. While thin sections of a wide variety of different membranes from fixed and embedded specimens invariably show the trilaminar "unit" pattern, freeze-fracturing allows a distinction to be made between membranes of different protein–lipid composition and the visualization, in great detail, of the respective domains occupied by proteins and lipids. Moreover, it makes possible the detection of localized areas in the membrane with a specific macromolecular organization, as well as changes in the protein–lipid relationships caused by various experimental (physiological and pathological) conditions.

Technique of Freeze-Fracturing.   Freeze-fracturing consists of freezing a cell or a tissue specimen at low temperature ($\sim -150°C$), fracturing the frozen specimens with a cooled microtome blade, and shadow-casting the frozen-fractured surface with platinum and carbon.[15] Fracturing and shadow-casting are carried out in high vacuum (10^{-6} torr). Once the platinum carbon replica of the frozen surface has been made, the specimen is removed from the vacuum and digested in order to set free the thin metallic film of the replica which is to be observed in a transmission electron microscope.

The Membrane in Freeze-Fracture.   The striking interest of freeze-fracture lies in the fact that the inside of cellular membranes is exposed during fracturing (Fig. 5).[16] Accordingly, each membrane yields two complementary halves—or fracture faces—which both appear structurally differentiated into a smooth matrix interrupted by random globular protrusions.* It is generally agreed that the smooth matrix corresponds to the membrane phospholipidic domain, while the random globular protrusions, called the intramembrane particles, represent membrane proteins.[17] The membrane face of a plasma membrane associated with the cell cytoplasm (protoplasm) is labeled "P face," while the face associated

---

*It must be noted that in contradistinction to fixed and embedded cells where the "unit" structure of the membrane is best visible in thin sections perpendicular to the plane of the membrane, the characteristic freeze-fracture images of membranes are obtained when the fracture plane is parallel to the plane of the membrane.

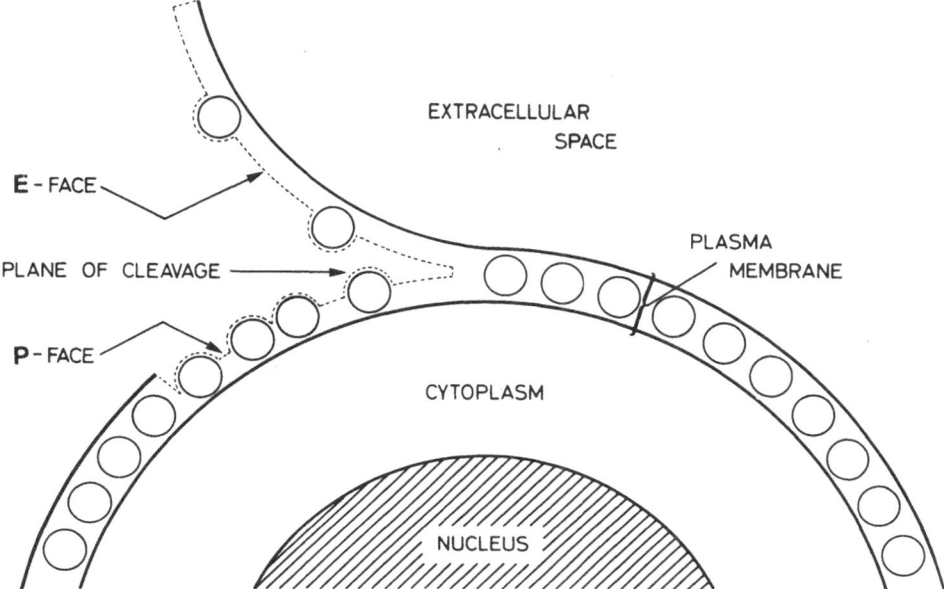

Figure 5. Schematic view of the process of membrane cleaving during freeze-fracture. The circles within the membrane, exposed by freeze-cleaving, represent the intramembrane particles (proteins).

with the extracellular (exoplasmic) space is labeled "E face" (see Fig. 5).[18]* In the case of intracellular membranes (i.e., a vacuole or a secretory granule) the P face is similarly associated with the cell cytoplasm, while the E face is on the inside (cavity) of the vacuole. In a given membrane, the P face usually contains more particles than the complementary E face. All these features can be observed in a suitably oriented replica of islet cells (Fig. 6). Large areas of intracellular membranes are revealed by a fracture plane across the cell cytoplasm, while comparable areas of plasma membranes become visible in a fracture plane running parallel to the cell surface.

Intracellular Membranes. The identification of the various intracellular membranes in a suitable freeze-fracture replica is based essentially on the recognition of the characteristic shapes of the organelles delimited by these membranes, as well as on their topographical location within the cell. In this respect, the sheet-like structure of the rough endoplasmic reticulum cisternae, the fenestrated plate-like nature of the Golgi stacks, the globular shape of secretory granules, and the pores of the nuclear envelope are characteristic and most helpful for identification (Figs. 7 and 8). As a first approach to the

*A terminology widely used before the one cited here was "A face," now called P face, and "B face," the present E face.[19]

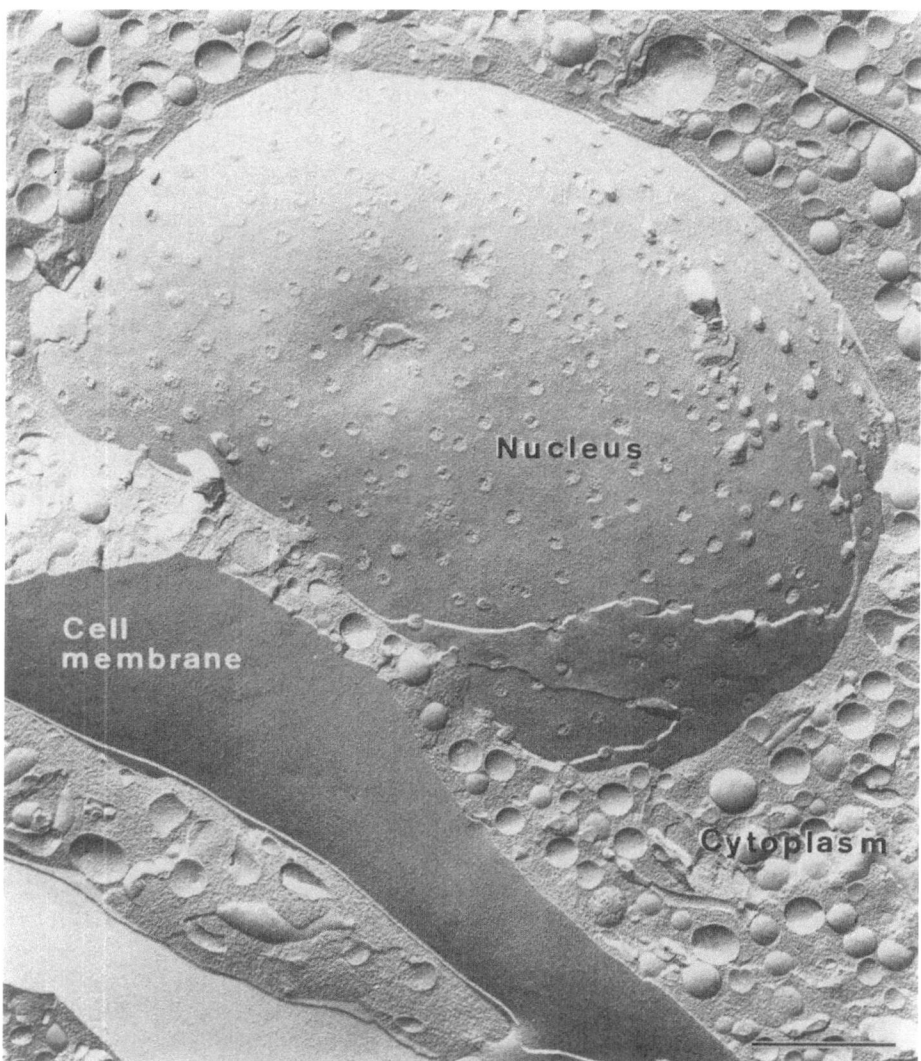

Figure 6. Freeze-fracture replica of a B cell from a nondiabetic Chinese hamster. The fracture face exposed three-dimensional views of the nucleus, of the cytoplasm, and of the cell (plasma) membrane. The small circles in the nuclear envelope represent the pores, while the concave or convex round profiles in the cytoplasm are mostly secretory granules whose limiting membrane has been exposed by the fracture process. ×19,000. The horizontal bar represents 1 μm. Courtesy of *Diabetologia,* Springer-Verlag.[49]

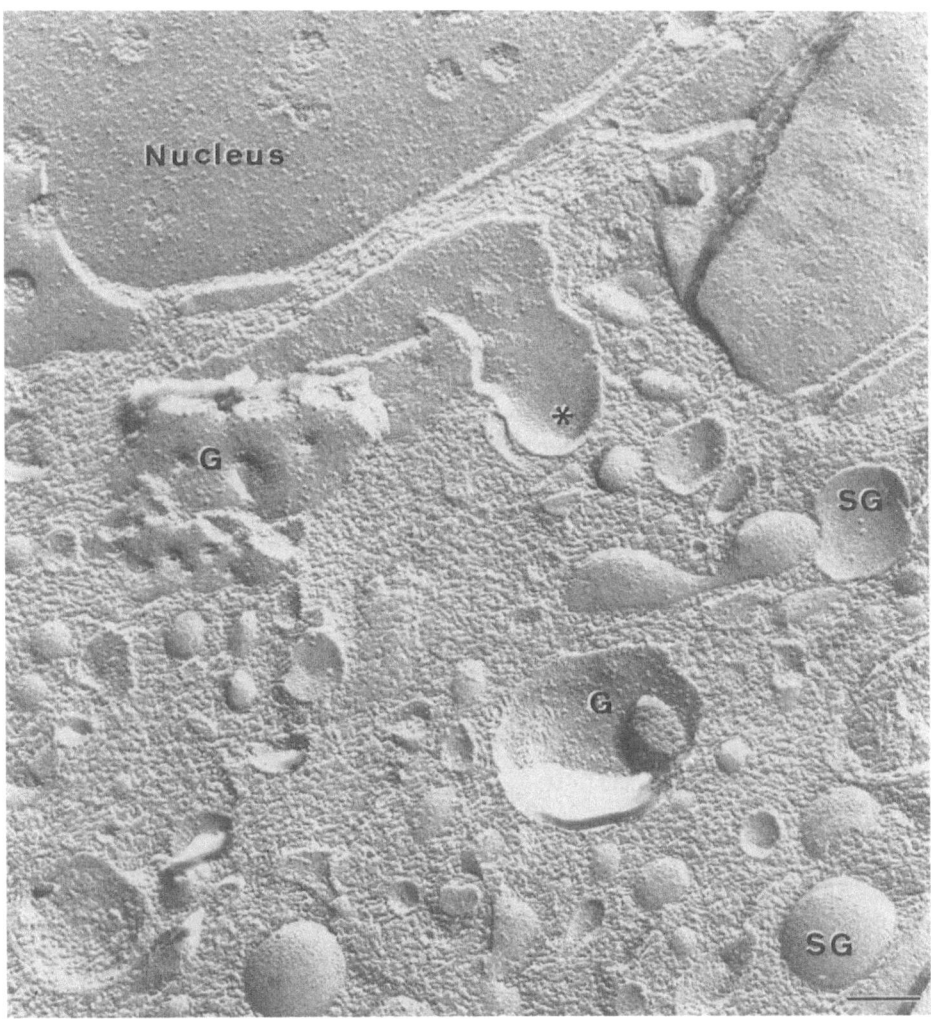

Figure 7. Freeze-fracture replica of the cytoplasm of an islet cell. The fracture face has exposed several membrane profiles in the granular cytoplasmic matrix. Among the easily recognizable profiles are parts of the nuclear membrane (nucleus), of the membrane of Golgi cisternae (G), and of that of secretory granules (SG). A striking feature in the upper Golgi profile is the abrupt rarefaction of intramembranous particles at one expanded end marked by the asterisk. The expanded end most probably represents the P face of a future secretory granule: Note that its content in intramembrane particles closely parallels the content of the P face of the free secretory granule (SG) seen in the middle right part of the picture. Secretory granule (SG) E face (lower right part of the picture) is practically particle free. ×49,000. The horizontal bar represents 0.2 μm.

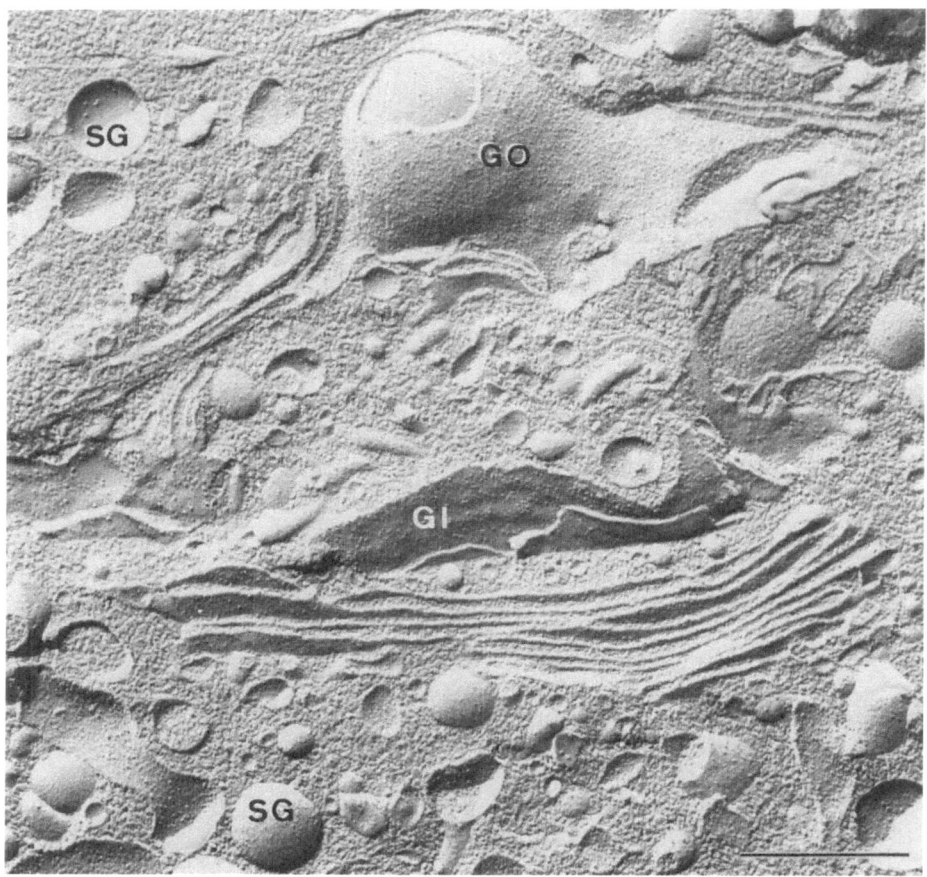

Figure 8. Freeze-fracture replica of an islet cell cytoplasm showing the difference in particle content between the P face of the membranes of the outer Golgi cisternae (GO) and those of the inner stacks (GI) (see also Table 1). Note that the P face of secretory granules (SG) (concave profile) has still fewer particles than inner Golgi stacks. The convex round profile (lower SG) represents a secretory granule E face. ×45,000. The horizontal bar represents 0.5 μm. Courtesy of *Diabetologia*, Springer-Verlag.[1]

morphological characterization of intracellular membranes, the average number and size of intramembrane particles (proteins) have been counted in unit areas (1 μm^2) of P and E faces in the rough endoplasmic reticulum, in the Golgi cisternae (outer and inner stacks), as well as in specific secretory granules (Table 1).* A striking feature emerging from both qualitative (see Figs. 7 and 8) and

*Unless specified, the descriptions and data in this paper apply to islet cells. Since freeze-fracture is a replicating technique, the usual criteria to distinguish between the main islet cell types (namely, B, A, and D cells), which are essentially the shape, size, texture, and electron density of the cores of specific secretory granules, are not valid. Thus, tentative identification of cell types in freeze-fracture relies either on indirect evidence (i.e., in the rat, B cells are situated mostly in the

Table 1. Number (± SEM) and Size (± SEM) of Intramembrane Particles in P and E Faces of Various Intracellular Membranes (Rough Endoplasmic Reticulum, Golgi Apparatus, and Secretory Granules)

Intracellular compartment	Number per square micrometer		Size (Å)	
	P face	E face	P face	E face
Rough endoplasmic reticulum	1953 ± 59	784 ± 30	124 ± 3	108 ± 2
Outer cisternae	3000 ± 83	—	111 ± 2	—
Golgi apparatus				
Inner cisternae	812 ± 171	—	106 ± 3	—
Secretory granules	250 ± 30	42 ± 8	137 ± 2	110 ± 2

quantitative (see Table 1) evaluation of replicas of intracellular membranes is that membranes of the rough endoplasmic reticulum are richly particulated, while those of secretory granules have a low particle content. The transition from high to low particle content appears to take place between the outer (convex) and inner (concave) cisternae of the Golgi apparatus. This important reorganization of the protein–lipid relationships in the Golgi membranes has to be correlated with the increase of approximately 20 Å in membrane thickness detected in thin-section studies.[3] What causes the drop in particle content, and why it occurs is not known; however, the low particle content of secretory granules is associated with drastic changes in the plasma membrane at the sites of exocytosis (see below).

Plasma Membrane. The plasma membrane of islet cells yields P and E fracture faces with a randomly distributed population of intramembrane particles, except at specific regions to be described later (Fig. 9). The plasma membrane belongs to a type relatively rich in particles, since in glutaraldehyde-fixed membranes P faces have an average of 2000 particles/μm², while E faces contain approximately 300 particles/μm² [extremes of particle number per square micrometer in P faces of various membranes are as low as 100 (myelin) and as high as 4000 (red blood cell)[21]]. Assuming that most of the intramembrane particles revealed by freeze-fracture span the membrane's thickness (integral proteins as defined in a recent model of membrane structure[22] are believed to do so, and they represent more than 80% of all membrane proteins[23]), one can describe, by the term "partition coefficient of particles" (K_p), the observation that particles are distributed unequally between the two complementary membrane faces[24]:

$$K_p = \frac{\text{Concentration of particles in P face } (C_P)}{\text{Concentration of particles in E face } (C_E)}$$

center of the islet[20]), on special cytological features of certain islet cells in certain animal species (see below), and/or on experimental manipulation of the cell content in secretory granules (i.e., sulfonylurea-induced degranulation of B cells, leaving mostly A and D cells well granulated). In this paper, most data are derived from rat islets and, according to the above-mentioned criteria, there is a high probability that they apply to B cells.

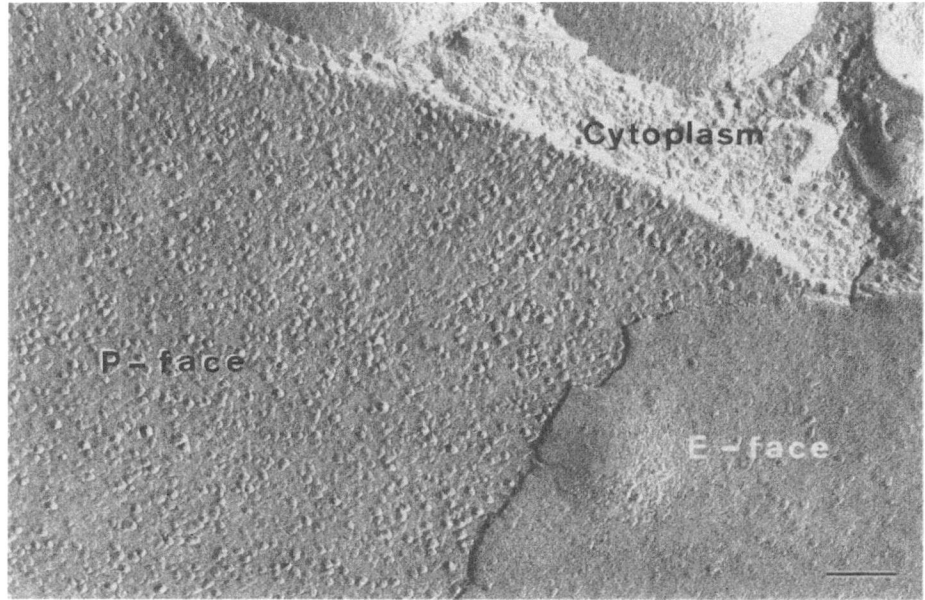

Figure 9. Freeze-fracture replica showing the P face and the E face of the plasma membranes of two adjacent islet cells. A part of the cytoplasm of the cell of which the P face is exposed is visible in the upper right corner. In fixed cells the P face has approximately six times more intramembrane particles than the E face (see Table 2). In this nonspecialized area of the membrane, all particles are randomly distributed (cf. Figs. 10 to 15). ×91,000. The horizontal bar represents 0.1 μm.

Table 2. Number (±SEM), Size (± SEM), and Partition Coefficient (K_p) of Intramembrane Particles in P and E Faces of Plasma Membranes of Fixed and Nonfixed Islet Cells

Plasma membrane	Number per square micrometer		Size (Å)		$K_p = C_P/C_E$
	P face	E face	P face	E face	
Fixed	1995 ± 45	300 ± 10	92 ± 6	95 ± 2	6.65
	$p^a < .001$	$p < .05$	NS	$p < .05$	
Nonfixed	1444 ± 11	365 ± 27	98 ± 4	111 ± 4	3.95

[a]Probability that the values are the same for fixed and nonfixed membranes. NS, not significant.

Among the facts which may influence K_p, one is the chemical fixation of the tissue before freeze-fracturing,[25] and it is customary to compare the same membrane system before and after chemical fixation. This has been carried out for islet cell plasma membrane by estimating the average number and size of intramembrane particles, as well as the K_p, in fixed and nonfixed islet cells. Chemical fixation affects the partition coefficient of particles of the islet cell plasma membranes by altering the number of particles in both P and E faces of the membrane. Moreover, there is an increase in the size of individual particles on E faces when islet cells are not fixed (Table 2). As stated before, intramembrane particles (proteins) appear usually distributed at random in the smooth phospholipidic matrix. There are important exceptions now to be described.

Intercellular Junctions. Regions in the membrane face where particles are not distributed homogeneously occur at the level of intercellular junctions.

Tight Junction. On P faces, elevated ridges or fibrils (complementary grooves or furrows on E faces) (see Fig. 11a,b) have been shown to correspond to the fused outer leaflets of adjoining plasma membranes in a tight junction.[13] As documented by studies in developmental systems, the ridge on the membrane P face would result from the coalescence and eventual coating of rows of individual intramembrane particles.[26] In support of such a mechanism is the observation that any tight junction presents segments in which the continuous ridge is replaced by chains of individual particles (see Figs. 10b and 11a). Tight junctions are well represented between all islet cells. However, they differ from those found in cavitary or tubular epithelia[27] in that they are never found to form continuous belts around cells. In their lesser form, they appear as short segments of individual ridges, with few branchings (Fig. 10a). In their most developed form (apart from experimental situations to be described below in which tight junctions appear widely increased), tight junctional ridges may form sizable networks with a radial, rather than longitudinal, development on the membrane face (Figs. 10b and 11a,b). The presence of tight junctions between islet cells prompted much speculation. By the fact that the fusion of outer leaflets of adjoining plasma membranes acts as a block on intercellular diffusion, continuous tight junctions in cavitary epithelia have been attributed the function of separating two environments which are not to mix freely (i.e., the urine in the lumen of the collecting tubules with the extracellular fluid bathing the lateral and basal poles of the cells); studies in which the transepithelial permeability (measured as electrical conductance) of a given epithelium is compared with the development of its tight junctions show that a low transepithelial permeability is associated with a highly developed tight junctional network.[28,29] How do these findings relate in the case of islet cells? The restricted. focal character of islet cell tight junctions seems to rule out the scheme established for tubular epithelia. However, if one tries to scale down the data obtained for the latter to individual islet cells sharing tight junctional networks of sizable radial development, one might propose the following hypothesis: Membrane fusion in a given network may delimit microenvironments, keeping

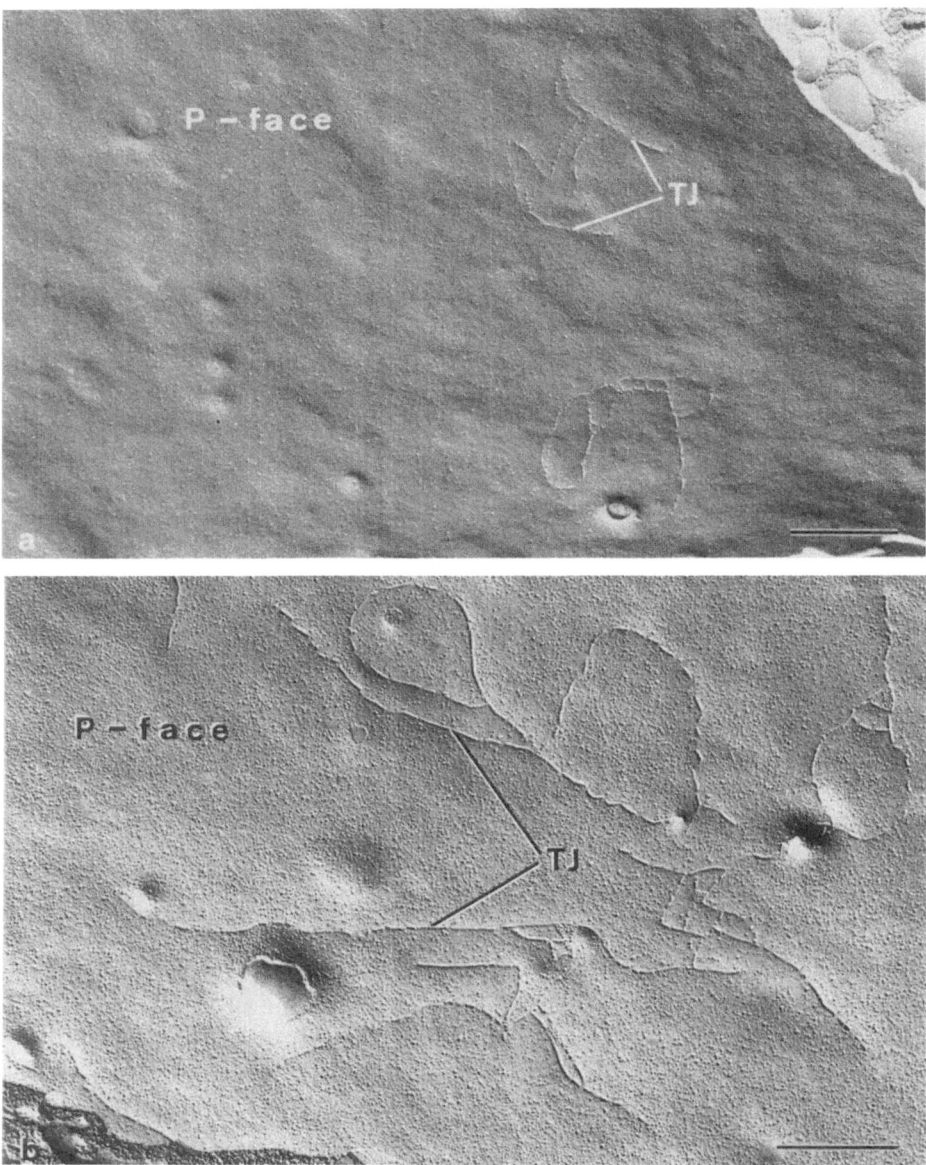

Figure 10. (a) P face of an islet cell plasma membrane showing a diminutive tight junctional network (TJ). (b) Islet cell plasma membrane (P face) containing moderately developed tight junctional elements (TJ). In both cases, note the irregular pattern formed by tight junctional ridges. (a) ×28,000, (b) ×32,000. (a, b) The horizontal bar represents 0.5 μm.

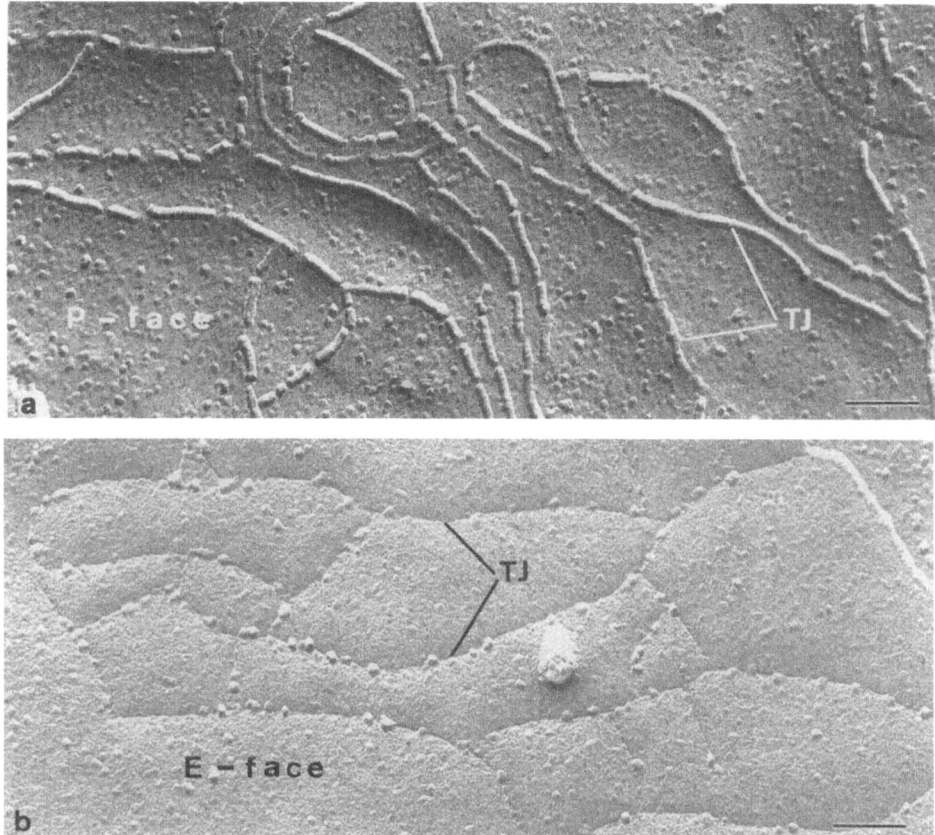

Figure 11. (a) P face of an islet cell plasma membrane showing the characteristic morphology of tight junctional elements (TJ). Each element, a ridge or a fibril superimposed on the smooth phospholipidic background, corresponds to a zone in which the outer leaflets of two adjoining plasma membranes are fused (cf. Fig. 4b). Outside the tight junctional elements, one sees the usual random intramembrane particles. Note the variegated pattern of the tight junctional network, as well as the zones of discontinuity in individual fibrils. (b) On the E face of the plasma membrane, tight junctional elements appear as interconnected grooves or furrows imprinted in the fracture face (TJ). In the same membrane, the furrows are complementary to fibrils. Several intramembrane particles adhere to the furrows. (a,b) ×100,000. (a,b) The horizontal bar represents 0.1 μm.

them from mixing with others, just as the lumen of a cavitary organ is partially or totally prevented from communicating with the outside of the tube. In this way, an islet cell could be provided with a means of selectively opening or closing certain membrane areas—say fitted with receptors—to substances (i.e., hormones) diffusing into the extracellular fluid. The existence of such mechanisms remains, of course, to be demonstrated, but the plasticity of tight junctional ridges, which can be assembled or disassembled in various experimental conditions (see below), renders them at least feasible.

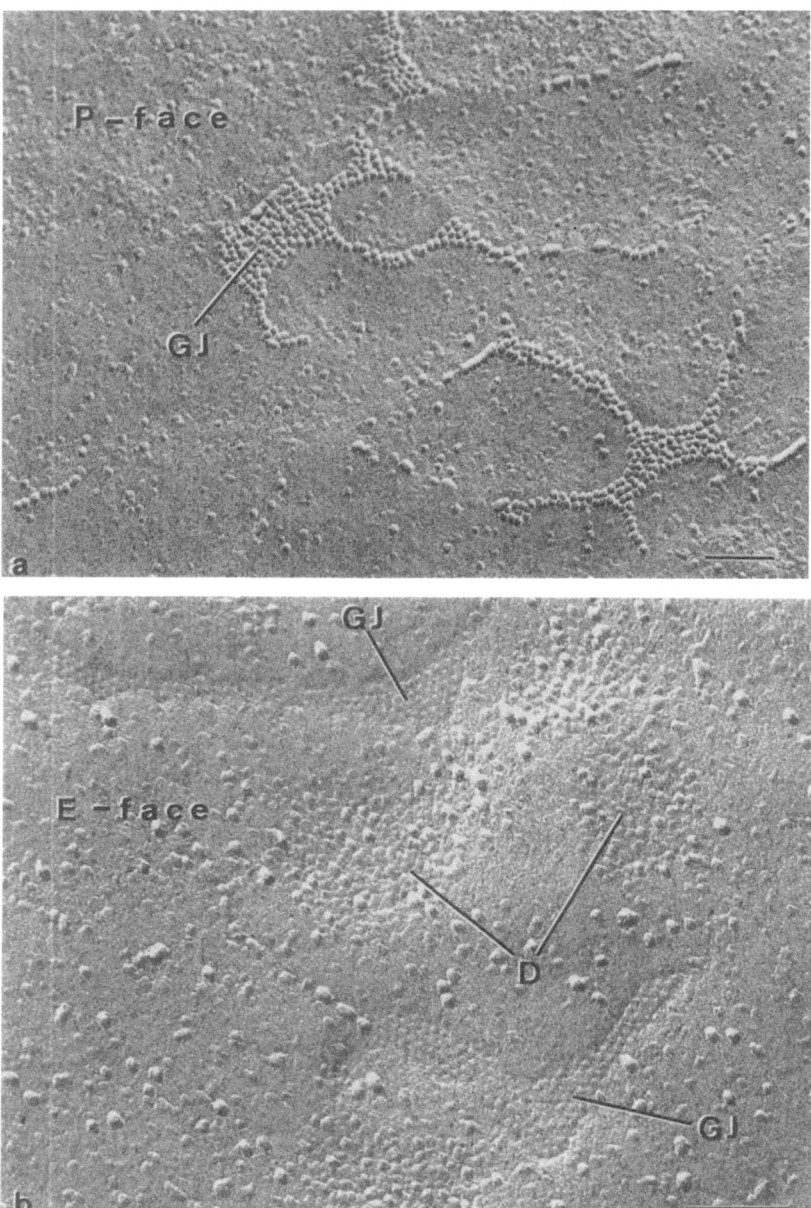

Figure 12. (a) Freeze-fracture of an islet cell plasma membrane showing the characteristic morphology of gap junctions on the P face. Gap junctions (GJ) appear as closely-packed aggregates of intramembrane particles. The shape of individual aggregates is extremely variable (see also Fig. 13a, b). Outside the gap junction arrays, the intramembrane particles are randomly scattered. (b) On the E face of the membrane, gap junctions appear as aggregates of closely-packed pits (GJ). Pits in the E-face are complementary to particles in the P face. Between the gap junctional aggregates, one sees the freeze-fracture counterparts of two desmosomes (D). (a) ×91,000, (b) ×135,000. (a,b) The horizontal bar represents 0.1 μm.

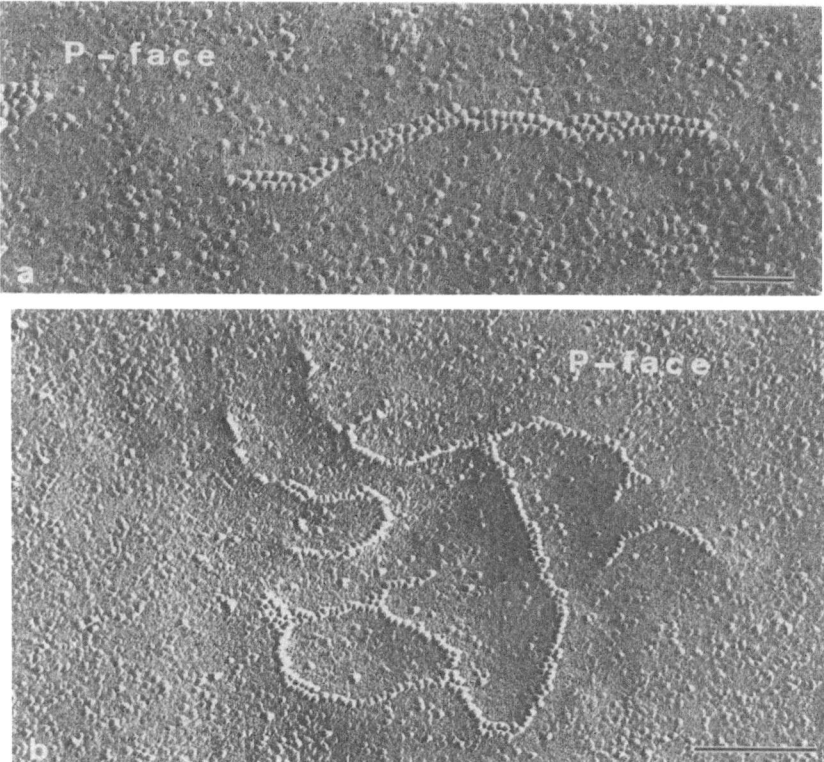

Figure 13. (a) Diminutive form of a gap junction on a P face. In this case, the junction is formed by two strands of closely-packed particles. (b) Another variation in gap junction morphology showing a linear pattern of intramembrane particle aggregates. (a) ×105,000, (b) ×79,000. The horizontal bar represents (a) 0.1 μm and (b) 0.2 μm.

Gap Junction. The other intercellular junction showing a characteristic morphological appearance in freeze-fracture is the gap junction. Gap junctions consist of focal aggregates of closely packed intramembrane particles on P faces, with corresponding aggregates of closely packed pits on the complementary E face (Fig. 12a,b).[13] Gap junction aggregates are of extremely variable shape and size (Fig. 13a,b), and they are frequently associated with tight junctional ridges (or grooves) on the same spot of membrane (Fig. 14).[27] An examination of gap junction particles at high magnification allows one to recognize small central pits in many of them (Fig. 15). Such pits, observed originally in the particles of the large gap junctions of the heart muscle cells,[19] could correspond to parts of hydrophilic channels which are assumed to bridge the cytoplasms of the two cells sharing the junction.[13] These channels are probably responsible for the exchange of ions and small molecules (up to 500 mol wt) which has been demonstrated to occur across gap junctions in suitable tissues.[30] Although the direct demonstration of exchange of ions or small molecules (a process termed, respectively, ionic or metabolic coupling)[31] between islet cells has not yet been obtained unambiguously, the detailed examination of gap junctions in these cells has led to an important finding: By screening membrane faces at high magnification, one could recognize numerous intramembrane particles not associated with gap junction aggregates, but which showed also a central pit (see Fig. 15). The pitted particles, recognized later in a wide variety of plasma membranes in different tissues, as well as in intracellular membranes, have been tentatively interpreted as the possible morphological counterparts of hydrophilic pores.[32] It is widely assumed in membrane models[33] that such pores would be responsible for the diffusion of hydrophilic molecules across the membrane bilayer.

As far as the possible functions of gap junctions between islet cells are concerned, one has to admit the same degree of uncertainty as for the functional role of tight junctions. Among the suggestions which can be proposed, one is that intercellular coupling would participate in the probably very complex regulatory mechanisms which allow the islet, an inhomogeneous endocrine microorgan from the standpoint of both its constituting cells and of its hormonal output, to maintain glucose homeostasis within tightly constricted limits. In this context, it may be worthwhile to recall that gap junctions (and tight junctions) are obligatory differentiations of the plasma membrane of islet cells in all animal species, including the human, studied so far and that they occur not only between homologous but also between heterologous cells.[34]

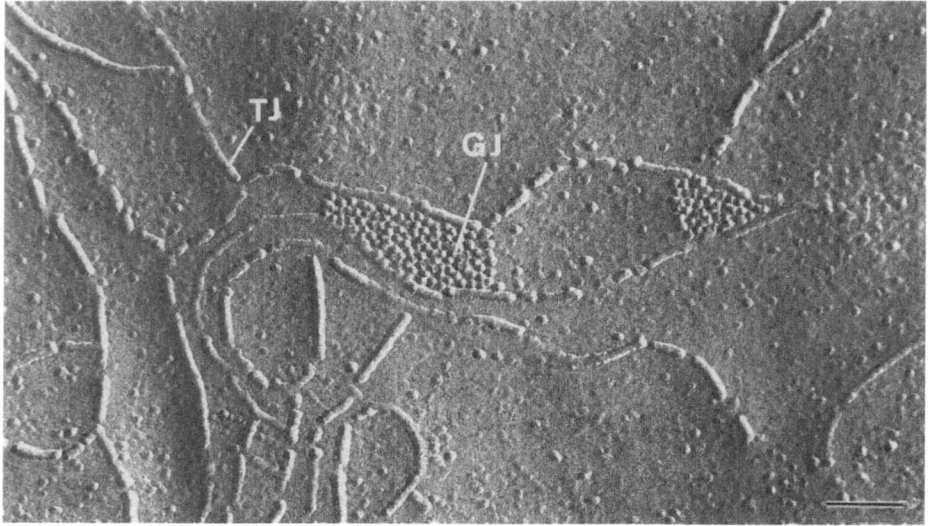

Figure 14. Association of characteristic tight junctional fibrils (TJ) with gap junction aggregates (GJ) on the P face of an islet cell plasma membrane. ×105,000. The horizontal bar represents 0.1 μm.

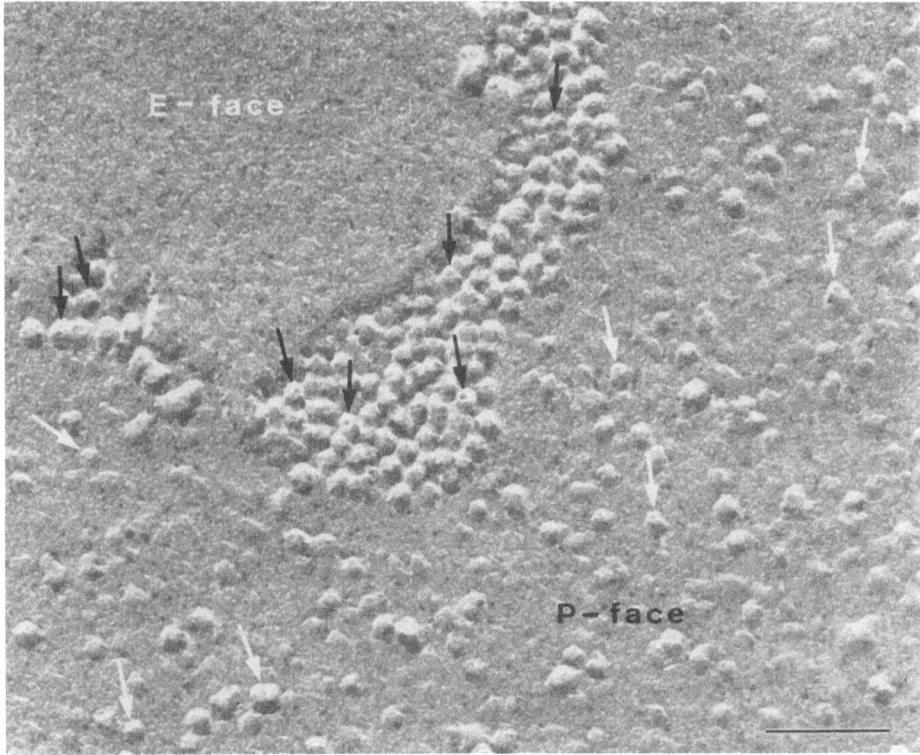

Figure 15. High-magnification picture of a freeze-fracture replica showing pits in individual gap junction particles (black arrows) as well as in particles outside the gap junctional area (white arrows). In both cases, pits may represent parts of hydrophilic channels piercing the particles. The particle aggregates on the P face are partially covered by a piece of adhering E face from the plasma membrane of the other islet cell sharing the gap junction. ×341,000. The horizontal bar represents 0.05 μm.

Receptors and Binding Sites at the Plasma Membrane

From the above discussion, it is clear that the problem of how islet cells regulate their secretion is overwhelmingly complex and constitutes a major issue in the possible understanding of pathological alterations of islet function. It has been suggested that intercellular junctions may participate in the regulatory processes, but it appears certain that they are not the sole factors involved. Intensive research in the last few years has identified specific sites in the membranes as possible candidates for regulatory functions in a wide variety of cells. These sites have been detected by their properties to bind selectively molecules which may be hormones or certain plant derivatives (lectins), and it has become customary to call such sites receptors if they bind selectively a hormone, or binding sites if they fix plant lectins. The hypothesis underlying receptor activity is that upon binding with the specific molecule, the receptor interacts with the membrane and triggers some sort of response from the cell. Chemically, receptors and binding sites are thought to be proteins or lipids with glucidic residues (glycoproteins or glycolipids) extended at the cell surface, and great interest has been generated by the discovery that the use of labeled molecules rendered possible the localization of binding sites and receptors at the ultrastructural level.[35] Binding studies at the ultrastructural level have thus attempted to define the topographical distribution of receptor sites on the cell surface, as well as to assess quantitatively the number of such sites in a given membrane.[6] In islet cells, the interest of carrying out such experiments was double: On the one hand, it was useful to establish the topography of certain binding sites at the cell surface; on the other hand, it was thought that through the use of such labeling techniques at the ultrastructural level one could eventually determine whether or not islet cells possess receptors to their own hormones. In this perspective, it seemed logical first to localize binding sites of the B cell membrane to plant lectins. Plant lectins have a strong affinity for carbohydrate residues of the cell surface (cell coat), and a variety of lectins are available, each of which seems to show a specificity for certain sugar residues [i.e., concanavalin A (Con A) attaches specifically to mannose and glucose residues, while ricin binds preferentially to galactose residues[36]]. The demonstration of lectin binding sites at the cell surface implies several preparatory steps, which will be briefly described. The first step consists of attaching the lectin to a dense marker molecule with a shape and/or size easily detectable by electron microscopy (both in thin sections or in shadow-cast replicas of the cell surface). Ferritin, with its dense iron core and a size of approximately 120 Å, as well as hemocyanin, a respiratory, copper-containing protein from invertebrate blood with a characteristic size (350 Å), shape (cylindrical), and electron density are widely used as markers.[37,39,40] The second step is to incubate the cells to be tested with a solution of the lectin–ferritin or lectin–hemocyanin complex* under various experimental conditions and then to process the treated cells for either conventional thin-section electron microscopy or for shadow-casting. The latter technique consists of dehydrating the fixed cells and replicating the outer surface of the cell membrane with platinum.† The application of the lectin-marker complex succeeds best on suspension of isolated cells or on thinly spread cells such as those obtained in monolayer cultures. Although it seems that lectin–ferritin complexes are able to reach the surface of cells in an intact, isolated islet,[38] most of the experiments to be reported have been carried out on monolayer cultures of neonatal rat endocrine pancreas.[39,40]

Lectin Binding Sites. Concanavalin (Con A) binding sites have been visualized in both thin-section and shadow-cast replicas with hemocyanin as a marker. While thin section allows the detection of binding sites in the cross-sectioned

---

*In the case of hemocyanin and Con A, the lectin is first made to react with binding sites, then the hemocyanin is applied to Con A already bound to glucidic residues.

†The shadow-casting technique is different from the freeze-fracture technique in that the former enables one to visualize the true outer surface of the membrane. As said before, freeze-fracturing consists of replicating the inside (hydrophobic region) of the membrane. A technique which combines the advantages of both shadow-casting and freeze-fracturing is deep-etching.[39,40]

membrane (Fig. 16), shadow-cast replica gives an idea of the three-dimensional distribution of the sites (Fig. 17a,b). With the latter technique, it is possible to observe that Con A binding sites are distributed in discrete patches on the cell surface when the tissue is incubated at 37°C. The patchy distribution is abolished by either incubation at low temperature (4°C) or by fixing the cells chemically (glutaraldehyde) before exposure to Con A and hemocyanin. In these conditions, Con A binding sites are randomly distributed. Such findings[39,40] indicate, in accord with similar studies carried out in different systems, that Con A binding sites are probably random in the native islet cell membrane and that patching is induced by Con A which may cross-link binding sites.[41]

The specificity of Con A binding to glucidic residue at the cell surface is demonstrated by incubating cells with both Con A and α-methyl glucoside or α-methylmannoside before hemocyanin treatment. In such conditions, Con A binding is inhibited, and practically no hemocyanin molecules are seen on the cell surface.[37,39,40] A similar result is obtained when hemocyanin alone is used to incubate the cells. In thin-sectioned material, other binding sites of the islet cell surface have been demonstrated, namely ricin binding sites (Fig. 18) and wheat germ agglutinin binding sites.[38] In these cases, a lectin–ferritin complex was used. Ferritin, in contrast to hemocyanin, is first bound to the lectin before the latter is made to react with the cells. Taken as a whole, the results obtained with lectins clearly demonstrate the feasibility of ultrastructural binding studies with islet cells, and work is now in progress with electron-dense complexes of insulin and glucagon to detect receptors for these hormones.

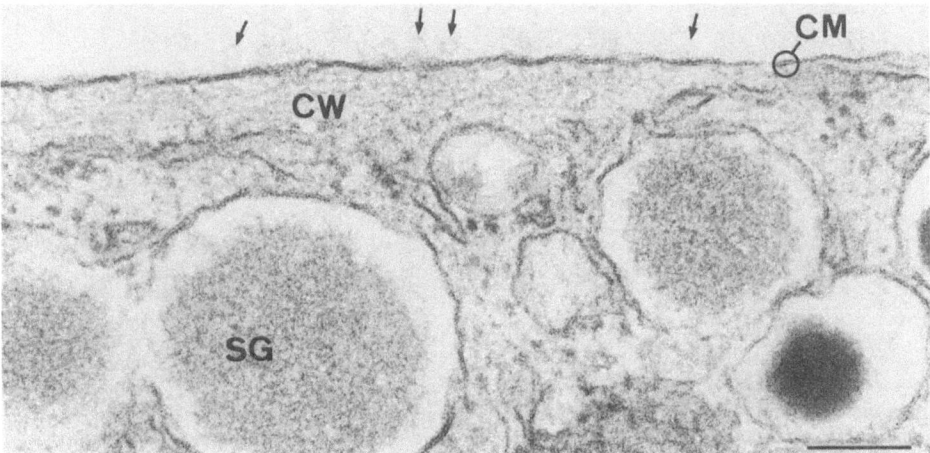

Figure 16. Thin section of the periphery of a B cell incubated in the presence of Con A and hemocyanin before fixation. Several small circles (arrows), representing individual hemocyanin molecules, can be seen at the outer aspect of the cell (plasma) membrane (CM) and reveal the sites where Con A is bound to glucoside residues of the cell surface. The cell membrane is underlined by the cell web (CW). SG, secretory granule. ×68,000. The horizontal bar represents 0.2 μm.

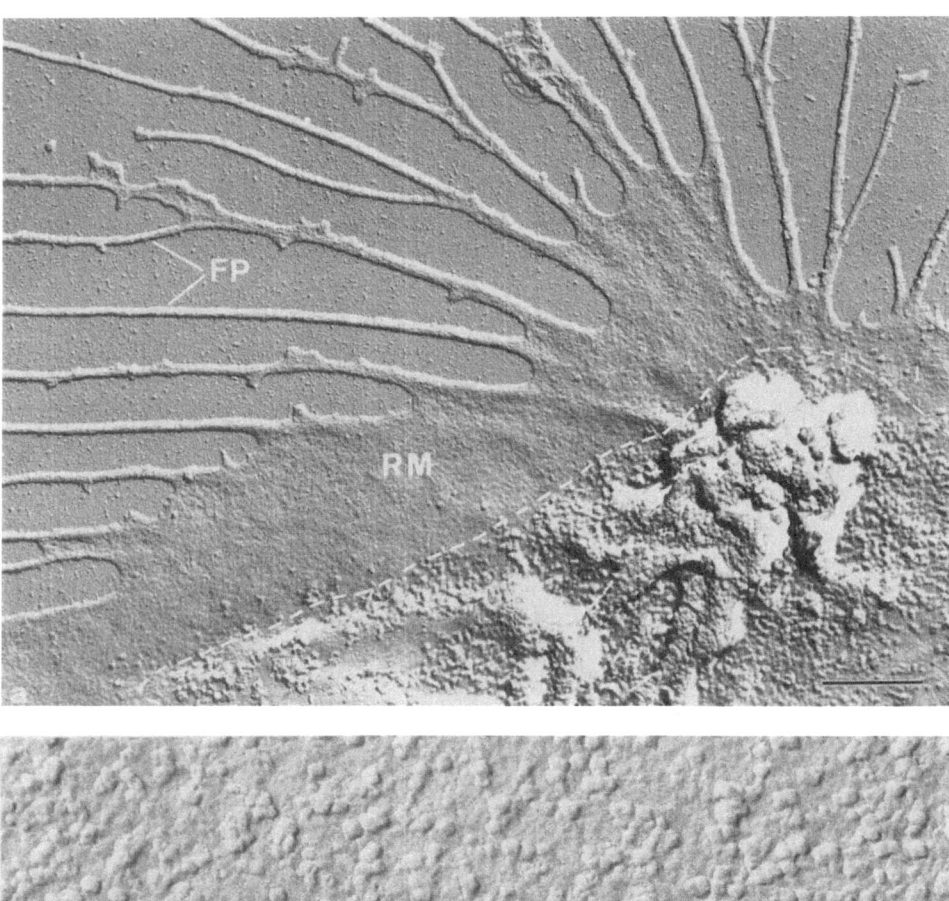

Figure 17. (a) Shadow-cast replica of the periphery of a pancreatic endocrine cell in monolayer culture treated with Con A and hemocyanin at 37°C before fixation. Under these conditions, the hemocyanin molecules which appear as dots protruding over the cell surface (see part b), are absent from the outermost periphery of the cell (ruffling membrane, RM) as well as from filopodia (FP) extending from the cell periphery. The boundary between the ruffling zone and the remainder of the cell membrane covered with hemocyanin molecules is indicated by the dotted line. (b) High magnification of a field of an islet cell plasma membrane treated with Con A and hemocyanin after fixation. The hemocyanin molecules are regularly arranged over the cell surface. (a) ×13,000, (b) ×52,000. The horizontal bar represents (a) 1 μm and (b) 0.2 μm.

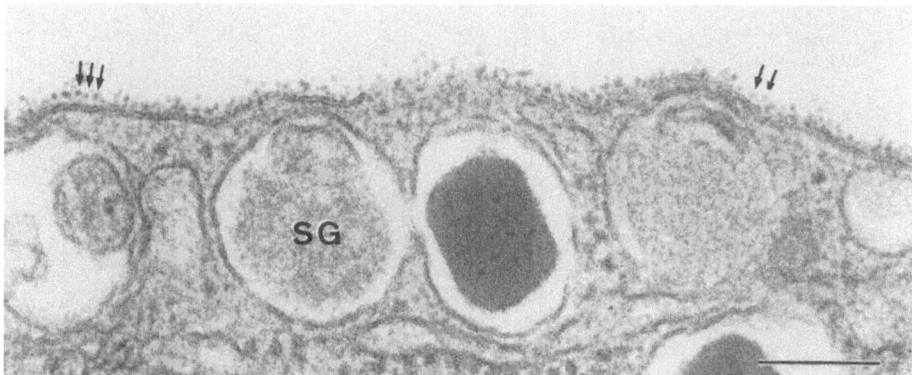

Figure 18. Thin section of the periphery of a B cell in monolayer culture incubated with a ricin–ferritin complex before fixation. In suitable orientations of the section plane, individual molecules of ferritin (arrows) can be seen close to the outer aspect of the cell membrane. SG, secretory granule. ×82,000. The horizontal bar represents 0.2 μm.

As reported above, Con A binding sites have different topographical distribution when incubation with Con A is done at 37°C, at 4°C, or after fixation. The fact that binding sites can be aggregated in patches at the cell surface, a phenomenon amply observed in lymphoid cells whose surface immunoglobulins have been cross-linked by divalent antibodies,[42] has two important implications: First, it stresses the fluid character of the membrane as proposed in a recent model where proteins are allowed to diffuse laterally into the plane of the phospholipid matrix[22]; second, it raises the question of whether there is any sort of control of the mobility of surface molecules. Recent experimental evidence indicates that redistribution of surface receptors as observed in lymphocytes can be perturbed by pretreatment of the cells with substances such as colchicine or cytochalasine B, which alter cytoplasmic microtubules and cytoplasmic microfilaments, respectively (for review, see Yahara and Edelman[11]). These and other data point to these nonmembrane organelles as possible candidates for the topographical modulation of surface receptors, and a direct interaction between the membrane and microtubules and/or microfilaments has been sought at the ultrastructural level. In islet cells, microtubules were not seen, so far, directly in contact with the plasma membrane (inner leaflet), although they may approach the membrane to within less than 500 Å. In contrast, by their subplasmalemmal distribution, the peripheral microfilaments of the cell web are better candidates for entering into some sort of relationship with the membrane and, in fact, selected images do show a contiguity between microfilamentous structures and the inner leaflet of the plasma membrane, both in thin-section and in freeze-fracture replicas (Fig. 19a–c). Of course, the exact nature of this relationship is entirely unknown at present, as is how microfilaments and microtubules may interact in the control of surface topog-

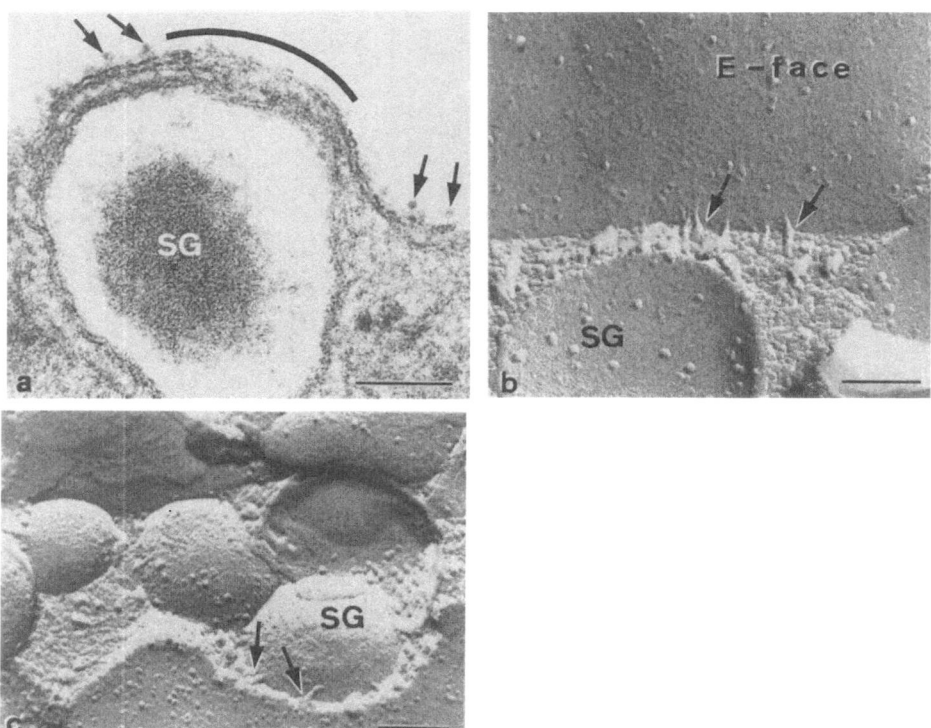

Figure 19. (a) High magnification of the periphery of a B cell in monolayer culture treated with a ricin–ferritin complex before fixation. Several ferritin molecules (arrows) label discrete areas of the cell surface but leave other regions unmarked (indicated by the black line). Part of the unlabeled region is bulging over a secretory granule (SG) close to the cell membrane. Between the cell membrane and the granule's limiting membrane, there is evidence for filamentous structures apparently in register with ferritin molecules. (b) Freeze-fracture replica showing filamentous structures (arrows) emerging from the cytoplasmic matrix and reaching the plasma membrane (E face); SG, secretory granules (P face). (c) Similar filamentous structures (arrow) are seen apparently bridging the cell membrane (P face) and the secretory granule membrane (SG) (E face). In both parts b and c, the filamentous structures may represent elements of the cell web possibly inserted into the plasma membrane matrix (in relationship with membrane subunits?). (a) ×128,000, (b) ×105,000, (c) ×90,000. The horizontal bar represents 0.1 μm throughout.

raphy. In closing these remarks, it must be acknowledged that in most—if not all—nucleated cells studied so far, the movement of surface receptors could not be related to a parallel movement of intramembrane particles (proteins) as revealed by the freeze-fracture technique. Possible explanations for this discrepancy have been given by Bretscher and Raff.[43]

Alterations of the Plasma Membrane during Normal Functioning

Stimulation of B cells by glucose increases insulin release and induces morphological changes at the level of the plasma membrane. Changes comprise: (1) modification of the number and size of intramembrane particles; (2) modification of the development of tight junctions; and (3) redistribution of intramembrane particles in certain membrane areas as a result of exocytosis of secretory granules. Except for alterations caused in the plasma membrane by exocytosis, the former two are of low amplitude and are detected only by a quantitative approach.

Changes in Intramembrane Particles

After 60 min stimulation of isolated islets by 300 mg/100 ml glucose, the plasma membranes of unfixed islet cells show a significant decrease in the number of intramembrane particles per square micrometer in P- and E-fracture face as compared with control islets incubated at low glucose (50 mg/100 ml) (1418 ± 92 vs. $1161 \pm 93 : p < .01$; 439 ± 23 vs. $353 \pm 19 : p < .01$). While the significance of such decrease is totally unknown at present, it does point again to the fluidity of the cell membrane organization under various influences; among the possible mechanisms responsible for the decrease in particle number, a removal of particles may come into question, as well as a dilution of particles due to exocytosis (see below).

Changes in Tight Junctions

Morphological changes affecting tight junctions during insulin release were observed by incubating isolated islets for 180 min in various concentrations of glucose (0, 50, and 300 mg/100 ml). Replicas of plasma membranes of B cells (P faces) were then analyzed by morphometry[44] for assessing the development of tight junctional elements. The results, expressed in arbitrary morphometrical units measuring the density of boundary length of tight junctions, show that a significant increase in the development of tight junctions is induced by glucose stimulation (Fig. 20). This observation lends some support to the hypothesis concerning the functional role of tight junctions in islet cells according to which tight junctional networks may be highly mobile differentiations of the cell membrane regulating the access of certain areas to external influences.

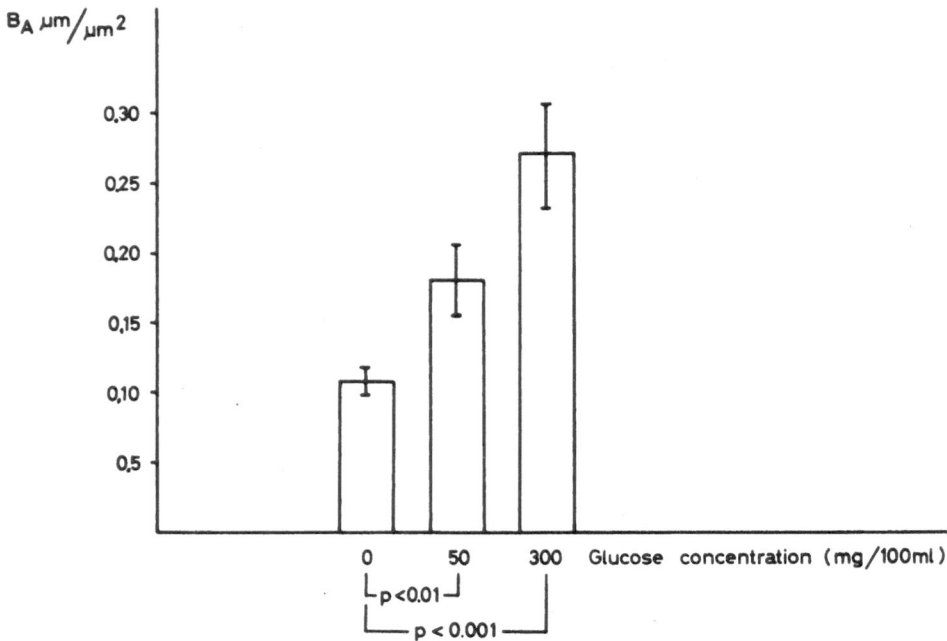

Figure 20. Density of boundary length (B_A) of tight junctions in plasma membrane area ($\mu m/\mu m^2$) of isolated islet cells incubated at different glucose concentrations. Data show that the incubation in increasing concentration of glucose significantly increases the density of boundary length of tight junctions.

Changes during Exocytosis

Much more evident than the decrease in the number of particles during glucose stimulation are the changes brought about by exocytosis. During this process, the granule's limiting membrane fuses with the plasma membrane and gets incorporated in the latter, allowing the granule core to be extruded into the extracellular space (Fig. 21b). By examining selected freeze-fracture replicas of glucose-stimulated B cells,[45,46] which show numerous exocytotic events, the following observations were made[46]: In areas of the plasma membrane (P face) which come into close relationship with the membrane of secretory granules (E face), an event which is considered preceding the actual fusion of the two membranes, intramembrane particles are lacking (Fig. 22a). Without clear-cut transition, these bare areas of the plasma membrane blend with the normally particulated surrounding regions. In other regions of the plasma membrane of stimulated cells, which are interpreted as harboring later stages of exocytosis (namely after the fusion has taken place) (Fig. 22c), granule cores of former secretory granules can be seen bulging in depressions of the plasma membrane.

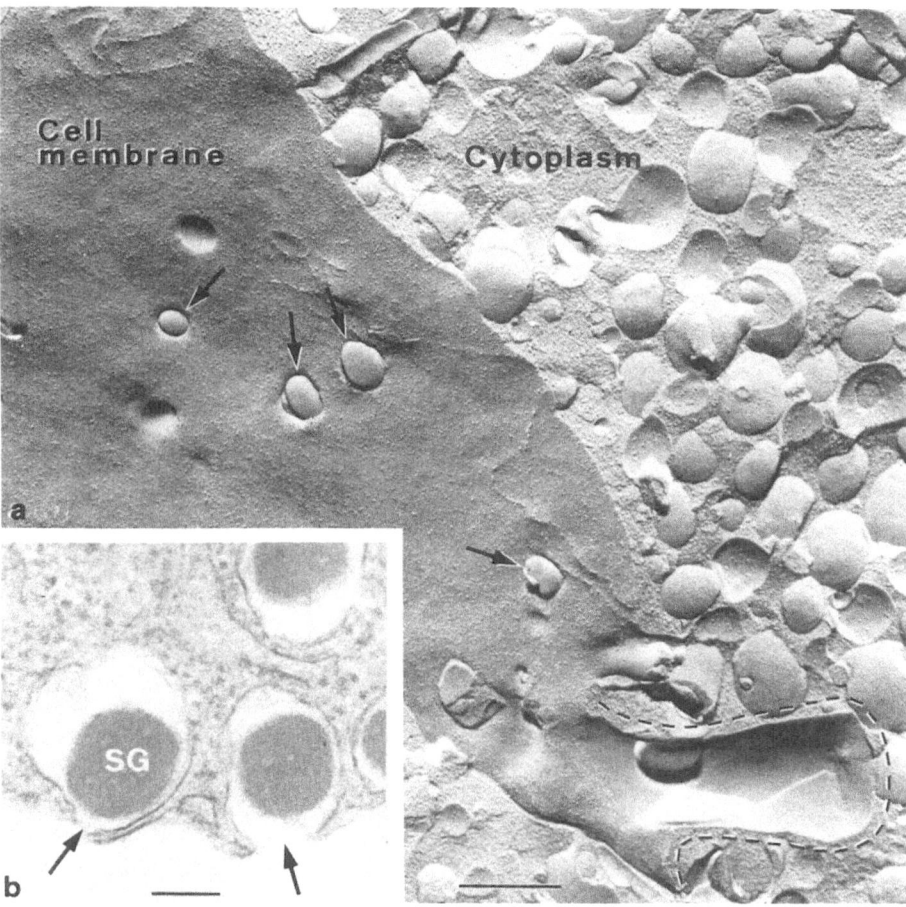

Figure 21. (a) Freeze-fracture replica of an islet cell stimulated with glucose and showing several exocytotic figures (arrows) on the P face of the cell (plasma) membrane. The exocytotic figures represent stages at which the granule core is being extruded after the fusion of the granule limiting membrane with the plasma membrane (see Fig. 22b). In the cross-fractured cytoplasm, one sees numerous profiles of secretory granule limiting membranes as well as a large concavity (outlined by a dotted line) merging with the cell membrane. Note that the membrane limiting the concavity (probably representing the membrane of several secretory granules fused together in a so-called chain release) is very smooth as compared with the richly particulated P face of the cell membrane. (b) Typical images of secretory granules (SG) undergoing exocytosis in a B cell. In this thin section, the arrows point to the opening of the inside of the granule in the extracellular space which occurs through fusion of the granule's limiting membrane with the cell (plasma) membrane. (a) ×13,000, (b) × 45,000. The horizontal bar represents (a) 1 μm and (b) 0.2 μm.

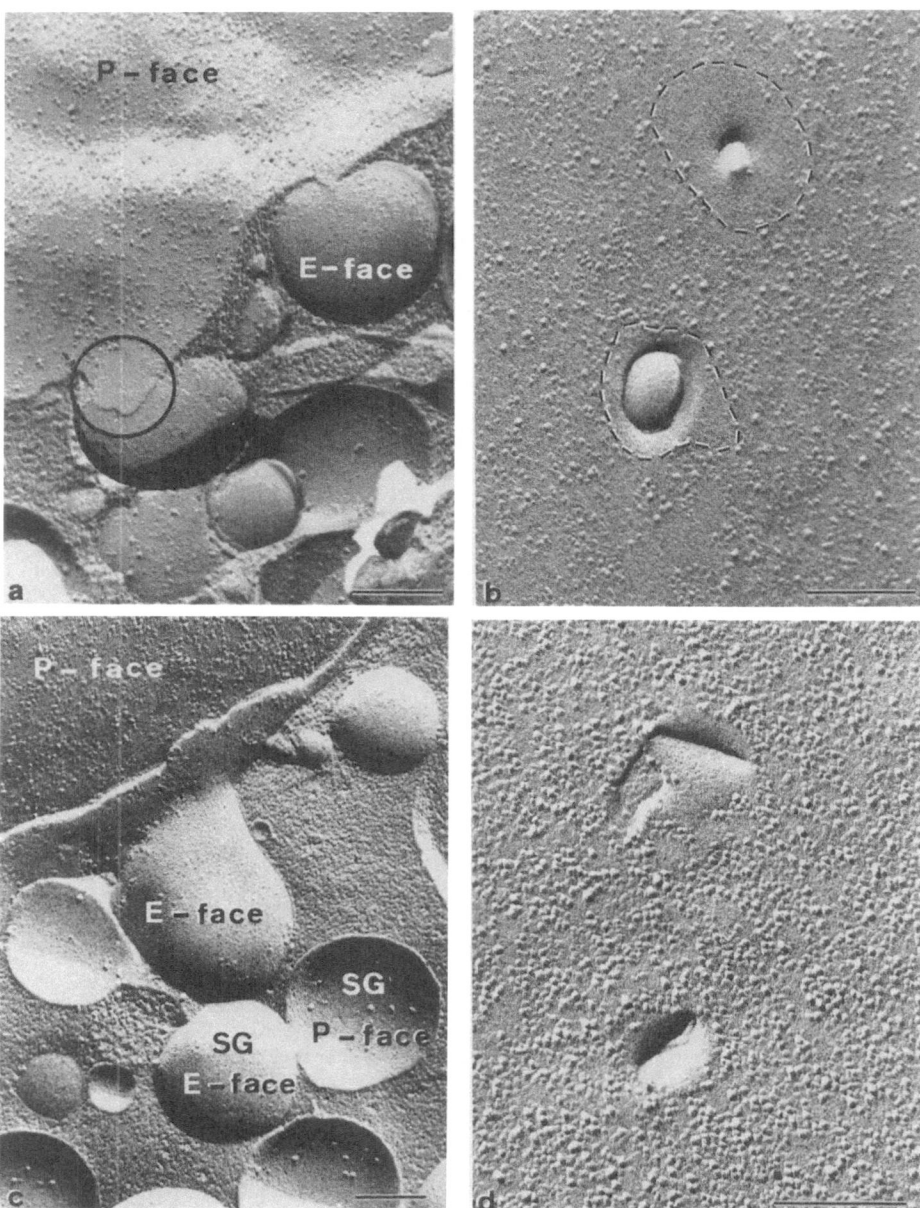

Figure 22. This set of figures illustrates four distinctive stages of exocytosis arranged in what is believed to be a time sequence. (a) Freeze-fracture replica involving the cytoplasm and the plasma membrane (P face) of an islet cell. At the point where the granule limiting membrane (E face) comes into close relationship with the plasma membrane (P face), an area devoid of intramembranous particles is seen in the latter membrane (encircled in black). (b) P face of an islet cell plasma

Again, the regions surrounding the granule cores are devoid of intramembrane particles (Figs. 21a and 22b). Finally, in images which are considered as terminal stages of exocytosis (after the dissolution of the granule core), one can see elongated depressions in the membrane similarly devoid of particles (Fig. 22d). As seen in the section dealing with the freeze-fracture appearance of intracellular membranes, the membranes of secretory granules are distinguished by their very low particle content, in contrast to the plasma membrane which has a high number of particles. Thus, the image shown in Fig. 22a may be interpreted as a remodeling of the richly particulated plasma membrane to accommodate the poorly particulated granule's limiting membrane, while images as shown in Figs. 22b and d may represent the actual granule membrane already incorporated into the plasma membrane. At no stage of exocytosis in islet cells could peculiar membrane differentiations such as "rosettes" of particles on plasma membrane and "annulus" on granule membrane[47] be detected. The particle-free areas of the plasma membrane are reversible modifications of the membrane structure, since a randomly distributed population of particles is found in cells which have been rested after glucose stimulation. The restoration of a normal distribution of intramembrane particles is thus rapid, emphasizing the fluid character of the membrane. Among the possibilities which may account for the reversibility of the particle clearing, the insertion of new particles in the membrane, as well as the selective removal, by endocytosis, of the bare patches of the membrane can be considered. In favor of the last mechanism is the fact that endocytosis is markedly increased by stimulation of B cells by glucose,[48] although which precise sites of the membrane are internalized is not known at present.

Alterations of the Plasma Membrane in Pathology

In the search for a possible cellular defect(s) underlying perturbations of glucose homeostasis, membranes are obvious candidates, given their fundamental role in many cell functions. Three different conditions will be reviewed here: (1) the spontaneous diabetic syndrome in Chinese hamster; (2) alloxan and streptozotocin intoxication; and (3) proteolytic digestion of islet cells *in vitro*.

---

membrane containing two depressed areas devoid of intramembranous particles (dotted lines). In the depression at the bottom of the picture, a bulging granule core is exposed by the fracture plane. (c) Cytoplasmic fracture showing the continuity of a granule limiting membrane (E face) with the E face of the plasma membrane. Both faces have a low intramembrane particle content. P faces of granule limiting membrane are seen as round concavities in the cytoplasm. (d) Islet cell plasma membrane (P face) showing two elongated depressions devoid of intramembrane particles. These images are believed to represent late stages in exocytosis, following the dissolution of the granule core in the extracellular space. (a) ×59,000, (b) ×72,000, (c) ×48,000, (d) ×89,000. The horizontal bar represents 0.2 μm throughout.

Diabetic Chinese Hamster

Chinese hamsters present well-characterized spontaneous diabetic states, and at the ultrastructural level their islet cells show unique features which render possible the direct differentiation of A cells from B cells in freeze-fracture replicas.[49] A quantiative analysis of the intramembrane particle content of plasma membranes in A and B cells of control, diabetic nonketotic, and diabetic ketotic Chinese hamsters shows a progressive decrease of particles in P and E faces (Table 3). On P faces of both A and B cells, the decrease is significant when control groups are compared with ketotic animals, as well as when nonketotic hamsters are compared with ketotic animals. In B cells, the decrease is significant between control and diabetic nonketotic animals as well; in addition, the decrease in the number of particles on P faces is accompanied by a significant increase of the particle mean size (Fig. 23) together with a tendency of the remaining particles to cluster.[49] Under the same conditions, a quantitative study of the freeze-fractured nuclear envelope in A and B cells showed a significant increase of the number of nuclear pores in both nonketotic (B cells) and ketotic (A and B cells) animals as compared with controls (see Table 3).

Alloxan and Streptozotocin Intoxication

A trend in plasma membrane reorganization similar to that found in Chinese hamsters is observed in islet cells which have been exposed *in vitro* to the diabetogenic drugs alloxan and streptozotocin.[50] In isolated islets incubated 5 min in the presence of alloxan (1 mg/ml) at low glucose concentration (20 mg/100 ml), P faces of endocrine cell plasma membranes show a significant decrease of their particle content; decrease continues steadily over 15 and 60 min incubation to reach 40% of control values at 60 min (Fig. 24). In the presence of streptozotocin, the drop of particles on P faces becomes significant only after 15 min of exposure. As with alloxan, however, it attains approximately 40% of control values after 60 min incubation (Fig. 24). In E faces, the quantitative assessment of particle number in both alloxan- and streptozotocin-treated islet cells gives no significant changes but a wide dispersion of the counts. This precludes interpreting the decrease in P face particles as resulting from an absolute diminution of the particle content of the membrane, from a change in the particle partition coefficient between P and E faces, or from both. A very interesting fact emerging from alloxan and streptozotocin studies is that conditions which are known biochemically to prevent the toxic effect of these drugs, i.e., a high glucose concentration in the incubation medium (300 mg/100 ml) or treatment of the tissue with nicotinamide (1.25 mg/ml), also fully prevent the ultrastructural alteration of the plasma membrane (Fig. 25).

Table 3.　Quantitative Data (Mean ± SEM) on Nuclear and Plasma Membranes in Pancreatic A and B Cells of Control (C), Nonketotic Diabetic (NK), and Ketotic Diabetic (K) Chinese Hamsters

	A cell						B cell					
	C	NK	K	C/NK[a]	C/K	NK/K	C	NK	K	C/NK	C/K	NK/K
Nuclear pores												
Number (per μm^2)	9.89	10.59	11.95	NS	<.005	<.02	8.93	9.94	10.15	<.1	<.02	NS
±SEM	0.46	0.46	0.27				0.26	0.55	0.32			
Surface area (% per μm^2)	7.46	7.99	9.01	NS	<.005	<.02	6.44	7.17	7.32	<.1	<.02	NS
±SEM	0.35	0.35	0.20				0.19	0.39	0.23			
Plasma membrane associated particles												
Number in P face (per μm^2)	1186	1071	920	NS	<.005	<.01	1217	948	767	<.005	<.005	<.05
±SEM	97	50	16				29	49	60			
Number in E face (per μm^2)	252	257	368	NS	NS	NS	248	194	298	NS	NS	NS
±SEM	50	67	82				25	28	94			
Mean size in P face (Å)	98.5	99.2	100.6	NS	NS	NS	95.0	96.5	102.1	<.1	<.005	<.001
±SEM	1.0	1.0	1.6				0.6	0.9	1.1			

[a]The statistical significance of differences between groups is indicated in each case (NS: $p > 0.15$). Courtesy of *Diabetologia*, Springer-Verlag.[49]

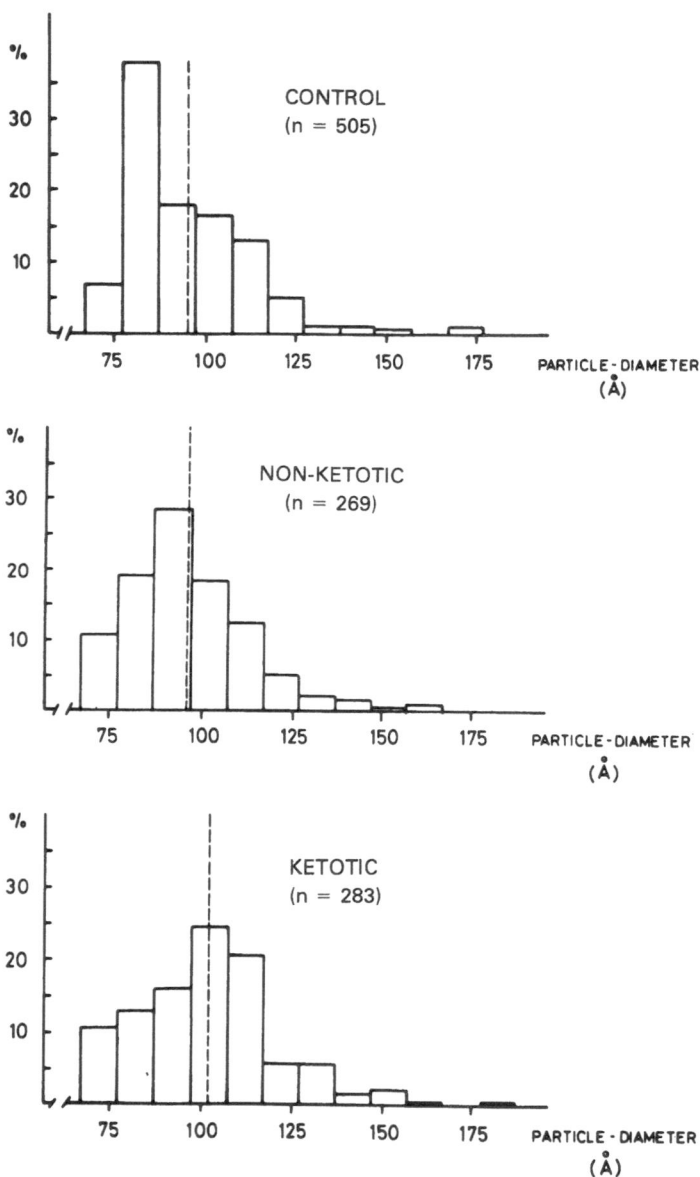

Figure 23. Frequency distribution (%) of particle sizes (Å) in the plasma membrane of B cells from control, diabetic (nonketotic), and ketotic Chinese hamsters. The data show a shift toward larger particle size during the course of diabetes. The mean size of particles in each condition is represented by the vertical dotted line. Courtesy of *Diabetologia,* Springer-Verlag.[49]

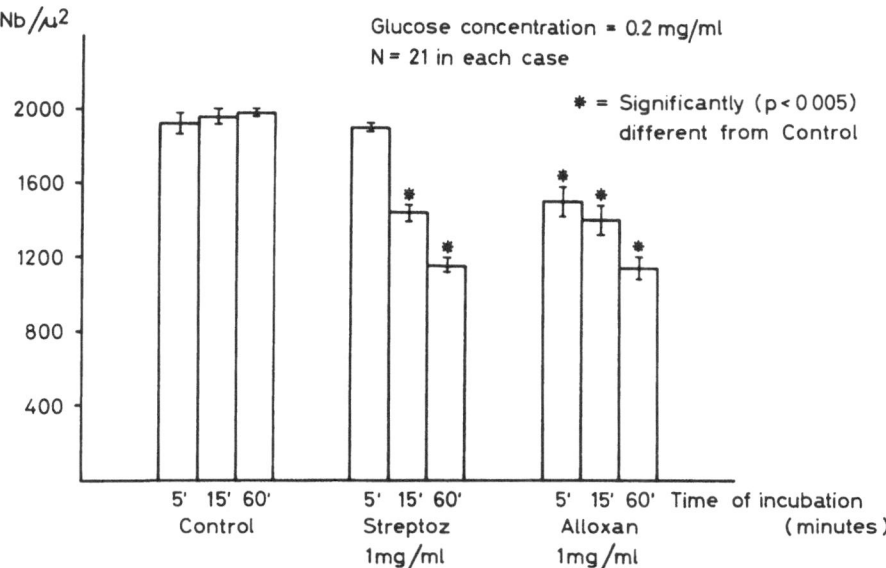

Figure 24. Mean number (±SEM) of intramembrane particles in P face (μm^2) of islet cells incubated at a low glucose concentration (0.2 mg/ml) and exposed to streptozotocin (1 mg/ml) or alloxan (1 mg/ml) for various periods of time. The number of individual observations equals 21 in each experimental condition. Asterisks indicate experimental values significantly ($p < .005$) different from control values. Courtesy of *Laboratory Investigation*.[50]

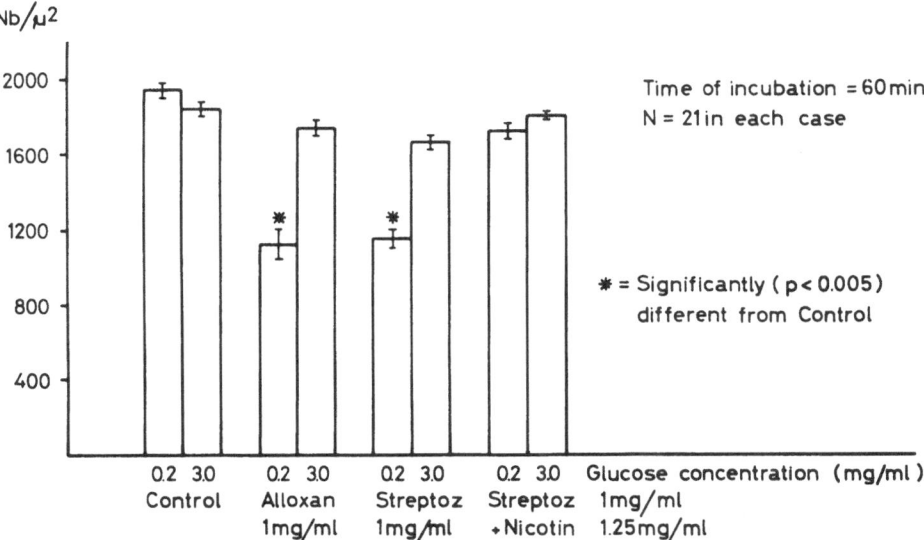

Figure 25. Mean number (±SEM) of intramembrane particles in P face of islet cells incubated for 60 min at a low (0.2 mg/ml) or high (3.0 mg/ml) glucose concentration in the absence or presence of alloxan (1 mg/ml), streptozotocin (1 mg/ml), or streptozotocin plus nicotinamide (1.25 mg/ml). The number of individual observations equals 21 in each experimental condition. Asterisks indicate experimental values significantly ($p < .005$) different from control values. Courtesy of *Laboratory Investigation*.[50]

Proteolytic Digestion of Islets

The last experimentally induced modulation of the islet cell plasma membrane to be reviewed has been obtained by a limited digestion of isolated islets in solutions containing proteolytic enzymes (trypsin, pronase).[4] Such treatment induces a sharp increase of the response of islet cells to stimulatory concentrations of glucose over periods of incubation ranging from 15 to 90 min[51] (Table 4). Concomitantly, in thin sections of pronase-treated and glucose-stimulated islets, there are numerous deformations of the plasma membranes of adjoining B cells enclosing extracellular masses, with polygonal shapes and an electron density similar to that of β granules (Fig. 26). Such images suggest that the secretory product released by B cells is trapped between the cells and/or prevented from being solubilized normally. Freeze-fracture replicas of such material reveal the counterpart of the plasma membrane deformations in the form of polygonal imprints (P face) or bulges (E face) in fracture face of islet cells (Fig. 27). Moreover, they show that most deformations occur within strikingly proliferated tight junctional networks (Figs. 27 and 28). The proliferation of tight junctions (see Fig. 28) assessed by the same morphometrical method as used for evaluating tight junctions during insulin release in untreated islets amounts to a fourfold increase of the density of boundary length (Fig. 29). While dense masses in the extracellular space are found only in glucose-stimulated pronase-treated islets, proliferated tight junctions occur both at low and high glucose concentrations. This result points to an independence of insulin release and

Table 4. Effect of Prior Incubation with Pronase (4 µg/ml) for 90 Min on Immunoreactive Insulin (IRI) Release during Incubation of Isolated Islets at Various Glucose Concentrations

Incubation time (min)	Glucose (mg/100 ml)	IRI release per five islets (ng/ml)				
		Controls			Pronase-treated (4 µg/ml)	
		Mean ± SEM	N^a	p^b	Mean ± SEM	N
15	0	0.77 ± 0.13	15	NS	0.92 ± 0.14	16
15	50	1.20 ± 0.33	15	NS	1.05 ± 0.17	16
15	300	3.06 ± 0.70	13	NS	4.75 ± 0.94	12
30	0	1.20 ± 0.23	15	NS	1.80 ± 0.24	16
30	50	1.18 ± 0.33	15	NS	1.72 ± 0.31	16
30	300	10.62 ± 0.97	13	<.001	20.44 ± 2.19	12
60	0	1.98 ± 0.32	11	NS	2.30 ± 0.37	16
60	50	1.52 ± 0.44	15	NS	2.43 ± 0.59	15
60	300	24.31 ± 2.50	13	<.001	46.67 ± 4.06	12
90	0	1.45 ± 0.21	14	<.001	2.86 ± 0.32	16
90	50	2.20 ± 0.63	15	=.05	3.97 ± 0.67	15
90	300	50.54 ± 4.06	13	<.01	72.12 ± 6.26	12

[a]Number of observations.

[b]The statistical significance of the difference between experimental and control values. Courtesy of *Science*.[51]

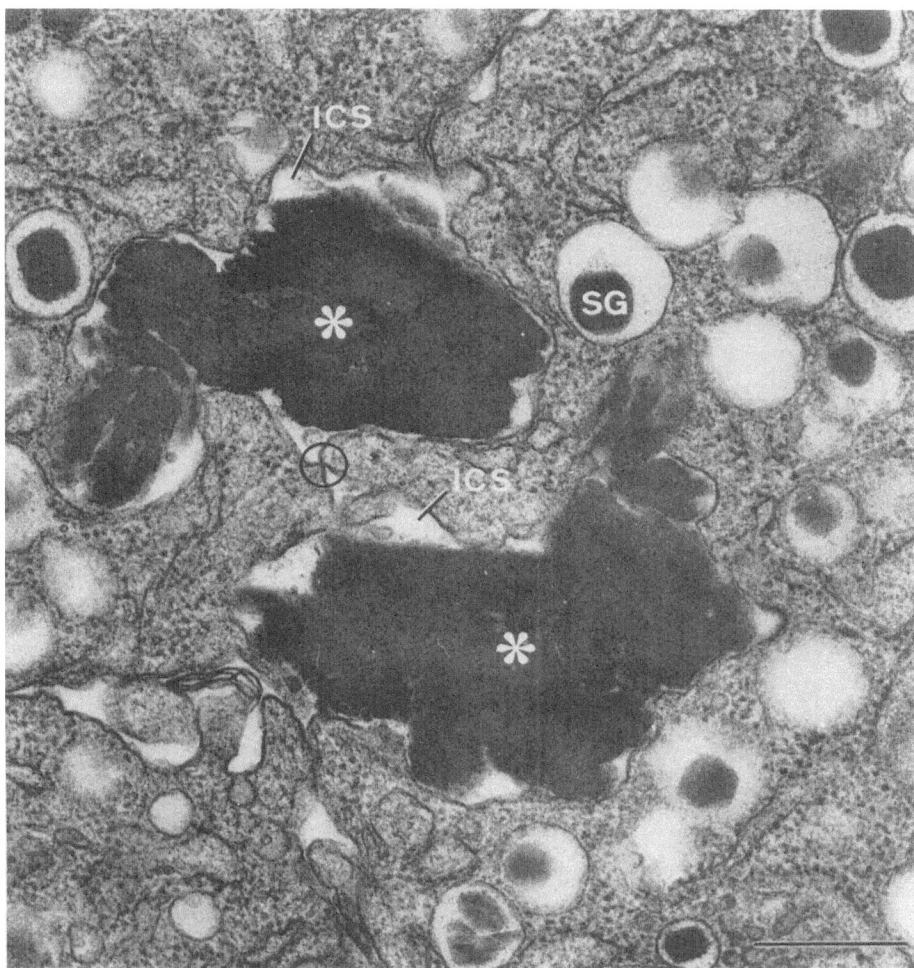

Figure 26. Thin section of isolated islet incubated in presence of 4 μg/ml pronase and stimulated with high glucose concentration (300 mg/100 ml). The intercellular space (ICS) between several B cells contains large irregular masses (*) of an electron density similar to that of the core of β secretory granules (SG). The masses induce deformation in the B cell plasma membranes. The small black circle outlines an area in which the plasma membranes of two adjacent B cells come into close contact, possibly through a tight junction (see Figs. 27 and 28). ×40,000. The horizontal bar represents 0.5 μm.

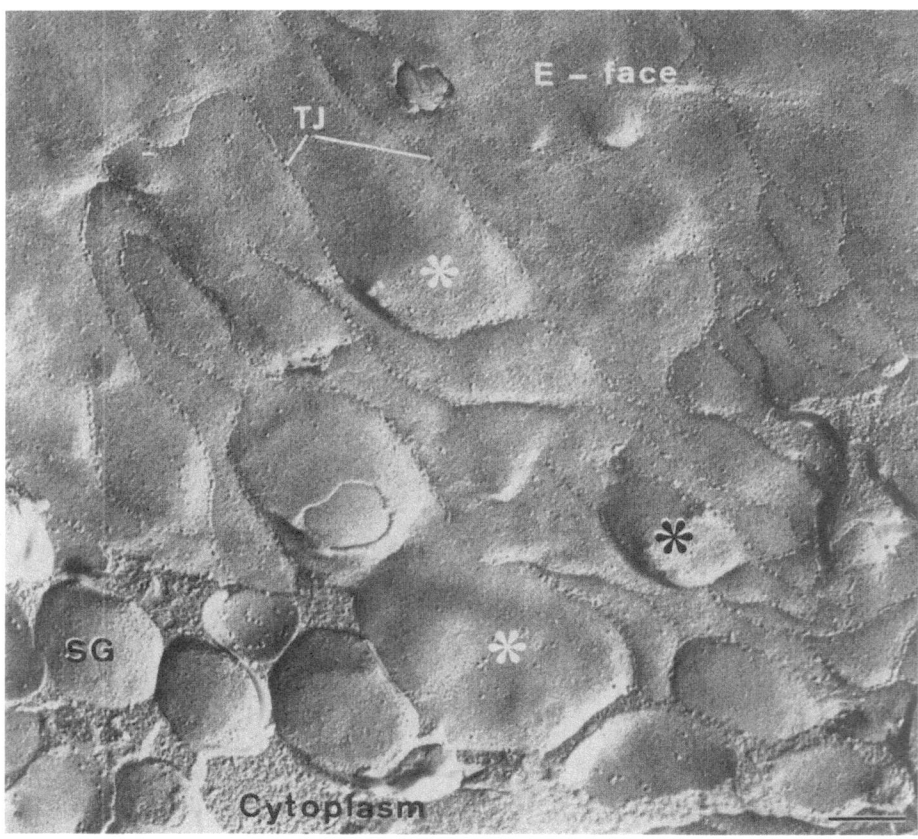

Figure 27. Freeze-fracture replica of an isolated islet treated with 4 μg/ml pronase and stimulated with a high glucose concentration (300 mg/100 ml). Part of an islet cell cytoplasm with secretory granules (SG) is exposed as is the E face of the plasma membrane. The membrane face contains variegated tight junctional furrows (TJ) delimiting deformations of the plasma membrane (*). The deformations are assumed to correspond to the imprints induced by the dense masses in the membrane (see Fig. 26). ×52,000. The horizontal bar represents 0.2 μm.

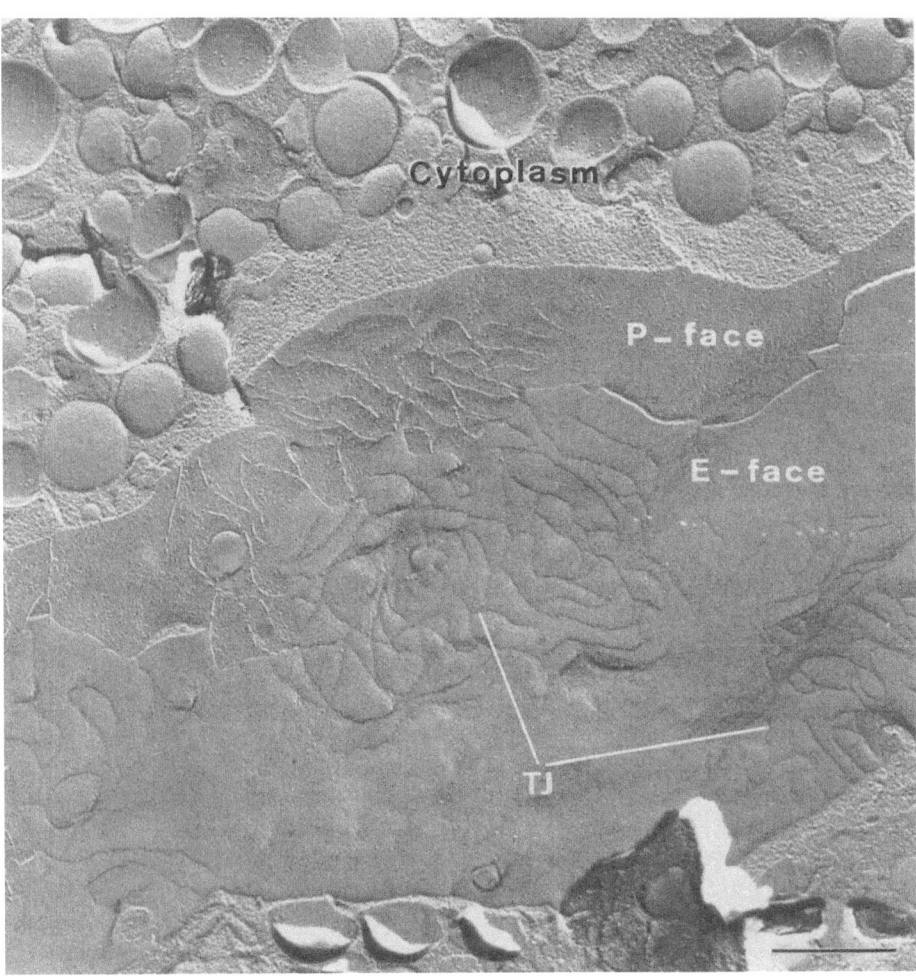

Figure 28. Freeze-fracture replica of isolated islet incubated with 4 μg/ml pronase and stimulated with a high glucose concentration (300 mg/100 ml). The fracture plane has exposed a large area of both the P and E face of two adjacent islet cells before breaking through the cytoplasm of the upper cell. P and E membrane faces display an extensive network of tight junctional elements (TJ). ×33,000. The horizontal bar represents 0.5 μm.

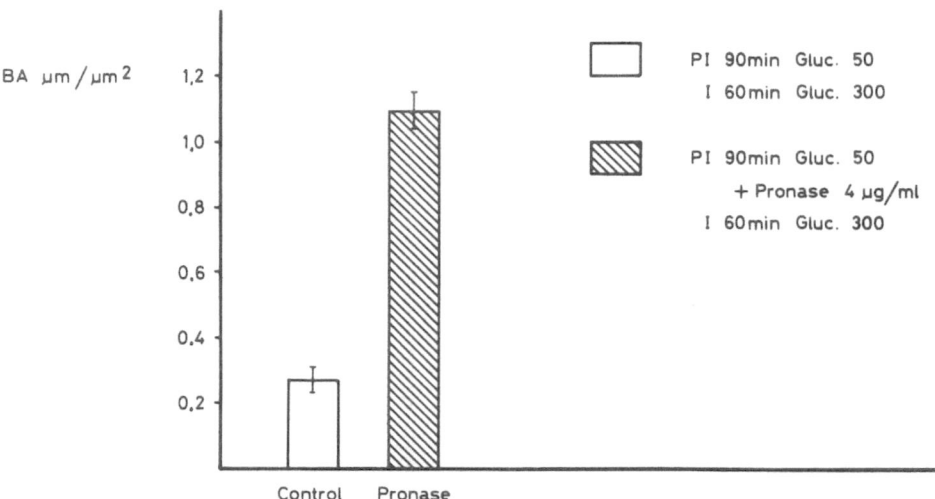

Figure 29. Density of boundary length (B_A) of tight junctions in control and pronase-treated isolated islets. Control and pronase-treated islets were preincubated (PI) for 90 min in 50 mg/100 ml glucose, then further incubated (I) for 60 min in high glucose concentration (300 mg/100 ml). The data show that pronase treatment induces a fourfold increase in the density of the boundary length of tight junctions.

tight-junction formation in pronase-treated islets, and it is compatible with the hypothesis that extracellular masses may form because the released secretory product is prevented by the proliferated tight junctions to diffuse and be solubilized. If true, this, in turn, may be a strong argument in favor of the view that tight junctions in islet cells serve to compartmentalize the extracellular space in contact with the plasma membrane.

Summary

An inquiry into the ultrastructure of membrane systems in pancreatic islet cells has allowed to establish, by several techniques of electron microscopy including thin-sectioning, freeze-fracture, shadow-casting, and surface labeling, a characteristic pattern of organization for both intracellular and plasma membranes. These techniques helped also to define, through the identification of intercellular junctions, specific relationships that exist between the different islet cell types. Several of these patterns of morphological organization were found to be altered in a variety of conditions of normal and pathological functioning of the islet, thus pointing to the fluidity of membrane structure as one of its most relevant characteristics.

Acknowledgment

These studies were supported by Grant No. 3,553,75 from the Swiss National Science Foundation. We wish to acknowledge the invaluable help of our colleagues at the Institute of Histology and Embryology—Dr. Mylène Amherdt, Dr. Francine Malaisse-Lagae, Dr. Mariella Ravazzola, Miss Isabelle Bernard, M. M. Bernard, and Mrs. Marthe Sidler—in various intellectual and technical aspects of the work reported here.

References

1. Orci, L.: *Diabetologia*, **10**:163, 1974.
2. Robertson, J. D.: *Biochem. Soc. Symp.*, **16**:3, 1959.
3. Dauwalder, M., Whaley, W. G., and Kephart, J. E.: *Subcell. Biochem.*, **1**:225, 1972.
4. Orci, L., Ravazzola, M., Amherdt, M., and Malaisse-Lagae, F.: In: *Proceedings of the Eighth Congress of the International Diabetes Federation.* Edited by W. J. Malaisse, and J. Pirart. Excerpta Medica, Amsterdam, 1974, p. 104.
5. Rambourg, A.: *Int. Rev. Cytol.*, **31**:57, 1971.
6. Nicolson, G. L.: *Biochim. Biophys. Acta*, **457**:57, 1976.
7. Lazarides, E., and Weber, K.: *Proc. Nat. Acad. Sci.*, **71**:2268, 1974.
8. Wessels, N. K., Spooner, B. S., and Luduena, M. A.: In: *Locomotion of Tissue Cells. Ciba Foundation 14.* Excerpta Medica, Amsterdam, 1973, p. 53.
9. Wessels, N. K., Spooner, B. S., Ash, J. F., Bradley, M. D., Luduena, M. A., Taylor, E. L., Wrenn, J. T., and Yamada, K. M.: *Science*, **171**:135, 1971.
10. Painter, R. G., Sheetz, M., and Singer, S. J.: *Proc. Nat. Acad. Sci.*, **72**:1359, 1975.
11. Yahara, I., and Edelman, G. M.: *Exp. Cell Res.*, **91**:125, 1975.
12. Revel, J. P., and Ito, S.: In: *The Specificity of Cell Surface.* Edited by E. D. Davis and L. Warren. Prentice Hall, New Jersey, 1967, p. 213.
13. McNutt, N. S., and Weinstein, R. S.: *Prog. Biophys. Mol. Biol.*, **26**:45, 1973.
14. Steere, R. L.: *J. Biophys. Biochem. Cytol.*, **3**:45, 1957.
15. Moor, H., and Mühlethaler, K.: *J. Cell Biol.*, **17**:609, 1963.
16. Branton, D.: *Proc. Nat. Acad. Sci.*, **55**:1048, 1966.
17. Branton, D.: *Phil. Trans. Roy. Soc. Lond. B.*, **261**:133, 1971.
18. Branton, D., Bullivant, S., Gilula, N. B., Karnovsky, M. J., Moor, H., Mühlethaler, K., Northcote, D. H., Packer, L., Satir, B., Satir, P., Speth, V., Staehelin, L. A., Steere, R. L., and Weinstein, R. S.: *Science*, **190**:54, 1975.
19. McNutt, N. S., and Weinstein, R. S.: *J. Cell Biol.*, **47**:666, 1970.
20. Ferner, H.: In: *Das Inselsystem des Pankreas.* G. Thieme, Stuttgart, 1952, p. 119.
21. Branton, D.: *Ann. Rev. Plant Physiol.* **20**:209, 1969.
22. Singer, S. J., and Nicolson, G. L.: *Science*, **175**:720, 1972.
23. Singer, S. J.: *Ann. Rev. Biochem.*, **43**:805, 1974.
24. Satir, P., and Satir, B.: *Exp. Cell Res.*, **89**:404, 1974.
25. Dempsey, G. P., Bullivant, S., and Watkins, W. B.: *Science*, **179**:190, 1973.
26. Montesano, R., Friend, D. S., Perrelet, A., and Orci, L.: *J. Cell Biol.*, **67**:310, 1975.
27. Friend, D. S., and Gilula, N. B.: *J. Cell Biol.*, **53**:758, 1972.
28. Claude, P., and Goodenough, D. A.: *J. Cell Biol.*, **58**:390, 1973.
29. Pricam, C., Humbert, F., Perrelet, A., and Orci, L.: *Lab. Invest.*, **30**:286, 1974.
30. Payton, B. W., Bennett, M. V. L., and Pappas, G. D.: *Science*, **166**:1641, 1969.
31. Gilula, N. B., Reeves, R. O., and Steinbach, A.: *Nature (London)*, **235**:262, 1972.

32. Orci, L., Perrelet, A., Malaisse-Lagae, F., and Vassalli, P.: *C. R. Acad. Sci. Paris*, **283**:1509, 1976.
33. Solomon, A. K.: *J. Gen. Physiol.*, **51**:335s, 1968.
34. Orci, L., Malaisse-Lagae, F., Ravazzola, M., Rouiller, D., Renold, A. E., Perrelet, A., and Unger, R. H.: *J. Clin. Invest.*, **56**:1066, 1975.
35. Nicolson, G. L., and Singer, S. J.: *Proc. Nat. Acad. Sci.*, **68**:942, 1972.
36. Sharon, N., and Lis, H.: *Science*, **177**:949, 1972.
37. Smith, S. B., and Revel, J. P.: *Dev. Biol.*, **27**:434, 1972.
38. Orci, L., Carpentier, J.-L., and Roth, J.: Unpublished observations.
39. Orci, L., Rufener, C., Malaisse-Lagae, F., Blondel, B., Amherdt, M., Bataille, D., Freychet, P., and Perrelet, A.: *Israel J. Med. Sci.*, **11**:639, 1975.
40. Orci, L.: In: *Peptides Hormones: Molecular and Cellular Aspects. Ciba Foundation Symposium 41.* Edited by R. Porter and D. W. Fitzsimons, Excerpta Medica, Amsterdam, 1975, p. 267.
41. Rosenblith, J. Z., Ukena, T. E., Yin, H. H., Berlin, R. D., and Karnovsky, M. J.: *Proc. Nat. Acad. Sci.*, **70**:1625, 1973.
42. Taylor, R. B., Duffus, W. P. H., Raff, M. C., and De Petris, S.: *Nature (New Biol.)*, **233**:225, 1971.
43. Bretscher, M. S., and Raff, M. C.: *Nature (London)*, **258**:43, 1975.
44. Weibel, E. R.: *Int. Rev. Cytol.*, **26**:235, 1969.
45. Orci, L., Amherdt, M., Malaisse-Lagae, F., Rouiller, C., and Renold, A. E.: *Science*, **179**:82, 1973.
46. Orci, L., Perrelet, A., and Friend, D. S.: *J. Cell Biol.*, 1977 (in press).
47. Satir, B., Schooley, L., and Satir, P.: *J. Cell Biol.*, **56**:153, 1973.
48. Orci, L., Malaisse-Lagae, F., Ravazzola, M., Amherdt, M., and Renold, A. E.: *Science*, **181**:561, 1973.
49. Orci, L., Amherdt, M., Malaisse-Lagae, F., Perrelet, A., Dulin, W. E., Gerritsen, G. C., Malaisse, W. J., and Renold, A. E.: *Diabetologia*, **10**:529, 1974.
50. Orci, L., Amherdt, M., Malaisse-Lagae, F., Ravazzola, M., Malaisse, W. J., Perrelet, A., and Renold, A. E.: *Lab Invest.*, **34**:451, 1976.
51. Orci, L., Amherdt, M., Henquin, J. C., Lambert, A. E., Unger, R. H., and Renold, A. E.: *Science*, **180**:647, 1973.

Chapter 8

The Physiology of Insulin Release

Paul E. Lacy

The β cells of the islets of Langerhans play a primary role in the pathogenesis of diabetes mellitus in man. Several lines of evidence obtained from clinical studies on diabetic subjects support this statement. Tolbutamide is an oral hypoglycemic agent which has been shown to stimulate insulin release from the β cell and to maintain normoglycemia in certain diabetic subjects. Thus tolbutamide apparently stimulates insulin secretion more effectively than glucose in these patients, which would suggest an impairment in glucose-induced insulin release in the β cells. Detailed studies on the pattern and rate of glucose-induced insulin secretion in maturity-onset diabetes and early stages of juvenile diabetes have shown a delay in the response of the β cells to glucose stimulation.[1] These findings also indicate an impairment in the ability of the β cell to recognize glucose and to translate this recognition into the release of insulin. Transplantation of the whole pancreas has been accomplished in diabetic patients.[2-4] During the period of survival of the transplant, the patients became normoglycemic and did not require exogenous insulin therapy, which clearly indicates that the primary defect is in the islet cells of the diabetic. The ultimate quest is to establish the identity of the defect or defects present in the β cells of diabetics. In order to search for these possible abnormalities, it is essential that basic information be obtained on the normal mechanisms for the formation, storage, and release of insulin by β cells. This chapter will be devoted to a review of the information available on the basic mechanism of insulin secretion as well as indicating potential sites for defects in this mechanism in diabetes mellitus.

Insulin Release

Glucose is the primary stimulus for the release of insulin in man and in most mammals. Long-chain fatty acids[5,6] and amino acids[7] will stimulate insulin release, however, *in vitro* studies indicate that their stimulatory effect is transitory unless the primary stimulus—glucose—is present. In ruminants, short-chain fatty acids are potent stimulators of insulin release,[8] and in sheep,

Paul E. Lacy • Washington University, St. Louis, Missouri.

butyrate is more effective than glucose.[9] Amino acids are more effective than glucose in stimulating insulin release from the fetal pancreas of rabbits.[10] Thus, β cells are responsive to the metabolic fuels of the body and vary in their responsiveness to these fuels in different species and in different stages of fetal development of the β cells.

In man and in those mammals in which glucose is the primary stimulus for insulin secretion, the sensitivity of the β cells to glucose stimulation may vary normally, or a variation in sensitivity can be produced experimentally. The 24-day fetal pancreas of the rabbit does not respond to glucose stimulation, whereas moderate stimulation occurs from day 29 of fetal life to 5 days postpartum, and normal response occurs by 6 weeks of age.[10] The 24-day fetal pancreas responds to stimulation with theophylline, but glucagon does not stimulate insulin release.

These findings indicate a maturation of the β cell which may involve the adenylate cyclase system and possibly other factors involved in the recognition of glucose. Experimentally, the sensitivity of β cells to glucose stimulation can be diminished by simply fasting rats for 48–72 hr.[11] The response of isolated islets from fasted rats to glucose stimulation can be enhanced by concomitant exposure of the islets to glucose and theophylline.[12] Adenylate cyclase activity and the cAMP content of the islets are markedly diminished in the fasted rat.[13,14] These findings also implicate the adenylate cyclase system and possible recognition factors for glucose as being responsible for the change in sensitivity of the β cell to glucose stimulation.

The pattern of insulin release from the β cell following glucose stimulation is biphasic.[15,16] Figure 1 illustrates this biphasic pattern of release from perifused, isolated rat islets maintained *in vitro*. The first phase of secretion reaches a maximum rate approximately 5 min after stimulation, and the second phase achieves a maximum level approximately 30 min after stimulation with glucose. Tolbutamide alone induces only a monophasic pattern of release, whereas tolbutamide in the presence of glucose (1.0 mg/ml) induces a monophasic pattern of release with a subsequent elevated basal rate of release.[16,17] The modified second phase or elevated basal secretion is apparently due to a synergistic action of glucose and tolbutamide.

The normal physiologic response of the β cell to a concentration of glucose greater than 1.0 mg/ml is a biphasic release of insulin. This simple statement encompasses numerous questions concerning the cellular mechanisms and intracellular events responsible for the secretion of insulin. How is glucose recognized by the β cell? Is the recognition and induction of release due to an interaction of glucose with glucoreceptors on the β cell, or is it due to the formation of specific metabolites or cofactors from the metabolism of glucose? How is insulin stored in the β cell? What are the intracellular, macromolecular, and biochemical mechanisms responsible for the release of stored insulin? Why does the β cell release insulin in a biphasic manner? How does glucose initiate the replenishment of insulin stored within the β cell? Do diabetic animal models exist with defects in this normal secretory mechanism? What are the sites for

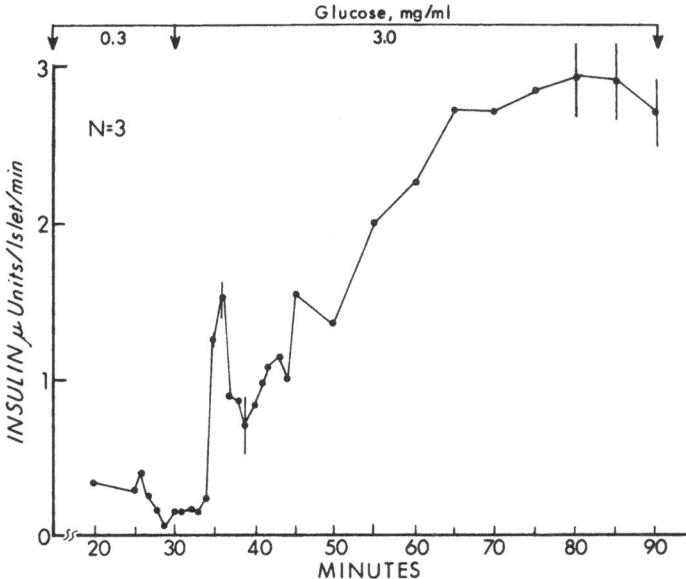

Figure 1. Biphasic pattern of insulin release from perifused, isolated rat islets. (Lacy *et al.*: *Diabetes*, **21**:987, 1972.)

potential defects in insulin secretion in β cells of human diabetics? These are the major questions which will be discussed in subsequent sections of this chapter.

Glucoreceptor or Glucose Metabolism?

At the present time, the two concepts concerning the mechanism by which glucose initiates insulin release are: (1) Glucose is metabolized with the formation of specific metabolites or cofactors which initiate insulin release; and (2) specific receptors for glucose exist on the β cell membrane. In 1963, Grodsky *et al.* compared the insulin release capacities of various sugars and suggested that only those which are metabolizable may stimulate insulin secretion.[18] Support for this suggestion was provided by studies on islet cell metabolism which demonstrated a close correlation between rates of utilization of glucose and mannose by the islets and their effects on insulin secretion.[19-21] The metabolism of glucose through the pentose cycle was also implicated in insulin release. Xylitol promoted insulin secretion in dogs, and the effect of several agents on insulin release could be correlated with their effects on the intraislet concentration of 6-phosphogluconate.[22,23]

A direct challenge to the metabolic theory of glucose action came from the quantitative studies of Matschinsky *et al.*[24] on determining the level of intermediates and cofactors of glucose metabolism within rat islets following stimulation with glucose. These investigators found that most of the metabolites and cofactors measured were unchanged during the first 5 min of glucose stimulation, even though insulin release could be detected within 1 min after injecting glucose. An increase in fructose diphosphate and triose phosphate did occur within 1 min, however, these metabolites also increased in conditions in which there was an absence of insulin release. Since the change in the metabolites of glucose in the β cell did not correlate with immediate insulin release, Matschinsky *et al.*[24] suggested that glucoreceptors may exist on the β cell membrane. Further evidence in support of this concept was the demonstration that glycolysis and glucose utilization could be inhibited with iodoacetate (0.2 mM), yet insulin release occurred in the presence of high concentrations of glucose with pyruvate as an alternate fuel.[25] A more elaborate model has been proposed which involves an initiator unit capable of binding glucose or mannose and a potentiator unit capable of binding a wider spectrum of agents which would not influence insulin release unless the initiator unit is stimulated.[26] These same authors also suggest a second model in which the metabolism of the initiator leads to the production of an intracellular agent which stimulates insulin release. Thus, the controversy has continued. Recently, other approaches have become available which provide additional indirect evidence in support of the existence of glucoreceptors on the β cell membrane. These indirect approaches have involved studies on the *in vivo* and *in vitro* action of alloxan.

Approximately 10 years after the discovery of the diabetogenic action of alloxan, it was found that the prior injection of either glucose or mannose would protect rats against the development of diabetes by alloxan.[27] Galactose had no protective action. These *in vivo* studies on the diabetogenic action of alloxan have been extended in recent years with the demonstration of a stereospecificity for the protective action of D-glucose.[28] The α anomer of D-glucose provides greater protection against the diabetogenic action of alloxan than the β anomer. The prior administration of 3-O-methyl-D-glucose also provides protection against the diabetogenic action of alloxan, and recent studies indicate a greater protection with the α anomer than with the β anomer.[29] These *in vivo* studies have lead to the suggestion that the protective site for glucose against alloxan is on the β cell membrane, and alloxan may be interacting with glucoreceptors on the membrane.[29,30]

An *in vitro* model has recently been developed for a direct study of the effect of alloxan on insulin secretion by isolated rat islets as well as determining the protective action of glucose and other agents on preventing this inhibitory action of alloxan.[31] In this model, isolated rat islets are perifused *in vitro* and exposed to alloxan (0.2 mg/ml) for a period of 5 min. Following exposure, the islets are stimulated with glucose (5.0 mg/ml). Exposure to alloxan produces a complete inhibition of subsequent glucose-induced insulin secretion, whereas the concomitant presence of glucose (5.0 mg/ml) during the period of exposure to alloxan provides complete protection of the islets (Fig. 2). Studies on the protective action of other hexoses revealed that D-glucose, D-mannose, and 3-O-methyl-D-glucose provide complete protection of the islets, whereas D-fructose, 2-deoxy-D-glucose, and D-galactose provide slight protection, and L-glu-

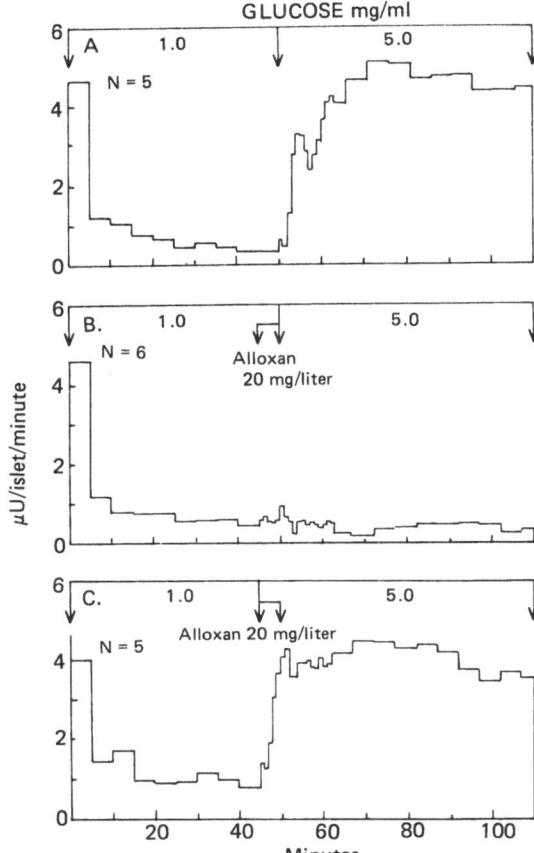

Figure 2. (A) Biphasic pattern of insulin release from perifused, isolated rat islets following stimulation with glucose. (B) Inhibition of glucose-induced insulin release following exposure of isolated islets to alloxan. (C) Protection of islets from alloxan by glucose (5.0 mg/ml). (Tomita *et al.*: *Diabetes,* **23**:517, 1974.)

cose provides no protection. A stereospecificity of protection was demonstrated since α-D-glucose provided greater protection than β-D-glucose.[32] It has also been shown that α-D-glucose is more effective in stimulating insulin release than β-D-glucose.[33,34]

In vitro exposure of the islets to alloxan for 5 min had no effect on subsequent tolbutamide-induced insulin release. This finding indicated that the islets were still viable and responsive to certain stimuli. Alloxan alone stimulates a monophasic release of insulin, apparently as a result of alloxan interacting with a specific initiating site on the β cell. The site of action of alloxan is not the hexose transport system in the β cell since the transport of glucose into isolated rat islets is normal following exposure to alloxan.[35] Barbituric acid, which is chemically similar to alloxan except for the substitution of two hydrogen groups on position C-5 instead of a carbonyl group, provides complete protection against the *in vitro* action of alloxan and accomplishes this action without being taken up by the islet cells.[36]

The interpretation of these findings at the present time is that alloxan is acting at the β cell membrane and the site of action must be adjacent to but not identical with the hexose transport site. This site of action on the β cell membrane probably involves glucoreceptors. The indirect evidence in favor of specific glucoreceptors on the β cell membrane includes the lack of correlation of metabolites of glucose with insulin release, the *in vivo* studies on the stereospecificity of glucose protection against the diabetogenic action of alloxan, and the *in vitro* studies on alloxan inhibition of subsequent glucose-induced insulin release. The indirect evidence strongly indicates the existence of glucoreceptors, however, direct evidence of binding of glucose and alloxan with specific sites on isolated plasma membranes of the islet cells will be needed before the existence of glucoreceptors can be completely accepted. If the interaction of glucose with glucoreceptors is responsible for the first step in the initiation of insulin release, glucose metabolism would still play a significant role in the intracellular events associated with the subsequent release of insulin from the β cell.

Calcium Metabolism

Extracellular calcium is an essential requirement for insulin secretion to occur.[37] Malaisse-Lagae and Malaise[38] and Malaisse[39] have measured the uptake of ^{45}Ca by isolated islets under a variety of experimental conditions. Glucose stimulates ^{45}Ca uptake, and the interrelationship between ^{45}Ca uptake and glucose concentration is characterized by a sigmoidal curve comparable to that for insulin release and glucose concentration. These studies reflect changes in bound ^{45}Ca, since the islets are washed several times prior to determining their radioactivity. A double-label isotope technique has been used to determine total accumulation of ^{45}Ca in isolated islets from obese hyperglycemic mice.[40] The double-label isotope technique has been used recently in our laboratory to study the acute effect of glucose on total ^{45}Ca accumulation in isolated rat islets.[41] As shown in Fig. 3, glucose (20 mM) stimulates a rapid accumulation of ^{45}Ca in the islets, which remains significantly greater than the calcium uptake with non-stimulatory levels of glucose for 70 min. Inhibition of insulin secretion with deuterium oxide had no effect on the stimulatory action of glucose with respect to acute calcium uptake. Thus, glucose directly initiates a change in the permeability of the β cell membrane to calcium.

A heterocyclic monocarboxylic acid antibiotic produced by *Streptomyces chartreuensis* has been observed to be a specific membrane carrier ionophore for divalent cations in plasma and organelle membranes.[42] A divalent cation ionophore, which transports calcium and magnesium across biological membranes, has been used to determine the effect of this ionophore on insulin release from perifused rat islets.[43] If the islets are perifused with the ionophore in the absence of glucose and calcium is added, a sudden spike of insulin release occurs. These findings clearly indicate that an increase in intracellular calcium alone can initiate insulin release. It is possible that calcium-specific ionophores may exist normally in biological membranes.[44] If this is established, then glucose

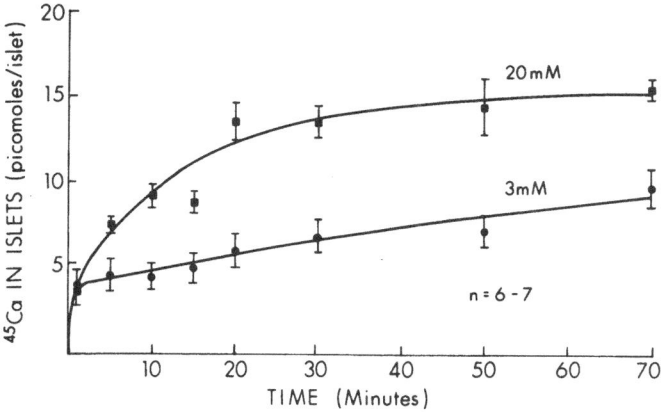

Figure 3. ^{45}Calcium uptake by isolated rat islets in the presence of low and high concentrations of glucose using the dual-label isotope technique. [^{3}H]Sucrose was used as the extracellular marker.

induction of the change in membrane permeability to calcium may involve ionophores or enzyme systems responsible for cation exchange across the plasma membrane.

Bound calcium in the β cell appears to be affected by cAMP.[39] Theophylline and DBcAMP promote an efflux of ^{45}Ca from perifused isolated islets containing bound ^{45}Ca. These agents will induce insulin secretion from isolated islets in the presence of a high concentration of glucose and extremely low levels of extracellular calcium.[45] Thus, agents which affect the level of cAMP in the β cell may affect insulin release in part through mobilization of calcium from bound pools within the β cell.

Adenylate Cyclase System

Recent studies have clearly demonstrated that the level of cAMP within the islets of Langerhans is increased following acute stimulation with glucose.[46,47] Measurements of adenylate cyclase activity in homogenates of rat islets demonstrated stimulation with glucagon, whereas glucose did not alter adenylate cyclase activity.[48] It will be necessary to obtain a plasma membrane fraction from the islets in order to determine whether glucose affects adenylate cyclase associated with the membranes. In contrast with other endocrine systems, cAMP does not appear to play the role of the second messenger in the β cell. The level of cAMP in the β cell can be increased markedly with a variety of agents (glucagon, theophylline, or DMcAMP) yet insulin secretion does not occur unless the primary stimulus—glucose—is present.

Adenylate cyclase activity and cAMP content of the islets can be diminished by fasting rats for 48–72 hr.[13,14] Under these conditions, glucose-induced insulin release is markedly impaired, whereas theophylline in conjunction with glucose will enhance the secretion of insulin. These same alterations in β cell secretion can be produced *in vitro* by using a long-term perifusion system for maintenance of isolated rat islets in a low concentration of glucose (0.5 mg/ml) for a period of 4 days.[49] As shown in Fig. 4, maintenance of the islets for 17 hr with low glucose will result in a marked impairment of insulin release and a blunting of the first phase of secretion as compared with controls. At the end of 4 days, the first phase of secretion is absent, with a gradually increasing rate of secretion during the second phase. The level of adenylate cyclase activity in the islets maintained in the presence of a low glucose concentration was approximately 50% of the levels present in normal islets. Stimulation of the islets with glucose and theophylline after 4 days of maintenance with low glucose will also return the insulin secretory activity of the islets toward normal. These *in vitro* studies would indicate that the primary factor in the fasting animal affecting the insulin secretory activity of the islets is the concentration of glucose. At the present time it is unknown whether this chronic effect of glucose is due to a change in glucoreceptors on the β cell membrane, a change in glucose metabolism within the β cell, a change in calcium metabolism, or an alteration in protein synthesis within the cell. The resolution of these fundamental questions will provide further insight into the mechanism of glucose induction of insulin secretion and the interrelationship of glucose and cAMP metabolism in the β cell.

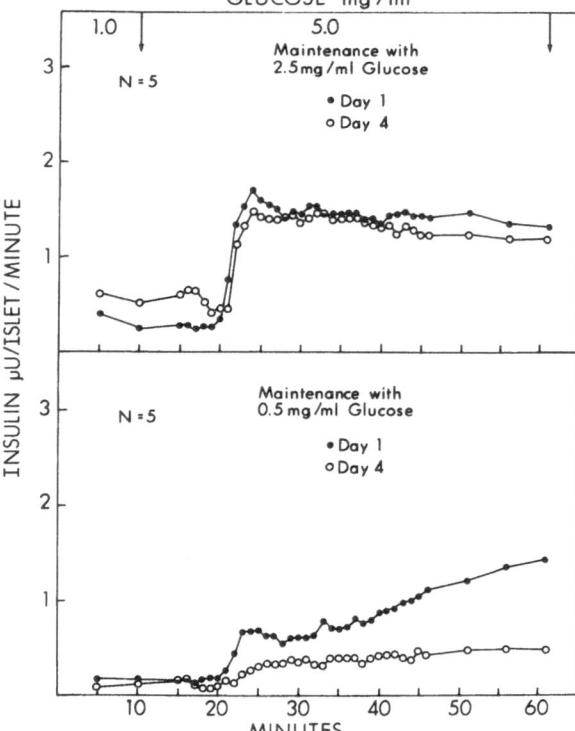

Figure 4. Effect of maintaining isolated rat islets with low (0.5 mg/ml) and high (2.5 mg/ml) concentrations of glucose on the pattern and rate of glucose-induced insulin released on day 1 and day 4. (Lacy *et al.: Diabetes,* **25**:484–493, 1976.)

Even though cAMP does not appear to be the second messenger responsible for insulin release, it does affect the intracellular events initiated by stimulation of the β cell with glucose. As discussed earlier, Malaisse[39] has suggested that cAMP may induce translocation of bound calcium to a free form which will result in insulin release. Recently, a sensitive method has been developed for quantitative studies on polymerized and depolymerized microtubulin in isolated islets.[50] Using this procedure, studies on the microtubulin content of islets from fasted rats have shown a significant decrease in the polymerized microtubulin or intact microtubules in the islets of these animals.[51] When the islets from the fasted rats were stimulated with glucose *in vitro,* no change in polymerized microtubulin occurred unless theophylline was present. When this agent was present, glucose-induced insulin secretion returned toward normal, and polymerized microtubules or intact microtubules were formed,

From the evidence available at the present time, it would appear that cAMP may have a modulating effect on insulin secretion by either liberating calcium from bound pools in the cell or by participating in the transformation of depolymerized microtubulin into intact microtubules, or by both of these mechanisms.

Microtubular–Microfilamentous System

The β cell has a microtubular–microfilamentous system similar to that present in many other types of cells. The microtubules are linear, hollow rods of varying lengths which have a diameter of approximately 200 Å. Microfilaments have a diameter of approximately 40–70 Å and are located predominantly beneath the plasma membrane of the β cell.[52] In tissue culture preparations of β cells in which the individual cells develop elongated cytoplasmic processes, columns of microtubules can be observed separating columns of β granules as shown in Fig. 5. The microtubules approach the plasma membrane and apparently become enmeshed in the microfilamentous web. Microfilaments contain actin as demonstrated by their interaction with heavy meromyosin.[53] Dynein is a protein associated with microtubules that is apparently involved in the induction of movement of flagella by the microtubules.[54]

The structure and function of microtubules can be altered by several different chemical agents. Colchicine, vinblastine, and vincristine alter the integrity of the microtubules, whereas deuterium oxide, hexylene glycol, and ethyl alcohol stabilize the microtubules but interfere with their function. *In vitro* studies on the effect of these agents on glucose-induced insulin secretion from isolated rat islets have demonstrated that each of these agents will inhibit glucose-induced insulin secretion.[55,56] In perifusion studies, it was demonstrated that these agents affect both the first and second phase of insulin secretion.[57] Since these agents had no effect on either calcium uptake or on insulin synthesis by the islets, it was postulated that the microtubular system was involved in the intracellular movement of β granules to the cell surface following glucose stimulation.[55,56]

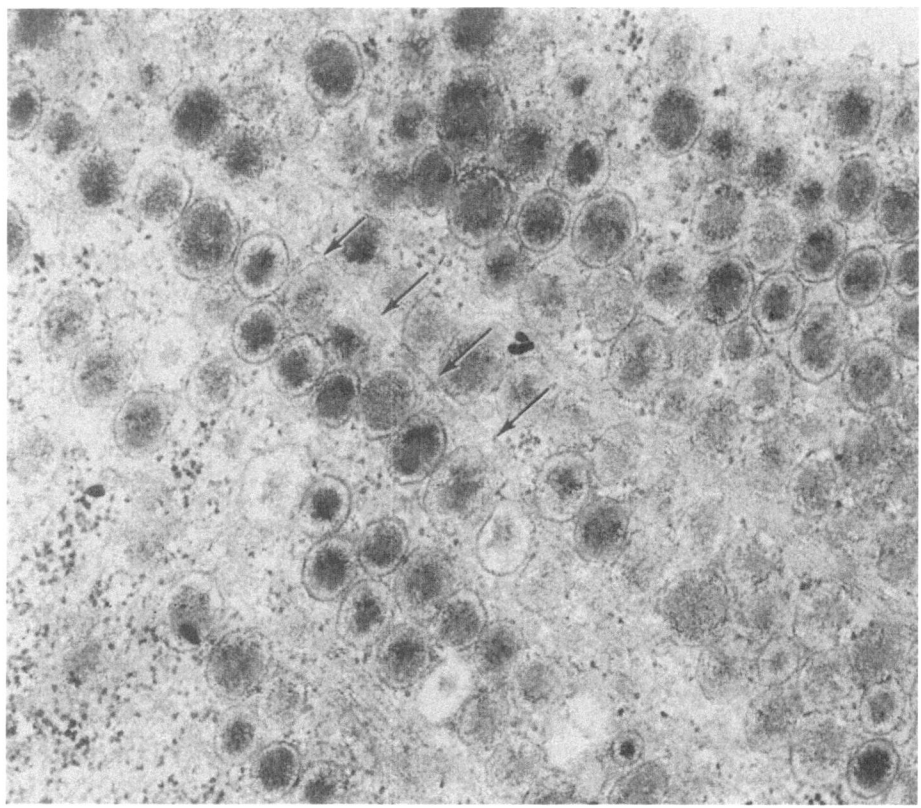

Figure 5. Electron micrograph of a β cell in a monolayer cell culture (2.5 days) of neonatal rat pancreas. Rows of microtubules (arrows) separate the linear columns of β granules in the β cell. ×36,700. (Orci *et al.*: *Ultrastruct. Res.,* **43**:270, 1973.)

The microfilamentous system can be affected by the cytochalasins, which are metabolites of molds. Following the addition of cytochalasin B to isolated islets, the microfilamentous web beneath the plasma membrane is altered with the formation of masses of felt-like accumulations of filaments at intervals beneath the membrane.[52] Cytochalasin B enhances glucose-induced and tolbutamide-induced insulin secretion. Orci *et al.*[52] have suggested that in the unstimulated β cell the microfilamentous web serves as a potential barrier to the β granules, and with glucose stimulation, the microfilaments assist in bringing the secretory granules to the β cell membrane. Cytochalasin B not only affects the microfilamentous system, but it also inhibits the hexose transport system of isolated islets[58] as well as in other cells.[59] These findings have raised questions concerning the primary site of action of cytochalasin B with respect to enhancement of glucose-induced insulin release. In recent studies in our laboratory, it has been shown that cytochalasin D does not affect the hexose transport system of isolated islets but does cause a redistribution of the microfilamentous system in the β cell similar to cytochalasin B and results in enhancement of glucose-induced insulin secretion.[60] These findings add further support to the original suggestion of Orci *et al.*[52] of the involvement of the microfilamentous system in insulin release from the β cell. Recently, Mirande *et al.*[61] have indicated that cytochalasin B and D may be inducing hypercontraction of microfilaments.

The hypothesis that the microtubular–microfilamentous system was involved in the translocation of β granules following glucose stimulation was based upon the assumption that granular movement actually occurred and that the movement was directional in nature. This assumption has been verified recently by cinemicrographic studies of movement of β granules in monolayer cultures of adult rat islet cells.[62] These studies demonstrated an increase in β granule movement following stimulation with glucose and a cessation of the movement when calcium was absent from the extracellular medium. The pathway and distance traveled of individual β granules were also determined. In one instance, a granule moved a total distance of 11.2 μm and accomplished this in three segments. In the first segment the granule moved at a rate of 1.2 μm/sec, paused for 2 sec, moved again for a distance of 3.8 μm, paused for 0.6 sec, and moved for a distance of 5.0 μm at a rate of 1.3 μm/sec. In this instance and in all of the granules measured, the movement was always unidirectional and occurred at a constant rate for each segment of movement. Rate of movement of individual granules ranged from 0.7–3.0 μm/sec, with an average rate of 1.5 μm/sec. This rate of movement is similar to the "fast" component of axoplasmic flow in nerve fibers. The addition of either vinblastine or deuterium oxide inhibited glucose-induced β granule movement, whereas cytochalasin B in the presence of a stimulating level of glucose produced a significant increase in β granule movement, and the amount of movement decreased when cytochalasin B was removed. These findings clearly indicated a directional movement of β granules, a rate of movement comparable to the "fast" component of macromolecular transport in nerve fibers, the requirement of intact microtubules for granule movement, and enhancement of movement when the microfilamentous system was affected by cytochalasin B.

Based upon observations such as the preceding, it has been proposed that the microtubular–microfilamentous system is responsible for the translocation of β granules to the cell surface following stimulation with glucose.[52,55,56,63] The microtubules could either serve as the guiding structure for the linear, unidirectional movement of the granules, or they could in some way provide the propelling force for the movement of the granules or microfilaments associated with the microtubules. The microfilamentous web beneath the plasma membrane could assist in bringing the granules to the final stage of their journey— the plasma membrane of the β cell. It has also been suggested that calcium may serve as the trigger for the induction of contraction of this system following glucose stimulation.[64,65] Further studies are needed to demonstrate anatomical or biochemical evidence of direct linkage of the secretory granules with the microtubular–microfilamentous system and identification of the propelling force for movement of the granules.

Emiocytosis

It has been shown by ultrastructural studies and *in vitro* studies on isolated secretory granules that the final step in the release of insulin from the β cell is by the simple process of emiocytosis.[66,67] The β granules are apparently translocated to the plasma membrane by the microtubular–microfilamentous system, and the membranous sacs encasing the granules fuse with the plasma membrane, rupture, and liberate the granules into the extracellular space where they dissolve. Orci *et al.*[68] have recently confirmed this release mechanism using freeze-etch electron microscopy by demonstrating a direct continuity of the plasma membrane with the membranous sac encasing a β granule.

One of the remaining problems in the process of emiocytosis is determining how fusion of the membranous sacs encasing the granules and the plasma membrane is initiated. In the adrenal medulla, the membranous sacs encasing medullary secretory granules contain lysolecithin which is absent or present in only small quantities in the plasma membrane of the medullary cell.[69] Since lysolecithin causes lysis of red blood cells, it has been suggested that lysolecithin in the membranous sacs of the medullary granules may be responsible for the fusion of the sacs with the plasma membrane in emiocytosis of chromaffin granules.[70] Studies are needed to determine the lipid composition of the membranous sacs of β granules and the plasma membrane as well as the *in vitro* conditions which will initiate or permit the fusion of the membranous sacs with plasma membrane fractions of the islets.

A second problem in the process of emiocytosis is the fate of the membrane encasing the β granule after it has been incorporated into the plasma membrane. Using peroxidase as an extracellular histochemical marker, Orci *et al.*[71] have demonstrated a recycling of plasma membrane of the β cell following glucose stimulation. In the presence of nonstimulating levels of glucose, the horseradish peroxidase remained at the cell surface, whereas following stimulation with glucose, microvesicles containing peroxidase could be demonstrated in the cytoplasm as well as in the Golgi complex and lysosomes of the β cells. Thus, some of the recycled membrane would appear to be reutilized in the Golgi area.

The continued incorporation of new membrane into the plasma membrane and recycling of portions of the plasma membrane raises interesting questions as to whether receptor proteins and enzymes associated with the β cell membrane are continually changing in distribution, whether intramembranous flow maintains a uniform anatomical distribution of these structures, whether specific removal of the newly incorporated membrane occurs, and whether the microtubular–microfilamentous system is involved in membrane recycling. These are important basic questions for future exploration.

Biphasic Pattern of Insulin Release

One of the intriguing aspects of insulin release is the biphasic pattern of secretion. This mode of secretion undoubtedly plays an important role in the rapid regulation of the level of blood sugar and maintenance of normoglycemia. Alterations of this normal biphasic response may also be of importance in the early stages of diabetes mellitus in man. An important question is what is the mechanism responsible for this biphasic pattern of insulin release?

An obvious suggestion for the biphasic pattern of release was that insulin released during the first phase temporarily inhibited secretion by a feedback mechanism. Acute *in vitro* studies have failed to demonstrate an inhibitory effect of massive quantities of insulin on the total amount of insulin released from isolated rat islets.[72] Perfusion studies have also failed to demonstrate an inhibitory effect of exogenous insulin on the biphasic pattern of release.[73] It does not appear that the biphasic pattern of release is due to a feedback mechanism, however, it is possible that chronic exposure of β cells to high concentrations of insulin might affect insulin release.

A second possibility is that individual β cells may have different levels of sensitivity with respect to glucose stimulation. The height and duration of the first phase of secretion is so constant in normal rat islets that it would seem unlikely that a stable pool of β cells would be initially resistant to glucose stimulation. Electrophysiologic studies of monolayer cultures of islet cells following glucose stimulation should provide information on the immediate response of individual cells, as well as determine whether recruitment of β cells occurs with time and whether it reaches a maximum in a finite period of time.

A third possibility is that a pool of insulin may be present in individual β cells which is immediately available for release following glucose stimulation. The microtubular–microfilamentous system could be responsible for the immediate availability of such a pool of insulin. Following glucose stimulation, β granules associated with the microtubular–microfilamentous system would be released initially, whereas other stored β granules and newly-formed granules would become associated with the system at later intervals, thus forming the second phase of secretion. Evidence in favor of this concept is the finding that the microtubular–microfilamentous system is involved in both phases of secretion, the demonstration of a decrease in intact microtubules with impaired insulin release from isolated rat islets following fasting, and the absence of a first phase of secretion as well as a diminution of the second phase of glucose-induced insulin release after maintenance of isolated islets *in vitro* for 4 days with a low concentration of glucose (Fig. 4).

Insulin Storage

Insulin is stored in the β cell in the form of secretory granules. Electron-microscopic, immunochemical studies have localized insulin to β granules.[74] Subcellular fractionation of the islets has also shown that insulin is present in the secretory granule fraction.[67] There is no evidence for the presence of insulin in the β cell other than in β granules.

Electron-microscopic, histochemical studies have also demonstrated zinc within β granules.[75] Ultrastructural studies of negatively stained preparations

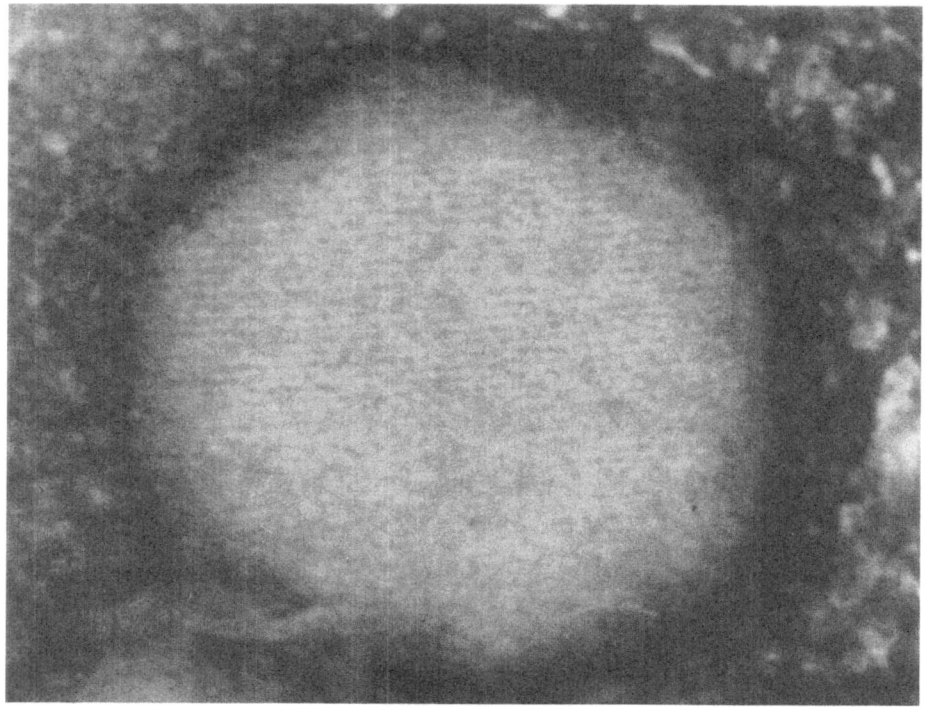

Figure 6. Electron micrograph of a negatively stained β granule demonstrating a 50 Å periodicity. ×247,000. Reproduced at 105%. (Greider *et al.: J. Cell Biol.*, **41**:162, 1969)

of β granules isolated by subcellular fractionation of isolated islets have revealed lines of repeating periodicity within the granule which are approximately 50 Å apart[76] (Fig. 6). This distance is consistent with the space required for the hexameric form of a zinc-insulin crystal. Therefore it would appear that the β granule represents a microcrystal of zinc insulin.

Ultrastructural studies have demonstrated a species difference in the appearance of β granules. In the dog and in man, the granules have rectangular crystalline profiles, whereas in the chicken the granules appear as bundles of crystalline plates, and in the rat the beta granules are round, homogeneous structures with a crystalline matrix.[77] The reason for this species variation in the storage form of insulin is not apparent at the present time. Ultrastructurally, β granules are surrounded by smooth membranous sacs with a space between the β granule and the wall of the sac. This space probably contains the C-peptide from proinsulin and possibly a small amount of proinsulin.

Insulin Biosynthesis

Proinsulin is a protein which is larger than insulin and is the precursor for the formation of insulin.[78] Stimulation of β cells with glucose initiates new formation of proinsulin in the endoplasmic reticulum of the β cell, and the newly-formed proinsulin is transported by an energy-requiring mechanism to the Golgi complex.[79] The mechanism of transfer of proinsulin from the endoplasmic reticulum to the Golgi complex has not been clearly delineated. Ultrastructurally, continuity of membranes of the endoplasmic reticulum with Golgi membranes has been demonstrated; thus it is possible that a direct transfer of proinsulin occurs or that microvesicles derived from the endoplasmic reticulum might be transported to the Golgi complex.

The single-chain proinsulin molecule is converted to the double-chain insulin molecule by the enzymatic removal of a connecting peptide segment which has been called the C-peptide. The enzyme or enzymes responsible for the removal of the C-peptide apparently are localized within the Golgi complex, and the conversion of proinsulin to insulin occurs in the Golgi area and continues in the β granules. The half-time for the conversion of proinsulin to insulin is approximately 60 min.[80]

In the Golgi complex, the newly-formed insulin is packaged into secretory granules, and the individual granules pinch off from the Golgi membranes. At some point in the process, zinc enters the membranous sacs encasing the β granules, complexes with insulin, and forms microcrystals of insulin. The C-peptide from proinsulin is secreted in equivalent amounts into insulin.[81] Since the beta granules are liberated by emiocytosis, it would appear that the C-peptide chains are present in the space between the β granules and the encasing membranous sacs. A small amount of proinsulin is also secreted with insulin, which probably reflects an incomplete conversion of proinsulin to insulin in the β granules.

The biochemical events linking glucose stimulation and initiation of proinsulin synthesis have not been clearly defined. Glucose apparently has a posttranscriptional effect, since it will increase insulin synthesis on previously existing messenger RNA.[82] Glucose also stimulates the overall rate of islet RNA synthesis and may affect the formation of messenger RNA for proinsulin production.[83]

The same question arises with respect to insulin biosynthesis as with insulin release from the β cell. Does glucose initiate insulin biosynthesis by reacting with a glucoreceptor or by metabolism of glucose in the β cell? Recent *in vitro* studies using alloxan indicate that alloxan will inhibit not only glucose-induced insulin release but also glucose-induced insulin biosynthesis.[84] This effect of alloxan on insulin biosynthesis can be prevented by glucose, and stereospecificity is indicated since the α anomer of D-glucose provided greater protection than the β anomer.

Model of Insulin Secretion

Figure 7 represents a model of insulin secretion based upon the information available at the present time. Certain aspects of the model are now firmly established, whereas other steps in the secretory process will require new information. The model serves an important function at the present time, since

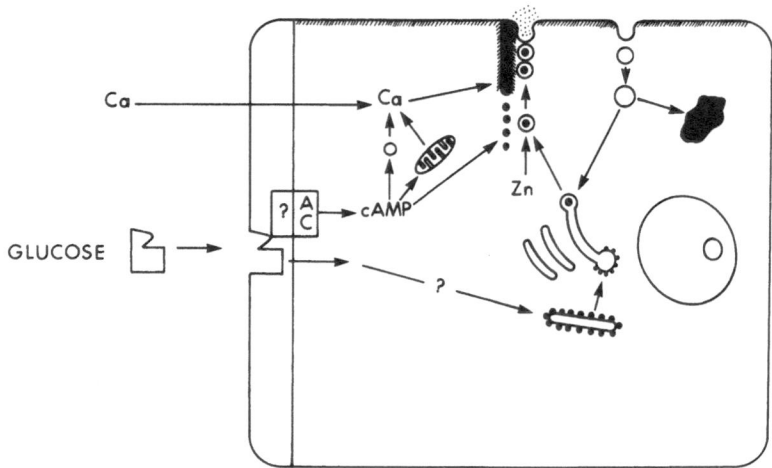

Figure 7. Model of β cell secretion. (See text.)

it provides a means of testing certain hypotheses and, as new information becomes available, various steps in the secretory process will undoubtedly become extremely complex before they become more simplified once again.

Insulin synthesis in the β cell is initiated either by the interaction of glucose with glucoreceptors on the β cell membrane or by the metabolism of glucose. This stimulatory action of glucose causes the initiation of proinsulin synthesis in the endoplasmic reticulum; proinsulin is transported to the Golgi complex by an energy-requiring mechanism; membrane-bound proteases in the Golgi complex initiate the conversion of proinsulin to insulin; the newly converted insulin and proinsulin are packaged into membranous sacs and liberated into the cytoplasm of the β cell; conversion of proinsulin to insulin continues, and zinc enters the membranous sacs, resulting in the formation of microcrystals of zinc insulin.

From the evidence available at the present time, it would appear that specific glucoreceptors for insulin release may well exist on the β cell membrane. The release of insulin from the β cell would be initiated by the interaction of glucose with the glucoreceptors. The receptors would appear to be close to but not identical with the hexose transport sites in the β cell membrane. As a result of the interaction of glucose with the receptor site, a change in membrane permeability to calcium occurs with the resultant accumulation of intracellular calcium. In addition, cAMP accumulation occurs in the β cell, presumably because of a direct stimulation of adenylate cyclase associated with the β cell membrane. Calcium initiates a contraction of the microtubular–microfilamentous system, resulting in the transport of β granules associated with this system to the cell surface where they are liberated by emiocytosis. This organized mechanism of transport could explain the biphasic pattern of insulin secretion, since those granules associated with the microtubular–microfilamentous system would be released in the first phase of secretion, whereas stored granules, and at a much later interval newly formed granules, would become associated with the system, resulting in the second phase of insulin release. The role of cAMP in secretion may involve two mechanisms; the first is the release of bound calcium from mitochondria and microvesicles in the β cell, and the second is the polymerization of microtubulin into intact microtubules. Recycling of portions of the plasma membrane is accomplished by formation of microvesicles which are transported either to the Golgi complex to be reutilized or to lysosomes where the membrane would be degraded. It is possible that the microtubular–microfilamentous system is involved in the recycling of membranes within the cell, although no definitive information exists to support this concept at the present time.

Potential Defects in Insulin Secretion in Diabetes

Based upon the present understanding of the normal mechanism of insulin secretion by the β cell, it is obvious that several potential sites for defects in this mechanism could be present in the diabetic individual. It would appear that the potential defects would most probably involve the insulin-releasing mechanism of the β cell rather than insulin biosynthesis, since no evidence exists at the present time for the presence of a defective or abnormal insulin in diabetic patients.

Glucoreceptors on the β cell membrane could be deficient in number or altered in structure with a resultant loss of sensitivity to stimulation by glucose. The adenylate cyclase system could be defective, with a resultant alteration in calcium metabolism and microtubular formation. Calcium flux across the β cell membrane could be defective, with a resultant impairment in insulin secretion. Deficiency in the microtubular–microfilamentous system could result in an impairment of glucose-induced insulin release. The final step in the release of insulin, the fusion of the membranous sacs with the plasma membrane, could be defective, with a resultant impaired insulin secretion. These alterations or defects could be due to a genetic abnormality in the β cell; an injury by an environmental agent, such as a viral infection; or the presence of auto-antibodies to certain components of the system, such as antibodies to glucoreceptors on the β cell membrane.

The spiny mouse is an animal model of diabetes which resembles many aspects of diabetes in man.[85] The β cells in these animals are sluggish in their responsiveness to glucose stimulation. The microtubular system of these animals has been studied ultrastructurally using vinblastine as a means of demonstrating microtubular protein within the cells. In comparison with normal animals, a marked deficiency in microtubular protein has been demonstrated.[86] It has been suggested that the microtubular deficiency could be responsible for the delay in insulin release. The generation and efflux of cAMP has been determined in islets isolated from spiny mice in the presence of different glucose concentrations.[87] The insulin response was deficient and a delayed, and markedly diminished, efflux of cAMP was observed from the islets of these animals.

Another experimental model which resembles certain forms of human diabetes is the fasted animal. As discussed earlier in this chapter, fasting of rats for a period of 48–72 hr results in an impaired insulin release following glucose stimulation, a diminished sensitivity to glucose stimulation, decrease in cAMP content and adenylate cyclase activity within the islets, and a decrease in polymerized microtubulin or intact microtubules in the islets. These findings are similar to the observations reported for the spiny mouse and raise the question as to whether the alterations produced by fasting reflect the primary defect or defects present in the β cells of the spiny mice, For example, the diminished cAMP content of islets of spiny mice and the diminished responsiveness in terms of cAMP production could affect the microtubular system the same as in the fasted animal. The possibility exists that in both of these experimental models the defect may be at an earlier site, such as glucoreceptors on the β cell membrane which have been altered either by fasting and hypoglycemia, or it may be on a genetic basis, as in the spiny mouse. The concept is purely speculative at the present time, since no information is available to validate it or deny it.

The continued studies of animal models and experimental conditions which will mimic certain forms of human diabetes should lead to definitive clues as to possible sites for defects in the β cells of diabetic patients. In addition, it is now possible to obtain human islets for *in vitro* studies similar to those accomplished with experimental animals. Islets can be isolated from the normal human pancreas, and the material can be obtained the same time kidneys are removed from recently expired patients for renal transplants. It is hoped that this same approach can be used in obtaining islets from recently expired diabetics for *in vitro* studies on insulin secretion and insulin biosynthesis.

References

1. Cerasi, E., and Luft, R.: *Diabetes,* **16**:615, 1967.
2. Kelly, W. D., Lillehei, R. C., Merkel, F. K., Idezuki, Y., and Goetz, F. C.: *Surgery,* **61**:827, 1967.
3. Barbosa, J., Burke, B., Buselmeier, T. J., Carpenter, A. M., Goetz, F. C. Harris, J., Kennedy, W. R., Kjellstrand, C. M., Michael, A. F., Najarian, J. S., and Recker, L.: *Kidney Int.,* **6(4)**:S32, 1974.
4. Gliedman, M. L., Tellis, V., Soberman, R., Rifkin, H., Freed, S. Z., and Veith, F. J.: *Kidney Int.,* **6(4)**:S164, 1974.
5. Crespin, S. R., Greenough, W. B. III, and Steinberg, D.: *J. Clin. Invest.,* **48**:1934, 1969.
6. Crespin, S. R., Greenough, W. B. III, and Steinberg, D.: *J. Clin. Invest.,* **52**:1979, 1973.
7. Floyd, J. C., Jr., Fajans, S. S., Conn, J. W., Knopf, R. F., and Rull, J.: *J. Clin. Invest.,* **45**:1487, 1966.
8. Manns, J. G., and Boda, J. M.: *Amer. J. Physiol.,* **212**:747, 1967.
9. Hertelendy, F., Machlin, L. J., Takahashi, Y., and Kipnis, D. M.: *J. Endocrinol.,* **41**:605, 1968.
10. Milner, R. D. G., Leach, F. N., Ashworth, M. A., Cser, A., and Jack, P. M. B.: *J. Endocrinol.,* **64(2)**:349, 1975.
11. Malaisse, W. J., Malaisse-Lagae, F., and Wright, P. H.: *Amer. J. Physiol.,* **213**:843, 1967.
12. Grey, N. J., Goldring, S., and Kipnis, D. M.: *J. Clin. Invest.,* **49**:881, 1970.

13. Selawry, H., Voyles, N., Gutman, R., Waide, A., Fink, G., and Recant, L.: *Diabetes*, **21**:329, 1972.
14. Howell, S. L., Green, I. C., and Montague, W.: *Biochem. J.*, **136**:343, 1973.
15. Grodsky, G. M., and Bennett, L. L.: *Proc. Soc. Exp. Biol. Med.*, **114**:769, 1963.
16. Grodsky, G. M., Curry, D., Landahl, H., and Bennett, L.: *Acta Diabetol. Lat.*, **6**:554, 1969.
17. Lacy, P. E., Walker, M. M., and Fink, C. J.: *Diabetes*, **21(10)**:987, 1972.
18. Grodsky, G. M., Batts, A. A., Bennett, L. L., Vcella, C., McWilliams, N. B., and Smith, D. F.: *Amer. J. Physiol.*, **205(4)**:638, 1963.
19. Ashcroft, S. J. H., Hedeskov, C. J., and Randle, P. J.: *Biochem. J.*, **118**:143, 1970.
20. Ashcroft, S. J. H., Bassett, J. M., and Randle, P. J.: *Diabetes*, **21**:538, 1972.
21. Ashcroft, S. J. H., Weerasinghe, L. C. C., and Randle, P. J.: *Biochem. J.*, **132**:223, 1973.
22. Montague, W., and Taylor, K. W.: *Biochem. J.*, **109**:333, 1968.
23. Montague, W., and Taylor, K. W.: In: *The Structure and Metabolism of the Pancreatic Islets*. Edited by S. Falkmer, B. Hellman, and L. B. Täljedal. Pergamon, Oxford, 1970, p. 263.
24. Matschinsky, F. M., Ellerman, J. E., Krzanowski, J., Kotler-Brajtburg, J., Landgraf, R., and Fertel, R.: *J. Biol. Chem.*, **246(4)**:1007, 1971.
25. Pace, C. S., Ellerman, J., Hover, B. A., Stillings, S. N., and Matschinsky, F. M.: *Diabetes*, **24(5)**:476, 1975.
26. Ashcroft, S. J. H., Chatra, L., Weerasinghe, C., and Randle, P. J.: *Biochem. J.*, **132**:223, 1973.
27. Bhattacharya, G.: *Science*, **117**:230, 1953.
28. Rossini, A. A., Berger, M., Shadden, J., and Cahill, Jr., G. F.: *Science*, **183**:424, 1974.
29. Rossini, A. A., Cahill, G. F., Jr., Jeanloz, D. A., and Jeanloz, R. W.: *Science*, **188**:70, 1975.
30. Scheynius, A., and Taljedal, I. B.: *Diabetologia*, **7**:252, 1971.
31. Tomita, T., Lacy, P. E., Matschinsky, F. M., and McDaniel, M. L.: *Diabetes*, **23**:517, 1974.
32. McDaniel, M. L., Roth, C. E., Fink, C. J., and Lacy, P. E.: *Endocrinology*, **99**:535, 1976.
33. Rossini, A. A., Soeldner, J. S., Hiebert, J. M., Weir, G. C., and Gleason, R. E.: *Diabetologia*, **10**:795, 1974.
34. Grodsky, G., Fanska, R., West, L., and Manning, M.: *Science*, **186**:536, 1974.
35. McDaniel, M. L., Anderson, S., Fink, J., Roth, C., and Lacy, P. E.: *Endocrinology*, **97**:68, 1975.
36. Weaver, D. C., McDaniel, M. L., and Lacy, P. E.: Site of protection of barbituric acid against alloxan inhibition of glucose-induced insulin secretion. Abstract. Presented at the Amer. Diabetes Assoc. Mtg., June, 1976.
37. Grodsky, G. M., and Bennett, L. L.: *Diabetes*, **15**:910, 1966.
38. Malaisse-Lagae, F., and Malaisse, W. J.: *Endocrinology*, **88**:72, 1971.
39. Malaisse, W. J.: *Diabetologia*, **9**:167, 1973.
40. Hellman, B., Sehlin, J., and Taljedal, I. B.: *Amer. J. Physiol.*, **221**:1795, 1971.
41. Naber, S. P., McDaniel, M. L., and Lacy, P. E.: Calcium-45 movements on isolated islets: Effect of glucose and D_2O. Abstract. Presented at the Amer. Diabetes Assoc. Mtg., June, 1976.
42. Reed, P. W., and Lardy, H. A.: *J. Biol. Chem.*, **247**:6970, 1972.
43. Charles, M. A., Lawecki, J., Pictet, R., and Grodsky, G. M.: *J. Biol. Chem.*, **250**:6134, 1975.
44. Warren, G. B., Toon, P. A., Birdsall, N. J. M., Lee, A. G., and Metcalfe, J. C.: *Proc. Nat. Acad. Sci.*, **71**:622, 1974.
45. Brisson, G. R., Malaisse-Lagae, F., and Malaisse, W. J.: *J. Clin. Invest.*, **51**:232, 1972.
46. Charles, M. A., Fanska, R., Schmid, F. G., Forsham, P. H., and Grodsky, G. M. *Science*, **179**:569, 1973.
47. Grill, V., and Cerasi, E. *J. Biol. Chem.*, **249**:4196, 1974.
48. Howell, S. L., and Montague, W.: *Biochim. Biophys. Acta*, **320**:44, 1973.
49. Lacy, P. E., Finke, E. H. Conant, S., and Naber, S.: *Diabetes*, **25**:484, 1976.
50. Pipeleers, D. G., Pipeleers-Marichal, M. A., Sherline, P., and Kipnis, D. M.: *J. Cell Biol.* (in press).
51. Pipeleers, D. G.: *Science*, **191**:88, 1976.
52. Orci, L., Gabbay, K. H., and Malaisse, W. J.: *Science*, **175**:1128, 1972.
53. Ishikawa, H., Bischoff, R., and Holtzer, H.: *J. Cell Biol.*, **43**:312, 1969.
54. Gibbons, B. H., and Gibbons, I. R.: *J. Cell Biol.*, **54**:75, 1972.
55. Lacy, P. E., Howell, S. L., Young, D. A., and Fink, C. J.: *Nature (London)*, **219**:1177, 1968.
56. Malaisse, W. J., Malaisse-Lagae, F., Walker, M. O., and Lacy, P. E.: *Diabetes*, **20**:257, 1971.
57. Lacy, P. E., Walker, M. O., and Fink, C. J.: *Diabetes*, **21**:987, 1972.

58. McDaniel, M. L., King, S., Anderson, S., Fink, J., and Lacy, P. E.: *Diabetologia,* **10**:303, 1974.
59. Kletzien, R. F., Perdue, J. F., and Springer, A.: *J. Biol. Chem.,* **247**:2964, 1972.
60. McDaniel, M., Roth, C., Fink, J., Fyfe, G., and Lacy, P. E.: *Biochem. Biophys. Res. Commun.,* **66(4)**:1089, 1975
61. Miranda, A., Godman, G., Deitch, A., and Tanenbaum, S.: *J. Cell Biol.,* **61**:481, 1974.
62. Lacy, P. E., Finke, E. H., and Codilla, R. C.: *Lab. Invest.,* **33(5)**:570, 1975.
63. Lacy, P. E.: *Amer. J. Pathol.,* **79(1)**:170, 1975.
64. Lacy, P. E.,: *Diabetes,* **19(12)**:895, 1970.
65. Malaisse-Lagae, F., Brisson, G. R., and Malaisse, W. J.: *Horm. Metab. Res.,* **3**:374, 1971b.
66. Lacy, P. E.: *Amer. J. Med.,* **31**:851, 1961.
67. Howell, S. L., Young, D. A., and Lacy, P. E.: *J. Cell Biol.,* **41(1)**:167, 1969.
68. Orci, L., Amherdt, M., Malaisse-Lagae, F., Rouiller, C., and Renold, A. E.: *Science,* **179**:82, 1973.
69. Blaschko, H., Firemark, H., Smith, A. D., and Winkler, H.: *Biochem. J.,* **104**:545, 1967.
70. Howell, J. J., and Lucy, J. A.: *FEBS Let.,* **4**:147, 1969.
71. Orci, L., Malaisse-Lagae, F., Ravazzola, M., Amherdt, M., and Renold, A. E.: *Science* **181**:561, 1973.
72. Malaisse, W., Malaisse-Lagae, F., Lacy, P. E., and Wright, P.: *Proc. Soc. Exp. Biol.,* **124**:497, 1967.
73. Grodsky, G. M., Fanska, R., and Schmid, F. G.: *Diabetes,* **22(4)**:256, 1973.
74. Misugi, K., Howell, S. L., Greider, M. H., Lacy, P. E., and Sorenson, G. D.: *Arch. Pathol.* **89**:97, 1970.
75. Pihl, E.: *Acta Pathol. Microbiol. Scand.,* **74**:145, 1968.
76. Greider, M. H., Howell, S. L., and Lacy, P. E.: *J. Cell Biol.,* **41**:162, 1969.
77. Lacy, P. E.: *Anat. Rec.,* **128**:255, 1957.
78. Steiner, D. F., Kemmler, W., Clark, J. L., Oyer, P. E., and Rubenstein, A. H.: In: *Handbook of Physiology.* Edited by D. F. Steiner and N. Freinkel. Williams & Wilkins, Baltimore, 1972, p. 175.
79. Howell, S. L.: *Nature (New Biol.),* **235**:85, 1972.
80. Steiner, D. F., Clark, J. L., Nolan, C., Rubenstein, A. H., Margoliash, E., Aten, B., and Oyer, P. E.: *Rec. Progr. Hormone Res.,* **25**:207, 1969.
81. Rubenstein, A. H., Clark, J. L., Melani, F., and Steiner, D. F.: *Nature (London),* **224**:697, 1969.
82. Permutt, M. A., and Kipnis, D. M.: *J. Biol. Chem.,* **247(4)**:1194, 1972.
83. Permutt, M. A., and Kipnis, D. M.: *J. Biol. Chem.,* **247(4)**:1200, 1972.
84. Niki, A., Niki, H., Miwa, I., and Lin, B. J., *Diabetes,* **25**:574, 1976.
85. Cameron, D. P., Stauffacher, W., Orci, L., Amherdt, M., and Renold, A. E.: *Diabetes,* **32**:1060, 1972.
86. Malaisse-Lagae, F., Ravazzola, M., Amherdt, M., Gutzeit, A., Stauffacher, W., Malaisse, W. J., and Orci, L.: *Diabetologia* **11**:71, 1975.
87. Cerasi, E., Grill, V., and Rabinovitch, A.: *Frontiers of Internal Medicine, 1974, 12th Int. Congr. Internal Med., Tel Aviv, 1974.* Karger, Basel, 1975, pp. 115–119.

Chapter 9

Idiopathic Diabetes

Bruno W. Volk and Klaus F. Wellmann

The manifestations of diabetes mellitus, because of their complex and diversified nature, make it often difficult to categorize the various types of the disease. It is not a single disease, but a syndrome which may be produced by a number of factors. It may result from extrapancreatic lesions, such as hyperplasia or tumors of the anterior pituitary gland or the adrenal cortex or medulla, or hyperthyroidism. In some cases diabetes may follow surgical removal of the pancreas, or its origin may be the destruction of the pancreatic islets resulting from pancreatic diseases which include hemochromatosis, pancreatitis, pancreatic lithiasis, and tumors of the pancreas.

However, in the majority of diabetes patients the etiology is not clear; in this case the term "idiopathic" is applied. According to the age of onset, and from a clinical viewpoint, the disease can be divided into the juvenile or growth-onset type of diabetes and the adult or maturity-onset type (Table 1). On the basis of many surveys of large populations it has been estimated that in the United States close to 10 million people are afflicted with diabetes.[1] It is believed that in some 40% of these the disease is unrecognized, owing to a variety of factors including the mildness or even absence of symptoms, inadequate medical care, or individual neglect.[1] While, according to the National Commission on Diabetes, "only" 35,000 deaths per year are directly attributable to diabetes, there is "strong evidence" that diabetes and its complications are responsible for more than 300,000 deaths per year, ranking it just behind heart disease and cancer as a cause of death in the United States. The Commission also found that the prevalence of diabetes in this country increased by more than 50% between 1965 and 1973. It was further calculated that at the current rate of increase, the number of deaths will double every 15 years. Juvenile diabetes has been estimated to comprise 5 to 8% of the total number of diabetics in the United States.[2–5] White,[6] in a study of 750 patients with juvenile diabetes, observed that the onset of the disease occurred before the age of 4 in 60%, while it was recognized before the age of 1 year in only 0.5%. In a survey of the material

Bruno W. Volk and Klaus F. Wellmann • Isaac Albert Research Institute of the Kingsbrook Jewish Medical Center, and Downstate Medical Center, State University of New York, Brooklyn, New York. Present address of B. W. V.: University of California, Irvine, California. Present address of K. F. W.: Beekman Downtown Hospital, New York, New York.

Table 1.   *Classification of Diabetes Mellitus in Man*

I.   Idiopathic diabetes (primary)
     (a) Maturity-onset (adult type)
     (b) Growth-onset (juvenile type)
II. Diabetes due to pancreatic pathology (secondary)
     (a) Pancreatitis with or without lithiasis (acute and chronic)
     (b) Extensive malignant tumors of pancreas
     (c) Hemochromatosis
III. Surgical removal of pancreas
IV. Disorders of endocrine glands other than the pancreas
     (a) Hyperplasia or tumors of adrenal cortex
     (b) Pheochromocytoma
     (c) Hyperfunction or tumors of the anterior pituitary gland
     (d) Hyperthyroidism

collected from the world literature, Schwartzman *et al.*[7] found that only 0.05% of the cases were diagnosed during the first month of life, while 0.5% were recognized within the first year after birth.

The morphologic changes in the diabetic pancreas are nonspecific and are not diagnostic for the disease. Such changes include insular fibrosis and hyalinization, arteriosclerosis and arteriolar sclerosis, and intra- and interacinar fibrosis.[8-14] Some of the lesions, such as hyalinization of the islets, which by the early authors have been considered characteristic of diabetes, have subsequently been observed also in nondiabetic individuals. Similarly, while quantitative studies have shown, in general, a reduction in the volume of islet tissue and a decrease in the relative numbers and weights of B cells existing in diabetic individuals, some diabetic pancreases have been observed to contain more islet tissue and B cell granulation than do those of nondiabetics.[15-18] In any case, the amount of B cell reduction seems to be in itself insufficient to account for diabetes, since in experimental animals 80 to 95% of the pancreas must be eliminated in order for the disease to develop. To make matters more complicated, it has been reported that the pancreas of a diabetic patient may contain certain amounts of extractable insulin,[19,20] and diabetic blood may contain insulin-like substances in concentrations similar to those found in nondiabetics.[21,22]

Thus, certain observations seemed to support the idea that extrapancreatic influences are the cause or precipitating factors of diabetes. These include various hormones,[23-25] trauma, emotional stress, obesity, viral infection,[26,27] or an autoimmune process.[28,29] Other possible extrapancreatic factors that may cause diabetes are heredity, excessive destruction of insulin and the presence of substances which are either of a protein nature or are associated with protein ("synalbumin")[30] which bind or hold insulin[31] and thus oppose its action. However, none of these hypotheses have been confirmed.

Recent developments in glucagon research suggested that the metabolic syndrome of diabetes mellitus may not only be the result of relative or absolute insulin deficiency per se, but it may require, in addition, the presence of glucagon.[32] Since glucagon is produced primarily by the A cells of the islets of Langerhans, diabetes, at least to some extent, can be considered to be a disease of the pancreas.

The chapters that follow will attempt to demonstrate the changes in the pancreas of diabetic patients, to emphasize the historical development of the recognition of these changes, and to correlate these changes within the framework of the modern concept of the pathophysiology of human diabetes.

Gross Pathology of the Pancreas

The changes of the pancreas in idiopathic diabetes are nonspecific. They consist primarily of a reduction of weight, accentuation of the lobular markings, and increased consistency. Weichselbaum[33] observed that the pancreatic weights of diabetics above the age of 20 may be as low as 28 g. Herxheimer[34] noted that diabetic pancreases were thin, small, or frequently infiltrated by fat. In 105 of 162 cases of diabetes mellitus he observed that the average weight of the diabetic pancreas varied from 40 to 50 g, with occasional values as low as 20 g. Similar low weights were described in adult diabetic pancreases by other authors.[14,35–37] Terplan[37] observed 8 out of 31 diabetic pancreases to be fatty. The weights ranged from 21 g in a 15-year-old child and 22 g in a 52-year-old adult to 110 g in the patient with the heaviest pancreas recorded. Maclean and Ogilvie[15] observed that 52% of pancreases in their study of adult diabetics weighed less than 50 g, while in a control group of nondiabetics only 20% of the pancreases weighed less. In their study of 27 juvenile diabetics,[38] the average weight of the pancreases with "acute" diabetes was 51.6 g, while that of 14 "chronic" diabetics was 38.3 g. In a series of 46 diabetic patients, varying in age from 14 to 77 years, Kraus[39] observed that the lowest pancreatic weight was 19 g. He also noted that in the majority of the patients with juvenile diabetes the pancreatic weight was particularly decreased, in many instances to half or less than half of that of the normal pancreas. Vartiainen,[40] in a study of diabetic patients of comparable sex and age, observed that 22 out of 166 pancreases weighed less than 40 g, while only two controls had pancreases below this weight. Terbrüggen[41] often found pancreases weighing from 17 to 40 g in juvenile diabetics. Warren and LeCompte,[42] in a study of 730 cases, observed 122 pancreases which were quite small and weighed less than 50 g. In 481 instances, the pancreas was normal or weighed between 50 and 100 g, and 127 cases showed a large organ which weighed 100 g or more. In a survey of 100 pancreases examined by Lazarus and Volk,[43] no significant differences between the pancreatic weights of diabetics and nondiabetics of similar age and sex were found. The weight of the pancreases of maturity-onset diabetics ranged from 40 to 160 g, with an average of 100 g, while 85% of these organs weighed between 80 and 110 g. The pancreatic weights of 100 nondiabetic controls ranged from 50 to 200 g, with an average of 99 g. The authors emphasized that the size or the weight of the pancreas may be misleading, since the presence of fatty infiltration or fibrosis may mask parenchymal atrophy which may be associated either with increased or decreased weight of the organ. Pancreases weighing 200 g may contain less parenchyma than those weighing only 50 g. The gross appearance of the pancreas is not indicative of the amount of islet tissue which may be present, despite extensive and diffuse destruction of the organ by acute pancreatitis, ductular obstruction, or carcinoma.

Nonspecific changes of the diabetic pancreas have been observed as early as 1894 by Hansemann,[44] who described 36 instances of "agranular atrophy" and in 3 cases of fibrous induration. Similar findings were observed by Simmonds[45] who found, in a study of 150 diabetic pancreases, that 45 were atrophic, 12 showed "coarse" fibrosis, and the rest were grossly normal, except for extensive fat infiltration.

Hyalinization of the Pancreatic Islets

Hyalinization of the islets has been generally considered to be the most common and probably the most typical lesion of the diabetic pancreas, although it is also found in nondiabetic individuals. It was reported independently and simultaneously by Opie[46] and Weichselbaum and Stangl[47] in 1901. Weichselbaum[11] observed hyaline degeneration in 28%, Seyfarth[48] and Allen[49] in 20%, and Kraus[39] in 10.5% of diabetic pancreases studied. Lazarus and Volk[50] noted hyalinization of the pancreatic islets in 25% of patients with maturity-onset diabetes. It was mild in 5%, moderate in 6%, and severe in 14% of their cases. Ehrlich and Ratner[51] observed hyalinization of the islets of Langerhans in 45 of 91 diabetic patients over 50 years of age (49.5%), an unusually high incidence.

Weichselbaum[11] observed hyalinization mostly in patients over 50 years of age and only rarely between the ages of 27 and 40 years. Bell[52] noted that hyalinization is rare in juvenile diabetics and that it shows a progressive increase in frequency and intensity with advancing age. He observed no hyalinization of the islets of patients under the age of 20 and found it in less than 10% of persons between the ages of 20 and 40. About one-fourth of those between the ages of 40 and 50 years, and 45.7% of those over 60 years of age displayed some hyalinization. Similarly, in a study of a series of patients over 50 years of age, Seifert[53] observed hyalinization in 50% of the diabetic pancreases as compared with 10% of those of nondiabetics. He also found that hyalinization of the islets occurred more frequently in diabetes than in its absence and emphasized that hyalinization develops without relation to severity and duration of the diabetes.

Warren *et al.*[54] stated that hyaline in the islets occurs more often in older diabetics, being relatively rare before the age of 40 (5.7%) and much more frequent after that age (34.5%). These authors, in a study of 481 cases of diabetes, noted that in those in whom the diabetes lasted 10 years or more, only 1 of 81 with onset of the diabetes prior to the 20th year showed hyaline, and in that case, only to a slight degree. On the other hand, in 341 cases whose age of onset of the diabetes was 35 years or more, 100 showed varying degrees of hyalinization. Legg[55] observed, in a study of 223 pancreases of diabetic patients, no instance of hyalinization in cases under the age of 40 years, while it was most frequent in patients over the age of 60.

While Opie[46] and Weichselbaum and Stangl[47] thought that hyalinization of the islets of Langerhans is typical for diabetes, it has subsequently been established that these changes can also be observed in nondiabetic individuals. In 1904 Ohlmacher[56] found extensive hyalinization of the islets in a 27-year-old nondiabetic individual. Saltykow[57] reported four cases with hyalinized islands in 21 pancreases of nondiabetic individuals. Similarly, Cecil[9] noted instances of hyalinized islets in nondiabetic patients. Milne and Peters[58] also mentioned hyaline changes in the islets of nondiabetic individuals. Seven of the cases reported by Wright[59] were people who were nondiabetic and over 50 years of age. In two instances the blood sugar values were not recorded, but the urine had traces of sugar. Ahronheim[60] observed hyalinized islets in 5 of 50 nondiabetics over 50 years of age. Arey[61] found hyalinization of the islets of Langerhans in 16.6% of nondiabetics and in 71.7% of diabetics 50 years and older. Warren,[62] in his monograph, *The Pathology of Diabetes Mellitus*, observed hyalinized islets also in nondiabetic individuals.

Bell,[63] in a study of 200 consecutive postmortem examinations of nondiabetic subjects who were 50 years or older, observed 5 cases with hyalinized islets. However, he noted that in none of these individuals were blood sugar determination or glucose tolerance tests carried out. Bell[64] also observed that a high proportion of nondiabetic persons over 80 years showed hyalinization of the islets. Moreover, these figures indicated that when hyalinized islets are found in elderly males there is only a 1 in 10 chance that the patient has clinical evidence of diabetes. In a study of over 4000 postmortem examinations on nondiabetic subjects, he[64] found mild hyalinization in 10% of those in the age group between 60 and 80 years, and 14 to 18% in the group between 80 and 100 years. Gepts[16] observed hyalinization of the islets in 4.2% of nondiabetic persons as compared with 41% in diabetics. Ehrlich and Ratner[51] noted an incidence of 3.9% of hyalinized islets in a series of 178 consecutive autopsies carried out on nondiabetic individuals. Hartroft[65] observed that the intensity of hyalinization of the pancreatic islets increases with age both in nondiabetic as well as in diabetic individuals, but that at any given age the severity is greater in the diabetic than in the nondiabetic patients.

The hyaline substance in the pancreatic islets is composed of an amorphous acellular material which appears between the islet cells and the intrainsular capillaries. In some islets it may be observed in small amounts surrounding the capillaries, while in others it may form a large mass which occupies most of the islets or completely replaces them. The hyaline material may contain spindle-shaped cells and in some islets may surround distinctly visible capillaries (Fig. 1). There is frequently an uneven involvement of the islets within the same pancreas. Thus, in some areas a large number of the islets are extensively or almost completely replaced by the hyaline, while in other areas only occasional

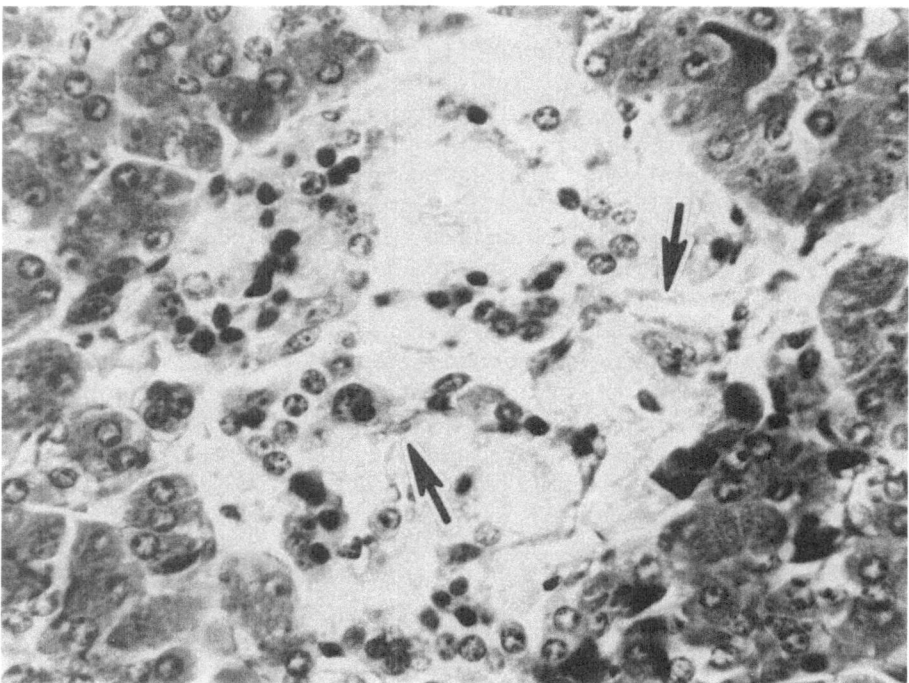

Figure 1. Hyalinized islet of pancreas of maturity-onset diabetic. The hyaline material appears fibrillar in character and contains capillaries (arrows), most of which appear compressed. Aldehyde fuchsin trichrome stain. ×650.

foci of partly hyalinized islets may be present. Despite the involvement of many islets, a good number of them may remain intact. Often, areas of the pancreas which contain many hyalinized islets also show concomitant fibrosis and atrophy of the exocrine parenchyma.

The hyaline material stains green with the aldehyde fuchsin trichrome method, although occasional areas may show a pale, bluish-green powdery hue. There are often irregularly shaped aldehyde fuchsin positive fibers seen which are sparsely distributed within the hyaline deposits. With the periodic acid Schiff trichrome method the hyaline material is negative and stains green. With phosphotungstic acid hematoxylin it is pale brown, and with the Masson trichrome procedure the hyaline substance stains sky blue and is traversed by strands of darker blue.

Opie[66] for the first time mentioned that there is a histologic resemblance of the hyalinized substance to amyloid, but he was unable to prove this observation with various amyloid stains. Similarly, Mallory[67] conjectured that the substance is closely related to amyloid. Gomori[68] also noted that amyloid deposits occasionally occurred in the islets of Langerhans in diabetic individuals. Bloom[69] observed congo-red-staining islets in a cat with spontaneous diabetes. Others[60,61,70] observed a substance giving a positive amyloid reaction with iodine green and methyl violet in human hyalinized islets and believed it to be amyloid. They found that it was localized in close proximity to the capillary walls and showed similar, but not identical, staining reactions to those of the spleen and liver in cases of generalized amyloidosis. Gellerstedt,[71] mainly on the basis of studies with the methyl violet reaction, suggested that the hyaline is actually amyloid and that the condition should be called "insular (para-) amyloidosis." He also felt that the hyaline within the islets represents a manifestation of senile amyloidosis which also commonly involves the brain and the heart. Arey[61] stated that the amyloid in the islets is an isolated feature and is usually not associated with amyloid in other tissues. Ehrlich and Ratner[51] noted distinct metachromasia with crystal violet and binding of Congo red in the hyalinized islets. When the Congo red material was examined in polarized light, it was seen to exhibit dichroic birefringence. They thought that the hyaline substance which they observed was localized between capillary walls and argyrophilic fibers and concluded from their observations that it was identical with amyloid. Schwartz,[72] using fluorescent dyes such as thioflavine-T, also felt that the hyaline material in pancreatic islets represents a manifestation of senile amyloidosis.

Lacy,[73] in electron-microscopic studies, observed that the hyaline material appears as masses of interlacing small fibrils which resemble closely the ultrastructure of amyloid. He also observed that the substance is not associated with the basement membranes but is deposited as foreign material between them. He pointed out that the picture is different from that of the homogeneous material observed in the capillaries of the skin and concluded that the hyaline material of the islets represents a pathologic entity which is separate from the thickening of the basement membranes of the small blood vessels. Porta *et al.*[74] observed, in electron-microscopic studies, deposits in islet cell adenomas that had tinctorial characteristics of amyloid.

Vascular Lesions

Hoppe-Seyler,[8] in 1884, observed considerable thickening of the walls of the arteries and arterioles in the pancreas of diabetic patients, with the changes predominant in the arterioles. Cecil[9] noted arteriosclerosis in 80% of 90 pancreases studied, In half of these cases, the small vessels also showed considerable sclerosis. He also observed that the incidence of vascular changes increases with age, 40% occurring between the ages of 20 and 30 years, and 77% between the 30th and 40th years. All except two pancreases displayed arteriosclerosis after the 40th year. Moritz and Oldt,[12] in a similar study, observed arteriosclerotic changes in the pancreas in 30% of diabetics aged 31 to 45 years, increasing to 55% after the age of 61. When hypertension was concomitantly present with the diabetes, 73% of the patients between the ages of 31 and 45 years, and 87% of individuals 61 years and older showed arteriolo- and arteriosclerosis of the pancreas. The presence of considerable arteriosclerotic changes in the pancreas was subsequently confirmed by other authors.[11,75,76] Moschcowitz[77] also noted arteriosclerosis in the diabetic pancreases which increased concomitantly with the age of the patients. On the other hand, he failed to observe vascular disease in the pancreas in six cases of juvenile diabetes. Warren *et al.*[78] reported severe sclerosis and calcification in 61 of their diabetic cases. They noted that although the splenic artery may show severe sclerosis and calcification, there was often little change in those branches which lead to the pancreas. Lazarus and Volk[79] observed considerable arteriolosclerosis in 66% of pancreases studied, while only 34% of the nondiabetic pancreases of patients of similar age showed arteriolosclerosis, and, in most instances, it was less severe than in the diabetic group. Moreover, the diabetic pancreases showed, in 52%, varying degrees of occlusive arteriosclerosis as compared with less severe alterations in 34% of the nondiabetic group.

The walls of the arterioles show thickening and hyalinization of the intima, which in many instances leads to almost complete occlusion of the lumina (Fig. 2). The extent of the involvement of the arterioles does not necessarily parallel the degree of sclerosis in the larger arteries. The latter, however, often show extensive sclerosis and, in some of the diabetic patients, may be almost or completely occluded. Lesions of the smaller blood vessels are frequently associ-

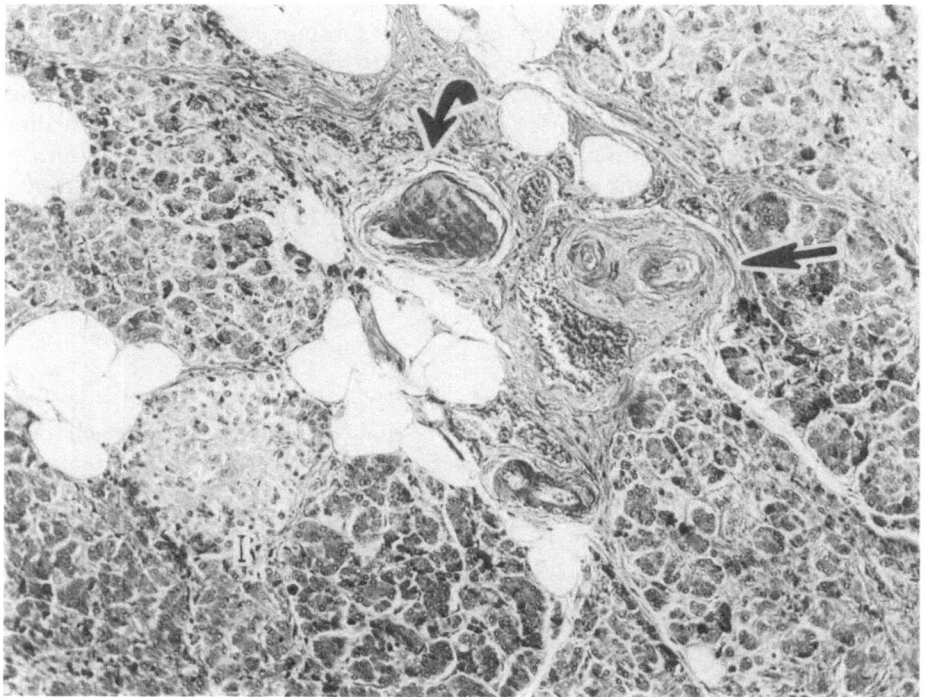

Figure 2. Portion of a diabetic pancreas showing arteriosclerosis (curved arrow) as well as arteriolar (straight arrow) sclerosis. Partially hyalinized islet (I) can be seen in the left lower corner. Periodic acid Schiff trichrome stain. ×650. Reproduced at 105%.

ated with interacinar fibrosis, with atrophy of the pancreatic parenchyma, and also, in some instances, with fibrosis of the islets. Those pancreases which contain large numbers of hyalinized islets also exhibit marked degrees of arteriosclerosis. These observations seem to be in agreement with those of Moschcowitz,[77] who also felt that arteriosclerosis may be of importance in the development of the hyalinization of the islets and as well as the cause of diabetes in the older age group of diabetic individuals. On the other hand, Warren *et al.*[81] felt that arteriosclerosis cannot be of outstanding importance in the production of diabetes, since they observed this lesion to a marked degree in only 7% of their diabetic pancreases.

Pancreatic Fibrosis

Fibrosis is the most frequently occurring change observed in the diabetic pancreas and has been known for many years. As far back as 1894 Hansemann[44] reported atrophy of the pancreatic parenchyma with replacement by a newly formed connective tissue and focal infiltration with round cells. He thought the diabetes was due to a disease of the exocrine pancreas and conjectured that, in some instances, it was the result of pancreatitis. Opie[46] believed that chronic interacinar pancreatitis was a symptom characteristic of diabetes mellitus. He conjectured that the connective tissue eventually engulfs the islets of Langerhans and thus produces islet fibrosis. Sauerbeck[80] found fibrosis of varying severity in 62% of 176 cases of diabetes. Hoppe-Seyler[8] observed extensive inter- and intraacinar connective tissue proliferation in a group of 18 diabetic pancreases. There was frequent involvement of the islets of Langerhans, eventually resulting in their complete obliteration. Cecil,[9] in a study of 90 diabetic pancreases, noted that 71% showed a distinct interacinar fibrosis. He also observed a correlation between the degree of these lesions and the age of the patient and noted that they occurred primarily in older persons. In his material, the interacinar fibrosis frequently implicated the pancreatic islets, resulting in their advanced sclerosis. Conversely, the severely sclerotic islets were always seen to be particularly involved in those areas where the exocrine pancreas was mostly fibrotic. Variainen[40] found 30 cases of gross fibrosis of the pancreas in a survey of 165 diabetics, while it was absent in a control series of the same number. Warren *et al.*[81] observed, in a group of 405 pancreases showing varying degrees of fibrosis, that 189 displayed slight fibrosis, the bulk being interacinar rather than interlobular, and 74 showed marked fibrosis, also predominantly of the interacinar type. There was no definite relationship between the islet lesions and interacinar fibrosis, with the exception of those instances where the islet fibrosis was severe. A moderate degree of interacinar fibrosis was usually noticeable. Lazarus and Volk,[82] in a group of 50 cases of maturity-onset diabetics, found varying degrees of fibrosis in 58% as compared to 42% in a control group of nondiabetic patients of similar age distribution with renal or cardiovascular disease. They observed that in every instance of insular fibrosis there was also parenchymal fibrosis present.

In the normal pancreas there is only a rather delicate fibrous tissue septum between the lobules of the pancreas, although occasionally more extensive fibrosis, both perilobular and interacinar, may be present. In the diabetic pancreas there are, in general, two noticeable, principal distributions of increased connective tissue. The more common type is interacinar fibrosis, which consists of diffuse proliferation of fibrous connective tissue between the acini (Fig. 3). Occasionally, the connective tissue is focally infiltrated by round cells, suggesting a possible inflammatory etiology (Fig. 4). The fibrosis may be diffuse, but quite often it is focally distributed. The connective tissue frequently engulfs and also may invade the islets, giving rise to insular fibrosis (Fig. 5), which, in some places, may be quite extensive. This manifests itself by the presence of periinsular bands of connective tissue proliferating into the islets along the course of the capillaries (Fig. 6). In many instances, the intrainsular proliferation may cause compartmentalization of the islets and frequently may result also in compression and loss of insular tissue. Most observers[11,39,48] agreed that intrainsular fibrosis occurs primarily in older diabetics, although the frequency varies considerably.

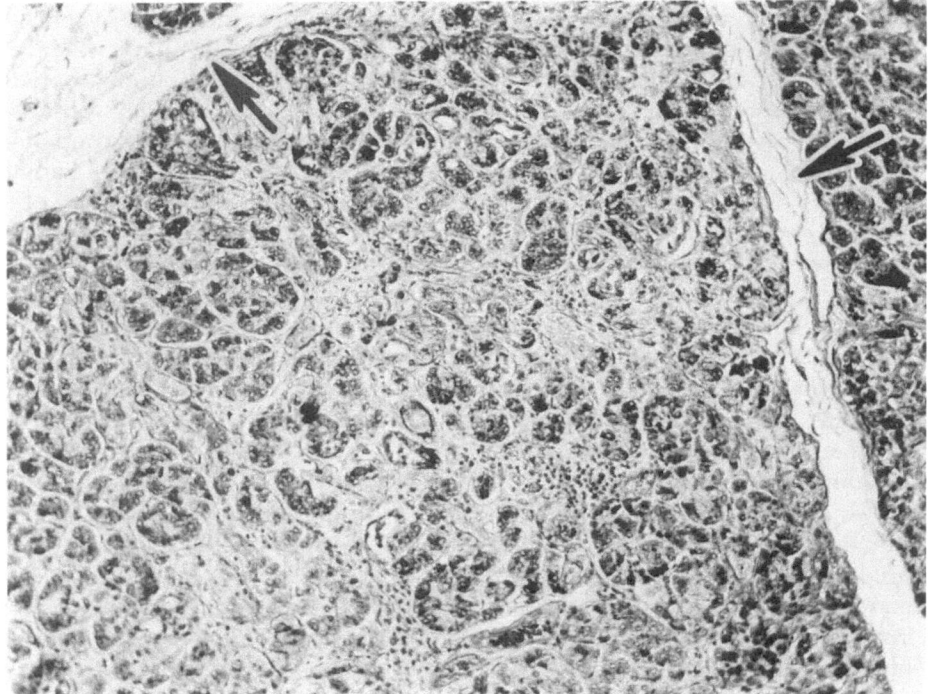

Figure 3. Diabetic pancreas showing marked interacinar fibrosis and parenchymal atrophy. There is absence of fibrosis of the interlobular septa (arrow). Periodic acid Schiff trichrome stain. ×125. Reproduced at 105%.

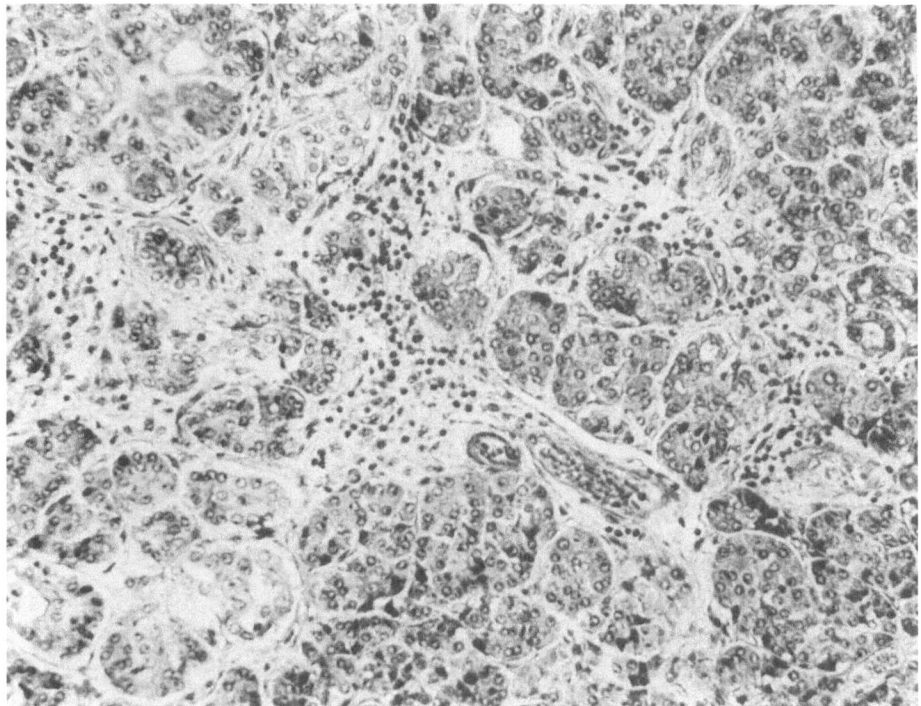

Figure 4. Pancreas of patient with maturity-onset diabetes showing interacinar fibrosis and diffuse infiltration with lymphocytes and plasma cells of the fibrous septa. Periodic acid Schiff trichrome stain. ×225. Reproduced at 105%.

The other type of increased fibrosis is perilobular in character and shows varying amounts of connective tissue bands, which separate lobules or groups of lobules (Fig. 7). In these pancreases, there may be augmentation of fibrous tissue between the acini. This increase may be less pronounced within the parenchyma than in the periphery. The exocrine pancreas usually displays varying degrees of atrophy, which may lead to focal proliferation and occasional dilatation of the ducts. The same pancreas may show fibrosis as well as hyalinization of the islets, and in some pancreases, the same islets may exhibit both lesions. In general, fibrosis, like hyalinization, occurs more often in older diabetics.

Hultquist and Olding[83] observed fibrosis of the pancreatic islets in 6 out of 10 infants born to diabetic mothers, 11 to 142 days after birth. The fibrosis covered an islet area of 5 to 10% in three cases, 10 to 20% in two cases, and more than 20% in one case. The three infants with the most pronounced islet fibrosis were heavier than normal at birth, and at least two of them were of "diabetic appearance." There was also enlargement of B cells, many of which contained hyperchromatic nuclei. Staining for amyloid was negative, and there

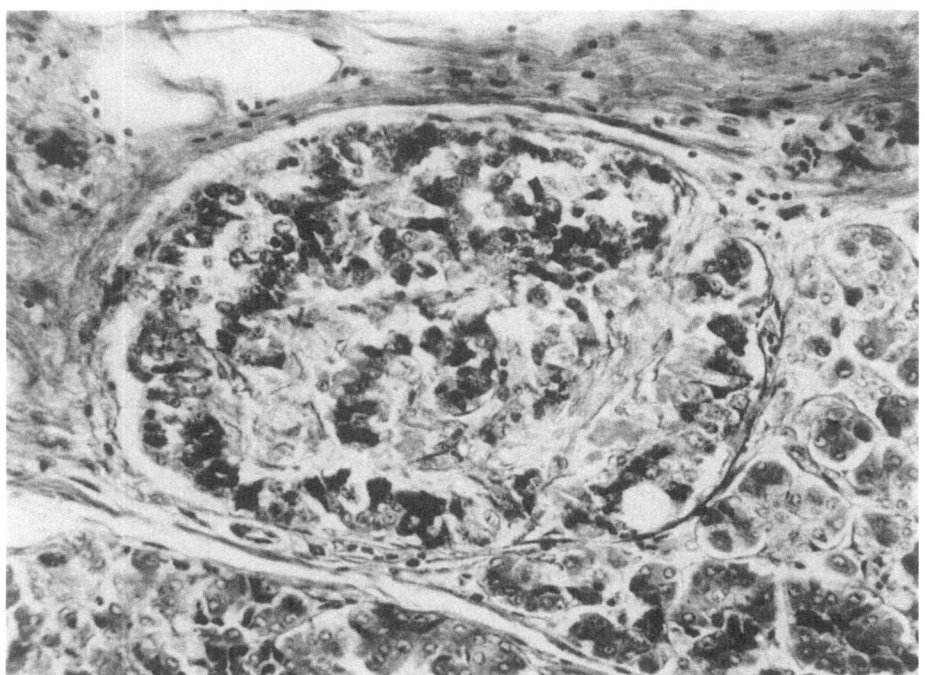

Figure 5. Early fibrosis of an islet of Langerhans. Fibrous strands cause beginning compartmentalization. Aldehyde fuchsin trichrome stain. ×280.

was absence of intra- and periinsular infiltration by inflammatory cells. The
authors believed that these changes are observed only in babies with maternal
diabetes, since they do not appear in infants of nondiabetic mothers.

The cause of fibrosis of the diabetic pancreas is difficult to explain.
Frequently in the perilobular type there is obstruction of the pancreatic ducts.
In general, in this type the islets usually are not involved. However, in some
instances, diabetes occurs when large numbers of islets are replaced by connective tissue. In a number of cases showing fibrosis of the pancreas a history of
previous gallbladder disease could be elicited. In all these instances, a thickened
fibrous capsule could be seen around many of the islets, an observation which
Otani[84] believed to be evidence of the pathological process. Another possible
cause for pancreatic fibrosis may be acute or chronic pancreatitis, as has
previously been suggested by several authors.[46,72,85-87] There is occasional
infiltration of the connective tissue with large mononuclear cells, lymphocytes,
and plasma cells, suggestive of a possible inflammatory etiology. These changes,
although they occur also in nondiabetic individuals, are encountered more
frequently in diabetic patients, after to a larger degree.[82] Chronic pancreatitis,
however, cannot account for the overwhelming majority of cases of pancreatic

arteriosclerosis. The pathogenetic factors may, therefore, be vascular impairment and ischemia, with focal atrophy and replacement of the exocrine pancreas.[88-90]

The vascular etiology of pancreatic fibrosis seems to be supported by the study of Cecil,[9] in which he found that arteriosclerosis is associated with interacinar fibrosis in 80% of the cases. He emphasized that conspicuous alterations were found in the small arteries, which frequently showed obliteration of their lumens. He further noted that fibrosis of the islets was, in general, associated with sclerosis of the small arteries of the pancreas. Hoppe-Seyler[8] also suggested that arteriosclerosis is the cause of interstitial fibrosis of the pancreas. These studies suggested that the exocrine cells become atrophic, partly because of ischemia resulting from narrowing of the arteriolar lumens, and partly because of shrinkage of the connective tissue surrounding the individual lobules. This author also felt that this type of pancreatic atrophy could be distinguished from atrophy of the pancreas in older individuals. He also noted that the fibrosis of the diabetic pancreas was far more conspicuous than in the nondiabetic and coined the term "pancreatitis interstitialis angiosclerotica" to indicate the type of fibrosis in the diabetic organ, which he

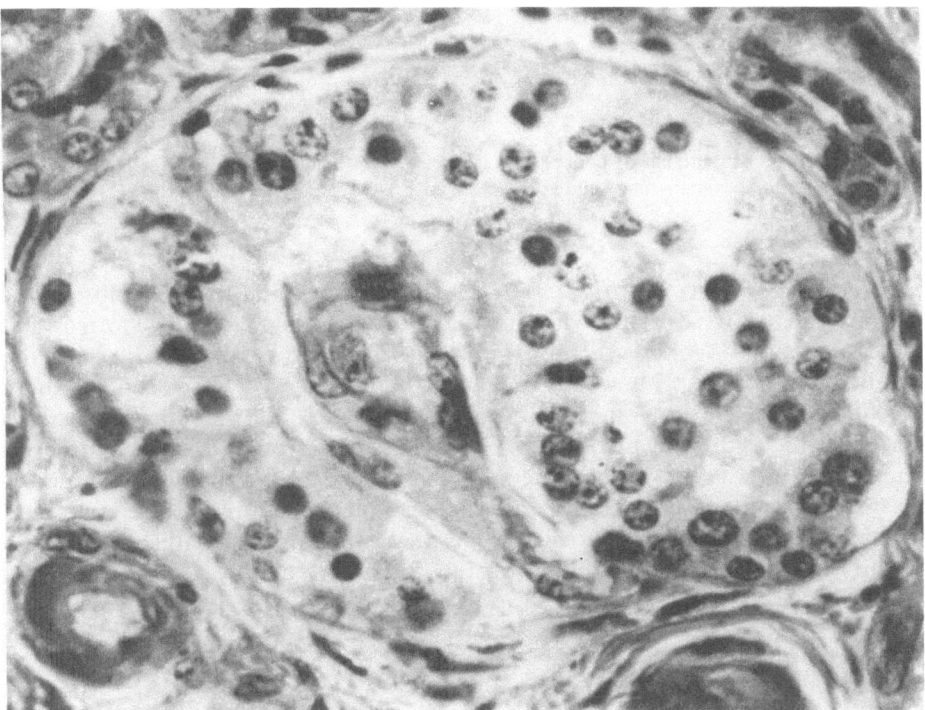

Figure 6. Islet of diabetic pancreas showing intrainsular pericapillary fibrosis. Aldehyde fuchsin trichrome stain. ×825. Reproduced at 105%.

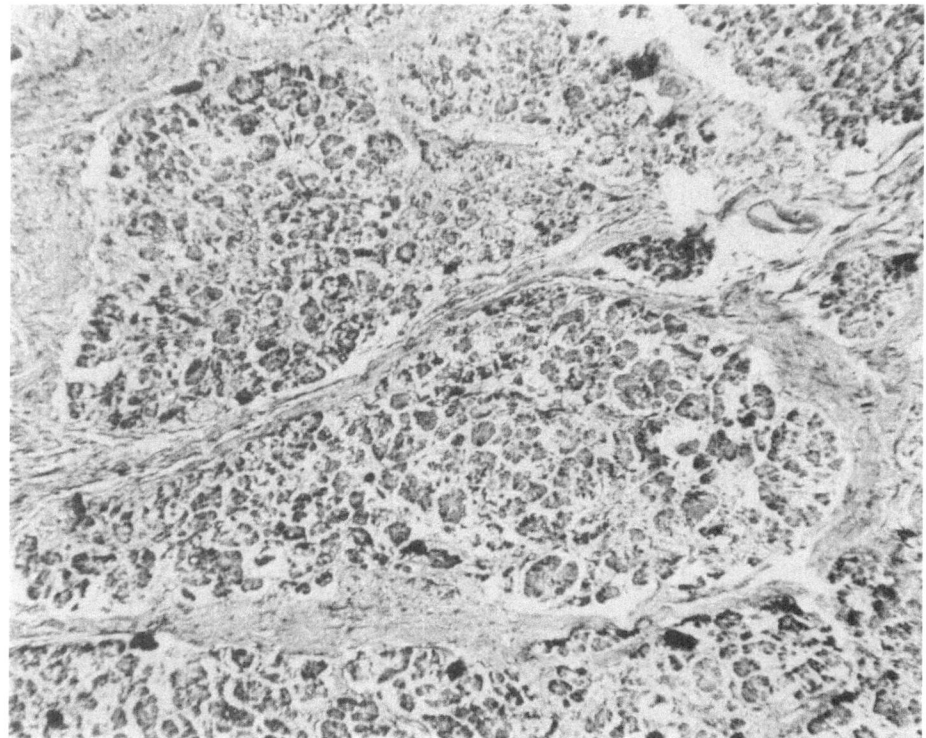

Figure 7. Portion of pancreas of patient with maturity-onset diabetes showing perilobular fibrosis and atrophy of the parenchyma. Aldehyde fuchsin trichrome stain. ×90. Reproduced at 110%.

believed was of vascular origin. The frequent association of arteriolosclerosis with interacinar fibrosis and with fibrosis of the islets suggested to Lazarus and Volk[82] that a pathogenetic relationship exists between vascular changes and the parenchymal lesions. They also observed that severe arteriosclerotic changes and, in some instances, complete or partial occlusion of large pancreatic vessels are associated with atrophy of the parenchyma and fibrosis, which also implies a cause and effect relationship. They therefore suggested that the frequency of fibrosis of the islets is related to a deficient vascular supply to the pancreas, primarily due to arteriolosclerosis, and also, in some instances, they believe it to be the result of sclerosis of the larger blood vessels.

Fatty Atrophy

The occurrence of fat in the pancreas of diabetic patients has been repeatedly discussed in the literature. Herxheimer[91] observed a combination of fatty changes, fibrosis, and acinar atrophy in many patients with diabetes of long duration. He noted that in the same organ there were foci of fatty changes with a severe degree of sclerosis alternating with marked atrophy of the gland. Gruber[92] noted fatty changes in diabetic pancreases and suggested that these alterations are often the site of arteriolosclerotic changes. He further observed the preservation of islets within the fat lobules and emphasized the frequently occurring association of areas of atrophy and fibrosis. Moreover, he observed these changes only in older individuals; they were never seen in younger persons or children. Fatty changes in the pancreas were also seen by a number of other workers. Dieckhoff[93] felt that lipomatosis of the pancreas is frequently associated with pancreatic lithiasis. He further observed that tumors of the pancreas may lead to atrophy, sclerosis, and lipomatosis of the distal portion of the organ. Priesel[94] reported a cystadenoma of the head of the pancreas. While in the area near the duodenum the pancreas was normal, the portions between the tumor and the spleen showed conversion of the pancreatic tissue into an appendage which was composed of fat tissue, containing only intact islets of Langerhans. Lang[95] reported a case in which an osteogenic sarcoma of the femur metastasized to the body and tail of the pancreas. The pancreatic tissue between the metastases became a mass of fat and connective tissue which contained accumulations of small and large islets of Langerhans, surrounded by small foci of exocrine tissue.

In the authors' study, 70 of 102 diabetic pancreases (71.4%) displayed varying degrees of fatty infiltration, as compared with 22 of 64 (34.4%) nondiabetic organs. The distribution of fat was usually focal and was frequently associated with atrophy and/or interacinar fibrosis. Often the fat was found within the septa separating the pancreatic lobes, or the picture alternated, with the atrophy predominant in other areas. Quite often, groups of islets were completely separated from the rest of the parenchyma by a zone of adipose tissue (Fig. 8). In many instances, these isolated islets showed conspicuous degrees of hyalinization. However, other areas of the same pancreas, not surrounded by fatty tissue, also exhibited sporadic hyalinized islets, although they were involved to a lesser degree. The impression of focal or lobular fatty infiltration of the pancreas was associated with vascular changes. This apparent cause and effect relationship seemed to be supported by the observation that atrophy, fibrosis, fatty changes, and hyalinization were often localized in the same area of fatty infiltration. Lazarus and Volk[96] hypothesized that ischemia resulting from sclerosis of the blood vessels produces a variegated pattern of response in the pancreas. In some instances, therefore, fibrosis and atrophy could be observed, while in other areas, fatty infiltration occurred in association with the above changes or alone. Eventually, in some pancreatic foci, the fatty changes may predominate. The authors were unable to explain why insular tissue may persist, even when the surrounding exocrine pancreas becomes atrophic. The foci of adipose tissue replacing the pancreatic parenchyma may possibly represent an *ex vacuo* proliferation of fat in an atrophic area. In what has been described as lipomatosis of the pancreas, the entire organ is converted into a mass of fat and, to a lesser degree, fibrous tissue, with only a few islets present.

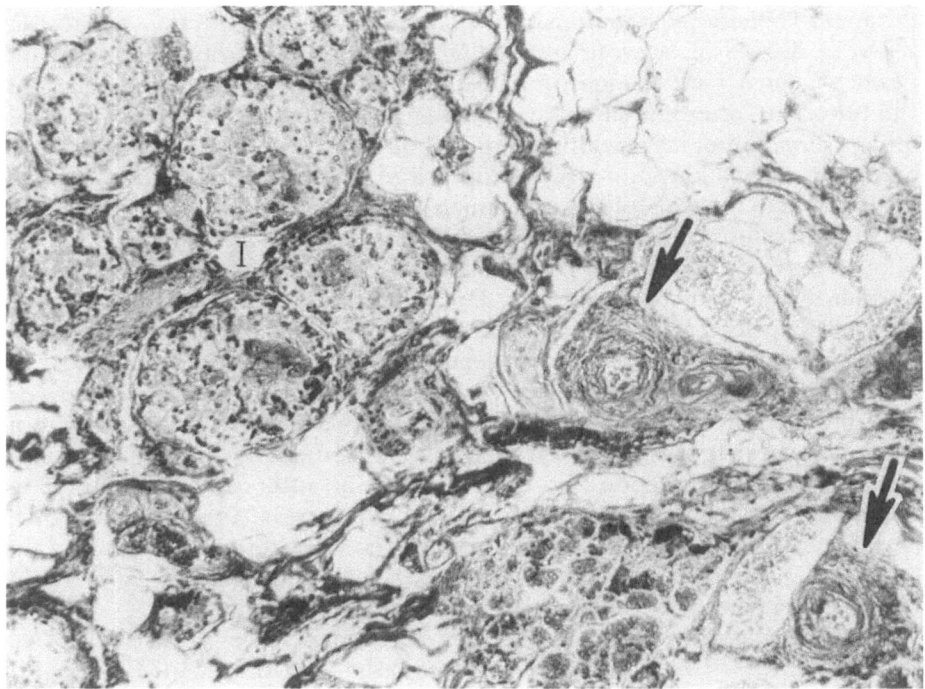

Figure 8. Portion of diabetic pancreas showing fatty atrophy. There are clusters of islets (I), most of which show conspicuous degrees of hyalinization. Several small arteries exhibit considerable sclerosis and marked narrrowing of the lumen (arrows). Periodic acid Schiff trichrome stain. ×115. Reproduced at 105%.

It is believed that pancreatic lipomatosis is associated with generalized obesity. No doubt, in some instances, the borderline between what may be called fatty atrophy and true lipomatosis is obscured. In the study of Lazarus and Volk,[96] one diabetic and two nondiabetic pancreases showed extensive or almost complete replacement of the exocrine portion by adipose tissue which contained well-preserved islets. They observed that this type of diffuse fatty infiltration of this organ usually can be found in markedly overweight individuals. On the other hand, these authors found that, although the nondiabetic pancreases displayed similar lesions, in most instances the degree of fatty infiltration was less severe.

Vacuolization ("Hydropic Degeneration") of the B Cells

In 1901 Weichselbaum and Stangl[47] described a lesion, later more elaborately discussed by Allen,[49] which consisted of a peculiar vacuolization of the pancreatic islets in comatose diabetic patients. Weichselbaum and Stangl termed these changes "hydropic degeneration" and interpreted them as being the result of liquefaction of the B cell granules, which eventually leads to atrophy of the B cells. They noted occasionally associated lymphocytic infiltration of the peri- and intrainsular connective tissue as well as a moderate increase of the intrainsular connective tissue and dilatation of the capillaries. Lymphocytic infiltration was also observed by Heiberg[97] and Fischer,[98] who believed it to represent a response to a degenerative process of the islet cells. In a later report, Weichselbaum[33] found vacuolization of the islets in 98 out of 183 diabetic patients (53%) to be one of the most frequent lesions in diabetics. Although these observations were confirmed by several authors,[99-101] albeit in smaller numbers (8 to 40%) than that of Weichselbaum, others[102,103] were unable to find these lesions in diabetic pancreases. Moreover, the vacuolization of the islets was observed by some in nondiabetic as well as in diabetic subjects.[104] Warren[62] observed vacuolization of the pancreatic islets in only 22 of 484 diabetic pancreases (4.5%). He warned that postmortem autolysis may be confused with this lesion. Gomori[105] found hydropic changes in the B cells in five nondiabetic patients. One of them had received large amounts of intravenous dextrose solution. On the other hand, he did not observe these changes in any of his diabetic patients. Hartroft,[106] using phase microscopy, reported vacuolization of the B cells in 8 of 46 diabetic patients (18%). Seifert[53] noted that 43% of diabetic pancreases in his study showed hydropic changes, in comparison with 5% of those of nondiabetics. Conroy[101] found hydropic changes in only 1 of 12 diabetic pancreases. Warren *et al.*[107] reported 36 cases with vacuolization of the B cells in a survey of 653 pancreases (2%). They felt that the rarity of such changes in their study was due to a large number of insulin-treated cases, since insulin, by reducing functional strain in these cells, decreases the frequency of these lesions. Their relation to the duration of diabetes is not entirely clear. However, in several instances, vacuolization has been reported in fulminant cases of diabetes of relatively short duration. Weichselbaum[33] observed a close correlation between hydropic degeneration and age. Nakamura[99] and Kraus[108] found these lesions more often in older individuals, while they never observed them in juvenile diabetics.

The possibility exists that vacuolization of the B cells occurred more frequently in the preinsulin era. Warren[62] described its presence in pancreatic duct epithelium in 73% of diabetic patients who had complicating infections and who had not been treated with insulin. However, Warren *et al.*,[107] in a study of pancreases from preinsulin patients with diabetes of short duration, who died in coma, and pancreases from mild diabetics who died from arteriosclerosis or intercurrent infection after 25 to 30 years of illness, observed that neither group showed evidence of hydropic B cell changes. However, in two of their cases, these lesions were observed in a control series of nondiabetic individuals.

It is believed that vacuolization of the B cells is due to glycogen infiltration during the course of the diabetic state. Toreson[109] observed vacuolization in 11 of 26 pancreases (42.3%) of diabetic patients. In 2 of these, glycogen was present in large amounts, while it was observed in small quantities in 6. Glycogen infiltration was found always in association with vacuolization of the B cells in the cytoplasm. However, glycogen infiltration in the human duct epithelium of the pancreas is apparently rare.

Lazarus and Volk[110,111] have shown in dogs that glycogen infiltration of the pancreatic B cells and so-called "ballooning" degeneration are independent phenomena. They believed that in those animals in which diabetes was induced by growth-hormone administration, the hydropic changes were reversible processes and independent degenerative lesions, as indicated by the integrity and preservation of the nuclei.

During the early phase of hydropic changes the B cell granules are usually replaced by small vacuoles which increase in size and eventually occupy all or most of the cytoplasm. The nuclei usually remain intact and are surrounded by glycogen. In a number of instances, these cells display basophilic cytoplasmic masses which have been called "Körnchen" by Weichselbaum[33] and were shown by Gepts[112,113] to be RNA. The glycogen first accumulates diffusely in the B cells and then collects into focal masses as shown by electron microscopy.[114,115] Lazarus and Volk[116] believed that glycogen infiltration is the result of distention and vacuolization of the endoplasmic reticulum, indicative of increased secretory activity. During the earlier phase, it seems that the vacuolization is apparently reversible. However, later the cytoplasm becomes atrophic and the cells eventually disappear.

Bastenie[117] observed vacuolization in a patient after 2 weeks of steroid treatment. Lazarus and Volk[118] similarly noted glycogen infiltration and vacuolization of the B cells in one diabetic patient and in one woman who developed diabetes during steroid therapy for breast cancer. In this patient the cytoplasm of the B cells, although vacuolated, contained intact nuclei. Vacuolization and glycogen infiltration were also observed in nondiabetic patients because of prolonged glucose administration prior to death.[119]

Hypertrophy of the Islets

True hypertrophy of the pancreatic islets has been observed in diabetic and nondiabetic individuals. In some instances, most of the islets may be considerably enlarged, but usually only a few are truly hypertrophied.[9] Pancreatic islets are considered to be hypertrophied when the diameter exceeds 300^{120} or 400^{121} μm. At times they may be so large that it becomes impossible to distinquish them from small adenomata. In general, there is no obvious reason to account for insular hypertrophy. However, it has been shown that the so-called giant islets are the result of fusion and coalescence of several small islets.[122]

Hypertrophy of the islets of Langerhans is not infrequent. Cecil[9,123] observed two types of hypertrophy of the islets: one, a small increase in the size of the islets without alterations in the character of the individual cells; the other, a change of the cells to a columnar or "ribbon" type in which the nuclei are located in the center. These are arranged in snakelike columns or coils, exhibiting an entirely different picture from that of the normal cell pattern, although the relationship between the cells and the capillaries is maintained. He observed 34 instances of hypertrophy and probable regeneration in 100 diabetic autopsies, while there were none in 33 cases of chronic pancreatitis, and only 1 in 17 instances of carcinomatous involvement of the pancreas. The two types of hypertrophy can, according to Cecil, be easily distinguished from each other. Ogilvie,[124,125] in a special study on hypertrophy of the islets, observed enlarged islets mainly in obese persons and considered them to be due to a pancreotropic factor of the pituitary. Maclean and Ogilvie[38] noted that hypertrophy of the islets occurs relatively frequently in young early diabetic patients. LeCompte[126] believed that the ribbonlike pattern in the B cells is characteristic of insular hypertrophy. He found that in many diabetic pancreases, especially those from juvenile diabetics, the ribbons are made of small cells with scanty cytoplasm which apparently are A cells. Hüttl[127] observed large islets at autopsy in those diabetic individuals on whom a pancreatic ligation has been performed. Warren *et al.*[128] reported 64 pancreases with hypertrophied islets in a study of 1376 diabetic organs. They were able to easily distinguish the two types of hypertrophy. The coiling, snakelike columns of cells were quite different from the typical sinusoidal structures, although the close relationship between the cells and capillaries is maintained. The epithelial cells of the islets were somewhat altered and tended to form a columnar, rather than the usual polyhedral cuboidal pattern. There were frequent irregular projections among the acini at the periphery of the islets. In this study, only a moderate proportion, and by far not all, of the islets, were hypertrophied, although occasionally the majority was considerably enlarged. The authors observed no correlation between the insular hypertrophy and the severity and duration of the diabetes nor the age of the patients.

Inflammatory Lesions of the Islets

Inflammatory lesions of the islets of Langerhans were described by Cecil in 1909.[9] These changes, which were called "insulitis" by von Meyenburg,[129] were present in two-thirds of young diabetics who died after clinical development of the disease of less than 1 year.[113] They have not been observed in chronic juvenile diabetics, elderly diabetics, or nondiabetics.[130] The inflammatory lesions are seen in only a small number of islets and consist mainly of small lymphocytes, with an admixture of a few polymorphonuclear leucocytes and histiocytes. The involved islets may be atrophic or, in many instances, they may consist of easily recognizable A and B cells.[113] Occasionally a lesion is accompanied by fibrosis.[9,113,131-133] LeCompte *et al.*[131,134] suggested that lymphocytic infiltration of the islets is possibly the response to preexisting toxic injury or perhaps a mild reaction to necrosis of the islets. Most arguments are in favor of an infectious origin of this lesion. Gundersen[26] reported an increased incidence of deaths from diabetes 2 to 4 years after an epidemic of mumps. Barboni and Manocchio[135] found inflammatory lesions in the pancreas of cows which developed diabetes a short time after the onset of foot and mouth disease. Also, insulin-dependent diabetics within 3 months of onset of the disease were found to have high titers for Coxsackie B virus, particularly of type B4.[136] These observations seem to be supported by experiments suggesting that insulitis could result from an immunological process. Thus, Renold *et al.*[137] observed, in cows that were repeatedly injected with pork or beef insulin, biological evidence of immunization against insulin. In these animals, LeCompte *et al.*[134] found significant infiltration of the islets by lymphocytes and other mononuclear cells, with a diminution in the number of B cells and moderate fibrosis. Also, Toreson *et al.*[138] observed diabetes and severe inflammatory lesions in the islets of rabbits immunized against beef insulin. This subject will be more extensively discussed in Chapter 15.

Regeneration and Ductal Proliferation

Proliferation of ductules is often seen in diabetic as well as in nondiabetic pancreases.[139] These ductules may be either intrainsular or they may be contiguous with or encircle the islets. The proliferating duct epithelium may assume the shape or the appearance of an islet ("pseudoislet") (Fig. 9) or simulate a regenerating or hyperplastic islet. In order to avoid confusion between proliferating duct epithelium and "pseudoislets" with insular tissue, it appears neces-

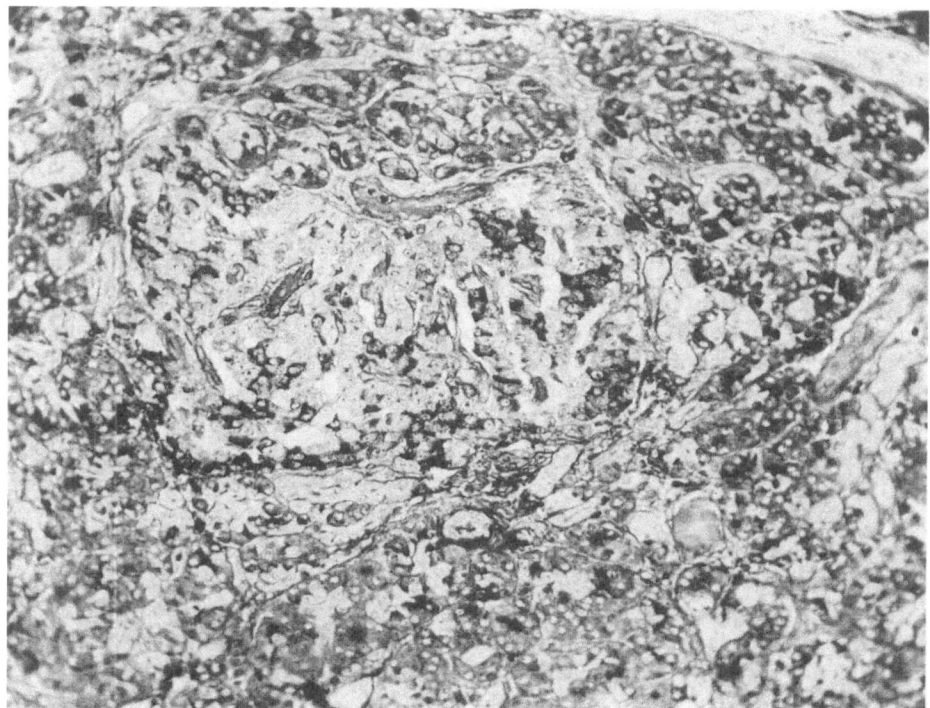

Figure 9. Portion of diabetic pancreas showing "pseudoislet" composed of proliferating ductular epithelium. Aldehyde fuchsin trichrome stain. ×190. Reproduced at 110%.

sary to utilize special staining techniques.[139] Regeneration of the islets has been believed to occur particularly in infants and children.[9,99,127,140,141] Weichselbaum[120] found these changes in 58 instances of a group of 183 pancreases, particularly in the head of that organ, and Cecil[123] observed islet regeneration and hypertrophy in a group of 100 diabetic pancreases. These changes were absent in 33 cases with chronic pancreatitis and in 17 cases with pancreatic malignancies.

Fat Deposits in B Cells

Dogiel,[142] in 1893, for the first time described the presence of fat deposits in the pancreatic islets. Subsequently, a number of other authors[48,99,129,143-146] reported the occurrence in the islets of fat droplets which, in some instances, were present in considerable amounts. Thus, Weichselbaum and Stangl[143] felt that the pancreatic islets of diabetics contained more fat than those of nondiabetics. Nakamura[99] similarly reported small and large fat droplets in pancreatic islets occurring in all diabetic patients. On the other hand, Symmers[144] and Seyfarth[48], while confirming the lesions prevailing in diabetic pancreases, noted also the occurrence of fat in various other conditions, particularly in patients who had a history of extended alcoholic intoxication. Wilder,[145] while observing the fatty infiltration more frequently in diabetics than in nondiabetic individuals, thought that these changes were probably the result, rather than the cause, of diabetes. He found marked fatty deposits in 11 patients and moderate ones in 15. Hartroft[147] observed fat droplets more frequently and in larger amounts in the islets of diabetic than of nondiabetic pancreases and suggested that their presence may be more significant than has been generally appreciated. Like[148] observed lipochrome (ceroid) granules in the B cells of nondiabetics in light- and electron-microscopic studies, and Deconinck *et al.*[149] in a study of the ultrastructure of the pancreatic islets, found lipid inclusions of varying sizes and shapes and, at times, vacuoles in the B cells of nondiabetic adults, but not in those of neonates.[150]

Calcium Deposits in the Islets of Langerhans

Calcium deposits in the cells of the pancreatic islets have been noted by several authors.[67,129] Fischer[98] observed in a diabetic pancreas white spots on gross examination, which upon microscopic studies turned out to be hypertrophied islets that were hyalinized and contained large amounts of calcium deposits.

Degranulation of B Cells

Bell[18] correlated the amount of B cell granulation with the diabetic state and observed a reduction of B cell granules, to some degree at least, in some diabetics. In a study of 995 diabetic pancreases, he observed complete or partial degranulation in those of all patients under the age of 20, of 79.5% of the patients between 20 and 40 years of age, of 48.2% between 40 and 60 years of age, and of 33.6% of those over 60 years of age. On the other hand, only 2 degranulated islets were found in a control group of 250 nondiabetic pancreases. Bell concluded that when degranulation occurs it is almost a confirmation of the diagnosis of diabetes.

Wrenshall et al.[19] observed that the B cell granules in the islets and the extractable insulin in the pancreas correlated on a one to one basis. They also noted that the extractable insulin averaged about 3 units/g of pancreas wet weight. It is noteworthy that the extractable insulin does not disappear after death, even though shortly after death the B cell granules become autolyzed. Warren et al.,[151] in a study of 223 consecutive diabetic cases, using specific stains, observed poor granulation of the B cells in 14 instances. They felt that the decrease of B cell granules is not sufficiently characteristic for diabetes in view of the fact that there is frequently considerable degranulation of B cells noticeable in autopsied pancreases and that the decrease of granules parallels the time interval between death and postmortem examination.

Quantitative Changes of the Islets of Langerhans

Since the beginning of the century, attempts have been made to estimate quantitatively the number, the weight, and the volume of the pancreatic islets of diabetic patients. However, the evaluation of quantitative changes in the endocrine pancreas rests on unstable ground because of technical difficulties. Moreover, the differences in the number of islets in various parts of the pancreas also have to be taken into consideration. All quantitative examinations of the islet tissue depend on more or less numerous fragments of tissue, which are taken from different areas of the pancreas, and, in comparison with the total mass of the organ, represent only a very minute portion of the organ. However, there is general agreement that there is usually a decline in the number as well as in the area of the islets of diabetic patients.

Weichselbaum and Stangl,[47] in a study of 18 diabetic pancreases, observed only few islets. Ssobolew[152] found considerable diminution of the islets in 13 diabetic patients, and in 4 individuals no islets were present at all. Sauerbeck[80] also noted a marked decrease in the number of islets in diabetics as compared with nondiabetics, and in a group of 90 cases, Cecil[9] observed 20 pancreases which showed a marked decrease of islets.

These early authors drew their conclusions by inspection of individual sections. However, other investigators attempted to determine the amount of islet tissue by measuring the number of islets present in the pancreas. Kraus[39] found that the number of islets per 50 cm² of pancreas in 20 diabetic patients ranged from 8.7 to 128, with an average of 54.1. He also observed a ratio of 2.4:1 between the normal and the diabetic pancreas. He further reported that in many diabetics the decrease of islets can be sufficiently conspicuous to be observed even without counting. Complete or almost complete absence of islets in diabetics has been described by other investigators.[7,18,153–157] Moore[154] reported a case of aplasia of the islets occurring in a 13-year-old girl who had had diabetes for at least 6 years. Many sections of the pancreas showed absence of normal islets, and only a few small cell groups suggestive of insular cells were present. Gepts[158] reported a marked decrease in the number of islets in young diabetics. In view of these findings, it seems that in most cases the absence of islet tissue reported by the earlier workers actually represents cases of juvenile diabetes.

Estimation of Islet Volume

The majority of investigators dealing with this subject attempted to relate the measurement of the area of the islets to the rest of the pancreas. Heiberg[159] was one of the early workers who used planigraphic measurements to compare the area of the islet tissue with that of the exocrine pancreas. Neumann[160] calculated the volume of the pancreatic islets and observed that it was markedly decreased in most diabetic pancreases. Susman[161] estimated, in a study of 200 pancreases, 55 of which were diabetic, that the islet tissue comprised 0.9 to 3.5% of the total pancreatic mass. In 60% of the diabetic cases the insular mass was less than 0.9%. In the remaining 40% of the diabetic organs, the values of the insular mass were within normal limits. Maclean and Ogilvie,[15] using a grid in the microscope to estimate the insular area, calculated the weight of the islets in 30 diabetic patients of varying age and sex distribution as ranging from 0.019 to 1 g, with a mean of 0.45 g, as compared with a range of 0.57 to 1.89 g and a mean of 1.06 g for an equal number of nondiabetic controls. In a later study, Maclean and Ogilvie[38] examined the weights of the islets of 41 young diabetic patients, 18 of whom had died within a period of 8 weeks after onset of the disease and were classified as acute cases. The remaining 23 who died at ages ranging from 9 months to 19 years after onset were considered as chronic. The mean weight of the islets was 0.70 g in 8 acute cases and 0.21 g in 19 chronic cases, as compared with 1.19 g in a series of 22 nondiabetic controls. The size of the islets in the acute cases was also bigger than in the chronic cases. The authors further calculated that while in the chronic group the mean proportion of islet tissue was 0.67%, it was 1.54% in the acute group, as compared with 2.45% in the nondiabetic controls. In a few instances in which the authors estimated the A:B ratio, the proportion of B cells was greater in the acute than in the chronic cases. Gepts,[16] using planimetric measurements of islets in 200 sections of each pancreas, calculated the weight of the average islet in a series of 28 diabetic patients, all of whom were 50 years and older, to be 0.765 g, as compared with the average islet weight of 1.358 g in 31 nondiabetic individuals. It is noteworthy that there is considerable overlap of the values, although there are significant differences between the average weight of the islets of nondiabetics as compared with those of diabetic individuals. Hellman,[162] using Wicksell's formula in his study of the distribution of the islets, thought that in diabetic as well as in nondiabetic humans there is a uniform mathematical relationship between the total islet volume and the islet diameter, so that a symmetrical volume distribution curve can be obtained, which indicates that a balance is retained between the number of small and large islets. Hellman and Angervale[163] observed a symmetrical volume distribution curve in maturity-onset diabetes with slight asymmetry in two instances, attributed to hyalinized islets, as well as in cases of insulinoma and acromegaly, and also in two patients with chronic juvenile diabetes. In the instances of juvenile diabetes, this asymmetry was believed to be due to the smallness and scarcity of the islets.

Differential Counts of the Islets of Langerhans

Although the two main cell types of the islets have been known since the beginning of the century, estimations of the proportion of the islet cells in the diabetic patient have been undertaken only relatively recently. These studies only became possible with the development of improved staining methods which permitted the identification of the different cellular types of the islets. The techniques generally used were the chrome alum hematoxylin and phloxine method of Gomori and the silver impregnation procedure of Gros–Schultze. However, because of various pitfalls in both techniques, a clear-cut delineation of the various islet constituents is fraught with error. Creutzfeldt[164,165] and Creutzfeldt and Theodossiou[166] emphasized the capriciousness of the Gros–Schultze procedure and demonstrated that different results could be obtained by slight variations of this method. He further showed that with this technique, in addition to A cells, other cell types, including B and D cells, could also be stained. He believed that the variations of the results of subsequent authors may be owing in part to difficulty in counting the cells in thick frozen sections as are used for the Gros–Schultze method and may also be the result of differences in staining techniques. Similarly, with Gomori's method, the phloxine may stain both the A and D cells. Therefore, when counting the A cells, using the procedure, additional cellular elements may be included.

Gomori,[68,167] in differential counts of 59 nondiabetic and 11 diabetic pancreases, using his chrome alum hematoxylin and phloxine method, found in several cases of diabetes a definite reduction in the B:A ratio. Ferner,[168–173] applying the Gros–Schultze silver stain to frozen sections of the diabetic pancreas, found an increase in the proportion of A cells ranging from 35 to 100%. He noticed in a 4-year-old child with diabetes many islets as well as islet "buds" ("Inselsprossen") consisting almost exclusively of silver-positive cells, which he believed to be A cells. On the basis of this information he hypothesized that diabetes, especially the juvenile form, is basically a result of failure of the silver cells, which he considered to be immature ("unreife" or "inselpotente") cells, to ripen into B cells. He further concluded that in most pancreases of juvenile diabetics a higher proportion of A cells exists than can be found in older diabetics. He believed that the increase of A cells is associated with a simultaneous reduction in B cells and interpreted this to be an attempt at regeneration.

He therefore felt that the A cells are precursors of B cells and that human diabetes is the result of the arrest of the transformation of A to B cells, thought to be the normal maturation process. Hess,[174] in agreement with Ferner's conclusions and also using the Gros–Schultze method, found a mean B:A cell ratio of 8.6:9.9 in 9 normal pancreases and 2.1:4.8 in 10 diabetic organs. He thought that these figures in the diabetic patients were closely grouped, while in normal patients they showed a greater spread of distribution. Von Meyenburg[175] also observed a low B:A cell ratio in diabetic pancreases. Hultquist *et al.*[176] found 41 to 50% silver cells in two diabetic organs, while in a series of 16 nondiabetic pancreases, they observed 27 to 40% silver cells, with an average varying from 33 to 35%. These authors noted that the patients who had 50% silver cells had severe diabetes. On the other hand, they noted that 5 of the 16 nondiabetic pancreases also had 40 to 47% silver cells. Terbrüggen,[41,177] using primarily a modification of Bensley's acid fuchsin methyl-green technique, confirmed the observations of the previous investigators and found an A:B ratio of 1:3 to 1:5 for most nondiabetic pancreases and one of 1:1 to 1:3 in 80% of the diabetic pancreases. He noted a distinct decrease of B cells and a concomitant increase of A cells in juvenile diabetics, with the A:B ratio varying from 1:1 to 1:2 (rarely, 1:3). Seifert,[178] using the same technique, observed an A:B ration of 1:1.3 to 1:4.6 in nondiabetic control pancreases and 1:1 to 1:2.5 in a group of diabetic organs. He felt that the low ratio was nonspecific because of the considerable overlap of figures between the diabetic and nondiabetic organ.

Bürkl,[179] Bürkl and Kovac,[180] and Creutzfeldt[164,165] were unable to confirm the observations of Ferner or of the other authors who used the silver impregnation technique. Gepts,[16,17] using a modification of Holmes' silver impregnation technique on thin paraffin sections, compared the cell count obtained with this procedure on the same pancreases with Gomori's chrome alum hematoxylin and phloxine method. He also found consistently higher values for the A cells with the silver method, and therefore, in agreement with Creutzfeldt, concluded that some of the B cells were also impregnated. Gepts[158] emphasized that there is no absolute increase in A cells in the diabetic and that the increase of these cells is rather due to a decrease in B cells occurring in many diabetics. This author also observed, in juvenile diabetics who died less than 6 months after onset of their symptoms, between 100 and 1000 B cells per cm², as compared with nondiabetic individuals of the same age group in whom the count varied from 1000 to 10,000. Warren *et al.*,[181] using granule stains for differential counts on islet cells, observed that the ratio of B:A cells was 1.8 in diabetic pancreases as compared with 8.2 in the nondiabetic organ.

Quantitative Estimation of Islet Tissue

Various authors attempted to study the weights of the islets as well as those of their cellular components and found, in general, a marked decrease in diabetic pancreases, although there was often considerable overlap between the figures observed in diabetic as well as in nondiabetic organs. Maclean and Ogilvie[15] estimated the weights of the islet tissue in pancreases of 30 diabetic patients of varying age and sex distribution and observed values of 0.02 to 1 g in the diabetic organs as compared with 0.51 to 2.89 g in the nondiabetic control group. The mean for the diabetic islets was 0.45 g, and that for the controls was 1.06 g. In a later study, Ogilvie[124] observed that the number of islets per gram of pancreas averaged 7130 and 14,000 in a group of 30 diabetic and 30 control pancreases, respectively. The A:B cell ratio was on the average 1:1.5 in the diabetics and 1:3 in the controls. Ogilvie[124] also observed that the mean weights of the islet tissue, the A cells, and the B cells were 0.1, 0.04, and 0.05 g in the growth-onset diabetics as compared with 0.5, 0.17, and 0.25 g, respectively, in the maturity-onset diabetics. In other words, the mean weight of the B cells was markedly reduced in both maturity- and growth-onset diabetics, but it was substantially lower in the latter. Moreover, he observed that the weights of the A and B cells were seemingly lower in the group aged 40 to 60 years than in the group over 60.

Since obesity is a common antecedent to diabetes and is often regarded as a prediabetic state, Ogilvie[182] studied the proportion of islet tissue and the size of islets in 19 obese persons, as well as in 19 control (lean) subjects. The percentage of islet tissue ranged between 0.74 and 5.71 and averaged 3.19 in the obese, whereas it varied from 0.80 to 3.84 with a mean of 2.05 in the control group. The average size of the islets, measured in square centimeters at a magnification of 120, ranged between 1.46 and 5.78 and averaged 2.59 in the obese, and from 0.99 to 2.22 with a mean of 1.57 in the controls. The proportion of islet tissue and the size of the islets were thus greater in the obese than in the controls by 56 and 65%, respectively.

Gepts,[16] in his study of 31 nondiabetic and 28 diabetic pancreases, observed that the mean total weight of the islet tissue was 1.358 g in the nondiabetic. The calculated mean weight of the B cells was 0.754 g and that of the A cells was 0.341 g in the nondiabetic organ. In the diabetic group the mean total weight of the islets was 0.765 g, whereby the mean mass of the B cells was 0.301 g and that of the A cells was 0.319 g.

References

1. Marble, A.: In: *Joslin's Diabetes Mellitus.* Edited by A. Marble, P. White, R. Bradley, and L. P. Krall. Lea & Febiger, Philadelphia, 1971, p. 1.
2. White, P.: *Diabetes in Childhood and Adolescence.* Lea & Febiger, Philadelphia, 1932, p. 60.
3. Boyd, J. D.: In: *Practice of Pediatrics.* Edited by J. Brennemann. W. F. Prior, Hagerstown, Md., 1946.
4. Danowski, T. S.: *Diabetes Mellitus, With Emphasis on Children and Young Adults.* Williams & Wilkins, Baltimore, 1957.
5. White, P.: *Diabetes,* **9**:345, 1960.
6. White, P.: In: *Diabetes.* Edited by R. H. Williams. Paul B. Hoeber, New York, 1960, p. 381.
7. Schwartzman, J., Crusius, M. E., and Beirne, D. P.: *Amer. J. Dis. Child.,* **74**:587, 1947.

8. Hoppe-Seyler, G.: *Dtsch. Arch. Klin. Med.,* **81**:119, 1904.

9. Cecil, R. L.: *J. Exp. Med.,* **11**:266, 1909.

10. Opie, E. L.: *Diseases of the Pancreas.* J. B. Lippincott, Philadelphia, 1910, p. 317.

11. Weichselbaum, A.: *Wien. Klin. Wochenschr.,* **24**:153, 1911.

12. Moritz, A. R., and Oldt, M. B.: *Amer. J. Pathol.,* **13**:679, 1937.

13. Neumann, F.: Cited by E. J. Kraus: In: *Handbuch der spez. Path. Path. Anat.* Edited by F. Henke, and O. Lubarsch. Julius Springer, Berlin, Vol. V/2, 1929, p. 689.

14. Lazarus, S. S., and Volk, B. W.: *The Pancreas in Human and Experimental Diabetes.* Grune & Stratton, New York. 1962, p. 196.

15. Maclean, N., and Ogilvie, R. F.: *Diabetes,* **4**:367, 1955.

16. Gepts, W.: *Ann. Soc. Roy. Sci. Méd. Nat. Brux.,* **10**:5, 1957.

17. Gepts, W.: *Endokrinologie,* **36**:185, 1958.

18. Bell, E. T.: *Diabetes,* **2**:376, 1953.

19. Wrenshall, G. A., Bogoch, A., and Ritchie, R. C.: *Diabetes,* **1**:87, 1952.

20. Wrenshall, G. A., Hartroft, W. S., and Best, C. H.: *Diabetes,* **3**:444, 1954.

21. Bornstein, J.: *J. Endocrinol.,* **7**:59, 1953.

22. Bornstein, J.: *Diabetes,* **2**:23, 1953.

23. Houssay, B. A.: *Amer. J. Med. Sci.,* **193**:581, 1937,

24. Long, C. N. H., and Lukens, F. D. W.: *J. Exp. Med.,* **63**:465, 1936.

25. Young, F. G.: *Lancet,* **2**:372, 1937.

26. Gundersen, E.: *J. Infect. Dis.,* **41**:197, 1927.

27. Gamble, D. R., Kinsley, M. L., Fitzgerald, M. G., Bolten, R., and Taylor, K. W.: *Brit. Med. J.,* **3**:627, 1969.

28. Pav, J., Jezkova, Z., and Skrha, F.: *Lancet,* **3**:221, 1963.

29. Chetty, M. P., and Watson, K. C.: *Lancet,* **1**:67, 1965.

30. Vallance-Owen, J.: *Diabetes,* **13**:241, 1964.

31. Antoniades, H. N., Gundersen, K., Beigelman, P. M., Pyle, H. M., and Bougas, J. A.: *Diabetes,* **11**:261, 1962.

32. Unger, R. H., and Orci, L.: *Lancet,* **1**:14, 1975.

33. Weichselbaum, A.: *Sitzungsbd. Akad. Wissensch. Math. Naturwiss. Kl.,* **119**:73, 1910.

34. Herxheimer, G.: *Verh. Dtsch. Ges. Verdau. Stoffwechselkr.,* **11**:112, 1933.

35. von Halasz, A.: *Wien. Klin. Wochenschr.,* **22**:1481, 1909.

36. Seyfarth, C.: *München Med. Wochenschr.,* **67**:617, 1920.

37. Terplan, K.: Personal communication to S. Warren, P. M. LeCompte, and M. A. Legg: *The Pathology of Diabetes Mellitus.* Lea & Febiger, Philadelphia, 1966, p. 113.

38. Maclean, N., Robertson, F., and Ogilvie, R. F.: *Diabetes,* **8**:83, 1959.

39. Kraus, E. J.: In: *Handbuch der speziellen pathologischen Anatomie und Histologie.* Edited by F. Henke and O. Lubarsch. Julius Springer, Berlin, Vol. V/2, 1929, pp. 662–727.

40. Vartiainen, I.: *Acta Med. Scand.,* **118**:536, 1944.

41. Terbrüggen, A.: *Virchow's Arch.,* **315**:407, 1948.

42. Warren, S., and LeCompte, P. M.: *The Pathology of Diabetes Mellitus.* Lea & Febiger, Philadelphia, 1952, p. 73.

43. Lazarus, S. S., and Volk, B. W.: *The Pancreas in Human and Experimental Diabetes.* Grune & Stratton, New York, 1962, p. 196.

44. Hansemann, D.: *Ztschr. Klin. Med.,* **26**:191, 1894.

45. Simmonds, F.: *Dtsch. Med. Wochenschr.,* **38**:1020, 1912.

46. Opie, E. L.: *J. Exp. Med.,* **5**:397, 1900–01.

47. Weichselbaum, A., and Stangl, E.: *Wien. Klin. Wochenschr.,* **14**:968, 1901.

48. Seyfarth, C.: *Verh. 32 Kongr. Inn. Med.,* **32**:178, 1920.

49. Allen, F. M.: *J. Metab. Res.,* **1**:5, 1922.

50. Lazarus, S. S., and Volk, B. W.: *The Pancreas in Human and Experimental Diabetes.* Grune & Stratton, New York, 1962, p. 209.

51. Ehrlich, J. C., and Ratner, I. M.: *Amer. J. Pathol.,* **38**:49, 1961.

52. Bell, E. T.: *Diabetes,* **1**:341, 1952.

53. Seifert, G.: *Verh. Dtsch. Ges. Pathol.,* **18**:50, 1959,

54. Warren, S., LeCompte, P. M., and Legg, M. A.: *The Pathology of Diabetes Mellitus.* Lea & Febiger, Philadelphia, 1966, p. 60.
55. Legg, M. A.: Quoted in: Warren, S., LeCompte, P. M., and Legg, M. A.: *The Pathology of Diabetes Mellitus.* Lea & Febiger, Philadelphia, 1966, p. 60.
56. Ohlmacher, J. C.: *Amer. J. Med. Sci.,* **128**:287, 1904.
57. Saltykow, O.: *Cor.-Bl. Schweiz. Aerzte,* **39**:625, 1909.
58. Milne, L. S., and Peters, H. L.: *J. Med. Res.,* **26**:405, 1912.
59. Wright, A. W.: *Amer. J. Pathol.,* **3**:461, 1927.
60. Ahronheim, J. H.: *Amer. J. Pathol.,* **19**:873, 1943.
61. Arey, J. B.: *Arch. Pathol.,* **36**:32, 1943.
62. Warren, S.: *The Pathology of Diabetes Mellitus.* Lea & Febiger, Philadelphia, 1938, p. 31.
63. Bell, E. T.: *Amer. J. Pathol.* **35**:801, 1959.
64. Bell, E. T.: *Diabetes Mellitus.* Charles C Thomas, Springfield, Ill., 1960, p. 55.
65. Hartroft, W. S.: *Diabetes,* **5**:98, 1956.
66. Opie, E. L.: *J. Exp. Med.,* **5**:527, 1900–01.
67. Mallory, F. B.: *The Principles of Pathologic Histology.* W. B. Saunders, Philadelphia, 1914, p. 521.
68. Gomori, G.: *Arch. Pathol.,* **36**:217, 1943.
69. Bloom, F.: *N. Engl. J. Med.,* **217**:395, 1937.
70. Van Beek, C. C.: *Nederl. Tijdschr. V. Geneesk.,* **83**:646, 1939.
71. Gellerstedt, N.: *Beitr. Z. Pathol. Anat. Allg. Pathol.,* **101**:1, 1938.
72. Schwartz, P.: *Trans. N.Y. Acad. Sci.,* **27**:393, 1965.
73. Lacy, P. E.: In: *Aetiology of Diabetes and Its Complications.* Edited by M. P. Cameron and M. O'Connor. *Ciba Foundation Coloquia on Endocrinology.* Little, Brown, Boston, Vol. 15, 1964, p. 84.
74. Porta, E. A., Yerry, Y. R., and Scott, R. F.: *Amer. J. Pathol.,* **41**:623, 1962.
75. Herxheimer, G.: In: *Handb. Inneren Sekretion.* Edited by M. Hirsch. Berlin, 1925.
76. Seyfarth, C.: In: *Verh. Deutsch. Ges. Pathol.* G. Fischer, Verlag, Stuttgart, 1950.
77. Moschcowitz, E.: *Ann. Int. Med.,* **34**:1137, 1951.
78. Warren, S., LeCompte, P. M., and Legg, M. A.: *The Pathology of Diabetes Mellitus.* Lea & Febiger, Philadelphia, 1966, p. 106.
79. Lazarus, S. S., and Volk, B. W.: *The Pancreas in Human and Experimental Diabetes.* Grune & Stratton, New York, 1962, p. 199.
80. Sauerbeck, E.: *Erg. Path. Path. Anat.,* **8**:538, 1902.
81. Warren, S., LeCompte, P. M., and Legg, M. A.: *The Pathology of Diabetes Mellitus.* Lea & Febiger, Philadelphia, 1966, p. 102.
82. Lazarus, S. S., and Volk, B. W.: *The Pancreas in Human and Experimental Diabetes.* Grune & Stratton, New York, 1962, p. 202.
83. Hultquist, G. T., and Olding, L. B.: *Lancet,* **2**:1016, 1975.
84. Otani, S.: *Amer. J. Pathol.,* **3**:1, 1927.
85. Comfort, M. W., Gambill, E. E., and Baggenstoss, A. H.: *Gastroenterology,* **6**:239, 1946.
86. Maimon, S. N., Kirsner, J. B., and Palmer, W. L.: *Arch. Int. Med.,* **81**:56, 1948.
87. Popper, H.: *Gastroenterology,* **19**:183, 1952.
88. Robbins, S. L.: *Textbook of Pathology.* W. B. Saunders, Philadelphia, 1957, p. 870.
89. Blumenthal, H. T., and Probstein, J. G.: *Pancreatitis: A Clinical–Pathologic Correlation.* Charles C Thomas, Springfield, Ill., 1959.
90. Hranilovich, G. T., and Baggenstoss, A. H.: *Arch. Pathol.,* **55**:443, 1953.
91. Herxheimer, G.: *Virchow's Arch.,* **183**:228, 1906.
92. Gruber, G.: In: *Handb. Path. Path. Anat.* Edited by F. Henke and O. Lubarsch. Julius Springer, Berlin, Vol. V/2, 1929, p. 211.
93. Dieckhoff, C.: *Beiträge Path. Anat. Pankreas. Med. Inaug.-Diss.,* Rostock, 1894.
94. Priesel, R.: *Frankfurt Ztschr. Pathol.,* **26**:453, 1922.
95. Lang, F. J.: *Virchow's Arch.,* **257**:246, 1925.
96. Lazarus, S. S., and Volk, B. W.: *The Pancreas in Human and Experimental Diabetes.* Grune & Stratton, New York, 1962, p. 204.
97. Heiberg, K. A.: *Centralbl. Allg. Path. Path. Anat.,* **221**:532, 1911.
98. Fischer, B.: *Frankfurt Ztschr. Pathol.,* **17**:218, 1915.

99. Nakamura, N.: *Arch. Pathol. Anat.*, **253**:286, 1924.
100. Martius, K.: *Franfurt Ztschr. Pathol.*, **17**:276, 1915.
101. Conroy, M. J.: *J. Metab. Res.*, **2**:367, 1922.
102. Karakascheff, K. I.: *Dtsch. Arch. Klin. Med.*, **82**:60, 1904–05.
103. Thoinot, L., and Delamare, G.: *Arch. Méd. Exp. Anat. Pathol.*, **19**:176, 1907.
104. Sauerbeck, E.: *Virchow's Arch.*, **177**:1, 1904.
105. Gomori, G.: *Amer. J. Pathol.*, **17**:395, 1941.
106. Hartroft, W. S.: *Proc. Amer. Diabetes Assoc.*, **10**:46, 1950.
107. Warren, S., LeCompte, P. M., and Legg, M. A.: *The Pathology of Diabetes Mellitus*. Lea & Febiger, Philadelphia, 1966, p. 73.
108. Kraus, E. J.: *Virchow's Arch.*, **247**:1, 1923.
109. Toreson, W. E.: *Amer. J. Pathol.*, **27**:327, 1951.
110. Lazarus, S. S., and Volk, B. W.: *The Pancreas in Human and Experimental Diabetes*. Grune & Stratton, New York, 1962, p. 102.
111. Volk, B. W., and Lazarus, S. S.: *Diabetes*, **13**:60, 1964.
112. Gepts, W.: In: *The Structure and Metabolism of the Pancreatic Islets*. Edited by S. Brolin, B. Hellman, and H. Knutson. Macmillan, New York, 1964, p. 513.
113. Gepts, W.: *Diabetes*, **14**:619, 1965.
114. Williamson, J. R., and Lacy, P. E.: *Arch. Pathol.*, **72**:637, 1961.
115. Volk, B. W., and Lazarus, S. S.: *Diabetes*, **12**:162, 1963.
116. Lazarus, S. S., and Volk, B. W.: *Arch. Pathol.*, **71**:44, 1961.
117. Bastenie, P.: *Cortico-Surrénale et Diabète Humain*. Masson et Cie, Paris, 1956, p. 148.
118. Lazarus, S. S., and Volk, B. W.: *The Pancreas in Human and Experimental Diabetes*. Grune & Stratton, New York, 1962, p. 106.
119. Gomori, G.: *Bull. N.Y. Acad. Med.*, **21**:99, 1945.
120. Weichselbaum, A.: *Sitzungsber Akad. Wiss., Wien. Math.-Naturw. Kl. Wien.*, **117**:211, 1908.
121. Warren, S., LeCompte, P. M., and Legg, M. A.: *The Pathology of Diabetes Mellitus*. Lea & Febiger, Philadelphia, 1966, p. 80.
122. Eder, M.: *Beitr. Path. Anat. Allg. Path.*, **115**:157, 1955.
123. Cecil, R. L.: *J. Exp. Med.*, **14**:500, 1911.
124. Ogilvie, R. F.: In: *Aetiology of Diabetes and Its Complications*. Edited by M. P. Cameron, and M. O'Connor. *Ciba Foundation Coloquia on Endocrinology*. Little, Brown, Boston, Vol. 15, 1964, p. 69.
125. Ogilvie, R. F.: *Endinburgh. Med. J.*, **51**:460, 1944.
126. LeCompte, P. M.: In: *Diabetes*. Edited by R. H. Williams, Paul B. Hoeber, New York, 1960, p. 309.
127. Hüttl, T.: *Beitr. Z. Klin. Chir.*, **163**:206, 1936.
128. Warren, S., LeCompte, P. M., and Legg, M. A.: *The Pathology of Diabetes Mellitus*. Lea & Febiger, Philadelphia, 1966, p. 80.
129. Von Meyenburg, H.: *Schw. Med. Wochenschr.*, **21**:554, 1940.
130. Deconinck, J., Potvliege, P. R., and Gepts, W.: In: *Handbook of Physiology*. Sect. 7, *Endocrinology*. Vol. 1, *Endocrine Pancreas*. Edited by R. O. Greep, E. B. Astwood, D. F. Steiner, N. Freinkel, and S. R. Geiger. Williams & Wilkins, Baltimore, 1972, p. 295.
131. LeCompte, P. M.: *Arch. Pathol.*, **66**:450, 1958.
132. Warren, S.: *JAMA*, **88**:99, 1927.
133. Stansfield, O., and Warren, S.: *N. Engl. J. Med.*, **198**:686, 1928.
134. LeCompte, P. M., Steinke, J., Soeldner, J. S., and Renold, A. E.: *Diabetes*, **15**:586, 1966.
135. Barboni, E., and Manocchio, I.: *Arch. Vet. Ital.*, **13**:477, 1962.
136. Gamble, D. R., Kinsley, M. L., Fitzgerald, M. G., Bolton, R., and Taylor, K. W.: *Brit. Med. J.*, **3**:627, 1969.
137. Renold, A. E., Soeldner, J. S., and Steinke, J.: In: *Aetiology of Diabetes and Its Complications*. Edited by M. P. Cameron and M. O'Connor. *Ciba Foundation Coloquia on Endocrinology*. Little, Brown, Boston, Vol. 15, 1964, p. 122.
138. Toreson, W. E., Lee, J. C., and Grodsky, G. M.: *Amer. J. Pathol.*, **52**:1099, 1968.
139. Lazarus, S. S., and Volk, B. W.: *The Pancreas in Human and Experimental Diabetes*. Grune & Stratton, New York, 1962, p. 212.

140. Gutman, C.: *Virchow's Arch. f. Path. Anat.,* **172**:493, 1903.
141. Schmidt, M. B.: *München Med. Wochenschr.,* **49**:51, 1959.
142. Dogiel, A. S.: *Arch. Anat. Entwicklungsgesch.,* **2**:117, 1893.
143. Weichselbaum, A., and Stangl, E.: *Wien. Klin. Woechenschr.,* **15**:969, 1902.
144. Symmers, D.: *Arch. Int. Med.,* **3**:379, 1909.
145. Wilder, R. M.: *S. Med. J.,* **19**:241, 1926.
146. Gibb, W. F., and Logan, V. W.: *Arch. Int. Med.,* **43**:376, 1929.
147. Hartroft, W. B.: In: *Diabetes.* Edited by R. H. Williams, Paul P. Hoeber, New York, 1960, p. 350.
148. Like, A. A.: *Lab. Invest.,* **16**:937, 1967.
149. Deconinck, J. F., Potvliege, P. R., and Gepts, W.: *Diabetologia,* **7**:266, 1971.
150. Deconinck, J. F., Van Assche, F. A., Potvliege, P. R., and Gepts, W.: *Diabetologia,* **8**:326, 1972.
151. Warren, S., LeCompte, P. M., and Legg, M. A.: *The Pathology of Diabetes Mellitus.* Lea & Febiger, Philadelphia, 1966, p. 62.
152. Ssobolew, L. W.: *Virchow's Arch.,* **168**:91, 1902.
153. Herzog, M.: *Virchow's Arch.,* **168**:83, 1902.
154. Moore, R. A.: *Amer. J. Dis. Child.,* **52**:627, 1936.
155. Dieckhoff, G.: *Beitr. Z. Wissensch. Med., Festschrift.* Theodor Thierfelder, Leipzig, 1895, p. 97.
156. Bence, J.: *Wien. Klin. Wochenschr.,* **20**:721, 1907.
157. Potter, N. B., and Milne, L. S.: *Amer. J. Med. Sci.,* **143**:46, 1911.
158. Gepts, W.: In: *Handbook of Diabetes Mellitus.* Edited by E. F. Pfeiffer. J. F. Lehmann, München, Vol. II, 1971, pp. 3–39.
159. Heiberg, K. A.: *Anat. Anz.,* **29**:49, 1906.
160. Neumann, F.: Cited by E. J. Kraus.: In: *Handbuch der Spez. Path. u. Path. Anat.* Edited by F. Henke and O. Lubarsch, Julius Springer, Berlin, Vol. V/2, 1929, p. 689.
161. Susman, W.: *J. Clin. Endocrinol.,* **2**:97, 1942.
162. Hellman, B.: *Acta Pathol. Microbiol. Scand.,* **51**:95, 1961.
163. Hellman, B., and Angervale, L.: *Acta Pathol. Microbiol. Scand.,* **53**:230, 1961.
164. Creutzfeldt, W.: *Beitr. Path. Anat.,* **113**:133, 1953,
165. Creutzfeldt, W.: *Ztschr. Inn. Med.,* **37**:217, 1956.
166. Creutzfeldt, W., and Theodossiou, A.: *Beitr. Path. Anat.,* **117**:235, 1957.
167. Gomori, G.: *Bull. N.Y. Acad. Med.,* **21**:99, 1945.
168. Ferner, H.: *Ztschr. Mikr. Anat. Forsch.,* **44**:451, 1938.
169. Ferner, H.: *Virchow's Arch.,* **309**:87, 1942.
170. Ferner, H.: *Deutsche Ztschr. f. Verdauungskr.,* **6**:21, 1942.
171. Ferner, H.: *Dtsch. Med. Wochenschr.,* **72**:540, 1947.
172. Ferner, H.: *Virchow's Arch.,* **319**:390, 1951.
173. Ferner, H.: *Das Inselsystem des Pankreas.* Georg Thieme Verlag, Stuttgart, 1952, p. 149.
174. Hess, W.: *Schweiz. Ztschr. Path. u. Bakt.,* **9**:46, 1946.
175. Von Meyenburg, H.: *Schweiz. Med. Wochenschr.,* **76**:207, 1946.
176. Hultquist, G., Dahlen, M., and Helander, C. G.: *Schweiz. Ztschr. Path. u. Bakt.,* **11**:570, 1948.
177. Terbrüggen, A.: *Klin. Wochenschr.,* **24–25**:434, 1947.
178. Seifert, G.: *Virchow's Arch.,* **325**:379, 1954.
179. Bürkl, W.: *Acta Anat.,* **12**:358, 1951.
180. Bürkl, W., and Kovac, W.: *Mikroskopie,* **6**:283, 1951.
181. Warren, S., LeCompte, P. M., and Legg, M. A.: *The Pathology of Diabetes Mellitus.* Lea & Febiger, Philadelphia, 1966, p. 97.
182. Ogilvie, R. F.: *J. Pathol. Bacteriol.* **37**:473, 1933.

Chapter 10

Pathogenetic Considerations of Idiopathic Diabetes

Bruno W. Volk and Klaus F. Wellmann

The hypothesis that idiopathic diabetes is a result of insufficient secretion of insulin seemed to be confirmed by many earlier experimental studies carried out around the turn of the century. This viewpoint was based on the studies of Von Mering and Minkowski[1] who, in 1889, were the first to observe that removal of the pancreas causes diabetes in the dog. The discovery of insulin by Banting and Best[2] in 1922 seemed to support this hypothesis, since the administration of pancreatic extracts could correct the metabolic abnormalities in diabetes. This was in keeping with the frequently observed atrophy of the pancreatic islets,[3–7] the decrease of extractable insulin[8–10] in pancreases of juvenile diabetics, and the occurrence of interacinar fibrosis, insular fibrosis, and hyalinization in the pancreases of maturity-onset diabetics.[11] Moreover, quantitative studies by various authors indicated a relative increase of A cells in many diabetic pancreases associated with a concomitant decrease of the B cells.[7,12–14]

A review of the histologic studies of the pancreatic islets has so far failed to uncover the cause for the progressive decrease of B cells in diabetic individuals. It is not clear whether the reduction in the number of these cells is congenital or whether it is the result of a progressive deterioration of insular tissue that may have gone on for a long time without notice during the preclinical phase of diabetes. The apparent specificity of these findings, however, seemed to have been contradicted by reports that the A:B ratio in the islets of Langerhans in a significant number of diabetic individuals appears normal,[7,12–15] while on the other hand, hyalinization, fibrosis, and vacuolization may also occur in nondiabetic pancreases, albeit to a lesser degree.[11]

The amount of B cell reduction seems to be in itself insufficient to account for the diabetes, since in experimental animals 80 to 90% of the pancreas must be removed in order for the disease to develop. The complexity of the problem

Bruno W. Volk and Klaus F. Wellmann • Isaac Albert Research Institute of the Kingsbrook Jewish Medical Center, and Downstate Medical Center, State University of New York, Brooklyn, New York. Present address of B. W. V.: University of California, Irvine, California. Present address of K. F. W.: Beekman Downtown Hospital, New York, New York.

is magnified by the demonstration that in some diabetic patients similar amounts of B cell granules,[15] extractable insulin,[1-10] and circulating insulin-like substances[16,17] can be found as are present in nondiabetic patients. The fact that the sulfonylureas which stimulate the secretion of pancreatic insulin are effective in lowering the blood sugar in many maturity-onset diabetics seems, furthermore, to indicate that these patients have a sufficient insulinogenic reserve.[18,19]

On the other hand, the observation that in some elderly diabetics the pancreas contains only 50% of the normal amount of insulin appears to contradict the above consideration,[20] since this indicates a functional deficiency of the B cells in these individuals. This decrease of insulin content cannot be explained by prolonged hyperglycemia to which the B cells have been subjected, since it has been shown experimentally that under chronic stimulation normal B cells can maintain a normal level of insulin reserve by compensating with enhanced hormonal synthesis and release.[21,22] Thus, the cause of secretory dysfunction of elderly diabetics remains obscure.

Moschcowitz[23] pointed out that arteriosclerosis may be of importance in leading to the hyalinization of islets and causing diabetes in the older age group. In keeping with Moschcowitz's suggestion, Lazarus and Volk[24] have shown that the diabetic pancreas is the seat of severe vascular disease which seems to be the most likely cause of the interacinar fibrosis, acinar atrophy, as well as intrainsular pericapillary fibrosis and hyalinization which are commonly observed. However, although these lesions may contribute to the reduction in the number of B cells and interfere with the insulin output from these cells, their presence probably does not sufficiently explain the development of disturbance in carbohydrate metabolism. They could possibly present a supplemental pathogenetic factor by altering normal B cell physiology and could also explain the development of diabetes in those instances where the pancreas shows comparatively well-organized and intact islets. This hypothesis, however, seems to be at variance with the general view that vascular changes follow rather than precede the diabetic state.

These contradictory results obtained from studies of the pancreas pointed to extrapancreatic factors which may play a role in the pathogenesis of diabetes, including trauma, emotional stress, obesity, and infection. With the exception of obesity, none of these factors appear to be precipitating causes, and the link between obesity and diabetes awaits clarification. Other extrapancreatic influences suggested to be causes of diabetes have been the secretions of some of the endocrine glands. The interest in this problem began when Houssay,[25] in 1937, demonstrated the effect of the secretion of the pituitary gland on carbohydrate metabolism. His studies were followed by the work of Long and Lukens[26] on the effect of the adrenal cortex on blood sugar homeostasis and by the observation of Young[27] that permanent diabetes could be produced in normal dogs by repeated injections of extracts of the anterior pituitary gland. Despite the importance of these observations, morphologic studies of the hypophysis or adrenals in diabetic patients were disappointing, and it has, as yet, not been possible to show in man that hormones are causative factors in cases of idiopathic diabetes.

Over the years several other concepts concerning the pathogenesis of idiopathic diabetes have been proposed. One of them is that a person destined to become diabetic inherits a defect which may lead to, or allows the development of, forces antagonistic to the action of insulin.[28] Another hypothesis was that there are substances either protein in nature or associated with protein[29] ("synalbumin") which hold or bind insulin,[30] and thus oppose its action. It has also been suggested that the difficulty lies not in the binding of insulin, but in a defect at the cellular level, i.e., insensitivity to insulin.[31,32] It has also been proposed that an autoimmune process may be a factor in the pathogenesis of diabetes by the mechanism of islet cell damage. However, there is no clear evidence to support these ideas.[33-36]

Most of these theories suggested that the pancreas is stimulated to increase insulin production in the attempt to compensate for the antagonistic forces to maintain normal blood sugar homeostasis. Thus, despite its effort, the insulin secretory mechanism eventually suffers, and the ability of the pancreas to produce sufficient amounts of insulin is reduced. However, this approach to the problem appeared to be contradicted by the findings in human diabetes, where often no obvious qualitative or quantitative alterations can be observed in the islets of Langerhans. Moreover, it has so far been impossible to produce experimental diabetes without changes in the B cells.

As the result of the introduction of methods which permitted an accurate measure of insulin content in the blood by Yalow and Berson,[37] it became possible to demonstrate that in the majority of patients with idiopathic diabetes insulin is not decreased. Moreover, it was shown that insulin activity in diabetics is, in some instances, higher than in nondiabetics.[37,38] Furthermore, Yalow and Berson[37] and Renold and Steinke[39] have observed in maturity-onset diabetics that insulin secretion after glucose administration occurs frequently at a slower rate than in nondiabetics. Even in juvenile diabetics, who for a long time have been considered the human counterpart to depancreatized animals, there is frequently an increase of insulin demonstrable, particularly during the early phase of the disease.

Furthermore, Seltzer and Harris[40] and Seltzer *et al.*[41] observed that the high levels of serum insulin noted in many diabetics are in reality lower than those found in nondiabetic persons for a corresponding level of hyperglycemia. In keeping with these observations, Cerasi and Luft[42-45] measured the secretory response of the B cells by analog computation of the glucose and insulin levels in the blood during continuous infusion of glucose, and they found the initial rise in serum insulin to be lacking or considerably diminished in all diabetic individuals, and the total response to be less than normal. This functional deficiency of the B cells occurred in patients with overt diabetes as well as in persons with genetic prediabetes, and even in approximately 20% of healthy individuals. Cerasi and Luft[42-45] concluded from these observations that the secretory deficiency of the B cells is the inherited factor that is responsible for diabetes and that in the majority of cases diabetes will occur only under the effect of added diabetogenous factors, with which the genetically deficient B cells are incapable of coping.

Recent studies suggested that the other hormone produced in the islets of Langerhans seems to play an important role in the pathogenesis of diabetes. Murlin et al.,[46] Kimball and Murlin,[47] and Collens and Murlin[48] observed, 1 year after the discovery of insulin, that transitory hyperglycemia occurs after the injection of extracts of insulin into animals. This blood sugar raising factor, which was called glucagon by these authors, was suggested to originate in the pancreatic A cells, an observation which was substantiated by the experiments of Van Campenhout and Cornelis.[49] As a result of these findings Ferner,[50-53] in 1952, maintained that the hyperglycemia in diabetes is due to hyperplasia of the pancreatic A cells with associated increase of their secretory product, glucagon.

On the basis of various experiments, it has more recently been postulated that the diabetic abnormalities in glucose homeostasis are the consequence of a bihormonal disorder in which a relative or absolute deficiency of insulin and a relative or absolute excess of glucagon both play etiologic roles. The idea that glucagon is an essential cofactor in the development of endogenous hyperglycemia is based on the observation that endogenous hyperglycemia has never occurred in the absence of glucagon. It has thus been observed that the hyperglycemia (diabetic and nondiabetic) in man[54-63] as well as under experimental conditions[64-71] is accompanied by a relative or absolute hyperglucagonemia. It has been shown,[72-74] furthermore, that hyperglucagonemia occurs in depancreatized dogs not treated with insulin and that extrapancreatic plasma glucagon, like pancreatic glucagon, is stimulated by arginine infusion.[72,74,75] The extrapancreatic glucagon is believed to be secreted by A cells in the gastric fundus and duodenum which are ultrastructurally indistinguishable from pancreatic A cells. Unger and co-workers have shown that "true" gut glucagon is biologically, immunometrically, and physicochemically identical with pancreatic glucagon and differs from so-called "glucagon-like immunoreactivity" of the postduodenal intestine.[78-80]

The fact that glucagon plays a role in blood sugar homeostasis seems to be supported by the discovery by Brazeau et al.[81] of somatostatin, which has been shown to be capable of inhibiting the release of growth hormone as well as of both glucagon and insulin.[82-86] It has been demonstrated that hyperglycemia fails to occur[81,82,87-90] unless glucagon levels are restored to normal by the concomitant infusion of exogenous glucagon.[88-90] This is followed by an immediate 50 mg/100 ml increase in glycemia,[75] almost certainly reflecting an increase in hepatic glucagon production. When glucagon is stopped, the hyperglycemia decreases rapidly.[75] The immediate rise in glucagon, however, is not prevented by insulin. These results are in agreement with *in vitro*[91,92] and *in vivo*[93,94] studies which demonstrated the considerable importance of glucagon in relation to insulin in the control of hepatic glucose production.

It has been implied on the basis of immunocytochemical methods that somatostatin is either synthesized or stored in cells of the islets of Langerhans, probably in the D cells,[95,96] and that cells believed to be D cells, which produce somatostatin or a somatostatin-like peptide, seemingly are arranged in a way which suggests an inhibitory action of these cells on A cell secretion.[97]

Unger and Orci[79] concluded from the results obtained in humans as well as in animals that glucagon plays an important role in diabetics: First, it has been observed that an increase in the secretion of glucagon occurs in association with every type of increase in the blood sugar concentration in animals as well as in humans; second, when the secretions of both glucagon and insulin are suppressed, hyperglycemia is not observed unless the concentration of glucagon is restored to normal by the concomitant administration of glucagon; and third, the somatostatin-induced suppression of glucagon release in diabetic animals and humans decreases or restores the blood sugar concentration to normal and alleviates certain symptoms in diabetes.

The conclusions made by Unger and Orci, however, were seemingly contradicted by the observations of other authors. Thus, Albisser *et al.,*[98] using an "artificial pancreas" in insulin-requiring diabetic patients, concluded that the "balancing" amount of glucagon appears unnecessary for blood sugar homeostasis. They believed that it is unlikely that the small amounts of insulin used had an effect on the supposedly high glucagon levels of the diabetic patients who were out of control at the beginning of the experiment. In a study of 38 insulin-dependent diabetic patients, Barnes *et al.*[99] evaluated the role of glucagon in the everyday regulation of carbohydrate and lipid metabolism. These authors were unable to find significant changes in the levels of glucagon, even after insulin was withdrawn for several hours; nor was there any correlation between the initial fasting levels of plasma glucagon and the measurements of plasma glucose and ketone bodies. Judging from these observations, the authors concluded that glucagon is unlikely to play a role of primary importance in blood glucose homeostasis or ketone body metabolism in ambulant insulin-dependent diabetic patients. Furthermore, Tasaka *et al.,*[100] in a study of insulin and glucagon in relation to plasma glucose over a period of 24 hr of normal food ingestion in four young people, observed the expected rise and decline in immunoreactive insulin and glucose occurring concomitantly with meals which indicated a regulatory relationship. On the other hand, the immunoreactive pancreatic glucagon levels failed to show significant variations related to meals or to sleep. Sherwin *et al.*[101] infused glucagon in "physiologic increments" into normal and nondiabetic obese subjects and noted that hyperglucagonemia caused only a transient increase of 5 to 10 mg/100 ml in basal glucose levels and had no effect on oral glucose tolerance or plasma insulin in normal or in obese nondiabetic persons. In patients with adult- and with juvenile-onset diabetes treated with insulin, hyperglucagonemia maintained for 2 to 4 days caused neither change in plasma nor in ketone concentrations. On the other hand, the hyperglucagonemia caused significant hyperglycemia during insulin withdrawal in diabetic patients. The authors concluded from these observations that glucagon has a diabetogenic effect only when insulin deficiency exists.

In a recent careful study to evaluate the relative roles of insulin and glucagon in carbohydrate homeostasis, Felig *et al.*[102] examined the effect of physiologic increments in insulin and/or glucagon and of somatostatin in normal and diabetic subjects. They concluded that glucagon contributes to glucose production via glycogenolysis as well as gluconeogenesis during fasting and in the protein–fat state. They further observed that insulin alone regulates inhibition of splanchnic glucose output and disposal of small or large glucose loads, and finally, that in diabetes, insulin deficiency is the primary defect and that hypoglucagonemia fails to improve glucose disposal, while hyperglucagonemia intensifies diabetes only if there is insulin lack.

On the basis of these experiments, Levine,[103] in a recent editorial, concluded "that glucagon is a potent diabetogenic factor in the absence of insulin, but that physiologic amounts of insulin can overcome or prevent the effects of appreciably increased glucagon levels, at least in man."

The conclusions derived by Unger and Orci, furthermore, were not borne out by the observations of Barnes and Bloom,[104] who, in a study of totally depancreatized patients, observed that hyperglycemia does occur in the absence of glucagon. They therefore suggested that this hormone is probably not of primary importance in the hyperglycemia of insulin-dependent diabetics.

There is no doubt that the recent work contributed significantly to the better understanding of the disturbance of blood sugar homeostasis in the diabetic state. However, it seems unlikely that the opposing effects of insulin and glucagon are the final answer to the question of the pathogenesis of diabetes mellitus. While the clinical observations seem to make the older morphologic studies concerning the cellular changes in the islets of Langerhans of diabetic individuals obsolete, the fact remains that quantitative and qualitative changes exist in pancreatic A and B cells which cannot be properly explained by the aforementioned physiologic and pathophysiologic studies. Attempts will have to be made to establish a correlation between the endocrinological abnormalities and the morphological changes occurring in the islets of Langerhans in diabetics with the help of newer, refined biochemical, histochemical, and immunocytochemical techniques and by studying the genetic potential of B cell division and the kinetics of islet cell proliferation.

References

1. Von Mering, J., and Minkowski, O.: *Arch. Exp. Pathol. Pharmakol.,* **26**:371, 1889–90.
2. Banting, F. G., and Best, C. H.: *J. Lab. Clin. Med.,* **7**:464, 1922.
3. Kraus, E. J.: *Virchow's Arch.,* **247**:1, 1923–24.
4. Nakamura, N.: *Arch. Pathol. Anat.,* **253**:286, 1924.
5. Moore, R. A.: *Amer. J. Dis. Child.,* **52**:627, 1936.
6. Schwartzman, J., Crusius, M. E., and Beirne, D. P.: *Amer. J. Dis. Child.,* **74**:587, 1947.
7. Maclean, N., and Ogilvie, R. F.: *Diabetes,* **8**:83, 1959.
8. Wrenshall, G. A., Bogoch, A., and Ritchie, R. C.: *Diabetes,* **1**:87, 1952.
9. Wrenshall, G. A., Hartroft, W. S., and Best, C. H.: *Diabetes,* **3**:444, 1954.
10. Hartroft, W. S., and Wrenshall, G. A.: *Diabetes,* **4**:1, 1955.
11. Lazarus, S. S., and Volk, B. W.: *The Pancreas in Human and Experimental Diabetes.* Grune & Stratton, New York, 1962, p. 196.

12. Gomori, G.: *Amer. J. Pathol.*, **17**:395, 1941.
13. Gepts, W.: *Ann. Soc. Roy. Sci. Méd. Nat. Brux.*, **10**:5, 1957.
14. Gepts, W.: *Endokrinologie*, **36**:185, 1958.
15. Bell, E. T.: *Diabetes*, **2**:125, 1953.
16. Bornstein, J.: *J. Endocrinol.*, **7**:59, 1953.
17. Bornstein, J.: *Diabetes*, **2**:23, 1953.
18. Bertram, F., Bendfeldt, E., and Otto, H.: *Dtsch. Med Wochenschr.*, **80**:1455, 1955.
19. Beaser, S. B.: *Metabolism*, **5**:933, 1956.
20. Gepts, W., and Gregoire, F.: In: *Recent Progress in Quantitative Microhistochemistry.* Edited by U. C. Dubach. Hans Huber, Bern/Stuttgart, 1972, p. 300.
21. Malaisse, W.: *Étude de la Secretion Insulinique In Vivo.* Editions Arscia, Brussels, 1968.
22. Malaisse, W., Malaisse-Lagae, V., Geritzen, G. G., Dulin, W. E., and Wright, P. M.: *Diabetologia*, **3**:109, 1967.
23. Moschcowitz, E.: *Ann. Int. Med.*, **34**:1137, 1951.
24. Lazarus, S. S., and Volk, B. W.: *The Pancreas in Human and Experimental Diabetes.* Grune & Stratton, New York 1962, p. 197.
25. Houssay, B. A.: *Amer. J. Med. Sci.*, **193**:581, 1937.
26. Long, C. N. H., and Lukens, F. D. W.: *J. Exp. Med.*, **63**:465, 1936.
27. Young, F. G.: *Lancet*, **2**:372, 1937.
28. Rimoin, D.: *Diabetes*, **16**:346, 1967.
29. Vallance-Owen, J.: *Diabetes*, **13**:241, 1964.
30. Antoniades, H. N., Gundersen, K., Beigelman, P. M., Pyle, H. M., and Bougas, J. A.: *Diabetes*, **11**:261, 1962.
31. Randle, P. J., Garland, P. B., Hales, C. N., and Newsholme, E. A.: *Lancet*, **1**:785, 1963.
32. Randle, P. J., Garland, P. B., Hales, C. N., Newsholme, E. A., Denton, R. M., and Pogson, C. I.: *Rec. Progr. Horm. Res.*, **22**:1, 1966.
33. Pav, J., Jezkova, Z., and Skrha, F.: *Lancet*, **2**:221, 1963.
34. Chetty, M. P., and Watson, K. C.: *Lancet*, **1**:67, 1965.
35. Deckert, T.: *Acta Med. Scand. Suppl.*, **476**:30, 1967.
36. Mancini, A. M., Zampa, G. A., Vecchi, A., and Costanzi, G.: *Lancet*, **1**:1189, 1965.
37. Yalow, R., and Berson, S.: *J. Clin. Invest.*, **39**:1157, 1960.
38. Steinke, J., Camerini, R., Marble, A., and Renold, A.: *Metabolism*, **10**:707, 1961.
39. Renold, A. E., and Steinke, J.: In: *Fortschritte der Diabetesforschung.* Edited by K. Oberdisse and J. Jahnkes. Georg Thieme Verlag, Stuttgart, 1963, p. 1.
40. Seltzer, H. S., and Harris, V. L.: *Diabetes*, **13**:6, 1964.
41. Seltzer, H. S., Allen, E. W., Herron, Jr., A. L., and Brennan, M. T.: *J. Clin. Invest.*, **46**:323, 1967.
42. Cerasi, E., and Luft, R.: *Acta Endocrinol.*, **55**:278, 1967.
43. Cerasi, E., and Luft, R.: *Acta Endocrinol.*, **55**:305, 1967.
44. Cerasi, E., and Luft, R.: *Acta Endocrinol.*, **55**:330, 1967.
45. Cerasi, E., and Luft, R.: *Diabetes*, **16**:615, 1967.
46. Murlin, J. R., Clough, H. G., Gibbs, C. B., and Stokes, A. M.: *J. Biol. Chem.*, **56**:253, 1933.
47. Kimball, C. P., and Murlin, J. R.: *J. Biol. Chem.*, **58**:337, 1933.
48. Collens, W. S., and Murlin, J. R.: *Proc. Soc. Exp. Biol. Med.*, **26**:485, 1929.
49. Van Campenhout, E., and Cornelis, G.: *C. R. Soc. Biol.*, **145**:933, 1951.
50. Ferner, W.: *Z. Mikrosk. Anat. Forschung*, **44**:451, 1938.
51. Ferner, W.: *Virchow's Arch.*, **309**:87, 1942.
52. Ferner, W.: *Dtsch. Ztsch. f. Verdauungskr.*, **6**:21, 1942.
53. Ferner, W.: *Das Inselsystem des Pankreas.* George Thieme Verlag, Stuttgart 1952, p. 74.
54. Aguilar-Parada, E., Eisentraut, A. M., and Unger, R. H.: *Amer. J. Med. Sci.*, **257**:415, 1969.
55. Unger, R. H., Aguilar-Parada, E., Muller, W. A., and Eisentraut, A. M.: *J. Clin. Invest.*, **49**:837, 1970.
56. Muller, W. A., Faloona, G. R., Aguilar-Parada, E., and Unger, R. H.: *N. Engl. J. Med.*, **283**:109, 1970.
57. Unger, R. H., Madison, L. L., and Muller, W. A.: *Diabetes*, **21**:301, 1972.

58. Frankel, B. J., Gerich, J. E., Ryoko, H., Fanska, R. E., Gerritsen, G. C., and Grodsky, G. M.: *J. Clin. Invest.*, **53**:1637, 1974.
59. Assan, R., Hautecouverture, G., Guillemant, S., Douchy, E., Protin, P., and Derot, M.: *Pathol. Biol.*, **17**:1095, 1969.
60. Buchanan, K. D., and McCarrol, A. M.: *Lancet*, **2**:1395, 1972.
61. Felig, P., Pozefsky, T., Marliss, E., and Cahill, G. F., Jr.: *Science*, **167**:1003, 1970.
62. Gerich, J. E., Langlois, M., Noacco, C., Karam, J. H., and Forsham, P. H.: *Science*, **182**:171, 1973.
63. Kalkhoff, R. K., Gossain, V. V., and Mature, M. L.: *N. Engl. J. Med.*, **289**:465, 1973.
64. Muller, W. A., Faloona, G. R., and Unger, R. H.: *J. Clin. Invest.*, **50**:1992, 1971.
65. Meier, J. M., McGarry, J. D., Faloona, G. R., Unger, R. H., and Foster, D.: *J. Lipid Res.*, **13**:228, 1972.
66. Katsilambros, N. Y., Abdel, R., Minz, M., Fussganger, K. E., Schroder, K. E., Straug, K., and Pfeiffer, E. F.: *Horm. Metab. Res.*, **2**:268, 1970.
67. Amherdt, M., Harris, V., Renold, A. E., Orci, L., and Unger, R. H.: *J. Clin. Invest.*, **54**:188, 1974.
68. Samols, E., Tyler, J. M., and Kajinuma, H.: In: *Proceedings of the Seventh Congress of the International Diabetes Federation.* Edited by R. R. Rodriguez and J. Vallance-Owen. Excerpta Medica, Amsterdam, 1971, p. 636.
69. Lindsey, C. A., Santeusanio, F., Braaten, J., Faloona, G. R., and Unger, R. H.: *JAMA*, **227**:757, 1975.
70. Willmore, D. W., Lindsey, C. A., Faloona, G. R., Moylan, J., Pruitt, B., and Unger, R. H.: *Lancet*, **1**:73, 1974.
71. Willerson, J. T., Hutcheson, D., Leshin, S. J., Faloona, G. R., and Unger, R. H.: *Amer. J. Med.*, **57**:747, 1974.
72. Pek, S., Vranic, M., and Kawamori, R.: *Program of the Fifth Annual Meeting of the Endocrine Society, 1974, A176.*
73. Matsuyama, T., and Foa, P. M.: *Diabetes*, **23**:344, 1974.
74. Mashiter, K., Harding, P. E., Chou, M., Mashiter, G. D., Stout, J., Diamond, D., and Field, J. B.: *Endocrinology*, **96**:678, 1975.
75. Dobbs, R. H., Sakurai, H., Sasaki, H., Faloona, G. R., Valverde, I., Baetens, D., Orci, L., and Unger, R. H.: *Science*, **187**:544, 1975.
76. Orci, L., Pictet, R., Forssmann, W. G., Renold, A. E., and Rouiller, C.: *Diabetologia*, **4**:56, 1968.
77. Polak, J. M., Bloom, S., Coulling, I., and Pearse, A. G.: *Gut*, **12**:311, 1971.
78. Sasaki, A., Faloona, G. R., and Unger, R. H.: *Gastroenterology*, **67**:746, 1974.
79. Unger, R. H., and Orci, L.: *Lancet*, **1**:14, 1975.
80. Sasaki, H., Rubalcava, B., Baetens, D., Blazquez, E., Srikant, C. B., Orci, L., and Unger, R. H.: *J. Clin. Invest.*, **56**:135, 1975.
81. Brazeau, P., Vale, W., Burgus, R., Ling, N., Butcher, M., Rivier, J., and Guillemin, R.: *Science*, **179**:1973.
82. Mortimer, C. H., Turnbridge, W. M. G., Carr, D., Yeomans, L., Lind, T., Coy, D. H., Bloom, S. R., Kastin, A., Mallinson, C. N., Besser, G. M., Schally, A. V., and Hall, R.: *Lancet*, **1**:697, 1974.
83. Koerker, D. J., Ruch, W., Chideckel, E., Palmer, J., Goodner, C. J., Ensinck, J., and Gale, C. C.: *Science*, **184**:482, 1974.
84. Johnson, D. G., Ensinck, J., Koerker, D. J., Palmer, J., and Goodner, C. J.: *Diabetes (Suppl. 1)*, **23**:374, 1974.
85. Iversen, J.: *Scand. J. Clin. Lab. Invest.*, **33**:125, 1974.
86. Efendic, C., Luft, R., and Grill, V.: *FEBS Lett.*, **42**:169, 1974.
87. Alberti, K. G., Christensen, N. J., Christensen, S. E., Hansen, A. P., Iversen, J., Lundbaek, K., Seyer-Hansen, K., and Orskov, H.: *Lancet* **2**:1299, 1973.
88. Goodner, C. J., Ensinck, J. W., Chideckel, E., Palmer, J., Koerker, D. J., Ruch, W., and Gale, C. C.: *J. Clin. Invest.*, **53**:28a, 1974.
89. Sakurai, H., Dobbs, R. E., and Unger, R. H.: *J. Clin. Invest.*, **54**:1395, 1974.
90. Alford, F. P., Bloom, S. R., and Nabarro, J. D. N.: *Lancet*, **2**:974, 1974.

91. Glinsman, W. H., and Mortimore, G. E.: *Amer. J. Physiol.,* **215**:553, 1968.
92. Mackrell, D. J., and Sokal, J. E.: *Diabetes,* **18**:724, 1969.
93. Vranick, M.: In: *Insulin Action.* Edited by I. B. Fritz. Academic Press, New York, 1972, p. 529.
94. Liljenquist, J. E., Bomboy, J. D., Lewis, S. B., Sinclair-Smith, B. C., Felts, P. W., Lacy, W. W., Crofford, O. B., and Liddle, W.: *J. Clin. Invest.,* **53**:190, 1974.
95. Pelletier, G., Leclerc, G., Arimura, A., and Schally, A. V.: *J. Histochem. Cytochem.,* **23**:699, 1975.
96. Orci, L., Baetens, D., Dubois, M. P., and Rufener, C.: *Horm. Metab. Res.,* **7**:400, 1975.
97. Orci, L., and Unger, R. H.: *Lancet,* **2**:1243, 1975.
98. Albisser, A. M., Leibel, B. S., Ewart, T. G., Davidovac, Z., Botz, C. K., Zingg, W., Schipper, H., and Gander, R.: *Diabetes,* **23**:397, 1074.
99. Barnes, A. J., Bloom, A., Crowley, M. F., Tuttlebee, J. W., Bloom, W. R., Alberti, K. G. M. M., Smythe, P., and Turnell, D.: *Lancet,* **2**:734, 1975.
100. Tasaka, Y., Sekine, M., Wakatsuki, M., Ohgawara, H., and Shizume, K.: *Horm. Metab. Res.,* **7**:205, 1975.
101. Sherwin, R. S., Fisher, M., Hendler, R., and Felig, P.: *N. Engl. J. Med.,* **294**:455, 1976.
102. Felig, P., Wahren, J., Sherwin, R., and Hendler, R.: *Diabetes, Suppl. 1,* **25**:323, 1976.
103. Levine, R.: Editorial. *N. Engl. J. Med.,* **294**:494, 1976.
104. Barnes, A. J., and Bloom, S. R.: *Lancet,* **1**:219, 1976.

Chapter 11

Hormonal Diabetes

Bruno W. Volk and Klaus F. Wellmann

Pituitary Diabetes

The close association between pituitary hyperfunction and the occurrence of diabetes derives from the classical clinical observation of the frequency of a disturbed glucose tolerance and overt hyperglycemia in acromegaly. To explain the absence of pancreatic pathology in cases of diabetes mellitus, suggestions have been made for many years that a disease of the pituitary gland may be the cause for a number of instances of diabetes.

In 1884, Loeb,[1] who was probably the first to do so, noted that glycosuria occurs in patients with pituitary tumors. Subsequently, Marie[2-4] recognized the clinical entity which he called acromegaly. Diabetes occurred in two of his four cases. He also diagnosed several cases as acromegaly which had previously been reported by others under different names. Despite the recognition of pituitary-induced diabetes, Loeb[5] later conjectured that the glycosuria was of neurogenic origin, owing to the fact that hypophyseal tumors, frequently observed in these cases, produced glycosuria by pressure on the neighboring "Zuckerzentrum." Marie[2] was the first to observe that the hyperglycemia associated with acromegaly was accompanied by excessive thirst and urinary output, symptoms which occur frequently in diabetes. Hansemann[6] and Dallemagne[7] reported cases where acromegaly was associated with diabetes and in which the pancreases appeared diseased at postmortem examination. They believed that this was the cause of acromegaly. Various other authors[8-23] noted that glycosuria occurred rarely in patients with tumors of the hypophysis without acromegaly and suggested that the glycosuria in instances of acromegaly was the result of excess secretion of the pituitary hormone. They also observed that hyperglycemia, glycosuria, and a lowered glucose tolerance usually occurs during the early phases of acromegaly, while during the late stages an increased glucose tolerance, often considerably above the normal, could be noted. Cushing,[11] particularly on the basis of clinical observations and experiments, noted the association

Bruno W. Volk and Klaus F. Wellmann • Isaac Albert Research Institute of the Kingsbrook Jewish Medical Center, and Downstate Medical Center, State University of New York, Brooklyn, New York. Present address of B. W. V.: University of California, Irvine, California. Present address of K. F. W.: Beekman Downtown Hospital, New York New York.

of glycosuria with excess secretion of the hypophysis and, conversely, the association of an abnormally high carbohydrate tolerance with hyposecretion.

The incidence of diabetes in cases of acromegaly varied with different investigators (Table 1). Hansemann[6] observed an incidence of 12.3% of hyperglycemia in a series of 97 cases with acromegaly. Hindsdale[9] found 14 diabetic cases in a series of 130 acromegalic patients (10.7%), and Williamson[12] observed 6 instances of diabetes in a group of 21 patients with acromegaly (28.5%). Borchardt[8] and Rosenberger[14] noted an incidence of approximately 40% who developed diabetes. Shepardson[15] observed that 6 out of 15 cases (40%) with acromegaly had diabetes. Ander and Jameson,[13] in a group of 88 acromegalics, noted concomitant diabetes in 16 (18.2%). On the other hand, Yater[16] and Wilder[17] reported an incidence of diabetes in 7.5 and 9.2%, respectively, in their reported cases of acromegaly, the lowest incidence among various serial observations. Wilder[17] emphasized that this figure may be exceedingly high, since in 7 of these 218 cases documented by Yater[16] and himself,[17] the diagnosis of diabetes could be considered doubtful, owing to the fact that it was based on alimentary glycosuria. If these doubtful cases were excluded, the incidence of diabetes in this series of acromegalic patients would be even less (6%).

Cushing and Davidoff[18] observed an incidence of 25% in a study of 100 patients with acromegaly. Coggeshall and Root,[19] in a review of 153 cases of acromegaly, including the 100 cases previously reported by Cushing and Davidoff,[18] observed an incidence of diabetes in 17% and of glycosuria in 35.9%, which compares with the incidence of diabetes in the general population of approximately 1.5 to 2%. McCullagh[20] found an incidence of 27.6% (21 cases) of

Table 1. *Incidence of Diabetes Mellitus in Acromegaly*

Authors	Number of cases of acromegaly	Number of cases with diabetes	Percentage
Hansemann (1897)[6]	97	12	12.3
Hinsdale (1898)[9]	130	14	10.7
Williamson (1898)[12]	21	6	28.5
Borchardt (1908)[8]	176	71	40.3
Rosenberger (1911)[14]	196	82	41.8
Ander and Jameson (1914)[13]	88	16	18.2
Cushing and Davidoff (1927)[18]	100	25	25.0
Yater (1928)[16]	79	6	7.5
Coggeshall and Root (1940)[19]	153	26	17.0
Wilder (1940)[17]	218	20	9.2
Shepardson (1944)[15]	15	6	40.0
McCullagh (1956)[20]	76	21	27.6
Hamwi et al (1960)[23]	27	11	40.0
Gordon et al (1962)[24] [a]	100	18	18.0
Total	1,476	334	22.6

[a]In 82 patients without diabetes, 29 had decreased glucose tolerance (35.3%).

diabetes in a study of 76 acromegalic patients, and Miller,[21] who compiled a study of 500 acromegalic patients from the literature, found an overall incidence of diabetes in 25% of the cases.

It has been suggested that the incidence of diabetes in acromegalics would increase significantly if glucose tolerance tests were carried out in each patient.[20,21] Following this idea, Hamwi *et al.*[23] studied the glucose tolerance in a group of 27 patients with acromegaly and observed 4 cases with overt diabetes and 7 instances of prediabetes. Therefore, 40% of these patients had impairment of carbohydrate metabolism. Gordon and associates[24] reported 18 cases of diabetes in a study of 100 acromegalics. In the 82 patients without diabetes, 29 had a decreased glucose tolerance (Table 1). In a series of 800 cases of acromegaly collated from the literature, Kozak[25] found an incidence of diabetes in 19% of the patients. He noted that by inclusion of additional patients with mild or intermittent glycosuria and impaired glucose tolerance, the incidence of impaired carbohydrate metabolism may well be 35 to 50%. On the other hand, Wilder,[17] while studying the incidence of acromegaly in 9377 diabetic patients, found only 20 cases of diabetes associated with acromegaly (0.21%), which actually represents only one instance of acromegaly in 500 patients with diabetes.

Marie[2] first reported that the diabetes associated with acromegaly is similar to idiopathic diabetes. Other authors, however,[14,20,26-32] noted that the diabetes associated with acromegaly frequently runs an atypical or irregular course, or that there is an unusual variability in the severity of the disease in these patients. While some[14,17,20-24,26-33] had the impression that the diabetes in acromegalics is mild and stable, others[20-22,33,34] reported that insulin resistance occurred more frequently in those conditions than in idiopathic diabetes. It has also been reported that in diabetes associated with acromegaly, fluctuations of sugar tolerance or glucosuria occur quite often.[8,35,36] According to some reports, diabetes in acromegalic patients may progress even despite an apparent arrest of acromegaly resulting from radiation treatment of the hypophysis.[37] On the other hand, spontaneous temporary or permanent recovery of the diabetes has been noted.[19,26,32,38-42] Plasma hyperinsulinism has also been described in acromegalics.[25,43] Several authors observed a considerable decrease of insulin requirements in diabetic patients who underwent hypophysectomy.[44-46] However, in nondiabetic patients, human growth hormone was found to reverse the increased sensitivity to insulin.[47] Since the development of methods for determination of growth hormone levels in blood and urine, acromegalic patients have been found to have higher levels than normal adults,[48-50] but there is no definite evidence that this is the case in diabetics.[49]

The evaluation of the role of growth hormone in causing diabetes mellitus has been approached from another angle by several investigators. Thus, Ehrlich and Randle,[51] measuring growth hormone concentration in sera of diabetics by immunoassay, found it to be elevated in 7 untreated, overweight diabetics and in 8 of 17 diabetics with retinopathy, but normal in most diabetics with ketoacidosis and weight loss. Berson and Yalow[52] presented data indicating that growth hormone, in large amounts, can induce impaired glucose tolerance and insulin resistance, and in small amounts, it appears to play an essential permissive role in the development of diabetic ketoacidosis. In fact, Berson and Yalow[52] noted lower plasma growth hormone levels in diabetics than in nondiabetics. Sönksen and associates,[53] in an investigation of the pathogenesis of diabetes in acromegaly, concluded that two possible intermediary stages in the development of diabetes associated with acromegaly exist. The first is the stage of "hyperinsulinism," with a normal or borderline glucose tolerance. In the second stage, the peak insulin response is delayed, and glucose tolerance may be within normal limits or impaired. This stage, the authors feel, would appear potentially reversible following adequate treatment. In the third stage, seen only with established diabetes, the pancreatic response appeared to be maximal in the fasting state, and no further rise in insulin concentration occurred after glucose injection.

Prolonged administration of growth hormone leads to hyperglycemia.[54-56] In some cases glycosuria in addition to hyperglycemia, insulin resistance, minimal ketonuria, and an impaired glucose tolerance have been noted after injection of this hormone.[57-61] Several authors reported that the administration of growth hormone to hypophysectomized patients with controlled diabetes causes a significant exacerbation of the diabetic state.[62,63]

The time interval between the occurrence of symptoms of acromegaly and the discovery of diabetes varies considerably. In most instances, the symptoms of acromegaly precede the diagnosis of diabetes.[33] Goldberg and Lisser[64] observed a range varying from 1 to 20 years between the onset of acromegaly and diabetes. In an analysis of 29 cases, Coggeshall and Root[19] observed that the average interval between the onset of acromegaly and that of diabetes was 9.5 years, but there were intervals from 1 to 22 years, with a majority of the cases of diabetes occurring within 15 years. In McCullagh's study,[20] acromegaly and diabetes were present in 1 case when the diagnosis was made. In another patient the hypophyseal symptoms were found to precede the diagnosis of diabetes by 15 years. In the acromegaly study of Gordon and associates,[24] the diagnosis of diabetes and acromegaly was made at the same time in 5 cases, in 12 cases the diabetes appeared some years after acromegaly became manifest, and in 1 patient it seemed to precede the onset of acromegaly. In general, the relationship between the onset of diabetes and the symptoms of acromegaly seems to vary between the reported extremes.

A family history of diabetes was obtained in 6 of 29 patients in the study of Coggeshall and Root,[19] whereas in the acromegalics without diabetes, a family history of diabetes was found in only 3 of 124 patients. This would be in keeping with the observations of Fraser,[65] who reported that the acromegalic subjects with diabetes more often have a family history of diabetes than do those without diabetes (21 and 2%, respectively). He also observed that the characteristic retinopathy is absent in the vast majority of acromegalics.

The Houssay phenomenon[66] of amelioration of diabetes was found as a counterpart in the human for the first time in a report by Lyall and Innes,[67] who reported a case of diabetes with intercurrent pituitary lesions and concomitant improvement of the diabetes. During the following year, Chabanier *et al.*[68]

reported on the surgical ablation of a normal pituitary gland in a patient with severe diabetes. Other observations of the effects of hypophysectomy,[44-46] of spontaneous destruction of the pituitary gland,[67,69-78] of radiation therapy to the skull and cord,[79] after basilary meningitis,[80] or after section of the pituitary stalk[81] indicated improvement of the diabetes. In most instances there was a decrease of insulin requirement as well as improvement of the albuminuria. Moreover, in several patients improvement of existing retinopathy occurred.[82-86] In another group of patients, reversal of the diabetes in 5 acromegalic cases was noted following long-continued therapy with estrogen.[20]

The relationship of pituitary hormones to carbohydrate metabolism has also been borne out by morphologic studies of the pituitary gland. Warren *et al.*[87] observed a more frequent occurrence of pituitary infarcts in diabetics than in nondiabetics. They conjectured that the increase of pituitary infarcts in diabetic patients is possibly the result of disease of the small blood vessels in the diabetic group, which led to a greater susceptibility of diabetic pituitaries to ischemia than was previously described.[88,89]

So far no consistent changes have been observed in the pancreases of acromegalic patients. The alterations reported by various authors[6,7,14,90-97] involve fibrosis, atrophy of the exocrine portion and hyalinization, sclerosis, and occasionally fatty degeneration of the islets of Langerhans. Kraus,[90-93] in an extensive study of the pancreas in acromegalic patients with diabetes, noted a considerable diminution of the number of islets. While the islets usually were small and composed of smaller than normal cells, the same pancreas also showed, in some areas, normal appearing or large islets. Occasionally there were hydropic changes of the B cells which he interpreted as an expression of decreased functional activity. In some instances, there was also intrainsular connective tissue proliferation. Kraus also found atrophy of the exocrine portion of the pancreas, as well as intra- and interacinar connective tissue proliferation. However, Kraus and Reisinger[92] observed a similar picture also in two acromegalic patients without diabetes. Other investigators[98-100] found marked hyperplasia of the islets, and in one case[99] the islets displayed adenomatous proliferation of the B cells. Lazarus and Volk[101] observed in a few cases moderate atrophy of the pancreatic acini and interacinar fibrosis as well as occasional periinsular fibrosis. The islets themselves appeared unchanged.

Warren *et al.*[102] reported a case of a 38-year-old man who died 6 weeks postoperatively and also developed diabetes insipidus following operation. One-third of the patient's anterior pituitary was necrotic and partly organized. The islets of Langerhans were small and formed of nongranulated or undifferentiated cells. Of two other women who had hypophysectomy following oophorectomy because of metastasizing carcinoma of the breast, one, who died 6 weeks after ablation of the hypophysis, had a normal A:B ratio of the islets, and the B cells were well granulated. The other patient, who died 11 months after hypophysectomy, showed also a normal A:B ratio, but there was partial degranulation of the B cells.

It is well known that acromegaly is the result of increased secretory activity of the eosinophilic cells of the anterior pituitary, which may be due to the presence of an eosinophilic tumor or, less frequently, to hyperplasia of these cells without an actual tumor. Several investigators, therefore, examined the hypophysis of patients with idiopathic diabetes, in order to find an explanation for the relationship between the pituitary and the disturbance of carbohydrate metabolism. Thus, Fry[103] studied 8 diabetic patients, 3 patients with acute pancreatitis, and 1 with carcinoma of the pancreas, and found in the cases of diabetes adenomatous masses of eosinophilic cells, "colloid invasion" of the anterior pituitary lobe as well as areas of cellular degeneration. In the patients with acute pancreatitis or carcinoma of the pancreas, the hypophysis showed no significant alterations. Kraus,[104] in a study of 23 diabetic cases, observed in some a decrease in the weight of the pituitary as well as a reduction in the number and size of eosinophils in most cases, in addition to infarcts and areas of fibrosis. In his cases of juvenile diabetes he observed that the average weight of the gland was 0.54 g as compared with a normal pituitary of approximately 0.65 g, and in 8 of 27 older diabetics the weights ranged from 0.4 g to 0.47 g. In these patients the eosinophils of the anterior pituitary lobe were decreased in number and smaller, and they often had pyknotic nuclei. Two patients showed vacuoles in the basophil cells which were similar to the hydropic changes in the islets of Langerhans. He called these alterations "diabetic changes of the hypophysis." In these juvenile diabetics he often observed small foci of what he termed "fetal cells," which consisted of undifferentiated cells in columnar palisaded arrangement usually seen in the anterior pituitary lobe. Labbé and Petresco[105] noted similar changes in the hypophysis to those described by Kraus. Cunz[106] found, in 11 of 15 diabetic patients between the ages of 37 and 83 years, an increase in the number of chief cells, while there was a concomitant reduction in eosinophils. He also observed in several patients an increase of the interstitial connective tissue. Kraus[107] observed that hyperfunction of the pancreatic islets causes changes in the hypophysis, such as hyperplasia and adenomas.

Hawking[108] observed a slight increase in the number of basophils in 1 out of 6 cases of diabetes. Heskel[109] did differential counts in 23 diabetic patients and observed an increase in the ratio of the maximally granulated basophils to intermediate mucoid cells which was similar when compared with 5 controls. Marchi[110] believed that a relationship exists between the severity of diabetes and an increase in acidophil cells in the hypophysis. Steiner,[111] in a study of the pituitary of 6 unstable juvenile diabetic patients, observed an increase of the acidophil cells with a mean of 59.4% as compared with an average of 40.3% in patients with stable, mild diabetes and in nondiabetic controls. Russfield[112] observed no typical histologic picture in the anterior lobe of diabetic patients, but he noted an increased growth hormone content in bioassays in the pituitary in 6 of 9 diabetics. However, other observers were unable to confirm the presence of changes in the hypophysis of diabetic patients.[113,114]

The fact, then, that an exceedingly low incidence of acromegaly can be observed in diabetics as well as the lack of significant abnormalities in the pituitary gland of diabetic patients seem to negate an influence of the hypophyseal hormones on the etiology of idiopathic diabetes mellitus.

Steroid Diabetes

It has been known for a long time that changes in carbohydrate metabolism occur with the destruction of the adrenal cortex. Porges,[115] as early as 1910, pointed out the frequency with which hypoglycemic episodes occurred in patients with Addison's disease and that similar episodes could be observed in adrenalectomized dogs. In 1913, Kraus[116] observed the frequent association of diabetes with hyperadrenalism, and in 1921, Achard and Thièrs[117] reported the first observation of coexisting hirsutism and diabetes in a 71-year-old female patient and related this syndrome to hyperplasia of the adrenals detected at autopsy. The fact that the adrenal cortical hyperactivity causes diabetes, which is comparatively mild and relatively insulin insensitive, was evidenced by the occurrence of hyperglycemia in Cushing's syndrome.[118] While Cushing,[119] in his original publication, observed basophilic adenomas of the pituitary in 3 out of 8 patients afflicted with this disorder, it has since been established that Cushing's syndrome is usually due to tumors or hyperplasia of the adrenal cortex and only seldom is associated with lesions of the pituitary gland.[33] The relationship between the adrenal cortical functions and blood sugar homeostasis was not appreciated prior to the studies of Hartman and Brownell[120] and Long and Lukens.[121] Long *et al.*[122] showed that diabetes is ameliorated by removal of the adrenal cortices and exacerbated by the administration of large amounts of 11-oxygenated steroids. Lukens,[123] in an early report, found that among 55 patients with proven tumor or hyperplasia of the adrenal cortex, carbohydrate tolerance was impaired in 49% and glycosuria occurred in 35% of the cases. In a study on the natural history of Cushing's syndrome, Plotz *et al.*[124] mentioned distinct diabetic curves in 94% of their cases. However, in less than one-fourth of the patients was glycosuria present, and only 5 of their own 33 cases had clinically obvious diabetes. Soffer and co-workers,[125] in a study on carbohydrate metabolism in a group of 50 patients with Cushing's syndrome, observed laboratory evidence of disturbance in blood sugar homeostasis in 42 cases; two of the remaining 8 had a flat glucose tolerance curve, and 6 had normal curves. The fasting blood sugar was determined in all patients, and in 15 it was found to vary from 135 to 200 mg/100 ml. Miller,[126] in collecting 174 patients from the literature, observed that 33 (19%) had a normal glucose tolerance, 96 (55%) had impaired glucose tolerance, and 45 (26%) had frank diabetes. Kozak,[25] in a similar compilation of 274 patients with Cushing's syndrome, observed that 67 patients had normal and 207 had abnormal glucose tolerance tests. Clinical diabetes was observed in 67 (24%) cases. While hyperadrenocorticism causes disturbances of the blood sugar homeostasis, the diabetes observed in a large number of patients with Cushing's syndrome usually disappears after extirpation of the adrenal tumor or subtotal resection of adrenal cortical tissue.[116,127,128]

In the nondiabetic the administration of steroids or adrenocorticotrophic hormones causes usually mild glycosuria and increased resistance to insulin.[127-133] The hyperglycemia disappears rapidly after steroid treatment is withheld.[134] If such treatment is maintained, the diabetes is usually well controlled with insulin, rarely with oral hypoglycemic drugs.[135,136] It has further been shown that the hyperglycemia and reduced glucose tolerance are transient and may disappear even when steroid treatment is continued.[137] Sprague *et al.*[138] emphasized the resistance of man to the diabetogenic action of cortisone. They found that protracted administration of cortisone acetate in doses of 100 to 200 mg caused a slight decrease in the glucose tolerance in 4 of 27 patients. In contrast to the high incidence of diabetes found in Cushing's syndrome, diabetes developed in less than 1% of the patients given continuous ACTH or cortisone for therapeutic reasons.[139] Moreover, in most of these cases there is either a family history of diabetes or an incidence of glycosuria prior to treatment.[139]

While hyperadrenocorticism causes hyperglycemia and glycosuria, conversely, in patients with Addison's disease, cortisone corrects the defect in carbohydrate metabolism and, in some instances, may cause diabetes.[140,141] Cortisone may also intensify existing diabetes and may cause increased resistance to insulin.[141] In the rare cases where diabetes and Addison's disease coexist, amelioration of the diabetic state may occur with the onset of adrenal cortical insufficiency.[142–145] Such patients have been observed to be extremely sensitive to insulin.[146,147]

Lukens *et al.*,[148] in a study of 55 cases with tumor or hyperplasia of the adrenal cortex, saw impaired carbohydrate homeostasis in 49% and significant glycosuria in 35%. Russi *et al.*,[149] in a review of 9000 routine autopsy cases, observed benign cortical adenomas in 1.45%. Of 131 patients with cortical adenomas, 21 had diabetes, but 19 of these also had hypertension. The incidence of diabetes in these cases as a whole was 3%. The authors felt that cortical nodules are easily overlooked and that the actual incidence of adenomas of the adrenal cortex is probably higher. Soffer *et al.*[150] observed, in a group of 33 patients with Cushing's syndrome, 10 cases with carcinoma, 8 with benign adenomas, and 5 with hyperplasia of the adrenal cortex. Plotz *et al.*,[124] also studying the adrenal pathology in Cushing's syndrome, observed in a series of 97 cases, 16 carcinomas, 11 benign adenomas, and 58 instances of hyperplasia of the adrenal cortex. Vartiainen,[151] examining the weight of the adrenals in his diabetic cases, found no change. Smith *et al.*[152] reported nodular hyperplasia of the adrenal cortex occurring in one-third of all their autopsies. Warren *et al.*,[153] in a series of 1036 autopsies on diabetic patients who died from 1948 through 1963, encountered a total of 38 instances with adrenal cortical nodules. In most cases the enlargement of the adrenals was slight, and only 6 had an adrenal weight of 30 g or more. Two patients had a clinical picture of Cushing's syndrome. The authors concluded that in some cases with Cushing's syndrome, the adrenal cortical nodules are of importance in the diabetic state.

Most observations indicated that diabetes due to hyperadrenocorticism in man showed insufficient evidence of damage of the islets of Langerhans to account for the diabetic state. In his series of 8 autopsied cases Cushing[119] studied the pancreas in 6. He observed in one instance lipomatosis, and in another an area of acute pancreatic necrosis. One case appeared normal, and the pancreas of another was extremely autolyzed. Of the remaining 2 cases, the islets of Langerhans appeared questionably enlarged in 1 and in the other the islets were hyperplastic and showed a slight increase of connective tissue. In a series of 14 cases with pituitary basophilism and glycosuria, Lukens[123] found that the islets were normal in 6 and the pancreas was fatty in 2. The condition of the pancreas was not recorded in 6 cases. In patients with adrenal cortical adenomas, however, the islets were numerous, large, and "cellular." Shepardson and Shapiro,[154] in a study of 18 patients with Cushing's syndrome with diabetes in which the pancreas was examined in 8, found that the pancreas was normal in 4 and small but microscopically normal in 1. One pancreas showed hemorrhagic fat necrosis, another fibrosis, and a third organ contained a small abscess. Albright[118] observed, in a case with Cushing's syndrome, marked hyperplasia of the islets of Langerhans which also displayed mitotic figures.

Kepler *et al.*[155] observed the frequent occurrence of pancreatic fat necrosis in patients with Cushing's syndrome. Franckson *et al.*[156] and Hausberger and Ramsay,[157,158] in histologic studies of the pancreas of cortisone-treated subjects, observed the same histologic signs of increased B cell stimulation as has been noted in experimental animals submitted to glucosteroid administration. Similar observations were made by Lazarus and Volk,[159] who noted vacuolization of the B cells in the pancreas of a woman who was treated with 100 mg of cortisone for 50 days for carcinoma of the breast. In periodic acid Schiff stained sections, the vacuoles were seen to contain large amounts of glycogen.

Lukens and Dyer[160] examined a pancreatic biopsy from a patient with Cushing's disease in whom bilateral adrenalectomy was performed. The pancreatic specimen was removed at the time when the second adrenalectomy was carried out. The patient, who had diabetes prior to the first operation, had no glycosuria on leaving the hospital. The islets showed marked hyaline degeneration, and in some portions of the pancreas they appeared hyperplastic. However, the authors felt that it was impossible to draw conclusions concerning the effect of the adrenal lesions from the changes observed in the islets.

Although diabetes induced by steroid administration is transient and usually disappears when it is stopped, the hyperglycemia may cause changes in the exocrine pancreas. Thus, Carone and Liebow[161] noted acute pancreatitis, peripancreatic fat necrosis, or both, in 16 (28.5%) of 54 patients who were treated with various steroids such as cortisone, ACTH, hydrocortisone, prednisolone, prednisone, or combinations of these. Furthermore, 59% of the patients treated with the hormone displayed ectasia of the pancreatic acini, while this was observed in only 24% of a control group. In a group of 54 untreated patients of similar age with comparable major disease only 2 (3.7%) showed evidence of focal or mild acute pancreatitis, but fat necrosis was absent. Baar and Wolff[162] studied the pancreases of 2 children who died at the ages of 3 and 11 years during prolonged steroid treatment. There were severe diffuse hemorrhagic pancreatic necrosis, infiltration of the pancreas with polymorphonuclear leukocytes, peripancreatic fat necrosis, and calcium deposits present. In most reports there was no evidence of a relation between the intensity and duration of steroid treatment and the extent of the pancreatic lesions. The changes in the pancreases of these steroid treated patients were similar to those seen in rabbits after prolonged cortisone administration.[163-165]

The role of adrenal secretion in diabetes mellitus in the absence of frank adrenal disease has attracted considerable attention. The possibility exists that diabetes occurs only in patients whose pancreases cannot sufficiently cope with the adrenal hypersecretion. In fact, it has been shown that the adrenal cortical function may actually be decreased in idiopathic diabetes. Wilson *et al.*[166] have demonstrated that patients with Addison's disease respond with distinct diabetic symptoms to a dose of cortisone which would have minimal effect in normal individuals. They suggested that these patients are habituated to a relative islet cell insufficiency as a compensatory protection against the hypoglycemia. They also showed that not all patients with hyperadrenocorticism have overt diabetes, but that osteoporosis and an elevated excretion of 11-oxysteroids may be present, which seems indicative of a compensatory overactivity of the islets of Langerhans, in order to prevent the expected hyperglycemia. This would be in keeping with the observations of Thorn *et al.*[167] that the hyperfunction of the adrenal cortex causing hyperglycemia is compensated by increased insulin production of the pancreas. This seems to be also borne out by the observation that in nondiabetic children who received adrenocorticotrophic hormones, the insulin extracted from the pancreas was elevated,[168] and by experiments carried out on rats in which a rise of the pancreatic insulin content by 40% has been observed after administration of ACTH.[169,170]

The coincidence of Addison's disease and diabetes is relatively rare.[25,171] Solomon and associates,[172] in a review of 113 cases collected from the literature, observed that diabetes preceded Addison's disease in 63%, Addison's disease preceded diabetes in 23%, and there was a simultaneous onset in 10%. In the remaining 4% the sequence was not specified. The interval between the apparent onset of the two diseases was less than a year in 21% of the patients. Gittler and co-workers[173] observed that of 3 cases reported, Addison's disease preceded the development of diabetes by 15 years in 1 and by 9 years in another. Beaven and associates[174] collected 63 cases, including 8 of their own, of Addison's disease with coexisting diabetes. In 37 of these individuals diabetes preceded Addison's disease, in 21 Addison's disease preceded the diabetes, and in 5 the disorders seemed to appear simultaneously. In those patients in whom Addison's disease developed first, the average time interval was 3 years prior to onset of diabetes, and of the 37 patients in whom diabetes had developed first, one had hypothyroidism as well, and 4 had concomitant thyrotoxicosis.

A more striking clinical feature in diabetic patients who developed Addison's disease is the increased sensitivity to insulin.[175] This leads to decreased insulin requirement and improvement of the glucose tolerance.[176,177] Hinerman[178] reported that in Addison's disease the islets of Langerhans are uniformly hyperplastic and that while all cells appear larger, the A cells show the most conspicuous change. These observations could not be confirmed by Sloper,[179] who noted small islet cell adenomas in 2 of 17 cases with Addison's disease studied.

Pheochromocytoma and Diabetes

Functional pheochromocytomas have been known for many years. They are tumors of the medulla or of related chromaffin tissue which either continuously or intermittently secrete large amounts of catecholamines (epinephrine or norepinephrine). Fraenkel,[180] in 1886, for the first time recorded a case of an 18-year-old girl who gave a history of 1 year of short paroxysmal attacks, palpitation, dizziness, vomiting, pallor, and retinitis, associated with a noncompressible heart pulse. The patient died suddenly, and postmortem examination revealed bilateral adrenal tumors which, judging from the gross and microscopic descriptions, were consistent with pheochromocytoma. Von Neusser[181] reported several patients with hypertension associated with tumors of the adrenal gland, and in 1915 Cannon[182] established that hyperglycemia due to sudden stress is frequently the result of increased secretion of epinephrine. Manasse,[183] in 1893, for the first time, published the morphologic description of a pheochromocytoma, and in 1902 Kohn[184] observed that the tumors are derived from the chromaffin system. Helly,[185] in 1913, correlated the symptoms of hypertension and glycosuria with a pheochromocytoma. Labbé and his associates[186] mentioned that paroxysmal symptoms are associated with tumors of the adrenal. However, it was not until 1927 that Mayo[187] removed an epinephrine-secreting tumor from a patient with hypertension and hyperglycemia in whom the blood sugar declined to normal postoperatively. Since then a number of reports have appeared in which the diabetes apparently was cured with the removal of a pheochromocytoma.[188–192] Many of these patients had required insulin, some in large amounts before operation, but none was required afterward. Griessmann[190] reported a patient who had presented diabetic coma, but the glucose tolerance was normal after removal of the tumor. Kozak[42] reported his observations on 5 patients with pheochromocytoma between 1954 and 1969. In 1 patient, removal of a large tumor in 1938 had not been followed by a change in the severity of the diabetes up to the time of death in 1948. Three patients exhibited dramatic amelioration of hyperglycemia and hypertension which occurred with the onset of diabetes shortly before the diagnosis of pheochromocytoma. One patient with growth-onset diabetes was not affected by the removal of the pheochromocytoma. Joslin *et al.*[193] observed no improvement of the diabetes in 1 patient after the operation, and another patient reported by Goldner[194] still exhibited a mildly diabetic curve two years later. On the other hand, Staquet *et al.*[195] observed a case with mild diabetes which completely disappeared after removal of a 30 mg medullary adrenal tumor. In several instances, there was a family history of diabetes.[196]

Pheochromocytomas are rare tumors. However, since the advent of pharmacologic tests for their detection they have been diagnosed with increasing frequency. Graham[197] observed 8 pheochromocytomas in a series of 1700 patients with hypertension (0.47%) subjected to bilateral lumbo-dorsal splanchnicectomy. Kvale *et al.*[198] reported in a study of 900 patients with hypertension of various types, an incidence of 2% of the cases afflicted with pheochromocytoma. Minno *et al.*[199] found 15 cases (0.1%) in a series of 15,985 consecutive autopsies, and the diagnosis was suspected in only 3 of these. Smithwick and Graham[200] observed an incidence of 1 case in 200 hypertensive patients on whom sympathectomy was carried out.

The coexistence of pheochromocytoma with diabetes has been well established in the literature.[200-209] In a review of pheochromocytomas, Eisenberg and Wallerstein[210] observed that 11% of their cases were afflicted with diabetes. Smithwick and Graham[200] noted that 9% of their patients had a reduced glucose tolerance, and 10% had frank diabetes. De Vries *et al.*[189] observed hyperglycemia and glycosuria in 21 of 50 reported cases in the literature, including 2 of their own. Kvale,[208] in a group of 57 patients with pheochromocytoma, noted an elevated blood sugar level in 11 of 25 normotensive patients. In another series of 17 patients with persistent hypertension, the blood sugar level varied from 102 to 256 mg/100ml and it was 120 mg/100ml or more in 10 patients. Some of the patients with pheochromocytoma have considerable insulin resistance.[190,211] Others may show lack of signs or biochemical characteristics of diabetes, or the diabetes may be exceedingly severe, and advanced ketosis may be present.[190,210] Evans[212] observed, in a study of 13 patients with pheochromocytoma, that 8 had diabetes when first seen, and in 1, who had metastatic pheochromocytoma, the diabetes developed after the initial tumor was removed. Of the 13 patients 4 had hypertension but no diabetes, 7 had diabetes with sustained hypertension, and 2 with paroxysmal hypertension. In a review of 76 patients with pheochromocytoma, Gifford and associates[213] observed that two-thirds had persistent hypertension and hyperglycemia, and in three-fourths hypermetabolism was present. Hermann and Mornes[214] observed disturbances of carbohydrate metabolism in 22% of the patients with pheochromocytoma, and Jailer and Mornes[215] found that 10% had this complication.

The morphologic alterations of the pancreas in patients with pheochromocytoma associated with diabetes has been reported by several authors. Blacklock and associates[209] noted that in one of their patients the pancreatic islets were more numerous than usual, and proceeded to find 4 to 5 similar cases in the same high-power field. In another case, the islets appeared hyperplastic. Because of postmortem autolysis no special stains were performed. However, in another patient with pheochromocytoma in whom the blood sugar levels were not available, the pancreatic parenchyma showed diffuse interlobular fibrosis and hyalinization in the wall of the small arteries and the arterioles. The islets were more numerous and appeared larger than normal. Lukens[216] studied a biopsy specimen obtained from the pancreas which was excised during the removal of a pheochromocytoma of the right adrenal in a 43-year-old woman who had paroxysmal hypertension and elevated blood sugar levels which ranged from 114 to 200 mg/100ml. Glycosuria was also present. The patient received 5 to 10 units of insulin daily. The pancreas showed marked degranulation and questionable early vacuolization of the B cells. Lukens concluded from experiences with experimental work that the hydropic changes and the degranulation of the islets were due to hyperglycemia, but that the changes were mild enough to be reversible. Warren and LeCompte[217] encountered three cases of pheochromocytoma in their group of diabetic pancreases. All tumors were discovered unexpectedly at postmortem examination. All had diabetes for at least 6 years, and in no instance was the presence of neoplasm suspected clinically. There was no significant change in the pancreas. Lukens and Dyer[160] reported pancreatic biopsies of two diabetics with pheochromocytoma. In one case there was extensive degranulation or early vacuolization of the B cells. The diabetes, requiring 15 units of insulin daily, was "cured" by removal of the tumor, the glucose tolerance being normal after operation. In the other case, the islets showed little change from the normal, although 50 units of insulin daily had been required to control the diabetes. After removal of the tumor, the patient no longer needed insulin, but the glucose tolerance remained abnormal. These two cases showed fewer islet changes than those of the other patient, whose diabetes was cured. From the few available studies it can be concluded that no consistent relationship exists between the histologic appearance of the islets and the behavior of diabetes associated with pheochromocytoma.

The Thyroid and Diabetes

In hyperthyroidism, disorders of carbohydrate metabolism occur frequently, but they are relatively mild in the majority of cases. Glycemic levels are often within normal values; however, the average blood sugar is slightly increased.[218,219] Moreover, while the glucose tolerance is usually decreased in hyperthyroid patients,[220,221] it improves in some patients after thyroidectomy.[222] The abnormality of blood sugar homeostasis is thought to be due to the fact that the thyroid hormone increases the rate of absorption from the intestine of glucose.[223,224] Diabetes is more common in patients with hyperthyroidism than it is in the population at large.[17,225-228] Regan and Wilder[226] observed diabetes in 1.7% of the patients with toxic nodular goiter. However, some of these figures were recorded before the advent of antithyroid drugs and radioiodine, and thyrotoxicosis at that time was a severe disease, often of long duration.

The incidence of diabetes in patients with thyrotoxicosis has been studied by many investigators. Joslin and Lahey,[229] in a study of 500 patients with thyroid disease, reported an incidence of glycosuria associated with primary hyperthyroidism in 38.6%; with adenomatous goiter (toxic goiter) with hyperthyroidism in 27.7%; and with nontoxic goiter with hyperthyroidism in 14.8%. In a large control study, the incidence of glycosuria was 13.6%. Clinical diabetes was present in 2.5% of those with primary hyperthyroidism and in 4.3% of those having adenomatous toxic goiter with hyperthyroidism. Regan and Wilder[226] recorded the occurrence of diabetes in 3.2% in a study of 5353 patients with thyrotoxicosis, and they found diabetes in 1.7% of the cases with toxic nodular goiter. Kreines *et al.*[230] observed a high prevalence of diabetes mellitus in clinical hyperthyroidism. Glucose tolerance consistent with diabetes was found in 29 of 51 patients (51%) before and in 13 of 44 cases (30%) after antithyroid treatment. Diabetes was more common in older patients with toxic nodular goiter than in younger ones with Graves' disease. John[231] observed that there is no relationship between the disturbance of metabolism or the severity of hyperthyroidism and the degree of hyperglycemia. On the other hand, McGavac[232] pointed out that the disease has no influence on the course of thyrotoxicosis.

Pirart,[233] in a study of 2819 diabetics, found 26 cases in whom diabetes and hyperthyroidism coexisted, an incidence of 1%. In a study of a series of "true" diabetics seen between 1928 and 1965 at the Joslin Clinic, Kozak[25] observed 604 cases of hyperthyroidism, which represents a similar incidence of approximately 1.1%. Regan and Wilder[226] reported the prior appearance of hyperthyroidism in 52% and of toxic nodular goiter with secondary hyperthyroidism in 62%. Allan,[234] in a study of diabetic patients, noted that primary hyperthyroidism appeared prior to the diabetes in 54% and toxic nodular goiter preceded the onset of diabetes in 68% of the cases. Kozak[25] observed that only 6 out of 86 diabetics developed hyperthyroidism prior to the onset of diabetes. Diabetes preceded primary hyperthyroidism in 66% and toxic nodular goiter in 67% of the patients. Simultaneous onset was observed in 23%. The author noted diabetic heredity in 42% of the cases in comparison with earlier studies where an incidence of 52% was noted. Bowen and Lenzner[235] observed diabetic hereditary in 55% of diabetics with primary hyperthyroidism and in 40% with toxic nodular goiter.

In a study of 26 cases of coexisting thyrotoxicosis and diabetes, Bastenie[236] observed that in 8 patients the diabetes became manifest 2 years or more after the thyrotoxicosis was diagnosed. In 10 other cases both conditions appeared at the same time, while in the remaining 8 cases the diabetes preceded the thyrotoxicosis by more than 2 years. Kozak[25] pointed out that in most instances the diabetic patient with hyperthyroidism behaves in the same manner with this condition, whether the diagnosis is that of a primary hyperthyroidism or toxic nodular goiter with secondary hyperthyroidism.

There are a few studies dealing with the changes of the pancreas in patients with hyperthyroidism. Garrod[237] observed the occurrence of atrophic lesions in the pancreas in some cases of thyrotoxicosis. Holst[238] found no change in the pancreas in 4 of 10 of his cases of diabetes associated with hyperthyroidism, while in 6 instances, the pancreas was small, and in 4 of these the number of islets had considerably decreased. Warren *et al.*[239] observed no changes in the pancreas in a number of cases of severe and long-standing hyperthyroidism.

Kozak,[25] in a review of the literature, maintained that according to the experience of others as well as of the Joslin Clinic, hypothyroidism and diabetes "occur together no less, and perhaps even more frequently than their independent frequencies would indicate." Baron[240] observed 4 diabetics among 91 hypothyroid patients, and Bloomer and Kyle[241] noted 11 among 80 hypothyroid individuals. Bastenie[236] found a definite relationship between the two diseases. At a Brussels General Clinic he observed 1 hypothyroid patient for every 13,000 nondiabetic cases, while there were 5 hypothyroid individuals detected among 1587 diabetics. At the University Medical Clinics in Brussels, 11 cases of marked hypothyroidism were found among 2819 diabetics. On the other hand, of 80 documented patients with hypothyroidism admitted during a period of 20 years, 16 concerned diabetic subjects, 11 were frank diabetics, often of long standing, and 5 were latent diabetics. Kozak[25] observed, during a period of 8 years, 52 cases of primary hypothyroidism (0.24%) among 22,500 new diabetic patients. Hecht and Gershberg[242] observed 9 hypothyroid patients in a group of 530 diabetics (1.7%).

Untreated myxedema may reduce the severity of the diabetes and insulin requirement. However, it does not preclude the occurrence of severe uncontrolled diabetes, ketoacidosis, and coma.[25]

References

1. Loeb, M.: *Dtsch. Arch. Klin. Med.,* **34**:443, 1883–84.
2. Marie, P.: *Rev. Méd.,* **6**:297, 1886.
3. Marie, P.: *N. Iconog. Salpetrière,* **1**:173, 1888.
4. Marie, P.: *De Prog. Méd.,* **9**:189, 1889.
5. Loeb, M.: *Centralbl. Inn. Med.,* **19**:893, 1898.
6. Hansemann, D.: *Berl. Klin. Wochenschr.,* **34**:417, 1897.
7. Dallemagne, M.: *Arch. Med. Exp. Anat. Pathol.,* **7**:589, 1895.
8. Borchardt, L.: *Ztschr. Klin. Med.,* **66**:332, 1908.
9. Hinsdale, G.: *Acromegaly.* W. M. Warren, Detroit, 1898.
10. Goetsch, E., Cushing, H., and Jacobson, C.: *Bull. Johns Hopkins Hosp.,* **22**:165, 1911.
11. Cushing, H.: *The Pituitary Body and its Disorders.* J. B. Lippincott, Philadelphia, 1912, p. 23.
12. Williamson, E. T.: *Diabetes Mellitus.* G. J. Pentland, London, 1898.
13. Ander, J. M. and Jameson, H. L.: Amer. J. Med. Sci., **148**:323, 1914.
14. Rosenberger, F.: *Die Ursachen der Glykurien: ihre Verhütung und Behandlung.* Müller & Steincke, München, 1911.
15. Shepardson, H. C.: *J. Nerv. Ment. Dis.,* **99**:862, 1944.
16. Yater, W. M.: *Arch. Int. Med.,* **41**:883, 1928.
17. Wilder, R. M.: *Clinical Diabetes Mellitus and Hyperinsulinism.* W. B. Saunders, Philadelphia, 1940, p. 262.
18. Cushing, H., and Davidoff, L. M.: *Arch. Int. Med.,* **39**:673, 1927.
19. Coggeshall, C., and Root, H. F.: *Endocrinology,* **26**:1, 1940.
20. McCullagh, E. P.: *Diabetes,* **5**:223, 1956.
21. Miller, M.: In: *Diabetes.* Edited by R. H. Williams. Paul P. Hoeber, New York, 1960, p. 708.
22. Frank, E.: *Pathologie des Kohlenhydratstoffwechsels.* Schwabe, Basel, 1949, p. 48.
23. Hamwi, G. J., Skillman, T. G., and Tufts, K. C.: *Amer. J. Med.,* **29**:690, 1960.
24. Gordon, D. A., Hill, F. M., and Ezrin, C.: *Canad. Med. Assoc. J.,* **87**:1106, 1962.
25. Kozak, G. P.: In: *Joslin's Diabetes Mellitus.* Edited by A., Marble, P., White, R. F. Bradley, and L. P. Krall. Lea & Febiger, Philadelphia, 1971, p. 667.
26. Schlesinger, W.: *Wien, Klin. Rundsch.,* **14**:286, 1900.
27. v. Noorden, C. and Isaac, S.: *Handbuch der Pathologie des Stoffwechsels.* A. Hirschwald, Berlin, 1907, p. 46.
28. Froment, M. J.: *Rev. Neurol.,* **29**:649, 1922.
29. Macleod, J. J. R.: *Modern Medicine.* C. V. Mosby, St. Louis, 1920, p. 3.
30. Ellis, A. W. M., and Turnbull, H. M.: *Lancet,* **1**:1200, 1924.
31. Goetsch, E.: *Quart. J. Med.,* **7**:173, 1913–14.
32. Colwell, A. R.: *Medicine,* **6**:1, 1927.
33. McCullagh, E. P., and Alivisatos, J. A.: *Diabetes,* **3**:349, 1954.
34. Berg, B. N.: *Bull. Neurol. Inst.,* **6**:178, 1937.
35. Sternberg, N.: *Nothnagel's Path. Ther.,* **7**:1, 1897.
36. v. Noorden, C.: *Die Zuckerkrankheit und ihre Behandlung.* A. Hirschwald, Berlin, 1910, p. 48.

37. Darragh, J. H., and Shaw, W. M.: *Canad. Med. Assoc. J.*, **64**:146, 1951.
38. Labbé, M.: *A Clinical Treatise on Diabetes Mellitus.* Wood, New York, 1922, p. 195.
39. Finzi, G.: *Boll. Soc. Med. Bologna*, **8**:201, 1897.
40. Buday, K., and Janese, N.: *Dtsch. Arch. Klin. Med.*, **10**:385, 1898.
41. John, H. J.: *JAMA*, **85**:1629, 1925.
42. Balfour, W. M., and Sprague, R. E.: *Amer. J. Med.*, **7**:596, 1949.
43. Perley, M. and Kipnis, D. M.: *N. Engl. J. Med.*, **274**:1237, 1966.
44. Kinsell, L. W., Lawrence, L., and Weyand, R. D.: *J. Clin. Endocrinol.*, **15**:859, 1955 (Abst.).
45. Luft, R., Olivecrona, H., and Sjörgren, B.: *J. Clin. Endocrinol.*, **15**:391, 1955.
46. Luft, R., Olivecrona, H., Ikkos, D., Kornerup, T., and Ljunggren, H.: *Brit. Med. J.*, **2**:752, 1955.
47. Luft, R.: In: *On the Nature and Treatment of Diabetes.* Edited by B. S. Leibel and G. A. Wrenshall. Excerpta Medica, Amsterdam, 1965, p. 496.
48. Dominguez, J. M., and Pearson, O. H.: *J. Clin. Endocrinol.*, **22**:865, 1962.
49. Glick, S. M., Roth, J., Yalow, R., and Berson, S. A.: *Nature (London)*, **199**:784, 1963.
50. Geller, J., and Loh, A.: *J. Clin. Endocrinol.*, **23**:1107, 1963.
51. Ehrlich, R. M., and Randle, P. J.: *Lancet*, **2**:233, 1961.
52. Berson, S. A., and Yalow, R. S.: *Diabetes*, **14**:549, 1965.
53. Sönksen, P. H., Greenwood, F. C., Ellis, J. P., Lowry, C., Rutherford, A., and Nabarro, J. D. N.: *J. Clin. Endocrinol.*, **27**:1428, 1967.
54. Bondy, P. K.: *Yale J. Biol. Med.*, **26**:263, 1954.
55. Carballeira, A., Elrick, H., Mackenzie, K. R., and Browne, J. S. L.: *Proc. Soc. Exp. Biol. Med.*, **81**:15, 1952.
56. Kibler, R., Werk, E. E., Engel, F. L., and Myers, J. D.: *Proc. Soc. Exp. Biol. Med.*, **89**:446, 1955.
57. Kinsell, L. W.: *Protein Metabolism, Hormones and Growth.* Rutgers University Press, New York, 1953.
58. Kinsell, L. W.: *The Hypophyseal Growth Hormone, Nature and Actions.* McGraw-Hill, New York, 1955, p. 507.
59. Crispell, K. R., and Parson, W.: *J. Clin. Endocrin. Med.*, **12**:881, 1952.
60. Shorr, E., Carter, A. C., Kennedy, B. J., and Smith, R. W.: *Diabetes*, **3**:94, 1954.
61. Shorr, E., Carter, A. C., Smith, R. W., Kennedy, B. J., Havel, B. J., Roberts, T. N., Sonkin, L. L., and Livingstone, E. T.: *The Hypophyseal Growth Hormone, Nature and Actions.* McGraw-Hill, New York, 1955, p.522.
62. Ikkos, D., Luft, R., and Gemzell, C. A.: *Lancet*, **1**:720, 1958.
63. Luft, R., Ikkos, D., Gemzell, C. A., and Olivecrona, A.: *Lancet*, **1**:721, 1958.
64. Goldberg, M. B., and Lisser, H.: *J. Clin. Endocrinol.*, **2**:477, 1942.
65. Fraser, R.: *Brit. Med. Bull.*, **16**:242, 1960.
66. Houssay, B. A., and Biasotti, A.: *Arch Ges. Physiol.*, **227**:664, 1931.
67. Lyall, A., and Innes, J. A.: *Lancet*, **1**:318, 1935.
68. Chabanier, H., Puech, P., Lobo-Onell, C., and Lelu, E.: *Presse Méd.*, **44**:986, 1936.
69. Feldman, F., Roberts, J. B., Susselman, S., and Lipetz, B.: *Arch. Int. Med.*, **79**:322, 1947.
70. Kotte, J. H., and Vonderahe, A. R.: *JAMA*, **114**:950, 1940.
71. Marzullo, E. R., and Handelsman, M. B.: *J. Clin. Endocrinol.*, **11**:537, 1951.
72. Calder, R. M.: *Bull. Johns Hopkins Hosp.*, **50**:87, 1932.
73. Williams, F. W.: *Diabetes*, **1**:37, 1952.
74. Martin, M. M., and Pond, M. H.: *J. Clin. Endocrinol.*, **14**:1046, 1954.
75. Rothfeld, B., and Rodas, J. M.: *Ann. Int. Med.*, **41**:140, 1954.
76. Georas, C. S., Meissner, G. F., Dillon, J. A., and Calenda, D. G.: *N. Engl. J. Med.*, **263**:374, 1960.
77. Alexander, R. I.: *Brit. Med. J.*, **1**:416, 1953.
78. Harvey, J. C., and de Klerk, J.: *Amer. J. Med.*, **19**:327, 1955.
79. Cushing, H.: *Papers Relating to the Pituitary Body, Hypothalamus and Parasympathetic Nervous System.* Charles C Thomas, Springfield, Ill., 1932, p. 34.
80. Almy, T. P., and Shorr, E.: *J. Clin. Endocrinol.*, **7**:455, 1947.
81. Field, R. A., Schepens, C. L., Sweet, W. H., and Appels, A.: *Diabetes*, **11**:465, 1962.

82. Poulsen, J. E.: *Diabetes,* **2**:7, 1953.
83. Poulsen, J. E.: *Diabetes,* **15**:73, 1966.
84. Field, R. A.: *N. Engl. J. Med.,* **264**:689, 1961.
85. Luft, R.: Symposium on the Influence of Hypophysectomy and Adrenalectomy on Diabetic Retinopathy. *Diabetes,* **11**:461, 1962.
86. Pearson, O. H., Ray, B. S., McLean, J. M., Peretz, W. L., Greenberg, E., and Pazianos, A.: *JAMA,* **188**:116, 1964.
87. Warren, S., LeCompte, P. M., and Legg, M. A.: *The Pathology of Diabetes Mellitus.* Lea & Febiger, Philadelphia, 1966, p. 343.
88. Frey, H. M.: *J. Clin. Endocrinol.,* **19**:1642, 1959.
89. Frey, H. M.: *Acta Med. Scand.,* **175**:523, 1964.
90. Kraus, E. J.: *Beitr. Path. Anat. Allg. Path.,* **58**:159, 1914.
91. Kraus, E. J.: *Virchow's Arch.,* **228**:68, 1920.
92. Kraus, E. J., and Reisinger, A.: *Frankf. Ztschr. Path.,* **30**:68, 1924.
93. Kraus, E. J.: In: *Handb. Spec. Path. Anat. Histol.* Edited by F. Henke and O. Lubarsch. Julius Springer, Berlin, Vol. V/2, 1929, p. 622.
94. Brooks, H.: *Arch. Neurol. Psychopathol.,* **1**:485, 1898.
95. Herxheimer, G.: *Virchow's Arch. Path. Anat. Physiol.,* **183**:228, 1906.
96. Herxheimer, G.: *Verhandl. Dtsch. Path. Gesellsch.,* **11**:343, 1908.
97. Steiger, O.: *Ztschr. Klin. Med.,* **84**:269, 1917.
98. Norris, C.: *Proc. N. Y. Pathol. Soc.,* **7**:19, 1907.
99. Amsler, C.: *Berl. Klin. Wochenschr.,* **49**:1600, 1912.
100. Cecil, R. E.: *J. Exp. Med.,* **11**:266, 1909.
101. Lazarus, S. S., and Volk, B. W.: *The Pancreas in Human and Experimental Diabetes.* Grune & Stratton, New York, 1962, p. 166.
102. Warren, S., LeCompte, P. M., and Legg, M. A.: *The Pathology of Diabetes Mellitus.* Lea & Febiger, Philadelphia, 1966, p. 342.
103. Fry, A. J. B.: *Quart. J. Med.,* **8**:277, 1915.
104. Kraus, E. J.: *Virchow's Arch.,* **247**:1, 1923–24.
105. Labbé, M., and Petresco, M.: *Ann. Anat. Pathol.,* **11**:761, 1934.
106. Cunz, H.: *Schweiz. Med. Wochenschr.,* **25**:75, 1945.
107. Kraus, E. J.: *Urol. Cutan. Rev.,* **48**:417, 1944.
108. Hawking, F.: *J. Pathol. Bacteriol.,* **42**:689, 1936.
109. Heskel, M. M.: *J. Albert Einstein Med. Cent.,* **5**:189, 1957.
110. Marchi, P.: *Arch. De Vecchi Anat. Pathol.,* **25**:1, 1956.
111. Steiner, H.: *Virchow's Arch.,* **339**:171, 1965.
112. Russfield, A. B.: *Cancer,* **13**:790, 1960.
113. Parsons, R. J.: *Medical Papers Dedicated to Dr. Henry A. Christian.* New York, 1936, p. 366.
114. Crooke, A. C.: *J. Pathol. Bacteriol.,* **41**:339, 1935.
115. Porges, O.: *Ztsch. Klin. Med.,* **69**:341, 1909.
116. Kraus, E. J.: *Dtsch. Med. Wochenschr.,* **39**:2377, 1913.
117. Achard, C., and Thièrs, J.: *Bull. Acad. Med.,* **86**:51, 1921.
118. Albright, F.: *Harvy Lect.,* **38**:123, 1942–43.
119. Cushing, H.: *Bull. Johns Hopkins Hosp.,* **50**:137, 1932.
120. Hartman, F. A., and Brownell, K. A.: *Proc. Soc. Exp. Biol. Med.,* **31**:834, 1933–34.
121. Long, C. N. H., and Lukens, F. D. W.: *J. Exp. Med.,* **63**:465, 1936.
122. Long, C. N. H., Fry, E. G., and Thompson, K. W.: *Amer. J. Physiol.,* **123**:130, 1938.
123. Lukens, F. D. W.: *Amer. J. Med. Sci.,* **193**:312, 1937.
124. Plotz, C. M., Knowlton, A. I., and Ragan, C.: *Amer. J. Med.,* **13**:597, 1952.
125. Soffer, L. J., Iannaccone, A., and Gabrilove, J.: *Amer. J. Med.,* **30**:129, 1961.
126. Miller, M.: In: *Diabetes.* Edited by R. H. Williams. Paul B. Hoeber, New York, 1960, p. 708.
127. Sprague, R. G., Priestley, J. R., and Dockerty, M. B.: *J. Clin. Endocrinol.,* **3**:28, 1943.
128. Walters, W., Wilder, R. M., and Kepler, E. J.: *Ann. Surg.,* **100**:670, 1934.
129. Sprague, R. G., Kvale, W. F., and Priestley, J. R.: *JAMA,* **151**:629, 1953.
130. Conn, J. W., Louis, L. H., and Wheller, C. E.: *J. Lab. Clin. Med.,* **33**:651, 1948.

131. Forsham, P. H., Thorn, G. W., Prunty, F. T. G., and Hills, A. G.: *J. Clin. Endocrinol.,* **8**:15, 1948.
132. Boland, E. W., and Headly, N. E.: *JAMA,* **141**:301, 1949.
133. Baehr, G., Soffer, L. J., Boad, N. F., Levitt, M. F., and Gabrilove, J. L.: *Tr. A. Am. Phys.,* **63**:89, 1950.
134. Bastenie, P. A., Conard, V., and Franckson, J. R. M.: In: *Handbook of Diabetes Mellitus.* Edited by E. F. Pfeiffer. J. F. Lehmann, Munich, Vol. II, 1971, p. 888.
135. Creutzfeldt, W., and Schlagintweit, S.: *Dtsch. Med. Wochenschr.,* **82**:1539, 1957.
136. Forsham, P. H.: In: *Textbook of Endocrinology.* Edited by R. H. Williams, W. B. Saunders, Philadelphia, 3rd Ed., 1962, p. 282.
137. Conard, V., and Franckson, J. R. M.: *Diabetes,* **3**:205, 1954.
138. Sprague, R. G., Power, M. H., Mason, H. E., Albert, A., Mathieson, D. R., Hench, P. S., Kendall, E. C., and Polley, H. F.: *Arch. Int. Med.,* **85**:199, 1950.
139. Bookman, J. J., Drachman, S. R., Schaefer, L. E., and Adlersberg, D.: *Diabetes,* **2**:100, 1953.
140. Sprague, R. G., Power, M. W., Mason, H. E., and Cluxton, H. E.: *J. Clin. Invest.,* **28**:812, 1949.
141. Perara, G. A., Pines, K. L., Hamilton, H. B., and Vislockey, K.: *Amer. J. Med.,* **7**:56, 1949.
142. Simpson, S. L.: *J. Clin. Endocrinol.,* **9**:403, 1949.
143. Thorn, G. W., and Clinton, M., Jr.: *J. Clin. Endocrinol.,* **3**:335, 1943.
144. Faber, V., and Gronbaek, P.: *Acta Endocrinol.,* **22**:145, 1956.
145. Beaven, D. W., Nelson, D. H., Renold, A. E., and Thorn, G. W.: *N. Engl. J. Med.,* **261**:443, 1959.
146. Bartels, E. C., Fields, M. L., and Murphy, R.: *Lahey Clinic Bull.,* **10**:234, 1958.
147. Rhinds, E. G. G., and Wilson, A.: *Lancet,* **2**:37, 1941.
148. Lukens, F. D. W., Flippen, H. F., and Thigden, F. M.: *Amer. J. Med.,* **193**:812, 1937.
149. Russi, S., Blumenthal, H. T., and Gray, S. H.: *Arch. Int. Med.,* **76**:284, 1945.
150. Soffer, L. J., Eisenberg, J., Iannaccone, A., and Gabrilove, J. L.: In: *The Human Adrenal Cortex.* Little, Brown, Boston, 1955, p. 487.
151. Vartiainen, F.: *Acta Med. Scand.,* **118**:539, 1944.
152. Smith, E. B., Beamer, P. R., Vellios, F., and Schulz, D. M.: *Principles of Human Pathology.* Oxford University Press, New York, 1959.
153. Warren, S., LeCompte, P. M., and Legg, M. A.: *The Pathology of Diabetes Mellitus.* Lea & Febiger, Philadelphia, 1966, p. 335.
154. Shepardson, H. C., and Shapiro, E.: *Endocrinology,* **24**:237, 1939.
155. Kepler, E. J., Sprague, R. G., Mason, H. L., and Power, M. H.: *Rec. Prog. Horm. Res.,* **2**:345, 1948.
156. Franckson, J. R. M., Gepts, W., Bastenie, P. A., Conrad, V., Cordier, N., and Kovacs, L.: *Acta Endocrinol.,* **14**:153, 1953.
157. Hausberger, F. X., and Ramsay, A. J.: *Endocrinology,* **53**:423, 1953.
158. Hausberger, F. X., and Ramsay, A. J.: *Endocrinology,* **65**:165, 1959.
159. Lazarus, S. S., and Volk, B. W.: *The Pancreas in Human and Experimental Diabetes.* Grune & Stratton, New York, 1962, p. 161.
160. Lukens, F. D. W., and Dyer, W. W.: *Amer. J. Med. Sci.,* **231**:313, 1956.
161. Carone, F. A., and Liebow, A. A.: *N. Engl. J. Med.,* **257**:690, 1957.
162. Baar, H. S., and Wolff, O. H.: *Lancet,* **2**:812, 1957.
163. Stumpf, H. H., and Wilens, S. L.: *Amer. J. Pathol.,* **31**:563, 1955.
164. Stumpf, H. H., Wilens, S. L., and Somoza, C.: *Lab. Invest.,* **5**:224, 1956.
165. Bencosme, S., and Lazarus, S. S.: *Arch. Pathol.,* **62**:285, 1956.
166. Wilson, D. L., Frawley, T. F., Forsham, P. H., and Thorn, G. W.: *Proc. Amer. Diabetes Assoc.,* **10**:120, 1950.
167. Thorn, G. W., Forsham, P. H., Frawley, T. F., Hill, S. R., Roche, M., Staebelin, D., and Wilson, D. L.: *N. Engl. J. Med.,* **242**:783, 824, 865, 1950.
168. Wrenshall, G. A., and Ritchie, R. C.: *Pediatrics,* **9**:504, 1952.
169. Fraenkel-Conrat, H. L., Herring, H. L., Simpson, M. E., and Evans, H. M.: *Amer. J. Physiol.,* **135**:404, 1942.
170. Fraenkel-Conrat, H. L., Herring, H. L., Simpson, M. E., and Evans, H. M.: *Proc. Soc. Exp. Biol. Med.,* **55**:62, 1944.

171. Webster, B. H., and Hurt, J. E.: *Diabetes,* **6**:436, 1957.
172. Solomon, N., Carpenter, C. C. J., Bennett, I. L., and Harvey, A. M.: *Diabetes,* **14**:300, 1965.
173. Gittler, R. D., Fajans, S. S., and Conn, J. W.: *J. Clin. Endocrinol.,* **19**:797, 1959.
174. Beaven, D. W., Nelson, D. H., Renold, A. E., and Thorn, G. W.: *N. Engl. J. Med.,* **261**:443, 1959.
175. Fraser, R. W., Albright, F., and Smith, P. H.: *J. Clin. Endocrinol.,* **1**:297, 1941.
176. Crampton, J. H., Scudder, S. T., and Davis, C. D.: *J. Clin. Endocrinol.,* **9**:245, 1949.
177. Baird, I. M., and Munro, D. S.: *Lancet,* **1**:962, 1954.
178. Hinerman, D.: *Arch. Pathol.,* **51**:539, 1951.
179. Sloper, J. C.: *Arch. Pathol.,* **58**:294, 1954.
180. Fraenkel, F.: *Virchow's Arch.,* **103**:244, 1886.
181. Von Neusser, E.: *Die Erkrankungen der Nebennieren.* Alfred Holder, Vienna, 2nd Ed., 1910, p. 97.
182. Cannon, W. B.: *Bodily Changes in Pain, Hunger, Fear, and Rage.* Appleton, New York, 1915.
183. Manasse, P.: *Virchow's Arch.,* **133**:391, 1883.
184. Kohn, A.: *Ergeb. Anat. Entwicklngsgesch.,* **12**:253, 1902.
185. Helly, C.: *München Med. Wochenschr.,* **33**:1811, 1913.
186. Labbé, M. Tinel, J., and Doumer, F.: *Bull. Man. Soc. Méd. Hôp. Paris,* **46**:982, 1922.
187. Mayo, C. H.: *JAMA,* **89**:1049, 1929.
188. Biskind, G. R., Meyer, M. A., and Beadner, S. A.: *J. Clin. Endocrinol.,* **1**:113, 1941.
189. De Vries, A., Rachmilewitz, M., and Schumert, M.: *Amer. J. Med.,* **6**:51, 1959.
190. Griessmann, H.: *Zentralbl. Chir.,* **77**:1343, 1952.
191. Jorde, R.: *Acta Med. Scand.,* **154**:139, 1956.
192. Green, D. M.: *JAMA,* **131**:1260, 1946.
193. Joslin, E. P., Root, H. F., White, P., and Marble, A. M.: *The Treatment of Diabetes Mellitus.* Lea & Febiger, Philadelphia, 1952, p. 640.
194. Goldner, M. G.: *J. Clin. Endocrinol.,* **7**:716, 1947.
195. Staquet, M., Bonnyns, M., Thys, O., and Demanet, J. C.: *Acta Clin. Belg.,* **20**:340, 1965.
196. Freedman, P., Moulton, R., Rosenheim, M. L., Spencer, A. G., and Willoughby, D. A.: *Quart. J. Med.,* **27**:307, 1958.
197. Graham, J. B.: Quoted in Smithwick, R. H., and Graham, J. B.: *Int. Abst. Surg.,* **92**:105, 1951.
198. Kvale, W. F., Priestley, J. T., and Roth, G. M.: *Arch. Surg.,* **68**:769, 1954.
199. Minno, A. M., Bennett, W. A., and Kvale, W. F.: *N. Engl. J. Med.,* **251**:959, 1954.
200. Smithwick, R. H., and Graham, J. B.: *Int. Abst. Surg.,* **92**:105, 1951.
201. Herde, M.: *Arch. Klin. Chir.,* **117**:937, 1912.
202. Biebl, M., and Wichsel, P.: *Virchow's Arch.,* **257**:182, 1925.
203. Schröder, K.: *Virchow's Arch.,* **268**:291, 1928.
204. de Wesselow, O. L.: *Lancet,* **2**:636, 1934.
205. Strickler, C. W.: *South Surgeon,* **11**:193, 1942.
206. McCullagh, E. P., and Engel, W. J.: *Ann. Surg.,* **116**:61, 1942.
207. Duncan, L. E., Semans, J. H., and Howard, J. E.: *Ann. Int. Med.,* **20**:815, 1944.
208. Kvale, W. F.: *Minn. Med.,* **41**:291, 1958.
209. Blacklock, J. W. S., Ferguson, J. W., Mack, W. S., Shafar, J., and Symington, T.: *Brit. J. Surg.,* **35**:179, 1947.
210. Eisenberg, A. A., and Wallerstein, H.: *Arch. Pathol.,* **14**:818, 1932.
211. Watkins, D. B.: *J. Chronic Dis.,* **6**:510, 1957.
212. Evans, J. A.: *Med. Clin. N. Amer.,* **44**:411, 1960.
213. Gifford, R. W., Kvale, W. F., Maher, F. T., Roth, G. M., and Priestley, J. T.: *Mayo Clinic Proc.,* **39**:281, 1964.
214. Hermann H., and Mornes, R.: *Le phéochromocytomes. Endocrin. de langue francaise (Ve Réunion d').* Masson et Cie, Paris, 1959, p. 334.
215. Jailer, J. W., and Longson, D.: In: *Biochemical Disorders in Human Disease.* Edited by R. H. Thompson and E. J. King. Churchill, London, 1957, p. 277.
216. Lukens, F. D. W.: *Proc. Amer. Diabetes Assoc.,* **10**:103, 1950.
217. Warren, S., and LeCompte, P. M.: *The Pathology of Diabetes Mellitus.* Lea & Febiger, Philadelphia, 1952, p. 204.

218. Sanger, B. J., and Hun, E. G.: *Arch. Int. Med., 30*:397, 1922.
219. Gotta, H., and Yriart, M.: *C. R. S. Biol., 113*:454, 1933.
220. Althausen, T. L.: *JAMA, 115*:101, 1940.
221. Popper, H. L., and Hirschhorn, S.: *Klin. Wochenschr., 10*:1071, 1931.
222. John, H. J.: *J. Clin. Endocrinol., 2*:264, 1942.
223. Althausen, T. L., and Stockholm, M.: *Amer. J. Physiol., 123*:577, 1938.
224. Schneeberg, N. G., Likoff, W. B., and Meranze, D. R.: *Arch. Surg., 46*:581, 1943.
225. Foster, D. P., and Lowrie, W. L.: *Endocrinology, 23*:681, 1938.
226. Regan, J. F., and Wilder, R. M.: *Arch. Int. Med., 65*:1116, 1940.
227. Balfour, W. M., and Sprague, R. G.: *Amer. J. Med., 7*:596, 1949.
228. Abt, A. F.: *Metabolism, 11*:202, 1962.
229. Joslin, E. P., and Lahey, F. H.: *Amer. J. Med. Sci., 176*:1, 1928.
230. Kreines, K., Jett, M., and Knowles, H. C., Jr.: *Diabetes, 14*:740, 1965.
231. John, H. J.: *Amer. J. Med. Sci., 175*:741, 1928.
232. McGavack, T. H.: *The Thyroid.* Mosby, St. Louis, 1951, p. 510.
233. Pirart, J.: *Ann. Endocrinol., 26*:27, 1965.
234. Allan, F. N., Lahey, F. H., and Murphy, R.: *Tr. Am. A. Study Goiter,* 1947, p. 248.
235. Bowen, B. D., and Lenzner, A. R.: *N. Engl. J. Med., 245*:629, 1951.
236. Bastenie, P. A.: In: *Handbook of Diabetes Mellitus.* Edited by E. F. Pfeiffer. J. F. Lehmann, München, 1971, p. 872.
237. Garrod, A.: *Lancet, 1*:483, 1912.
238. Holst, J. E.: *Acta Med. Scand., 55*:302, 1921.
239. Warren, S., LeCompte, P. M., and Legg, M. A.: *The Pathology of Diabetes Mellitus.* Lea & Febiger, Philadelphia, 1966, p. 347.
240. Baron, D. N.: *Lancet, 2*:796, 1955.
241. Bloomer, H. A., and Kyle, L. H.: *Arch. Int. Med., 104*:234, 1959.
242. Hecht, A., and Gershberg, H.: *Metabolism, 17*:108, 1968.

Chapter 12

Pancreatitis, Pancreatic Lithiasis, and Diabetes Mellitus

Klaus F. Wellmann and Bruno W. Volk

In an earlier review of this topic, coauthored by the second author of this chapter in 1962, pancreatitis and pancreatic lithiasis in their relation to diabetes mellitus were dealt with in separate chapters.[1] During the past decade and a half, however, it has become evident that stone formation in the pancreas is nearly always a late phase in the course of chronic or chronic recurrent pancreatitis. Also, while in the past occasional authors[2] distinguished between intraductal and parenchymal pancreatic lithiasis, and while it may still be difficult to determine by radiologic means whether the stones lie within the ducts or without,[3,4] virtually all recent observers emphasize the exclusively intraductal location of pancreatic calculi.[5-16] Seemingly diffuse parenchymal calcifications merely reflect the presence of small amorphous calculi in the finer radicles of the pancreatic ducts; and while the epithelium that lines the radicles may perish due to stasis, pressure necrosis, and infection, careful histologic study will often succeed in demonstrating the presence of remnants of the ductular epithelium immediately adjacent to the concrements.[8,14] It is true that calcium deposits may also occur during and after the saponification of necrotic foci of pancreatic fat; however, these soaps, once formed, are absorbed and are not converted to inorganic calcium salts.[7] In summarizing these observations, Sarles et al.[10] concluded that to differentiate between (ductal) lithiasis and (parenchymal) calcifying pancreatopathy no longer appears justified.

This review, then, deals with the various interrelationships of pancreatitis, whether calcifying or not, and diabetes. For a detailed survey of the earlier literature, the reader is referred to Lazarus and Volk's 1962 monograph.[1]

Ever since the 1963 Marseille Symposium on the etiology and pathology of pancreatitis, the acute and the chronic forms of the disease have been looked upon as separate entities. While chronic pancreatitis is characterized by lasting damage, both functional and anatomical, acute pancreatitis is—at least poten-

Klaus F. Wellmann and Bruno W. Volk • Isaac Albert Research Institute of the Kingsbrook Jewish Medical Center, and Downstate Medical Center, State University of New York, Brooklyn, New York. Present address of K. F. W.: Beekman Downtown Hospital, New York, New York. Present address of B. W. V.: University of California, Irvine, California.

tially—reversible, a distinction that holds true for recurrent forms (acute or chronic) as well.[9,11,17,18] Nevertheless, there are cases on record of chronic pancreatitis developing after the acute variety of the disease occurs; Classen and Hooper[19] found such an event in 18 of 119 patients with acute pancreatitis, Creutzfeldt *et al.*[18] in 2 of 20, and Grott[20] in as many as 11 of 20. It is difficult for a reviewer to determine whether all of these actually were bona fide cases of acute pancreatitis, but it is of interest to note that Sarles, a leading authority in the field who initially[10] denied any relationship between acute and chronic forms, more recently[21] modified his stand by stating that acute pancreatitis may, in fact, progress into the chronic variety, if rarely so. For the purposes of the subsequent discussion, the distinction between acute and chronic pancreatitis (the first reversible, the other not) has been maintained.

Acute Pancreatitis and Diabetes

Acute hemorrhagic pancreatitis is neither very rare nor very common. Of all patients admitted to the medical departments of three Central European university hospitals, between 0.35% and 0.56% had acute pancreatitis,[18] and 172 of 47,700 adult patients (0.36%) treated over a 20-year span in the Department of Surgery of the University of Copenhagen fell into this category.[22] At autopsy, acute pancreatitis has been found in 0.3 to 0.6% of all cases.[23]

Disturbances of the carbohydrate metabolism occur frequently during or immediately after an attack of acute pancreatitis. Akzhigitov and Strygina[24] found hyperglycemia in 151 of 211 (71.7%) such patients, Bank *et al.*[25] in 50% of the cases, Barbier and colleagues[26] in 38 of 56 cases (67.9%), Bartelheimer[27] in up to 30%, Fomenko[28] in 156 of 690 patients (22.6%), Hayduk *et al.*[29] in 11 to 30% of all cases, Lozano Castañeda[30] in 25 to 50%, Nielsen and Simonsen,[31] in their review, in 10 to 79%, Silva Pozo[32] in 16 of 68 (23.6%), and Zakaraya[33] in 25 of 574 patients (4.4%); and of 104 persons with acute pancreatitis seen by Strohmeyer *et al.*,[34] 15 (14.4%) showed subclinical and another 15 (14.4%) overt diabetic values. The degree of hyperglycemia encountered is generally low; in most cases, concentrations of 130 to 200 mg/100 ml are recorded,[26,34] but occasionally much higher figures have been seen.[31]

Glucosuria is usually less often present in these patients. It was stated to occur in 30% of cases with acute pancreatitis by Bank and co-workers,[25] in 8 to 16% of cases by Barbier *et al.*,[26] in 11 to 31% of patients by Lozano,[30] in 8 to 25% in the series reviewed by Nielsen and Simonsen,[31] in 11% of cases by Pariente *et al.*,[35] and in 34 of 574 patients (5.9%) with acute pancreatitis investigated by Zakaraya.[33] These figures, and the ones on hyperglycemia recorded above, are similar to those in a review of the earlier literature on the subject.[1] Why there should be such great variations in the incidence of hyperglycemia and glucosuria between the studies of different authors remains unexplained.

Complicating any statistical evaluation such as the one presented is the fact that preexisting diabetes cannot always be ruled out in patients presenting acute pancreatitis. Indeed, it has been stated that pancreatitis occurs twice as often in diabetic than in nondiabetic persons.[36] The mechanism by which diabetes induces pancreatitis has not been determined, but it has been proposed that hyperlipemia,[32] a diminished resistance against infections,[37] and small vessel disease,[36] all common in diabetics, are among the factors responsible. Preexisting diabetes was noted in 10 of 684 patients (1.4%) by Akzhigitov and Strygina,[24] in 3 of 116 cases (2.6%) by O'Sullivan *et al.*,[38] and in 8 of 112 patients (7.1%) by Strohmeyer and co-workers.[34] Silva Pozo *et al.*[32] found preexisting diabetes in 16 of their 470 patients (3.4%) with acute pancreatitis, and they quote other studies with incidences ranging from 2.0 to 7.9%. Case reports recording acute pancreatitis in known diabetics usually concern adults.[39] However, Malone[40] described such an event in 4 children; in 2 other children with acute pancreatitis and diabetes observed by Cywinski *et al.*[41] there was no known preexisting diabetes or family history of this disease.

In the great majority of patients, the hyperglycemia and the glucosuria observed during or shortly after the onset of acute pancreatitis are only transitory disturbances, and most figures will return to normal within a few days or weeks,[1,25,26,30,32] although delayed recovery has once been recorded after as much as 4.5 months.[31] A progressive rise of the blood sugar values is an ominous sign,[26] and in a certain number of patients permanent diabetes will ensue. In a review of 27 published reports, Akzhigitov and Strygina[24] found that 210 of 5182 patients (4.0%) with acute pancreatitis had become diabetic; in their own material of 684 cases, the corresponding proportion amounted to 2.3%. Persisting diabetes may be seen in 3 to 10% of such cases according to Barbier *et al.*[26] and in 2% of patients according to Bank and his colleagues.[25] Derot *et al.*[42] observed such an outcome in three of 45 cases (6.7%), Johansen and Ørnsholt[43] in 2 of 22 (18%), and O'Sullivan *et al.*[38] in 7 of 116 patients (6.0%). Miller,[44] however, recorded it only twice among 2855 cases culled from published reports.

While most authors fail to state just how long after acute pancreatitis they tested their patients for diabetes, some have supplied these data. Thus, 12 years after the acute disease, Fomenko[28] found diabetic blood sugar values in 8 of 690 cases (1.2%). Grott[20] followed 20 patients for up to 14 years and saw as many as 5 of them (25%) become diabetic. After an average interval of 12 years, diabetes was noted in 11 of 162 cases (6.8%) recorded by Mathiesen and Rasmussen,[22] and of 115 patients studied by Zakaraya,[33] 2 months to 10 years after acute pancreatitis, 4 had remained diabetic (3.5%). In the series of Bank *et al.*,[25] an impaired glucose tolerance was observed in 10% of cases after 6 weeks. These authors also found that in the few patients that developed permanent diabetes, the exocrine pancreatic function tests were always grossly abnormal, and they suggested that these patients may either have had undiagnosed, preexisting chronic pancreatitis or may have suffered unusually extensive postnecrotic pancreatic fibrosis.

Permanent diabetes following acute pancreatitis is usually of a mild degree; many cases respond to diet alone,[38,45] although some patients do require insulin.[34,38] Bank and co-workers administer insulin only if the symptoms warrant it or if ketosis develops.[25] Low plasma insulin concentrations have been observed, both during the acute, pancreatitic stage [25,46] and in patients who had become permanently diabetic.[43,45] In the latter group, Bank *et al.*[25] also found elevated serum glucagon values.

Very little is known about the incidence of diabetic microangiopathy, and of other diabetic complications, in patients whose diabetes was caused by acute pancreatitis. On clinical grounds, Verdonk *et al.*[47] recently observed retinopathy or nephropathy in 4 of 22 of their patients (18%) within this category. They found the occurrence of microangiopathy significantly correlated with the duration of the diabetic state. Morphologic studies of such cases are yet to be recorded.

Although slight to moderate hyperglycemia and glucosuria are rather common in acute pancreatitis, as has been discussed, diabetic coma due to acute pancreatitis is distinctly rare. In a review of the literature written in 1961, Hughes[48] found 57 cases of diabetic coma in association with acute pancreatitis to which he added 1 case of his own. There was preexisting diabetes in 40 of these 58 patients, while the remaining 18 had not been diabetic. More recent reviews of this topic were published by Gülzow and Bibergeil,[37] Hayduk *et al.*,[29] a'nd Nielsen and Simonsen[31] ; the former authors added 7 personal cases, all patients without preexisting diabetes. Pertinent case reports[49-55] continue to be published, including some documenting an association of acute pancreatitis with hyperosmolar, nonketotic diabetic coma.[35,53,54,56-58] In these latter cases, a block in ketogenesis or the presence of liver cell damage have been suggested as pathogenetic mechanisms.[37]

Patients with coexisting acute pancreatitis and diabetic coma tend to have excessively high blood glucose values. The blood amylase activity is usually elevated, but cases with normal or even subnormal figures (attributed to necrosis of the entire pancreas) have been observed.[37] Furthermore, patients with diabetic coma not associated with pancreatitis also commonly show considerably enhanced amylase (but not lipase) values, thought to reflect an activation of liver amylase.[59] Although insulin will normalize the very high blood glucose concentrations in comatose, pancreatitic patients within 6 to 72 hr[37] the prognosis in such cases is very poor; only 6 of the 29 patients discussed in the review of Nielsen and Simonsen[31] survived, and 4 of the 6 became permanently diabetic. This represents a mortality rate of 79.3%; in contrast, acute pancreatitis alone is associated with a mortality ranging from 8 to 20%.[29]

Chronic Pancreatitis and Diabetes

It is not easy to determine how often chronic pancreatitis actually occurs. While the average incidence with which this condition was diagnosed on clinical grounds in the medical departments of three Central European university hospitals amounted to only 0.07% (with a range from 0.036 to 0.194%),[18] Haenel and Heuser,[60] on the other hand, termed chronic pancreatitis "one of the most common diseases" and found it in 169 (18.6%) unselected hospital patients. Their criterion for diagnosis was a urine amylase figure elevated to at least 256 Wohlgemuth units, but it would appear to be questionable whether this can simply be equated with "chronic pancreatitis." In autopsy studies, chronic pancreatitis has been found in 6 to 8% of the total,[23] but the histological criteria vary, and "the true incidence of pathologic changes in the pancreas depends on how carefully one looks for them."[23] Pancreatic fibrosis of varying degrees, frequently the endstage of chronic inflammatory disease, was present in 234 of 1000 consecutive autopsies (23.4%) examined by Woldman *et al.*[61] On the other hand, considerable arterio- or arteriolosclerosis can often be found in the pancreas associated with fibrosis, indicating a vascular, rather than inflammatory, basis for this lesion.[1]

In general, pancreatic lithiasis is of rare occurrence. Earlier autopsy studies reviewed by Lazarus and Volk[1] showed an incidence ranging from 0.0057 to 0.072%. More recently, somewhat higher figures have been recorded. Thus, Doerr[23] stated that no more than 1 case with pancreatic stones may be found for every 1000 autopsies performed; Shaper[13] encountered calculi in 4 of 3500 necropsies (0.11%), and Stobbe *et al.*[15] reported 43 cases in a series of 27,787 autopsies (0.15%). A much higher incidence of pancreatic lithiasis is found when the pancreas is examined for stones radiologically,[1] especially in certain parts of the world where many patients with diabetes due to chronic calcifying pancreatitis are seen; in Uganda, for example, Shaper[13] demonstrated the presence of pancreatic calculi in 8% of his diabetic cases.

The occurrence of diabetes mellitus in a patient with chronic calcifying pancreatitis has first been described in 1788 by Cawley.[62] During the past 15 years, the relationship of chronic pancreatitis and diabetes has been the subject of an ever increasing number of case reports from all parts of the world[63-80] as well as of numerous, more or less comprehensive review articles.[1,4,25,26,30,32,34,38,42,44,60,69,70,81-91] One is forced to suspect, from the sheer number of publications alone, that chronic pancreatitis is frequently associated with diabetes. But before the relationship between the two conditions will be explored in detail, it may be advantageous to briefly review what is known about the etiology of chronic pancreatitis.

In a survey of etiologic factors operative in pancreatitis, Colbert[17] distinguishes a "major" group (with cholelithiasis, alcoholism, the postoperative state, and idiopathic cases) from a "minor" one (to which hyperparathyroidism, hyperlipemia, trauma, pregnancy, drugs, and hereditary forms of the disease belong). Clark,[64] addressing himself specifically to possible causes of the calcifying variety of chronic pancreatitis, enumerated the following entities: alcoholism, malnutrition, hereditary pancreatitis with aminoaciduria, fibrocystic disease of the pancreas, hypercalcemia in hyperparathyroidism, abdominal trauma, and mumps virus infection. Most other authors offer similar, if not identical and usually shorter, lists, but some startling quantitative differences emerge as one moves around the globe.

In the industrialized countries of the Western world, alcoholism usually—but not invariably—tops the roster. In France, this has been confirmed in several series of cases,[9-11,21,70] especially for the calcifying form; thus, Sarles *et al.*[21] noted that at least 94 of 100 patients with radiologically determined pancreatic lithiasis were alcoholics. In Germany, Creutzfeldt and co-workers[18] found alcoholism in 9 of 20 cases of chronic calcifying pancreatitis, and cholelithiasis in 4; Haenel and Heuser,[60] on the other hand, implicated biliary tract disease in 47.5% of their patients. Alcoholism was of no major concern in one study of chronic pancreatitis recorded in Ireland[92]; there, it applied to only 4 of 53 cases (7.5%). In the United States, Minagi and Margolin[7] stated that 75 to 90% of all patients with calcifying pancreatitis are alcoholics, while Howard[86] put the figure at 80%; O'Sullivan *et al.,*[38] however, listed biliary tract disease in 37% of their patients and alcoholism in only 19%, but these authors combined cases of acute and chronic pancreatitis in their evaluation. Woldman and colleagues,[61] also in the United States, encountered bile duct disease in 87 of 234 patients (37.2%) with pancreatic fibrosis seen at autopsy, while they confessed uncertainty about the incidence of alcoholism in their material. An unusually large study of 900 South African cases of chronic pancreatitis has recently been analyzed by Bank *et al.,*[25,93] who listed alcoholism in 60% of all cases and in 90% of those with the calcifying variety; gallstones were present in 10%, miscellaneous causes in 16%, and no etiology could be determined in the remaining 14% of patients. Alcohol appears to play an important role in Japan, too; it affected 6 of 10 persons with pancreatic lithiasis observed by Horiuchi *et al.,*[85] as well as "some" of the 17 patients with pancreatic lithiasis examined by Funakoshi and co-workers.[94]

A situation different from that detailed above prevails in tropical countries. Of 100 patients with chronic calcifying pancreatitis from the state of Kerala in southern India, 98 were nonalcoholics, and the gallbladder proved normal each time it was examined.[5] No alcoholism existed in 45 Nigerian cases with this disease, while more than 90% of these patients gave a history of protein malnutrition.[90] Other reports from Nigeria[6,95] and some from Zaire,[14,96] Uganda,[13,97] and Indonesia[98] also emphasize the pivotal role of protracted protein deficiency in the causation of chronic relapsing pancreatitis in tropical regions. However, alcohol has been implicated as an important contributory factor in Uganda, where 19 of 36 Africans (53%) with the disease indulged in "episodic heavy drinking,"[97] and in Rhodesia, where most native patients observed by Wicks[99] and Wicks and Clain[100] consumed large quantities of home-brewed beer which has an alcohol concentration of 19 g/liter, and where evidence of childhood or adult malnutrition was meager.

In a discussion on the etiology and geographical distribution of chronic calcifying pancreatitis, Sarles[9] recently summarized the situation as follows: "The disease seems to be particularly related to two main conditions: alcoholism (specially in countries where individuals are fed a high-protein, high-fat diet), and malnutrition. A possible combination of alcoholism and malnutrition is not evident from the information provided." Howard[86] has emphasized the differences between alcoholic and gallstone pancreatitis. He found that the former was a disease of younger people, mainly males with an average age of 36 years, while gallstone pancreatitis affected mainly women whose mean age was 53 years; also, many if not most of the patients with alcoholic pancreatitis go on to develop pancreatic lithiasis, diabetes, and steatorrhea, while only few of those with gallstone pancreatitis do. The possible role of viruses in the pathogenesis of pancreatic disease and diabetes mellitus has recently been reviewed by Craighead[101] ; while he deemed it likely that the pancreas "is affected in viral disease far more commonly than is recognized clinically," those viruses that have been implicated in the causation of diabetes in man (mumps, rubella, and Coxsackie virus Group B) apparently damage the B cells of the islets of Langerhans directly and do not generally induce significant chronic pancreatitis. Both clinically and histologically, chronic pancreatitis on a familial basis does not differ from nongenetic types of the disease; the mode of transmission is non-sexlinked and appears to be autosomal dominant.[102]

Pancreatic calcification is common in persons with chronic pancreatitis. Bank *et al.*[25] found it in 235 of their 900 patients (26.1%) and Pelaez Redondo,[4] in a review paper, in 47 to 50% of all cases with this disease. The combined figures from 8 other published studies[11,18,26,32,34,84,103,104] indicate that 169 of 555 chronic pancreatitis patients, or 30.4%, had the calcifying form; the reported incidences range from a low of 9.4%[103] to a high of 74.4%.[11]

In general, chronic calcifying pancreatitis affects younger adults, and many more men than women. In Sarles' study in France,[21] there were 93 men and 7 women ranging in age from 22 to 67 years, with a mean age of 38.4 years. Creutzfeldt *et al.,*[18] in Germany, found the condition in 16 men (mean age 38.6 years) and 4 women (mean age 61.7 years). In 56 cases of chronic relapsing pancreatitis, 22 of them with calcifications, recorded by Gambill *et al.*[104] in the United States, the sex ratio was 4.3 to 1, male to female. Among 68 patients with calcifying pancreatitis collected in Japan,[105] there were twice as many men as there were women, and most patients were between 40 and 50 years old. Of the 100 patients of Geevarghese and co-workers[5] in India, 61 were less than 25 years old, and 64 were male. In the same country, Moorthy *et al.*[106] examined 11 men and 3 women with chronic calcifying pancreatitis; 10 of these patients were 30 years of age or younger. In Malawi, most Africans with this disease were in the fourth decade of their lives, most Asians in the fifth or sixth.[107] In Nigeria, Kinnear[6] observed 30 patients (19 males and 11 females) of whom 20 were less than 20 years old; also in Nigeria, 31 of 45 patients (26 males, 19 females) in Olurin and Olurin's study[90] were in that age group. Shaper,[97] in Uganda, found 28 male and 8 female patients with this condition; their ages ranged from 12 to 54 years (mean age 33 years). Reports from the Congo,[14,96] from Rhodesia,[99] and from Indonesia[98] indicate a similar age pattern and a comparable sex ratio.

Disturbances in carbohydrate metabolism ranging from abnormal glucose tolerance tests to overt diabetes are very common in patients with chronic pancreatitis, especially in those with the calcifying variety. The large body of data from the past 15 years documenting the frequency of this association will now be reviewed in geographical order. In France, Darnaud[83] found that 69 of 179 (39%) patients with chronic pancreatitis, culled from 12 different reports, were diabetic; Derot *et al.*[42] and Tutin[91] gave a ratio of 30 to 50%. Grott[20] saw 20 diabetics among 57 patients (35%) and stated that the longer the pancreatitis existed, the greater was the likelihood of developing diabetes (35% of his patients did so 6 to 10 years after acute or subacute exacerbation of their disease). Lescut[88,108] recorded disturbances of the carbohydrate metabolism in 66 of 115 cases (57.4%) of chronic pancreatitis; 32 of these (27.8%) displayed permanent, 20 (17.4%) "intermittent," and 14 (12.2%) latent diabetes. In the material of Potet et al.,[109] 8 of 16 histologically studied cases of chronic pancreatitis had a disturbance of the carbohydrate metabolism. Sarles et al.[11,12,21] analyzed 73 patients with the calcifying form of the disorder; 21 (28.8%) were overtly and 32 (43.8%) latently diabetic. Vachon and Abry[110] found 8 diabetics (34.8%) and 7 "paradiabetics" (30.4%) among 23 cases of calcifying chronic pancreatitis; of 61 patients with the noncalcifying type, only 2 (3.3%) had diabetes and 15 (24.6%) "paradiabetes." In Belgium, 21 of 41 chronic pancreatitis patients (51.2%) observed by Barbier et al.[26] were diabetic, but in 15 of them the fasting blood sugar values did not exceed 150 mg/100 ml. In Germany, Bartelheimer[27] recorded a lowered glucose tolerance in 28 of 202 patients with chronic pancreatitis (13.9%), while Ammann,[111] in Switzerland, found disturbances of the carbohydrate metabolism in as many as 31 of 35 (88.6%) patients suffering from this disease; of these, 10 (28.6%) showed an abnormal glucose tolerance test and 21 (60.0%) presented with overt diabetes. All but 1 of 20 persons (95.0%) with calcifying pancreatitis seen in Germany by Creutzfeldt et al.[18] were diabetics. Among the 43 cases with chronic pancreatitis reported by Strohmeyer and co-workers,[34] 16 (37.2%) had overt and 10 (23.3%) latent diabetes; 14 of the 19 patients (73.7%) with the calcifying form were diabetic. These authors also reviewed the literature prior to 1974 and found that the recorded incidence of diabetes in chronic calcifying pancreatitis ranged from a low of 9.2% to a high of 88.8%. Diabetes was present in 16 (7.9%), with a decreased glucose tolerance seen in another 57 (28.2%), out of 202 patients with chronic pancreatitis examined by Müller-Wieland,[112] and of 169 persons with chronic pancreatitis diagnosed by Haenel and Heuser,[60] 32 (18.9%) were listed as overtly and 107 (63.3%) as latently diabetic. In Switzerland, Dettwyler[84] and Martin and Dettwyler[89] stated that 9 of 28 cases (32.1%) with the disease had latent and 12 (42.9%) overt diabetes. Silva Pozo et al.[32] in Spain, found an incidence of 58.3% (14 of 24 patients were diabetic, including all 4 cases with the calcifying variety). Also in Spain, Pelaez Redondo[4] reviewed the literature in 1971 and recorded diabetes in 8 to 70% and latent diabetes in 27 to 75% of cases. While only 4 of 53 (7.5%) persons with chronic pancreatitis examined in Ireland by Fitzgerald et al.[28] were diabetic, 2 of the 5 patients (40.0%) with the calcifying form were so classified.

In the United states, Classen and Hooper[19] saw diabetes develop in 3 of 18 patients (16.7%) with chronic relapsing pancreatitis, while Gambill et al.[104] encountered this in 30 of 56 (53.6%) of their cases. Howard[86] culled 404 cases of pancreatic calcification from 118 different publications and calculated that 34% were associated with diabetes. Woldman[61] recorded 31 instances of diabetes among 234 cases of sclerosing pancreatitis found at autopsy (13.2%). In a review of the literature by Miller,[44] 41 of 322 patients (12.7%) with noncalcifying and 119 of 263 persons (45.2%) with calcifying pancreatitis had diabetes.

Sato and Saitoh[102] collected 70 patients (from 19 families) with familial chronic pancreatitis from the literature and encountered 22 (13.4%) diabetics among them. The Mayo Clinic data analyzed by Stobbe *et al.*[15] indicate that diabetes existed in 5 of 20 persons (25%) with chronic calcifying pancreatitis. In Brazil, 8 cases (61.5%) of overt and 2 (15.4%) of chemical diabetes were present in 13 patients with chronic pancreatitis investigated by Vaissman *et al.*[113] In South Africa, Bank and co-workers[25,93] found overt diabetes in 30%, abnormal glucose tolerance curves in another 20%, and normal glucose tolerance but low insulin reserves in 25% of 665 patients with noncalcific chronic pancreatitis; for the 235 persons with the calcifying form of the disease, the incidences were as follows: overt diabetes, 70%; abnormal glucose tolerance, 20%; normal glucose tolerance but reduced insulin reserve, 8%. In Japan, Funakoshi *et al.*[94] found diabetes in 15 of their 17 patients (88.2%) with chronic calcifying pancreatitis and in 50 to 70% of cases recorded in other Japanese publications. In another review of the literature of that country by Horiuchi and co-workers,[85] "at least" 62 of 102 patients (60.8%) with pancreatic lithiasis were overtly, and another 12 (11.8%) latently, diabetic. Disturbances of carbohydrate metabolism were encountered in 10 of 17 cases (58.8%) of chronic pancreatitis described by Hasamura *et al.*,[3] while 15 of 31 patients (48.4%) with the calcifying form surveyed by Makiyama and Kita[105] had diabetes. According to Oda,[114] 29% of cases with chronic pancreatitis show a disturbance of the carbohydrate metabolism, while 17% display glucosuria.

In the tropics, the incidence of diabetes mellitus in patients with chronic pancreatitis is at least as high as, if not higher than, that encountered in the industrialized countries of the world. All reports reviewed in this paragraph concern the calcifying form of the disease. Olurin and Olurin,[90] in Nigeria, recorded diabetes in 37 of 45 cases (82.2%), while Shaper,[13] in Uganda, diagnosed 12 instances (80.0%) of overt and 3 (20.0%) of latent diabetes among his 15 cases. In the lower Congo River region, Sonnet *et al.*[14] found 16 diabetics (75.0%) and 4 persons with prediabetes (25.0%) in a group of 20 such cases diagnosed radiographically. Finally, 6 of 7 Rhodesian patients (85.7%) investigated by Wicks[99] and 16 of 18 (88.9%) cases of calcifying chronic pancreatitis encountered in Indonesia by Zuidema[98] were listed as diabetics.

The authors of virtually all of the reports just reviewed tacitly assume that pancreatitis comes first, and that diabetes follows as a sequel. This supposition may not necessarily be true, as Dettwyler[84] has emphasized. For example, in 24 of 62 diabetics with pancreatic lithiasis reviewed by Horiuchi *et al.*[85] the presence of diabetes had been known before the pancreatic stones were demonstrated. It is still possible, and even likely, that pancreatitis in most of these patients antedated the development of diabetes, but it would follow, nevertheless, that the true incidence of diabetes secondary to chronic pancreatitis is probably somewhat lower than that reflected in the statistics quoted in the preceding paragraphs.

In the industrialized countries of the world, diabetes resulting from chronic pancreatitis constitutes only a small proportion of all cases of this disease. Canivet and Battesti,[115] in France, found 9 of 933 diabetics (0.96%) in that category, while Derot *et al.*[42] encountered 45 such cases among 2000 hospitalized patients with diabetes (2.25%) who were systematically investigated for the presence of radiologically demonstrable pancreatic calculi. Lescut[88,108] put the incidence at 1.6%. In Spain, Silva Pozo and colleagues[32] analyzed 470 cases of diabetes and encountered 14 with chronic pancreatitis (3.0%). The largest series evaluated in the United States is that of Sprague *et al.*,[116] who found 24 instances of diabetes following chronic pancreatitis in a total of 8000 diabetic patients (0.30%). It is pertinent to note here, however, that there was a positive family history for diabetes mellitus in 6 of the 14 cases of Silva Pozo *et al.*[32] and in 7 of the 24 patients of Sprague and co-workers[116] ; this, again, implies that some cases classified as pancreatogenic diabetes may actually belong to the category of genetically induced diabetes.

In the tropical countries, a much higher proportion of diabetes induced by chronic pancreatitis prevails. In southern India, the 100 cases of pancreatic lithiasis evaluated by Geevarghese *et al.*[5] constituted 14.5% of all diabetics encountered. However, in a second series from India, that of Moorthy and co-workers,[106] only 14 of 890 patients with diabetes (1.6%) had calcifying pancreatitis. In Nigeria, 74 of 830 diabetics (8.9%) seen by Osuntokun[95] and 30 of 226 such cases (13.3%) examined by Kinnear[6] displayed pancreatic calcification. In the Congo region, an incidence of 4.4% (3 of 68) was recorded by Bourgoignie *et al.*,[96] while Sonnet and colleagues[14] encountered calcifying pancreatitis in 10 of 65 diabetic Congolese Bantus (15.4%). Finally, in Rhodesia, Wicks and Clain[100] discovered no fewer than 25 chronic pancreatitis patients in a series of 107 consecutively examined African diabetics; the resulting incidence of 23.4% appears to be the highest on record.

Diabetes resulting from chronic pancreatitis has certain clinical characteristics that set it apart from the average case of genetic diabetes. Numerous authors[4-6,11-14,25-27,32,42,44,63,72,83,84,87,89,96,98,100,103,108,110,113,116-123] have addressed themselves in a more or less comprehensive manner to this subject, or to some aspect of it. What follows will be an attempt to briefly describe the composite picture that emerges from these clinical observations.

Since chronic pancreatitis, including the calcific variant, effects comparatively young, predominantly male individuals—a fact amply documented above—those persons that go on to become diabetic are also younger than the average patient with genetically determined, maturity-onset diabetes, and most of them are males. Ideally, a family history of diabetes is lacking, but diabetes in the family may fortuitously coincide with chronic diabetes in a given propositus, as has been noted. The data reviewed here, however, do not support Koch's[87] contention that "permanent diabetes will manifest itself in pancreatitis only if the patient is already genetically predisposed toward the development of diabetes."

How much time must elapse after the first bout of pancreatitis has occurred and before diabetes appears? Many authors found that diabetes is usually a late manifestation of the disease.[26,27,44,82] Dettwyler[84] was more specific and stated that diabetes occurs, on the average, 7 years after the first digestive symptoms of pancreatitis have been noted. Bank *et al.*[25] estimated that 2% of all patients will develop diabetes as early as after the very first attack of chronic pancreatitis; but they also reported that the last episode of pancreatitis-induced abdominal pain may antedate the onset of diabetes by as much as 1 or 2 decades. While calcifications become visible in radiographs 6 months to several years after the first signs of pancreatitis,[11] Lescut[99,108] recorded the advent of diabetes in 4 cases within less than 6 months after the onset of pancreatitis. Sprague *et al.*[116] listed the following intervals between first pancreatitic symptoms and diagnosis of diabetes: less than 1 year, five cases; 1 to 5 years, 4 cases; 6 to 10 years, 6 cases; 11 to 15 years, 3 cases; 16 to 20 years, 2 cases; and more than 20 years, 4 cases. In the experience of Vaissman *et al.*,[113] the average interval in 8 cases of overt diabetes amounted to 5.7 years. Finally, Vachon and co-workers[110,123] recorded cases with an early onset of diabetes (interval of 1 to 3 years) and some with a late manifestation of this complication (16 and 20 years); these authors also emphasized that the earlier the onset of diabetes, the more severe its manifestations tend to be.

Diabetes in patients with chronic pancreatitis has an insidious onset and tends to be slowly progressive.[25,83,84,89,118] In a few cases, diabetes is transient and may even disappear spontaneously,[26,89,118] possibly owing to insular tissue regeneration.[84] Sprague and co-workers[116] emphasized that the diabetes becomes more severe with flare-ups of the pancreatitis and ameliorates as the attacks subside. Polyuria is usually absent.[89] Blood sugar values rarely exceed 200 or 250 mg/100 ml[26,83,88,108,110,123] and the average daily loss of glucose in the urine is less than 20 to 30 g.[26,83,110,123] Of 44 cases of pancreatogenic diabetes reviewed by Darnaud,[83] 24 were classified as mild, 16 as moderate, and 4 as severe; of 7 cases evaluated by Baikalov *et al.*,[117] 2 were listed as mild, 4 as moderate, and 1 as severe. Other authors also characterized their cases as "mild"[26,27,118] or "moderate."[42,88,96,103,108]

While pancreatitis-induced diabetes is thus quite subdued in its clinical manifestations, it is, nevertheless, also characterized by its instability,[4,25,26,44,71,83,84,89] and wide variations of the blood glucose concentration may be encountered within the same patient. Ketoacidosis and coma have been observed[4,5,14,26,71,72,84,89] but, on the whole, coma is uncommon, possibly because of the nonavailability of fat stores in these patients,[25] many of whom are malnourished. Much more frequently seen is hypoglycemic shock,[13,14,25,26,84,89,112,119–121,124] especially after insulin injections. Factors that have been proposed as the causes of the hypoglycemia in these patients include: An unusual sensitivity to insulin,[4,25] a lack of pancreatic glucagon stores,[124] and islet cell neoformation and hyperplasia.[119–121] Bank *et al.*[25] also list such potential factors as insulin leakage from damaged β cells, trapped or unavailable hepatic glycogen stores, alcohol-induced hypoglycemia, and an irregular caloric supply secondary to alcoholism or variable absorption due to steatorrhea. While Bank and colleagues[25] stated that "the development of diabetes is the single most lethal event in the long-term prognosis of alcoholic chronic pancreatitis," it is hypoglycemic shock that provides the mechanism through which many of these patients actually die. Once hypoglycemia occurs, it tends to be severe and quite resistant to therapy[25,84,89] ; the patient whose pancreas is illustrated in Fig. 1 belonged into this category.

Laboratory examinations have added further data that help characterize the diabetic state secondary to chronic pancreatitis. Martin and Dettwyler[89] found no increase in the blood cholesterol and lipid values; 1 year later, Dettwyler[84] reported that as many as 40% of his cases of pancreatogenic diabetes, but only 8% of patients with the idiopathic form of the disease, had blood cholesterol concentrations of less than 180 mg/100 ml. In 1970, Joffe *et al.*[122] found significantly lower mean fasting cholesterol and phospholipid levels in 20 such patients; the mean fasting triglyceride values were also lower than in matched groups of essential diabetics and nondiabetic controls, but not significantly so. The blood amylase levels are of no value in assessing cases with chronic pancreatitis; while Dettwyler[84] recorded generally normal amylase activities in such patients, elevated activities of this enzyme have been found in

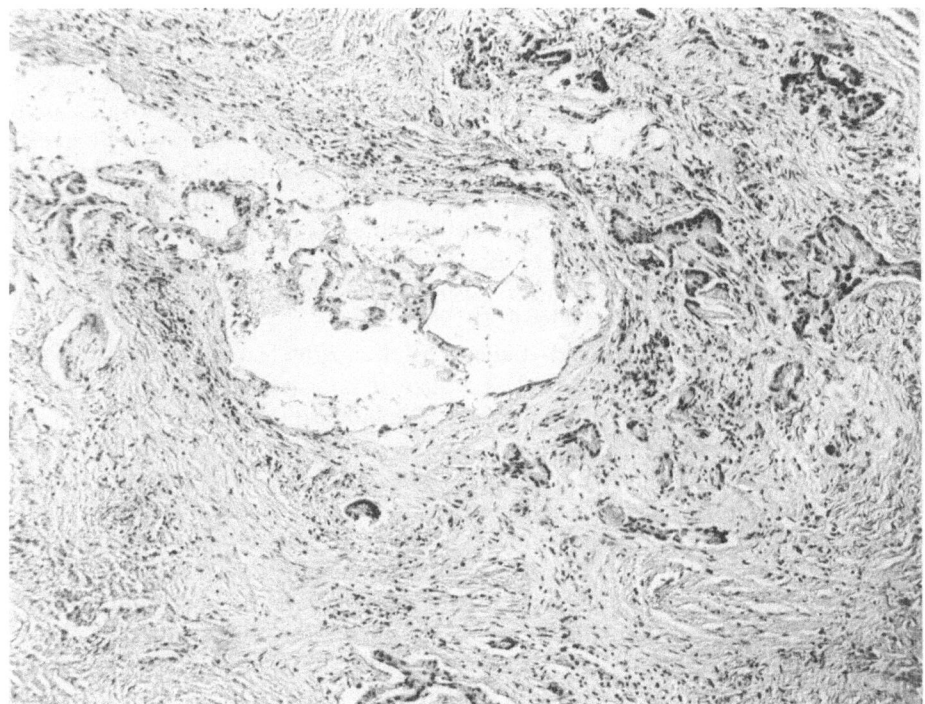

Figure 1. Pancreas of 47-year-old man with chronic relapsing pancreatitis. Most of the exocrine pancreatic glands have been replaced by dense fibrous tissue. Sparse round cell accumulations are present. Calcified detritus is visible in a dilated duct. The patient had been diabetic for at least 2 decades. There was no family history of diabetes and no personal history of alcoholism. The bile ducts were free of disease. The patient died in intractable hypoglycemic shock. Decalcified section, hematoxylin and eosin stain. ×95. Reproduced at 105%.

individuals with poorly controlled diabetes without any evidence of pancreatitis.[125]

Hormone assays have shown that while patients with pancreatogenic diabetes may have low,[25,126] normal,[3,25,87,127] or even elevated[3,87] fasting blood insulin values, there is no rise, or a decidedly subnormal one at best, in their insulin levels after maximal β cell stimulation with glucose, glucagon, secretin, pancreozymin, or tolbutamide.[25,34,82,126-128] In a study reported by Joffe *et al.*,[128] this pertained even to patients with normal glucose tolerance curves, for their maximum mean insulin output after stimulation (273 $\pm$ 80 μU/ml, at 40 min) was significantly below that of the control subjects (867 $\pm$ 79 μU at 35 min). Terms such as "acquired insulinopenia,"[128] "impaired insulin reserve,"[25] and "low-output diabetes"[51] have therefore been employed in order to characterize the diabetic state observed in cases of chronic pancreatitis. Furthermore, in studies conducted in South Africa, 16% of such patients were found to have severely reduced glucagon reserves,[25] and all of six individuals with diabetes secondary to chronic calcific pancreatitis responded to induced insulin hypoglycemia with significantly impaired peak human growth hormone levels.[129] The human growth hormone responses to arginine in these patients were also lower but were not significantly different from those in control subjects.

Since diabetes in persons with chronic pancreatitis is primarily characterized by reduced insulin stores, treatment with oral antidiabetic drugs—which is predicated upon the availability of sufficient insulin reserves in the islets of Langerhans—is not likely to be effective. This has, in fact, been found by a number of authors[14,26,89]; nevertheless, others reported satisfactory control with oral hypoglycemic agents in at least some[13,71,76,84,88,108,111,117] or even many[103] of their patients. Bank *et al.*[25] propose that oral treatment should be given a trial before insulin therapy is commenced since their endocrine studies have shown that the pancreas in these cases is still able to produce some insulin. For the majority of patients, however, insulin will be required; the recommended daily dosage is generally in the vicinity of 20 to 30 U, although values as low as 10 and as high as 50 U/day have been recorded,[14,26,44,84,88,89,96,108,113] In some of the tropical countries, many patients with calcifying chronic pancreatitis require as much as 65, 80, or even more units of insulin per day.[6,13,90] It is pertinent to note here that the South African authors[25,122] warn of the danger of inducing irreversible hypoglycemic shock and prefer to keep their patients hyperglycemic until and unless symptoms necessitate more vigorous treatment.

While ultrastructural studies of pancreatic changes in individuals suffering from pancreatogenic diabetes have not been recorded to date, the light-microscopic alterations in this organ (Fig. 1) have been the subject of a fairly large number of reports.[7,9,11-14,21,26,36,61,66,84,95,104,109,119,120,122,127] Always present is fibrosis of various degrees; in the earlier stages, fibrosis is predominantly perilobular and periductal, but in more advanced cases, interacinar fibrosis is readily demonstrable as well. At times, residual foci of necrosis[104] and chronic inflammatory infiltrates,[7,95,104] consisting in the main of lymphocytes, plasma cells, and histiocytes, may be seen, but signs of inflammation are more often than not rather subdued or altogether lacking.[11,13] Associated with the fibrotic process are distortion, dilatation, atrophy, and eventual disappearance of many of the exocrine acini in numerous lobules. The pancreatic ducts appear distended and soon contain eosinophilic proteinaceous material which subsequently calcifies; as mentioned in the first paragraph of this review, the epithelial cells lining such cystically dilated ducts often perish so that the intraductal location of the pancreatic calculi is no longer readily discernible. Pancreatic perineural inflammatory infiltrates and degenerative nerve lesions, as observed by Sarles,[9] may, in part, be responsible for the episodic attacks of pancreatalgia that characterizes chronic relapsing pancreatitis.[5,6,25,118] Also described were cases displaying hyperplasia of the centroacinar cells,[66] epidermoid metaplasia of the ductal epithelium,[66] or fatty, rather than fibrotic, replacement of the glandular acini.[13] Finally, Blumenthal *et al.*[36] found a fivefold increase in the incidence of proliferative lesions of the small (pancreatic and extrapancreatic) blood vessels (principally arteries and arterioles) in patients with preexisting diabetes who subsequently developed chronic relapsing pancreatitis; they postulate that small vessel disease may be at the root of the pancreatitic process, at least in these cases.

Histologic changes pertaining to the islets of Langerhans in patients with chronic pancreatitis and diabetes have also been recorded. Several authors have described hyperplasia, hypertrophy, or neoformation of islet cells.[11,13,26,84,119-121] The number of islets was found relatively increased in 19 and reduced in 33 cases studied by Sarles *et al.*[21] While Shaper[13] reported hydropic degeneration and fibrosis of the islets, neither degenerative alterations nor degranulation were observed in 8 cases carefully investigated by Potet and co-workers,[109] who also registered a relative decrease in the number of B cells in relation to the A cells of their patients. And yet, all authors appear to be unanimous in their opinion that there exists no correlation between the severity of the diabetic state, as observed clinically, and the extent or severity of either the endocrine[12,21,26,84] or exocrine[14,84,109,127] morphologic lesions in the pancreas.

Lazarus and Volk,[1] in an earlier review of this topic, concluded that "diabetes resulting from chronic pancreatitis differs from ordinary diabetes by the absence of the complicating diseases which are characteristic of the idiopathic type." During the past 15 years, however, it has become evident that such complicating diseases do occur, even though their incidence is lower than in genetically determined diabetes.[25,84,88,89,108,113,116,129-132] Among these complications, diabetic (poly)neuropathy is comparatively common[85,89]; it occurred in approximately 30% of the 900 chronic pancreatitis patients observed by Bank *et al.*,[25] in 1 of 14 cases (7.1%) seen by Moorthy and co-workers,[106] in 2 of 37 individuals (5.4%) surveyed by Olurin and Olurin,[90] in 5 of 20 cases (25%) reported by Shaper,[13] in 1 of 24 patients (4.2%) in the study of Sprague *et al.*,[116] and in 2 of 18 persons (11.1%) examined by Tutin.[91] A factor complicating the evaluation of the incidence of polyneuropathy in subjects with diabetes secondary to chronic pancreatitis is that alcoholism, present in many of them, may also induce neuropathy,[84,89] as may pancreatitis per se.[84] Nevertheless, an examination of the time relationship involved lead Bank *et al.*[25] to conclude that neuropathy in the great majority of their cases was secondary to diabetes and not to alcoholism.

None of the vascular complications observed in pancreatogenic diabetes is more frequently encountered than is retinopathy, even though Bour *et al.*[130] deemed it much less common than in idiopathic diabetes. It was seen in 10 of 62 patients (16.1%) investigated by Horiuchi *et al.*[85] in 4 of 66 cases (6.1%) recorded by Lescut,[88,108] in 1 of 14 persons (7.1%) examined by Moorthy and co-workers,[106] in 1 of 24 patients (4.2%) described by Sprague *et al.*,[116] and in 3 of Tutin's[91] 18 cases (16.7%). Clinically evident retinopathy or nephropathy was said to have been present in 20 of 146 individuals (13.7%) investigated by Verdonk and colleagues.[47] While 4 of 71 (5.6%) Nigerian diabetics with pancreatitis had diabetic retinopathy, this held true for 35 of 758 (4.6%) Nigerian diabetics who did not suffer from chronic pancreatitis.[8] In a South African study of this kind, however, the incidence was 7.4% (2 of 27) for diabetics with pancreatitis versus 30% in matched diabetics without this disease.[132]

The least commonly encountered vascular complication in diabetes following chronic pancreatitis is diabetic nephropathy. While some cases have been so classified on the basis of clinical data,[47,84,85,116] it appears that only 4 histologically proven examples of nodular (specific) intercapillary glomerulosclerosis (Kimmelstiel-Wilson) (Fig. 2) have thus far been recorded.[16,133–135] Five more instances have been described in an abstract published in 1969 by Ennis *et al.*,[136] but histological documentation of these cases has not appeared in print. The 5 cases of Ennis and co-workers were found in a series of 46 patients with chronic relapsing pancreatitis, which would give an incidence of 10.9%.

Occasionally, still other complications attributable to diabetes have been recorded in individuals with chronic pancreatitis. Thus, Clarke[64] described an instance of amyotrophy, and cataracts were found in 1 of 20 (5.0%) such patients investigated by Shaper[13] as well as in 4 of 37 (10.9%) persons examined by Olurin and Olurin.[90] It is perhaps also noteworthy that as many as 25% of the 900 patients surveyed by Bank *et al.*[25] had tuberculosis.

The question of why vascular complications are comparatively less prevalent in pancreatogenic diabetes has been of interest to many investigators.[25,42,47,84,89,122,129–131,137] The most obvious explanation given implicates the chronological factors involved. The development of vascular complications in diabetes is clearly related to time[8,42,47]; the necessary mean interval between the onset of pancreatogenic diabetes and the appearance of vascular complications was variously estimated, or calculated, to be 7,[130] 13,[84] or 10 to 15[89] years. Patients with diabetes secondary to chronic pancreatitis tend to be comparatively young, and they have a significantly reduced life expectancy[89]; in Dettwyler and Martin's study[84] death occurred after an average duration of 7.5 years so that many, if not most, of these patients never reach the age at which diabetic vascular complications ordinarily manifest themselves.

Other factors implicated in the reduced incidence of such complications in these patients include the deficient growth hormone levels recorded by Vinik *et al.*[129] and especially the low blood lipid concentrations observed in many of

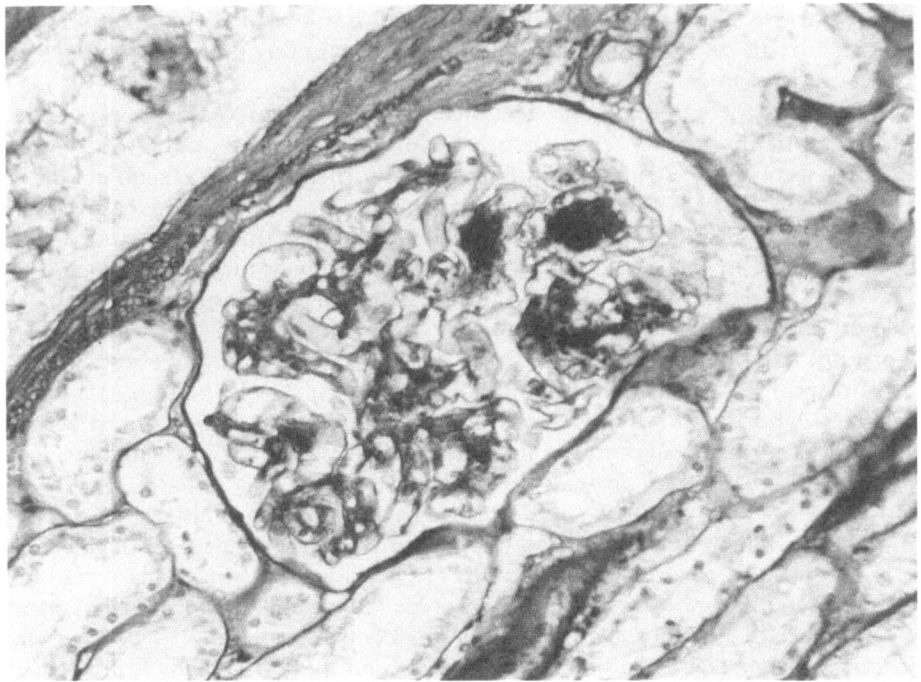

Figure 2. Renal cortical tissue of patient represented in Fig. 1. Nodular (specific) intercapillary glomerulosclerosis (Kimmelstiel–Wilson) as well as moderate thickening of the tubular basement membranes are present. Periodic acid Schiff and hematoxylin stain. ×375. Reproduced at 105%.

them; they may help retard the development of vasculopathy.[25,84,122] Low caloric intake because of diarrhea and steatorrhea secondary to exocrine pancreatic insufficiency has also been thought to be important.[25,131]

References

1. Lazarus, S. S., and Volk, B. W.: *The Pancreas in Human and Experimental Diabetes.* Grune & Stratton, New York, 1962, pp. 177 and 182.
2. Mahadeven, R.: *Brit. Med. J.,* 1:626, 1961.
3. Hasumura, Y., Sawabu, N., Hayakawa, H., Nishimura, K., and Hirose, S.: *Saishin Igaku,* 27:994, 1972.
4. Pelaez Redondo, J.: *Rev. Esp. Enferm. Apar. Dig.,* 34:289, 1971.
5. Geevarghese, P. J., Pillai, V. K., Joseph, M. P., and Pitchumoni, C. S.: *J. Assoc. Phys. India,* 10:173, 1962.
6. Kinnear, T. W. G.: *E. Afr. Med. J.,* 40:288, 1963.
7. Minagi, H., and Margolin, F. R.: *Amer. J. Gastroenterol.,* 57:139, 1972.
8. Osuntokun, B. O.: *Brit. J. Ophthalmol.,* 53:652, 1969.
9. Sarles, H., *Gastroenterology,* 66:604, 1974.
10. Sarles, H., Muratore, R., Sarles, J. C., Guien, C., and Camatte, R.: *Dtsch. Med. Wochenschr.,* 87:125, 1962.

11. Sarles, H., and Sarles, J. C.: *Verh. Dtsch. Ges. Inn. Med.,* **70**:773, 1964.
12. Sarles, H., Sarles, J. C., Pèze, R., Camatte, R., and Delmont, J.: *Arch. Mal. Appar. Dig.,* **51**:469, 1962.
13. Shaper, A. G.: *Lancet,* **1**:1223, 1960.
14. Sonnet, J., Brisbois, R., and Bastin, J. P.: *Trop. Geogr. Med.,* **18**:97, 1968.
15. Stobbe, K. C., ReMine, W. H., and Baggenstoss, A. H.: *Surg. Gynecol. Obstet.,* **131**:1090, 1970.
16. Tasaka, S., Arai, Y., Shibata, N., Onda, H., Tanaka, M., and Sekiguchi, E.: *Iryo,* **21**:616, 1967.
17. Colbert, R. C.: *Southwestern Med.,* **52**:6, 1971.
18. Creutzfeldt, W., Fehr, H., and Schmidt, H.: *Schweiz. Med. Wochenschr.,* **100**:1180, 1970.
19. Classen, J. N., and Hooper, J.: *Amer. Surg.,* **30**:391, 1964.
20. Grott, J. W.: *Journées Ann. Diab. Hôtel Dieu,* **10**:347, 1969.
21. Sarles, H., Sarles, J. C., Camatte, R., Muratore, R., Gaini, M., Guien, C., Pastor, J., and Le Roy, F.: *Gut,* **6**:545, 1965.
22. Mathiesen, F. R., and Rasmussen, E.: *Acta Chir. Scand.,* **129**:410, 1965.
23. Doerr, W.: *Verh. Dtsch. Ges. Inn. Med.,* **70**:718, 1964.
24. Akzhigitov, G. N., and Strygina, T. A.: *Klin. Med.,* Vol. 46, No. 4, p. 70, 1968.
25. Bank, S., Marks, I. N., and Vinik, A. I.: *Amer. J. Gastroenterol.,* **64**:13, 1975.
26. Barbier, P., Berge, S., and Jacobs, E.: *Acta Gastroenterol. Belg.,* **30**:329, 1967.
27. Bartelheimer, H.: *Verh. Dtsch. Ges. Inn. Med.,* **70**:759, 1964.
28. Fomenko, L. I.: *Klin. Khir.,* **1**:11, 1970.
29. Hayduk, K., Dürr, F., and Schollmeyer, P.: *Dtsch. Med. Wochenschr.,* **93**:913, 1968; *Germ. Med. Monthly,* **13**:432, 1968.
30. Lozano Castañeda, O.: *Rev. Invest. Clin. (Mexico),* **20**:221, 1968.
31. Nielsen, O. S., and Simonsen, E.: *Acta Med. Scand.,* **185**:459, 1969.
32. Silva Pozo, J., Martinez, P. M., Leon, J. V., Carnero, A. P., and Rodriguez, J. V.: *Rev. Esp. Enferm. Apar. Dig.,* **32**:373, 1970.
33. Zakaraya, K. A.: *Khirurgiia,* **41**:94, 1965.
34. Strohmeyer, G., Gottesburen, H., and Behr, C.: *Dtsch. Med. Wochenschr.,* **99**:1481, 1974.
35. Pariente, R., Bignon, J., Liot, F., Labram, C., Chrétien, J., and Brouet, G.: *Bull. Soc. Méd. Hôp. Paris,* **116**:897, 1965.
36. Blumenthal, H. T., Probstein, J. G., and Berns, A. W.: *Arch Surg.,* **87**:844, 1963.
37. Gülzow, M., and Bibergeil, H.: *Med. Klin.,* **62**:496, 1967.
38. O'Sullivan, J. N., Nobrega, F. T., Morlock, C. M., Brown, A. L., Jr., and Bartholomew, L. G.: *Gastroenterology,* **62**:373, 1972.
39. Pérez-Jiménez, F., Hita, J., Cosme, A., Muro, J., and Martinez-Fernandez, A.: *Rev. Clin. Españ.* **132**:171, 1974.
40. Malone, J. I.: *J. Ped.,* **85**:825, 1974.
41. Cywinsky, J. S., Walker, F. A., White, H., and Traisman, H. S.: *Acta Paed. Scand.,* **54**:597, 1965.
42. Derot, M., Bour, H., Tutin, M., and Guy-Grand, B.: *Diabète* **18**:93, 1970.
43. Johansen, K., and Ørnsholt, J.: *Metabolism* **21**:291, 1972.
44. Miller, M.: In: *Diabetes.* Edited by R. H. Williams, P. B. Hoeber, New York, 1960, p. 708.
45. Bagdade, J. D.: *Lancet* **II**:1041, 1969.
46. Rudyi, R. V., and Chaplinsky, V. V.: *Klin. Med.,* Vol. 43, No. 11, p. 77, 1965.
47. Verdonk, C. A., Palumbo, P. J., Gharib, H., and Bartholomew, L. G.: *Diabetologia,* **11**:395, 1975.
48. Hughes, P. O.: *Brit. J. Surg.,* **49**:90, 1961.
49. Andrews, J. T.: *Med. J. Austr.* **II**:582, 1960.
50. Delore, K., and Croizat, B.: *Lyon Méd.,* **215**:503, 1966.
51. Hayduk, K., Kaufmann, W., and Diem, R.: *Med. Welt,* p. 1936, 1968.
52. Maclean, D., Murison, J., and Griffiths, P. D.: *Brit. Med. J.,* **IV**:757, 1973.
53. Rømer, F. K.: *Ugeskr. Laeger,* **133**:1920, 1971.
54. Rømer, F. K.: *Nord. Med.,* **86**:1321, 1971.
55. Witzel, L., Böleskei, P., Porzelt, R., and Haasis, R.: *Med. Welt,* p. 838, 1971.
56. Davidson, A. I.: *Brit. Med. J.,* **I**:356, 1964.

57. Gordon, A. G.: *Brit. J. Clin. Pract.*, **19**:697, 1965.
58. Sjöberg, K. H.: *Läkartidningen*, **63**:2913, 1966.
59. Belfiore, F., and Napoli, E.: *Clin. Chem.*, **19**:387, 1973.
60. Haenel, U., and Heuser, R.: *Münch. Med. Wochenschr.*, **109**:1857, 1967.
61. Woldman, E. E., Fishman, D., and Segal, A. J.: *JAMA*, **169**:1281, 1959.
62. Cawley, T.: *London Med. J.*, **9**:286, 1788.
63. Chudzikiewicz, T.: *Polski Tydg. Lek.*, **19**:1335, 1964.
64. Clarke, S. W.: *Proc. Roy. Soc. Med.*, **59**:856, 1966.
65. Derouiche, F., El Aifa, K. N., Kallal, Z., and Doghri, T.: *Tunisié Méd.*, **52**:101, 1974.
66. Espejo y Gomez de Avellaneda, M.: *Diabète*, **18**:153, 1970.
67. Hirabayashi, H., and Nomura, M.: *Naika*, **20**:982, 1967.
68. Joseph, P. P.: *J. Indian Med. Assoc.*, **44**:35, 1965.
69. Justin-Besançon, L., Lamotte, M., Lamotte-Barrilon, S., Grivaux, M., and Colomb, G.: *Sem. Hôp. Paris*, **36**:753, 1960.
70. Legré, M., Vignoli, R., and Saint-Pierre, A.: *Arch. Mal. Appar. Dig.*, **51**:1447, 1962.
71. Lewis, T. D.: *Austral. New Zeal. J. Med.*, **4**:518, 1974.
72. Meoni, S.: *Atti Accad. Fisiocr. Siena (Medicofis.)*, **14**:501, 1965.
73. Mowar, S. N.: *J. Indian Med. Assoc.*, **45**:386, 1965.
74. Naomé, J.: *Rév. Med. Liège*, **18**:596, 1963.
75. Payet, M., Sankalé, M., Diop, B., Frament, V., Cave, L., Gombert, J., and Rahmi, R.: *Bull. Soc. Méd. Afr. Noire Lang. Franç.*, **11**:456, 1966.
76. Picq, J., and Consigny, P.: *Diabète*, **14**:301, 1966.
77. Shultsev, G. P.: *Klin. Med.*, Vol. 39, No. 6, p. 43, 1961.
78. Staniszewski, J., Tuszewski, F., and Szewczyk, Z.: *Wiad. Lek.*, **23**:2115, 1970.
79. Takaoka, Y.: *Nippon Rinsho*, **25**:2733, 1967.
80. Wenderlich, Z., and Nowak, W.: *Wiad. Lek.*, **25**:2149, 1972.
81. Anonymous: *Journées Ann. Diab. Hôtel Dieu*, **9**:417, 1968.
82. Anonymous: *Lancet*, **II**:1070, 1968.
83. Darnaud, C.: *Révue Int. Hépat.*, **5**:285, 1955.
84. Dettwyler, W.: *Sem. Hôp. Paris*, **40**:1676, 1964.
85. Horiuchi, N., Kitamura, T., Nakagawa, F., Sasaki, A., and Inui, H.: *Nippon Rinsho*, **29**:2146, 1971.
86. Howard, J. M.: In: *Surgical Diseases of the Pancreas*. Edited by J. M. Howard and G. L. Jordan, Jr., Pitman Med., London, 1960, p. 203.
87. Koch, E.: In: *Handbuch des Diabetes Mellitus*. Edited by E. F. Pfeiffer. Munich, 1971, p. 861.
88. Lescut, J., and Fourlinnie, J. C.: *Lille Méd.*, **12**:719, 1967.
89. Martin, E., and Dettwyler, W.: *Journées Ann. Diab. Hôt. Dieu*, **4**:55, 1963.
90. Olurin, E. O., and Olurin, O.: *Brit. Med. J.*, **IV**:534, 1969.
91. Tutin, M.: *Gaz. Méd. France*, **73**:17, 1966.
92. Fitzgerald, O., Fitzgerald, P., Fennelly, J., McMullin, J. P., and Boland, J. S.: *Gut*, **4**:193, 1963.
93. Marks, I. N., and Bank, S.: *S. Afr. Med. J.*, **37**:1039, 1963.
94. Funakoshi, A., *et al.*: *Nippon Rinsho*, **32**:3620, 1974.
95. Osuntokun, B. O.: *J. Neurol. Sci.*, **11**:17, 1970.
96. Bourgoignie, J., Sonnet, J., and Dechef, G.: *Ann. Soc. Belg. Méd. Trop.*, **42**:261, 1962.
97. Shaper, A. G.: *Brit. Med. J.*, **I**:1607, 1964.
98. Zuidema, P. J.: *Trop. Geogr. Med.*, **11**:70, 1959.
99. Wicks, A. C. B.: *Central Afr. J. Med.*, **19**:189, 1973.
100. Wicks, A. C. B., and Clain, D. J.: *Amer. J. Dig. Dis.*, **20**:1, 1975.
101. Craighead, J. E.: *Progr. Med. Virol.*, **19**:161, 1975.
102. Sato, T., and Saitoh, Y.: *Amer. J. Surg.*, **127**:511, 1974.
103. Fitzgerald, O., Fitzgerald, P. and McMullin, J. P.: *Rev. Surg.*, **21**:77, 1964.
104. Gambill, E. E., Baggenstoss, A. H., and Priestley, J. T.: *Gastroenterology*, **39**:404, 1960.
105. Makiyama, H., and Kita, K.: *Naika*, **22**:779, 1968.
106. Moorthy, S. S., Sankaran, K., Varghese, C. V. J., Jeyamitra, D., and Sen, S. B.: *J. Indian Meu. Assoc.*, **59**:57, 1972.

107. Goodall, J. W., and Pilbeam, S. T.: *Trans. Roy. Soc. Trop. Med. Hyg.,* **58**:575, 1964.
108. Lescut, J.: *Lille Méd.,* **13**:46, 1968.
109. Potet, F., Barge, J., and Duclert, N.: *Arch. Anat. Pathol.,* **18**:219, 1970.
110. Vachon, A., and Abry, M.: *Actual. Hépatogast. Hôtel Dieu,* 1964, p. 96.
111. Ammann, R.: *Dtsch. Med. Wochenschr.,* **95**:1, 1970.
112. Müller-Wieland, K.: *Dtsch. Med. Wochenschr.,* **93**:391, 1968.
113. Vaissman, I., Kamel, D., Manhaes H., Veloso, E., and Basser, H. W.: *Arq. Bras. Endocrin. Metab.,* **18**:35, 1969.
114. Oda, M.: *Nippon Rinsho,* **25**:299, 1967.
115. Canivet, J., and Battesti, J. P.: *Diabète,* **5**:191, 1961.
116. Sprague, R. G.: *Proc. Staff Meet. Mayo Clin.,* **22**:553, 1947.
117. Baikalov, L. K., Lemeshko, V. I., and Sokolovsky, A. N.: *Ter. Ark.,* Vol. 36, No. 9, p. 70, 1964.
118. Deuil, R., and Chavanat, B.: *Gaz. Méd. France,* **67**:2241, 1960.
119. Friedlander, E. O.: *Ann. Int. Med.,* **52**:838, 1960.
120. Gepts, W.: In: *14. Symposium der Deutschen Gesellschaft für Endokrinologie.* Springer Verlag, Heidelberg, 1960, p. 101.
121. Halmos, T., Korányi, L., Salamon, F., Szücs, L., and Tarjányi, M.: *Endokrinologie,* **63**:43, 1974.
122. Joffe, B. I., Krut, L., Bank, S., Marks, I. N., and Heller, P.: *Metabolism,* **19**:87, 1970.
123. Vachon, A., Cuffia, S., and Shaaban, M.: *Révue Int. Hépat.* **11**:311, 1961.
124. Joffe, B. I., Bank, S., and Marks, I. N.: *Lancet,* **II**:1038, 1968.
125. Malins, J., and Walsh, C. H.: *Brit. Med. J.,* **IV**:757, 1973.
126. Rogers, J. B., Howard, J. M., and Pairent, F. W.: *Amer. J. Surg.,* **119**:171, 1970.
127. Peters, N., Dick, A. P., Hales, C. N., Orrell, D. H., and Sarner, M.: *Gut,* **7**:277, 1966.
128. Joffe, B. I., Bank, S., Jackson, W. P. U., Keller, P., O'Reilly, I. G., and Vinik, A. I.: *Lancet,* **II**:890, 1968.
129. Vinik, A. I., Joffe, B. I., Joubert, S. M., and Jackson, W. P. U.: *J. Clin. Endocrinol. Metab.,* **31**:86, 1970.
130. Bour, H., Derot, M., Tutin, M., Kopf, A., and Cordelier, J. L.: *Sem. Hôp. Paris,* **47**:2403, 1971.
131. Creutzfeldt, W., and Perings, E.: *Acta Diabet. Lat., Suppl.,* **1**:432, 1972.
132. Sevel, D., Bristow, J. H., Bank, S., Marks, I., and Jackson, P.: *Arch. Ophthalmol.,* **86**:245, 1971.
133. Duncan, L. J. P., MacFarlane, A., and Robson, J. S.: *Lancet,* **I**:822, 1958.
134. Shapiro, F. L., and Smith, H. T.: *Arch. Int. Med.,* **117**:795, 1966.
135. Wellmann, K. F., and Volk, B. W.: *Diabetes,* **25**:713, 1976.
136. Ennis, G., Miller, M., Unger, F. M., and Unger, L.: *Diabetes* **18**:333, 1969.
137. Deckert, T.: *Acta Med. Scand.,* **168**:439, 1960.

Chapter 13

Cancer and Diabetes

Bruno W. Volk and Klaus F. Wellmann

The relationship of cancer and diabetes has been discussed for many years. Despite the large number of studies which have been carried out over the years, no unanimity of opinion has been expressed. Some investigators believed that cancer occurs more frequently in diabetics than in nondiabetic persons, with an incidence ranging from 3 to 10%.[1-4] Others,[5-7] using different figures, arrived at the conclusion that no association between these diseases exists. In 1934, Marble[5] studied the records of 10,000 patients with proven diabetes. Among these 256 (2.56%) had malignant disease. He also investigated the figures of insurance companies and felt that although certain evidence suggested that cancer was more common among diabetic individuals, it was not possible to draw any definite conclusions. In a study of associated causes of death of persons dying of cancer, in Massachusetts, during a 10-year period, Wilson and Maher[1] noted that diabetes and cancer occur together much more frequently than would be expected if the two diseases were independently studied. Ellinger and Landsman,[2] in a survey of 1280 diabetic patients seen at the Montefiore Hospital in New York City from 1933 to 1941, found 39 (3.04%) afflicted with malignant disease. This incidence of cancer was 6.5 times greater than that in the general population (0.46%) in the State of New York in 1941. Jacobson,[3] using data from certificates and matched hospital case histories in New York, concluded that cancer is more common among diabetics than nondiabetics.

While the earlier workers thus felt that cancer occurs more often in diabetic than in nondiabetic patients, more recent surveys indicated that cancer occurs no more frequently in persons with diabetes than in those without it. In a survey of 6317 autopsy records, Herdan[8] observed that malignant tumors occurred in only 10.1% of diabetics, whereas the incidence in nondiabetics was 19.5%. Aronson et al.[9] observed a smaller percentage of intracranial neoplasms in a group of 343 patients with clinically verified diabetes than among 1943 nondiabetic persons (2.9% vs. 11.4%). Furthermore, while gliomas were present in the nondiabetic group in 64 (3.2%), none was observed among the

Bruno W. Volk and Klaus F. Wellmann • Isaac Albert Research Institute of the Kingsbrook Jewish Medical Center, and Downstate Medical Center, State University of New York, Brooklyn, New York. Present address of B. W. V.: University of California, Irvine, California. Present address of K. F. W.: Beekman Downtown Hospital, New York, New York.

diabetic patients. The frequency of benign nongliomatous tumors was the same in both groups. Joslin *et al.,*[10] in 1958, in another study of carcinoma associated with diabetes during the period of 1937 to 1941 by utilizing a modified life table methodology, observed 67 cases, where the expected number was 74.3. In a study of 103,354 patients discharged from the hospital during the period from 1953 to 1961, Steele and Sperling[11] observed an incidence of 6.86% of cancer in 2171 diabetic patients, while the frequency of malignancy was only 2.88% of the total number of discharged individuals. In a series of 1854 diabetic patients on whom autopsies were performed, Warren *et al.*[12] observed 224 cases with carcinoma (12.1%). In view of the fact that according to the National Vital Statistics Division in 1962, cancer accounted for 16% of the total deaths in the United States, the authors concluded that malignancy is neither unduly prevalent nor rare in the diabetic population. Marble and Ramos[13] found that the ratio of deaths from cancer to total deaths in the general population of Massachusetts from 1950 to 1952 (17.0 to 17.6%) was greater than that in diabetic persons (10.7%) in 1956 to 1965. The authors concluded that the lower ratio from cancer associated with diabetes probably reflects the fact that at comparable ages, the life expectancy of diabetic persons is still less than that of individuals in the general population. From the accumulated data it could be concluded that the overall frequency of carcinoma in diabetic individuals appears to be less or does not seem to be significantly different from that in nondiabetic persons.

While there is divergence of opinions as to the coexistance of diabetes and cancer, the incidence of diabetes or impaired carbohydrate tolerance among persons with malignancies seems to be unquestionable. Freund,[14] in 1885, reported the occurrence of hyperglycemia in 62 of 70 patients with cancer. Marks and Bishop[15] observed that the rate of disappearance of glucose after intravenous injection was considerably slower in patients with cancer than that in the control group. Lisker and associates[16] found an abnormal glucose tolerance in 52% of 66 patients with malignant blood dyscrasias as compared with matched controls where the frequency of impaired blood sugar homeostasis was only 8.5%. Edmonson[17] observed impaired glucose tolerance and increased free fatty acid utilization in 20 cachectic patients with advanced cancer in comparison with 17 normal control subjects. Glicksman and associates[18,19] performed standard glucose tolerance tests in 950 consecutive unselected patients with a tissue diagnosis of cancer or with benign lesions. An abnormal blood sugar homeostasis was observed in 36.7% of 628 cancer patients as compared with 9.3% of the control group of 322 individuals having benign neoplasms; 13% of the cancer group and 4.4% of the control series were nondiabetics. When studying the distribution of types of cancer, these authors observed the high frequency of a diabetic response in 64% of 25 patients with cancer of the endometrium and 47% of 32 patients with skin cancer, 44.4% of 18 patients with cancer of the soft tissue, 45.5% of 33 patients with cancer of the floor of the mouth, 54.5% of 11 patients with lymphosarcoma, 50% of 16 patients with Hodgkin's disease, and 70% of 10 patients with cancer of the thyroid gland. Of 5 patients with cancer of the pancreas, 4 had abnormal glucose tolerance tests. Glicksman and associates[19] further observed that patients with endometrial carcinoma had a 64% incidence of abnormal glucose tolerance tests, while those with epidermoid carcinoma of the cervix had only a 16% incidence of impaired blood sugar homeostasis. Similarly, Benjamin and Romney,[20] in study of 50 patients with uterine cervical carcinoma, and 75 patients with carcinoma of the endometrium, observed a higher and statistically greater frequency of diabetes or disturbed glucose tolerance in endometrial carcinomas than in the control subjects without malignancies. The results were similar for two population groups studied, one in New York City and the other in Capetown, South Africa. Benjamin and Casper,[21] in a study of 18 randomly selected patients with carcinoma of the endometrium, observed abnormal glucose tolerance tests when performed before and after the intramuscular administration of 100 mg of progesterone. Of these 18 patients, 10 showed improvement of the glucose tolerance, which was considered to be the result of the action of progesterone in promoting the peripheral utilization of glucose. In a similar vein, Lynch and co-workers[22] observed that in a group of 154 patients with endometrial carcinoma, 42% had abnormal glucose tolerance.

Several authors, however, pointed out that the abnormal glucose tolerance in cancer patients must also take into account the age of the individuals, since abnormal results are frequently surprisingly high in healthy older persons in the general population.[23-25] It has also been pointed out that the results of such tests can be greatly influenced by previous diet, physical activity, and state of nutrition. Thus, Weisenfeld *et al.*[26] concluded, after performing oral and intravenous tests for glucose tolerance, glucagon response, tolbutamide response, and glucose-insulin sensitivity in a series of hospitalized patients, that 47 had cancer and 48 had no malignancy. All of them showed decreased glucose tolerance tests despite a normal fasting blood sugar level. The authors therefore concluded that the decreased tolerance to glucose given orally to patients with cancer is not a specific response to this disease, but rather to the underlying chronic illness.

It has often been stated that pancreatic carcinoma is more frequent in the diabetic than in the general population. In 1893, Mirallié[27] for the first time observed glycosuria occurring in 13 of 15 patients with pancreatic carcinoma. Other authors[28-38] also found in a significant percentage of their patients with primary pancreatic carcinoma fasting hyperglycemia, glycosuria, or impaired glucose tolerance. Among these, Eusterman[28] and Ranson[30] noted abnormalities of carbohydrate metabolism in 10.4 and 17.1%, respectively, of their patients. McKittrick and Root[39] observed that of 37 diabetics afflicted with malignancy, 32.4% had cancer of the pancreas. Of the patients with primary carcinoma of the pancreas, 77.5% had abnormal glucose tolerance tests. Dashiell and Palmer[40] noted impaired blood sugar homeostasis in 18 of 21 cases (85%). Levy and Lichtman[41] and Arry *et al.*[42] made similar observations. In a series of 435 cancers of varying sites in diabetic patients Warren *et al.*[12] observed here that 45 (10.3%) were primary tumors of the pancreas. On the other hand, in the autopsy material of 5673 cases of cancer, only 179 carcinomas of the pancreas (3.2%) were found. This would be in keeping with the observations of other investigators that in diabetic patients a greater frequency of cancer of the pancreas exists. Bell[43] also noted that carcinoma of the pancreas is twice as frequent in diabetics than in nondiabetic individuals. In collating the references from the literature he observed 30 diabetic patients among 390 cases with pancreatic carcinoma, an incidence of 7.7%. In a series of 256 diabetic patients with cancer reported from the Joslin Clinic in 1934 and in a series of 101 cases studied from 1940 to 1952, Marble and Ramos[13] observed that carcinoma of the pancreas comprised 13% in the first and 12% in the second. In a review of the records of 65 patients with primary carcinoma of the pancreas who had been seen during the period of 1955 to 1959, Clark and Mitchell[44] found that 10 (15.4%) had diabetes. In some of them the diabetes was discovered after hospital admission. Murphy and Smith[45] in a survey of 251 patients with primary pancreatic carcinoma, observed that 37.4% had abnormal glucose tolerance tests. They further noted that the often abnormal glucose tolerance in pancreatic carcinoma was not greater when the tumor was present in the body or tail than when it occurred in the head. On the other hand, Salmon[46] cited the records of patients without overt diabetes in whom the pancreas was almost totally replaced by tumor tissue.

Several authors studied the relationship of cancer of the pancreas to the duration of the diabetic state. Marble[5] observed that the average duration of diabetes was 2.6 years prior to the onset of symptoms relating to malignancy of the pancreas, with a total duration of diabetes of 3.4 years preceding that of the tumor. Bell[43] noted, in a study of pancreatic cancer, that the average duration of diabetes was 3.4 years and that in 10 instances the diabetes was diagnosed less than 1 year prior to symptoms relating to pancreatic malignancy. Schlesinger *et al.,*[47] in a series of 7 cases of primary pancreatic carcinoma associated with diabetes, observed that in 5 instances the diabetes appeared less than 2 years prior to the onset of symptoms of malignancy. In 4 of these cases, the family history was negative for diabetes. Green *et al.,*[48] in a review of 209 cases with primary carcinoma of the pancreas, observed that 4.3% had diabetes prior to symptoms referable to the carcinoma, while in 32 (15.3%) the diabetes occurred following the onset of abdominal symptoms. Warren *et al.,*[12] in a study of the duration of diabetes in relation to carcinoma of the pancreas, observed in a group of 45 cases including one islet cell carcinoma, that in about one-third the symptoms of the carcinoma preceded the signs of diabetes or occurred approximately simultaneously. They cautioned that this time relationship does not necessarily indicate a causal relation, but it makes it more likely.

The question of whether the diabetes is due to destruction of the islets by carcinoma of the pancreas has been repeatedly raised. Silver and Lubliner[49] observed 2 cases of diabetes in 57 carcinomas of the head and neck of the pancreas, while they noted 14 instances of diabetes in 43 cases with cancer of the body and tail of this organ. However, other investigators did not feel that the cause of diabetes is related to the encroachment by tumor on the islets of Langerhans. On the other hand, Gullick[50] noted in his study an equal incidence of hyperglycemia in tumors of the head, body, and tail. Berk,[51] in a survey of the literature, observed hyperglycemia in 27.3% of the cases with carcinoma of the pancreas and glycosuria in 9.4%. In his own group of 34 patients, 77.5% had impaired carbohydrate tolerance. Marble and Ramos[13] observed that in their 44 cases of carcinoma of the pancreas associated with diabetes, in practically all instances the tumor occupied the head of the organ. Bell[43] observed that in 85% of his cases glycosuria failed to develop, although the destruction of the pancreas was just as great in this group, as in that with glycosuria. He was impressed by the fact that the islets frequently persisted unless they were actually replaced by the neoplasm. In a number of instances, the B cells were well granulated, although they were embedded in tumor tissue. Bell[43] also conjectured that since the islets of Langerhans are surrounded by an atrophic exocrine pancreas and are embedded in cancer or connective tissue, the possibility must be considered that insulin may not have access to the circulation. Marble[52] pointed out that in cases of carcinoma of the pancreas, the decreased carbohydrate tolerance may not be specific in cancer patients of any type. He also noted that although glycosuria is often found in cases of pancreatic carcinoma, actual diabetes seldom occurs. He felt that in carcinomas of the pancreas the disturbance of carbohydrate homeostasis may possibly not be specific.

Levy and Lichtman[41] believed that the disturbance of blood sugar homeostasis in cases with carcinoma of the pancreas is different from that of patients with idiopathic diabetes and, furthermore, that it can be controlled less easily by insulin and diet. They also felt that the occasional improvement of the diabetic state, unrelated to insulin or diet, is not due to invasion by the tumor alone, but that variations in circulatory and pancreatic duct pressure may be contributory factors.

References

1. Wilson, E. B., and Maher, H. C.: *Amer. J. Cancer,* **16**:227, 1932.
2. Ellinger, F., and Landsman, H.: *N.Y. J. Med.,* **44**:259, 1944.
3. Jacobson, P. H.: *Millbank Mem. Fund. Quart.,* **26**:90, 1948.
4. Warren, S., and LeCompte, P. M.: *The Pathology of Diabetes Mellitus.* Lea & Febiger, Philadelphia, 1952, p. 268.
5. Marble, A.: *N. Engl. J. Med.,* **211**:339, 1934.
6. Seifert, G., and Eichler, R.: *Ztschr. Krebsforsch.,* **60**:200, 1954.
7. Ferner, W.: *Ztschr. Krebsforsch.,* **60**:399, 1955.
8. Herdan, G.: *Brit. J. Cancer,* **14**:449, 1960.
9. Aronson, S. M., Aronson, B. E., Okasaki, H., and Browder, E. J.: *Tr. Amer. Neurol. Assoc.,* **84**:155, 1959.
10. Joslin, E. P., Lombard, H. L., Burrows, R. E., and Manning, M. D.: *N. Engl. J. Med.,* **260**:486, 1959.
11. Steele, J. M., and Sperling, W. L.: *Guthrie Clin. Bull.,* **30**:63, 1961.
12. Warren, S., LeCompte, P. M., and Legg, M. A.: *The Pathology of Diabetes Mellitus.* Lea & Febiger, Philadelphia, 1966, p. 435.
13. Marble, A., and Ramos, E.: In: *Joslin's Diabetes Mellitus.* Edited by A. Marble, P. White, R. Bradley, and L. P. Krall. Lea & Febiger, Philadelphia, 1971, p. 696.
14. Freund, E.: *Wien. Med. Bull.,* **8**:268, 1885.
15. Marks, P. A., and Bishop, J.: *Proc. Amer. Assoc. Cancer Res.,* **2**:131, 1956.

16. Lisker, S. A., Brody, J. I., and Beizer, L. H.: *Amer. J. Med. Sci.,* **252**:282, 1966.
17. Edmonson, J. H.: *Cancer,* **19**:277, 1966.
18. Glicksman, A. S., and Rawson, R. W.: *Cancer,* **9**:1127, 1956.
19. Glicksman, A. S., Myers, W. P. L., and Rawson, R. W.: *Med. Clin. N. Amer.,* **40**:887, 1956.
20. Benjamin, F., and Romney, S.: *Cancer,* **17**:386, 1964.
21. Benjamin, F., and Casper, D. J.: *Amer. J. Obstet. Gynecol.,* **94**:991, 1966.
22. Lynch, H. T., Krush, A. J., Larsen, A. L., and Magnuson, C. W.: *Amer. J. Med. Sci.,* **252**:381, 1966.
23. Streeten, D. H. P., Berstein, M. M., Marmor, B. M., and Doisy, R. J.: *Diabetes,* **14**:579, 1965.
24. Crockford, P. M., Harbeck, R. J., and Williams, R. H.: *Lancet,* **1**:465, 1966.
25. Balodimos, M. C., Balodimos, P. M., Davis, C. B., Belleau, R., Joshi, P. C., and Kusakcioglu, O.: *Geriatrics,* **22**:159, 1967.
26. Weisenfeld, S., Hecht, A., and Goldner, M. G.: *Cancer,* **15**:18, 1962.
27. Mirallié, C.: *Gaz. Hôp.,* **66**:889, 1893.
28. Eusterman, G. B.: *Tr. Amer. Gastroenterol. Assoc.,* **25**:126, 1922.
29. Friedenwald, J., and Cullen, T. S.: *Amer. J. Med. Sci.,* **176**:31, 1928.
30. Ranson, H. K.: *Amer. J. Surg.,* **40**:264, 1938.
31. Franco, S. C.: *Amer. J. Digest. Dis.,* **8**:65, 1941.
32. Kiefer, E. D., and Moravec, M.: *S. Clin. North. Amer.,* **23**:738, 1943.
33. Arkin, A., and Weisberg, S. W.: *Gastroenterology,* **13**:118, 1949.
34. Elman, R., and Butcher, H. R.: *Gastroenterology,* **13**:285, 1949.
35. Broadbent, T. R., and Kerman, H. D.: *Gastroenterology,* **17**:163, 1951.
36. Brown, R. K., Moseley, V., Pratt, T. D., and Pratt, J. H.: *Amer. J. Med. Sci.,* **223**:349, 1952.
37. Smith, B. K., and Albright, E. C.: *Ann. Int. Med.,* **36**:90, 1952.
38. Country, J. C., and Foulk, R.: *U.S. Armed Forces Med. J.,* **4**:831, 1953.
39. McKittrick, L. S., and Root, H. F.: *Diabetic Surgery.* Lea & Febiger, Philadelphia, 1928, p. 250.
40. Dashiell, G. F., and Palmer, W. L.: *Arch. Int. Med.,* **81**:173, 1948.
41. Levy, H., and Lichtman, S. S.: *Arch. Int. Med.,* **65**:607, 1940.
42. Arry, M., Pallard, P., and Vadron, A.: *Rev. Lyon Méd.,* **12**:859, 1963.
43. Bell, E. T.: *Amer. J. Pathol.,* **33**:499, 1961.
44. Clark, C. G., and Mitchell, P. E. G.: *Brit. Med. J.,* **2**:1259, 1961.
45. Murphy, R., and Smith, F. H.: *Med. Clin. North Amer.,* **47**:397, 1963.
46. Salmon, P. A.: *Surgery,* **60**:554, 1966.
47. Schlesinger, F. G., Schwarz, F., and Wagenvoort, C. A.: *Acta Med. Scand.,* **166**:337, 1960.
48. Green, R. C., Jr., Baggenstoss, A. H., and Sprague, R. G.: *Diabetes,* **7**:308, 1960.
49. Silver, G. B., and Lubliner, R. K.: *Surg., Gynecol. Obstet.,* **86**:703, 1948.
50. Gullick, H. D.: *Medicine,* **38**:47, 1959.
51. Berk, J. E.: *Arch. Int. Med.,* **68**:525, 1941.
52. Marble, A.: In: *The Treatment of Diabetes Mellitus.* Edited by E. P. Joslin, H. F. Root, P. White, and A. Marble. Lea & Febiger, Philadelphia, 1959, p. 328.

Chapter 14

Hemochromatosis and Diabetes

Bruno W. Volk and Klaus F. Wellmann

Hemochromatosis is a rare disorder of metabolism characterized by the deposition throughout the body of abnormally large amounts of hemosiderin and, to a lesser degree, of hemofuscin, particularly in the liver, pancreas, and skin. The three cardinal signs of the disease are hepatomegaly with cirrhosis, diabetes mellitus, and abnormal pigmentation of the skin. In 1865 Trousseau[1] described the first case which seemed to have the characteristic symptoms, although no name was coined by him for this disease. The second case was reported in 1871 by Troisier,[2] who called the disease "Le cirrhose pigmentaire dans diabète sucré." Hanot and Chauffard,[3] 11 years later, believed that the diabetes associated with hemochromatosis was probably the primary disease and caused cirrhosis as well as pigmentation of the skin. They called the disease "Cirrhose hypertrophique pigmentaire dans le diabète sucré." Other authors[4-7] similarly considered the hyperglycemia as the primary cause of the disorder and thought that the disturbance of blood sugar homeostasis resulted from the changes in the liver and other organs. Hanot[5] coined the term "diabète bronzé." Von Recklinghausen,[7] in 1889, named the disease hemochromatosis and subsequent investigators[8-13] defined the clinical and pathological entity of this disease.

The various aspects of idiopathic hemochromatosis were extensively reviewed in the classic monograph by Sheldon[14] and by other investigators.[15-22] Hemochromatosis does not occur before the age of 10. The majority of cases are diagnosed in later life, usually between the ages of 40 and 60 (68%). Idiopathic hemochromatosis is observed about 10 times more frequently in males than in females, 90.4% versus 9.6% in the study of Finch and Finch.[19] The rarity of the disease in women has been explained by their ability to expel the absorbed iron by menstruation and pregnancy. In Sheldon's study[14] only 1 of 13 women (8%) was diagnosed as having hemochromatosis before the age of 45, in contrast to 108 of 279 men (39%). Hemochromatosis is a relatively rare disease, accounting, in general, for about 1 in 7000 hospital deaths.[19]

Diabetes is by no means associated with the disease in all cases. Bork,[23] in

Bruno W. Volk and Klaus F. Wellmann • Isaac Albert Research Institute of the Kingsbrook Jewish Medical Center, and Downstate Medical Center, State University of New York, Brooklyn, New York. Present address of B. W. V.: University of California, Irvine, California. Present address of K. F. W.: Beekman Downtown Hospital, New York, New York.

1928, observed 55 patients with diabetes (37%) among 111 cases with hemochromatosis. In Sheldon's[14] study of 311 collected cases of hemochromatosis, diabetes was present in 80% of the patients. Disturbances of carbohydrate metabolism were observed by Althausen and associates[24] in 18 of 23 patients (77%), by Heilmeyer[25] in 79% of a group of 36 patients, and by Stachewitsch[26] in 69% in a series of 83 patients afflicted with the disease. Creutzfeldt[27] found 6 cases of diabetes in a group of 20 patients with hemochromatosis in whom the diagnosis was done by liver biopsy.

Hemochromatosis in cases of diabetes is uncommon. John[28] observed only 1 case among 4490 diabetics, and Butt and Wilder[29] encountered at the Mayo Clinic only 30 cases over a period of 30 years. Marble and Baily[15] found 30 patients with proven hemochromatosis in a study of over 30,000 new cases at the Joslin Clinic from 1932 to 1951 (0.11%). Similarly, Jensen[30] observed 48 patients among 30,258 (0.16%) admissions at the New England Diaconess Hospital during the period of 1958 to 1965.

According to Sheldon,[14] the average duration of life in 89 instances of idiopathic hemochromatosis from the time medical advise was first sought to the time of death was 18.5 months. Diabetic coma was the cause of death in 50% and cirrhosis of the liver in 11%. The rest of the patients died from myocardial failure, infections, and carcinoma of the liver.

Boulin[31] found, in 70 cases, the average duration from the onset of diabetes to be 4 years with extremes varying from 1 to 20 years. Marble and Bailey[15] reported an average duration of 4.9 years in a study of 27 fatal cases. The duration of diabetes in the series of Warren *et al.*[32] ranged from 2 months to 25 years.

Jensen,[30] in his series of 48 patients seen at the Joslin Clinic from 1958 to 1968, noted that the diabetes developed in 82% of the patients with hemochromatosis during the course of the disease. It may appear rather suddenly, and the insulin requirements may increase during the early stages. The diagnosis of both diabetes and hemochromatosis was made at the time of admission to the hospital in 3 patients. The diagnosis of diabetes preceded that of hemochromatosis in the remaining cases. The time interval between the diagnosis of the diabetes and that of hemochromatosis varied from less than 1 year in 11 patients and from 1 to 5 years in 12 patients. The longest time interval between the diagnosis of diabetes and the onset of hemochromatosis was 20 years in 2 patients, and in 1 patient the duration was 16 years. The average time interval between the diagnosis of diabetes and hemochromatosis was 51 months.

Pathologically, the pancreas is usually enlarged, has a firm consistency, and is always markedly pigmented. The color ranges from reddish-brown to deep brown or chocolate. Histologically, there is usually considerable interlobular and interacinar fibrosis present (Fig. 1). The pigment, in general, is densely deposited in the duct cells, in the acinar cells, as well as in the connective tissue. During the progression of the disease the connective tissue and the deposited pigment appear to compress the cells until they become atrophic and are replaced by pigment granules. No definite relationship exists between the quantity of pigment and the extent of atrophy of the acinar cells. The changes

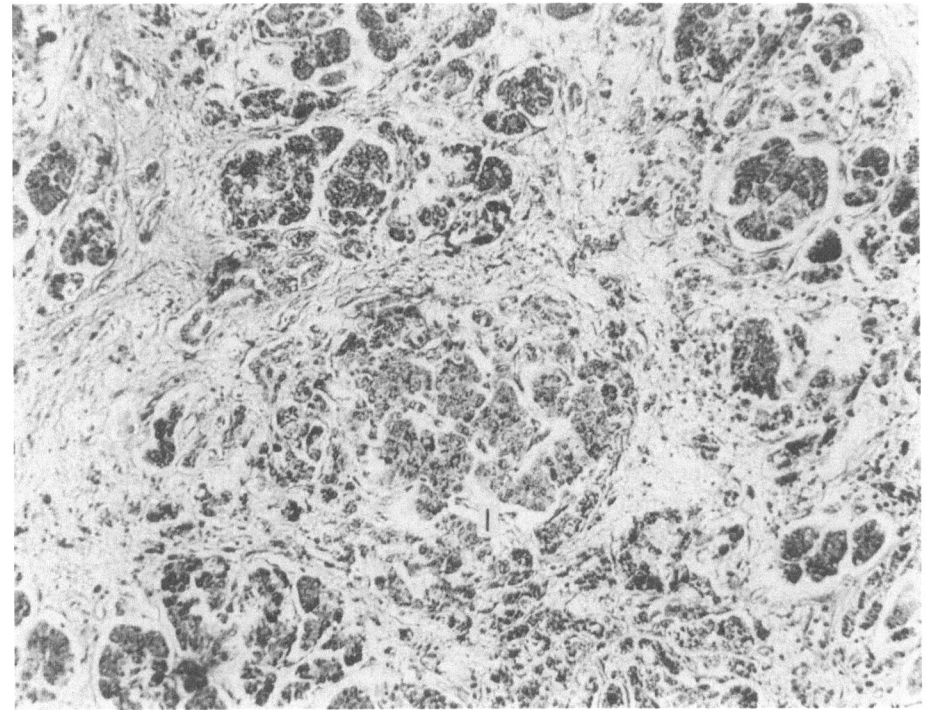

Figure 1. Pancreas of patient with hemochromatosis. There is very marked fibrosis causing distortion of the normal parenchymal architecture. Islet of Langerhans (I). Periodic acid Schiff trichrome stain. ×165. Reproduced at 105%.

eventually terminate in cirrhosis of the pancreas in approximately 90% of the patients.[14] In pancreatic cirrhosis the fibrous bands separating the atrophic exocrine pancreas are more abundant than those seen in maturity-onset diabetes (Fig. 1). Moreover, they are broader and more abundant and contain iron pigment. The amount of fibrous tissue in the pancreas varies considerably. It may be focally accumulated in some areas of the pancreas, or it may be eventually evenly distributed throughout the entire organ.[23,33,34] The extent of fibrosis does not necessarily parallel the degree of pigment.

Several authors reported an increase of fat in the pancreas of hemochromatosis.[35-41] Some felt that this increase was within the interlobular fat,[35,39] while others[40,41] believed it to be *ex vacuo* replacement by fat in an atrophic pancreas. The islets are involved in about 80% of the cases. They usually contain less pigment than the rest of the pancreas and, in many instances, have little or no pigment at all. Whenever present it may be intra- or extracellular. The islets are frequently large and prominent[23,33]; however, in many instances, their number is decreased, and they may be difficult to identify or even entirely absent.[23,42-46] They frequently may undergo fibrosis. The connective tissue may follow the path of the capillaries, and eventually the fibrous strands may transsect the islets and divide them into smaller compartments.[35]

Hartroft[48] and McGavran and Hartroft[49] observed that when iron is present in the islets of Langerhans it tends to accumulate in the B cells and that the A cells are markedly reduced in number. There is, in general, no relationship between the degree of pigmentation and B cell granulation,[50] although there is usually loss of granules observed. However, degranulation of B cells in some of the islets may occur without pigment deposition. Although the B cells are usually degranulated in hemochromatosis, in general, it is difficult to differentiate, as far as the pigmentation and morphology are concerned, between the islets of diabetics and nondiabetics.[17]

There are two pigments deposited in the pancreas. One, in which iron can be demonstrated, is hemosiderin, and the other, in which iron cannot be found, is hemofuscin.[14] Mallory[51] conjectured that hemosiderin is a product of the intracellular digestion of hemofuscin and that both are derived from blood pigment. Hemosiderin is usually present in overwhelming preponderance and can be observed in almost every case of the disease. It has not been established whether the iron-containing pigment is injurious to the pancreatic cells. In fact, pigmentation and fibrosis of the pancreas do not necessarily parallel each other. The pigmentation may be slight, while there is extensive fibrosis present. Various authors felt that the deposition of pigment and the fibrosis are independent processes.[52,53] This seems to be borne out by experiments in which the administration of huge amounts of iron to animals over prolonged periods of time has not reproduced the lesions of hemochromatosis as observed in the human.[54,55]

Within the connective tissue the deposition of the pigment may be intracellular or it may be free. It may be seen in varying sizes from small granules to large amorphous lumps which probably constitute conglomerations of necrotic cells. The pigment, furthermore, is not necessarily uniformly distributed throughout the pancreas, and occasionally it may be found to be focally deposited.[14,40,56,57]

In general, the extent of pigmentation in the pancreas is not as excessive as that found in the liver. According to Sheldon,[14] the morphologic basis for differentiation between idiopathic hemochromatosis and hemosiderosis is a predominance of hemosiderin in the liver, skin, and pancreas as well as in the epithelium of the gastrotestinal tract, in the choroid plexus, and in the endocrine glands. While hemofuscin is usually present in the blood vessels, particularly in the smooth muscles of the media of both arteries and veins and in the adventitia,[14] hemosiderin can be found within the stroma and interacinar cells of the pancreas and in the columnar cells lining the ducts, as well as in the pancreatic islets. Warren et al.[58] felt that the excess of iron per se does not explain the hemochromatosis. This hypothesis seems to be based on the observation that extensive fibrosis can only be found in the pancreas, liver, and spleen, while it is absent in other organs despite heavy deposits of iron.[14,52] Warren and Drake[59] rejected the diagnosis of hemochromatosis, if a known etiology, such as repeated hemolysis, could be elicited from the history.

Steinke,[60] who performed insulin assays on two pancreases from hemochromatosis patients of the study of Warren *et al.*, observed that these cases fall within the same range of insulin content as do the cases of nonhemochromatotic adult-onset diabetes.

The etiology of hemochromatosis is still unsettled, and several theories have been advanced to explain its involvement. Sheldon,[14] in a review of the literature, concluded that hemochromatosis should be considered as the "result of inborn error of metabolism," with the defect present in the cells of the body causing an increased avidity of all tissues for iron. This hypothesis, apparently supported by the occasional occurrence of the disorder in siblings,[61] suggests that the storage of iron continues throughout the life of the individual and does not reach a total quantity sufficient to produce symptoms until middle life, which would explain the age incidence of this disorder. Other theories include a defect in the complex regulatory mechanism of the serum iron level connected with increased saturation[62]; increased permeability of the sinusoids for red cells, subsequently removed by phagocytes[63]; increased intestinal absorption of iron owing to lowering of the mucosa in the intestine[64,65]; alterations of reticuloendothelial function so that these cells are incapable of returning iron to the circulation[66-68]; and altered innervation in the midbrain.[69,70] Crosby[71] thought that hemochromatosis is a hereditary disorder of iron metabolism which permits absorption of dietary iron in excess of requirement and in excess of the body's ability to excrete it. Iron, according to this theory, gradually accumulates, causing cirrhosis as well as injury of the various organs where it is deposited. On the other hand, MacDonald[72] suggested that the most probable explanation of hemochromatosis seems to be that it is acquired rather than inherited, that it is not a single disease entity with a single cause and single course, but a condition which came about by the coexistence of two factors; one, an excess of iron, and the other, a nutritional (especially folic acid) deficiency, often associated with the development of cirrhosis. The iron excess occurs from ingestion or parenteral administration. The author admits that the cause of cirrhosis with or without iron is not understood, but that it is not due to iron.

Finch and Finch[19] believed that there are no unique features of idiopathic hemochromatosis by which it may be distinguished pathologically from other iron storage diseases, such as dietary or transfusion hemochromatosis or hemosiderosis. Hemosiderosis is an increase in storage iron without associated tissue damage. These authors[19] estimated that there are approximately 20,000 persons with hemochromatosis in the United States of whom only a small fraction are in the symptomatic stage of their illness. Gillman and Gillman[73,74] believed that dietary deficiency plays a major role in the development of hemochromatosis in the Bantu in South Africa. These authors felt, after studying 400 liver biopsies in 120 patients with pellagra, that hemochromatosis can be regarded as one of the common sequelae of pellagra. They believed that the fundamental defect in this disease is a disturbance of intracellular metabolism which is induced by dietary imbalance, and they thought that both hemosiderin and hemofuscin have a common origin in the mitochondria. However, since this disease in South African pellagrins shows equal sex distribution, the question arises of whether it may not be different from the classic idiopathic hemochromatosis. Furthermore, it seems that hemosiderosis is not characteristic of pellagra as seen in the United States.[75,76] Bothwell *et al.*[77] have shown that clearcut differences exist between the distribution of iron in hemochromatosis, where the majority of the deposits occur in hepatic cells, and in the Bantu, where the material is deposited in phagocytic cells, primarily the Kupffer cells. Moreover, in the spleen the iron content is considerably greater in patients from South Africa.

MacDonald[53] believed that hemochromatosis is a variant of portal cirrhosis because of the increased storage of iron, which is also observed in cases of portal cirrhosis. He further believed that poor nutrition alone or in conjunction with alcoholism may be an important factor in the development of hemochromatosis. He observed pancreatic fibrosis in approximately 85% of the cases with uncomplicated portal cirrhosis and was skeptical of the familial nature of this disorder. MacDonald and Pechet[78] were able to produce lesions in rats which were similar to hemochromatosis in man by means of a high intake of iron associated with a high fat diet deficient in choline.

While the progression of diabetes in hemochromatosis usually runs parallel to the extent of islet involvement, there are instances where the fibrosis as well as the deposition of pigment are moderate and cannot provide an explanation for the disturbance of carbohydrate hemostasis.[14,79] The hypothesis has been advanced that the simultaneously occurring cirrhosis of the liver may make it difficult or impossible to obtain normal glycogen stores and that, therefore, the extensive hepatic involvement may contribute to the development of the diabetic state. It has also been conjectured that the fibrosis surrounding the pancreatic islets in patients with hemochromatosis acts as a barrier between the B cells and the blood stream and, therefore, may decrease the availability of glucose for normal metabolism and give rise to the diabetic state.[80]

References

1. Trousseau, A.: *Clinique Méd. d'Hôtel-Dieu de Paris,* 2nd Ed., Vol. 2, 1865, p. 663.
2. Troisier, M.: *Bull. Soc. Anat.,* **16**:231, 1871.
3. Hanot, V., and Chauffard, A.: *Rev. Méd.,* **2**:385, 1882.
4. Letulle, M.: *Bull. Mem. Soc. Méd. Hôp. Paris,* **2**:406, 1885.
5. Hanot, V.: *Brit. Med. J.,* **1**:206, 1896.
6. Hanot, V., and Schachmann, M.: *Arch. Physiol. Norm. Pathol.* **7**:50, 1886.
7. Von Recklinghausen, F.: *Naturforscher und Ärzte in Heidelberg,* 1889, p. 324.
8. Calmettes, J.: Contribution à l'étude de la cirrhose de diabète bronzé. Thèse de Paris, 1896.
9. Berg, H. W.: *Med. Record,* **56**:881, 1899.
10. Labbé, M.: *Arch. Appar. Dig. Nutr.,* **6**:403, 1912.
11. McCreery, A. H.: *Canad. Med. Assoc. J.,* **7**:481, 1917.
12. Zaleski, S.: *Virchow's Arch.,* **104**:91, 1886.
13. Kretz, R.: *Beit. Klin. Med. Chir.,* Heft 15, 1896.
14. Sheldon, J. H.: *Haemochromatosis.* Oxford University Press, London, 1935.
15. Marble, A., and Bailey, C. C.: *Amer. J. Med.,* **11**:590, 1951.
16. Marble, A., and Steinke, J.: *Medizinische,* **1**:19, 1959.

17. Bell, E. T.: *Diabetes,* **4**:435, 1955.
18. Dubin, I. N.: *Amer. J. Clin. Pathol.* **25**:514, 1955.
19. Finch, S. C., and Finch, C. A.: *Medicine,* **34**:381, 1955.
20. MacDonald, R. A., and Mallory, G. K.: *Arch. Int. Med.,* **105**:686, 1960.
21. Bothwell, T. H., and Finch, C. A.: *Iron Metabolism.* Little, Brown, Boston, 1962.
22. Beutler, E., Fairbanks, V. F., and Fahey, J. L.: *Clinical Disorders of Iron Metabolism.* Grune & Stratton, New York, 1963, p. 213.
23. Bork, K.: *Virchow's Arch.,* **269**:178, 1928.
24. Althausen, T. L., Doig, R. K., Weiden, S., Motteram, R., Turner, C. N., and Moore, A.: *Arch. Int. Med.,* **88**:553, 1951.
25. Heilmeyer, L.: *Acta Haematol.,* **11**:137, 1954.
26. Stachewitsch, A.: Cited by Creutzfeldt, W.: In: *Acta Hepatosplenol.,* **6**:156, 1959.
27. Creutzfeldt, W.: *Acta Hepatosplenol.* **6**:156, 1959.
28. John, H. J.: *JAMA,* **112**:2272, 1939.
29. Butt, H. R., and Wilder, R. M.: *Arch. Pathol.,* **26**:262, 1938.
30. Jensen, W. K.: In: *Joslin's Diabetes Mellitus.* Edited by A. Marble, P. White, R. F. Bradley, and L. P. Krall. Lea & Febiger, Philadelphia, 1971, p. 712.
31. Boulin, R.: *Press. Med.,* **53**:326, 1945.
32. Warren, S., LeCompte, P. M., and Legg, M. A.: *The Pathology of Diabetes Mellitus.* Lea & Febiger, Philadelphia, 1966, p. 365.
33. Potter, N. B., and Milne, L. S.: *Amer. J. Med. Sci.,* **143**:46, 1911.
34. Labbé, M., and Stevenin, H.: *Presse Méd.,* **30**:424, 1922.
35. Rosenthal, S. R.: *Arch. Pathol.,* **13**:83, 1932.
36. Elmer, W. P.: *Int. Med. J. (St. Louis),* **18**:912, 1911.
37. Hensel, O.: *Med. J. Rec.,* **127**:14, 1928.
38. Sprunt, T. P.: *Arch. Int. Med.,* **8**:75, 1911.
39. Blumer, G.: *N.Y. Med. J.,* **94**:922, 1911.
40. Hess, O. and Zurhelle, E.: *Ztsch. Klin. Med.,* **57**:344, 1905.
41. Cecil, R. L.: *J. Exp. Med.,* **14**:500, 1911.
42. Barber, H.: *Guy's Hosp. Rep.,* **79**:45, 1929.
43. Barber, H., and Bith, H.: *Bull. Mem. Soc. Méd. Hôp. Paris,* **33**:119, 1912.
44. Manning, D. F.: *J. Missouri Med. Assoc.,* **22**:390, 1925.
45. Ollivier, J.: La Cirrhose Pigmentaire (Étude Critique). Thèse de Paris, 1925, p. 47.
46. Roth, O.: *Dtsch. Arch. Klin. Med.,* **117**:224, 1915.
47. Seibert, P.: *Beitr. Path. path. Anat.,* **84**:111, 1930.
48. Hartroft, W. S.: *Diabetes,* **5**:98, 1956.
49. McGavran, M. H., and Hartroft, W. S.: *Amer. J. Pathol.,* **32**:631, 1956.
50. Warren, S., LeCompte, P. M., and Legg, M. A.: *The Pathology of Diabetus Mellitus.* Lea & Febiger, Philadelphia, 1966, p. 367.
51. Mallory, F. B.: *Amer. J. Pathol.,* **1**:117, 1925.
52. Herbut, P. A., and Tamaka, H. T.: *Amer. J. Clin. Pathol.,* **16**:640, 1946.
53. MacDonald, R. A.: *Arch. Int. Med.,* **107**:606, 1961.
54. Brown, E. B., Jr., Dubach, R., Smith, D. E., Reynafarje, C., and Moore, C. V.: *J. Lab. Clin. Med.,* **50**:862, 1957.
55. Brown, E. B., Jr., Smith, D. E., Dubach, R. and Moore, C. V.: *J. Lab. Clin. Med.,* **53**:591, 1959.
56. Abbott, M. E.: *J. Pathol. Bacteriol.,* **7**:55, 1901.
57. Donaldson, R.: *Guy's Hosp. Rep.,* **79**:28, 1929.
58. Warren, S., LeCompte, P. M., and Legg, M. A.: *The Pathology of Diabetes Mellitus.* Lea & Febiger, Philadelphia, 1966, p. 370.
59. Warren, S., and Drake, W. L., Jr.: *Amer. J. Pathol.,* **27**:573, 1951.
60. Steinke, J.: Quoted in: Warren, S., LeCompte, P. M., and Legg, M. A.: *The Pathology of Diabetes Mellitus.* Lea & Febiger, Philadelphia, 1966, p. 371.
61. Rogers, W. F., Jr.: *Amer. J. Med. Sci.,* **220**:530, 1950.
62. Gitlow, S. E., and Beyers, M. R.: *J. Lab. Clin. Med.,* **39**:337, 1952.

63. Rössle, R.: In: *Handbuch der Spez. path. Anat. u. Hist.* Edited by F. Henke and O. Lubarsch. Springer Verlag, Berlin, 1930, p. 243.
64. Granick, S.: *Bull. N.Y. Acad. Med.,* **25**:403, 1949.
65. Drabkin, D. L.: *Physiol. Rev.,* **31**:345, 1951.
66. Eppinger, H.: *Die Leberkrankheiten.* Springer Verlag, Berlin, 1937, p. 423.
67. Schmidt, M. B.: *Ergeb. Allg. Path. path. Anat.,* **35**:105, 1940.
68. Vannotti, A., and Delachaux, A.: *Metabolism and its Clinical Significance.* Grune & Stratton, New York, 1949, p. 15.
69. Regelsberger, H.: *Klin. Wochenschr.,* **21**:1122, 1942.
70. Brick, I. B.: *Arch. Int. Med.,* **96**:26, 1955.
71. Crosby, W. H.: *Controversy in Internal Medicine.* Edited by F. J. Ingelfinger, A. S. Relman, and M. Finland: W. B. Saunders, Philadelphia, 1966. p. 261.
72. MacDonald, R. A.: *Controversy in Internal Medicine.* Edited by F. J. Ingelfinger, A. S. Redman, and M. Finland: W. B. Saunders, Philadelphia, 1966, p. 261.
73. Gillman, J., and Gillman, T.: *Arch. Pathol.,* **40**:239, 1945.
74. Gillman, J., and Gillman, T.: *Gastroenterology,* **8**:19, 1947.
75. Eddy, W. H., and Dalldorf, G.: *The Avitaminosis.* Williams & Wilkins, Baltimore, 1944, p. 129.
76. Spies, T. D.: In: *Clinical Nutrition.* Edited by N. Jolliffee, F. F. Tisdall, and P. R. Cannon. Paul B. Hoeber, New York, 1950, p. 531.
77. Bothwell, T. H., Abrahams, C., Bradlow, B. A., and Charlton, R. W.: *Arch. Pathol.,* **79**:163, 1965.
78. MacDonald, R. A., and Pechet, G. S.: *Amer. J. Pathol.,* **46**:85, 1965.
79. Even, R.: *Étude Clinique et Experimentale.* Le Francois, Paris, 1932, p. 133.
80. Lazarus, S. S., and Volk, B. W.: *Arch. Pathol.,* **71**:44, 1961.

Chapter 15

The Pathology of Juvenile Diabetes

Philip M. LeCompte and Willy Gepts

Juvenile or "growth-onset" diabetes is sometimes arbitrarily defined to include all cases with onset before 15 years of age,[1-3] amounting to about 5% of the diabetic population. However, it has long been known that an additional 10% or so of adults have a clinically similar form of diabetes, likewise that children may occasionally exhibit a mild diabetes of "maturity-onset" type, which seems to have a different pattern of inheritance from the usual juvenile type.[4]

For the purpose of this chapter we shall utilize the clinical definition, the typical case having a sudden onset in a lean person and evolving into a labile or "brittle," ketosis-prone, insulin-dependent type of diabetes, with low plasma insulin and low extractable insulin in the pancreas. By contrast, the usual case of maturity-onset diabetes has an insidious onset in an obese person, is insulin-independent and relatively stable, with an appreciable amount of insulin in the plasma and pancreas. As will be seen below, the pathology of the pancreas is quite different in the two types.

Macroscopic Changes

The pancreas of juvenile diabetics is often small and reduced in weight.[5-9] This change does not result from a congenital hypoplasia as suggested by a few earlier authors[5] but is the consequence of a progressive atrophy which develops in the course of the disease. This is shown by the fact that, at the clinical onset, the pancreas of juvenile diabetics is of normal weight.[8] Doniach and Morgan,[10] on the basis of their figures on pancreatic weight, suggested that the pancreas seems to stop growing at the onset of juvenile diabetes.

Very rare cases with congenital malformations of the pancreas have been reported, such as complete agenesis[11] or the absence of the head or the tail.[12,13]

Except for some increased firmness due to fibrosis in chronic cases, the pancreas of juvenile diabetics shows no other distinctive gross abnormalities.

Philip M. LeCompte • Faulkner Hospital (formerly), and Harvard Medical School, Boston, Massachusetts. *Willy Gepts* • Universitair Ziekenhuis Brugmann, Vrije Universiteit Brussel, Brussels, Belgium.

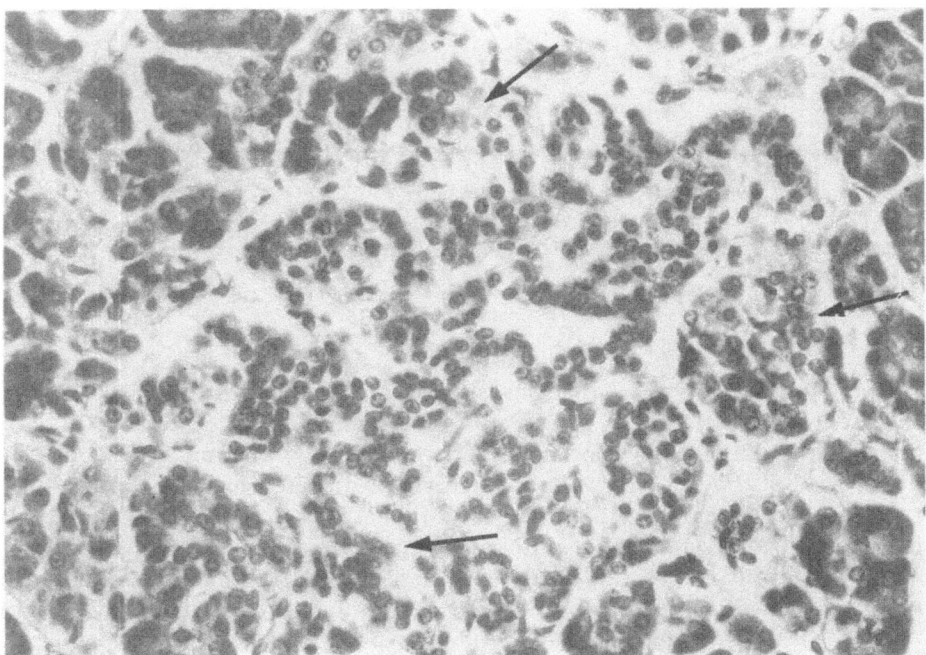

Figure 1. Chronic juvenile diabetic. "Atrophic" islet at a high magnification. It consists of narrow cords of small cells with scanty cytoplasm. The outlines are irregular, with localized continuity between islet cell cords and acinar tissue (arrows). Gomori's chromium hematoxylin–phloxine. ×450. Reproduced at 105%.

Microscopic Changes

The changes which can be observed in the pancreas of juvenile diabetics are qualitative and quantitative.

Qualitative Changes

General Appearance of the Islets The pancreas of juvenile diabetics shows two types of islets: apparently atrophic islets* and hyperactive islets. The atrophic islets (Fig. 1) predominate in all cases, whether acute or chronic. They are composed of small cells, with a small and dense nucleus, and scanty cytoplasm. These cells are grouped in thin cords and arranged in a fibrous stroma. Atrophic islets often have irregular outlines and sometimes show a continuity between groups of endocrine and acinar cells. With granule stains, B cells cannot usually be demonstrated; the small cells which compose these islets hardly ever show specific staining characteristics.

---

*These islets, which have always been considered as atrophic, are actually, according to present evidence, composed of active endocrine cells, see p. 350.

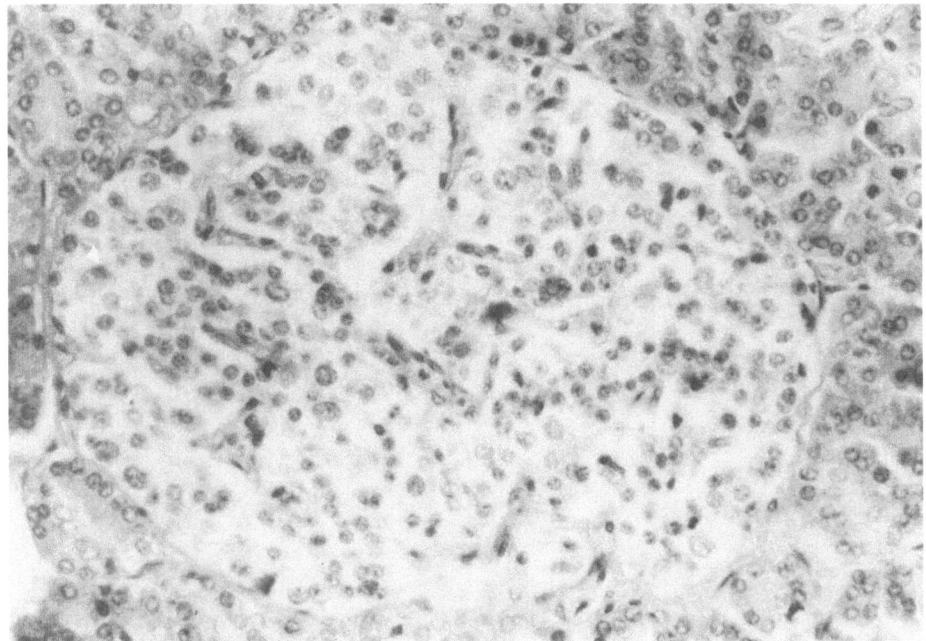

Figure 2. Recent-onset juvenile diabetic. Large, apparently hyperactive islet. Gomori's chromium hematoxylin–phloxine. ×350. Reproduced at 105%.

The hyperactive islets (Fig. 2) are much rarer that the atrophic, and are found mainly in young diabetics with a disease of short duration. They are larger than the others, and are sometimes even hypertrophic. They have distinct and regular outlines, and are composed of large cells, with a big nucleus. With granule stains (Fig. 3), these islets appear to be composed of A cells, mainly located at the periphery, and of a more or less large number of B cells, completely or almost completely degranulated. Their cytoplasm is clear, sometimes hydropic in appearance; it often contains small particles, with hazy contours, which stain blue with toluidine blue and red with pyronine; this staining is abolished by a previous treatment with ribonuclease. These particles were already described in 1909 by Weichselbaum,[14] who called them "Körnchen," but it has become evident that they are not secretion granules. From their histochemical characteristics, they appear to be composed of ribonucleic acid, and are indicative of a strongly developed endoplasmic reticulum and, therefore, of a secretory hyperactivity.

The relative proportion of atrophic and hyperactive islets varies from one case to another and also within the same case, from one area of the pancreas to another. A few lobules may show numerous hyperactive islets, whereas everywhere else only atrophic islets are found. Furthermore, hyperactive islets are difficult to find at all in the pancreas of very young diabetic children, under the age of 2 years.

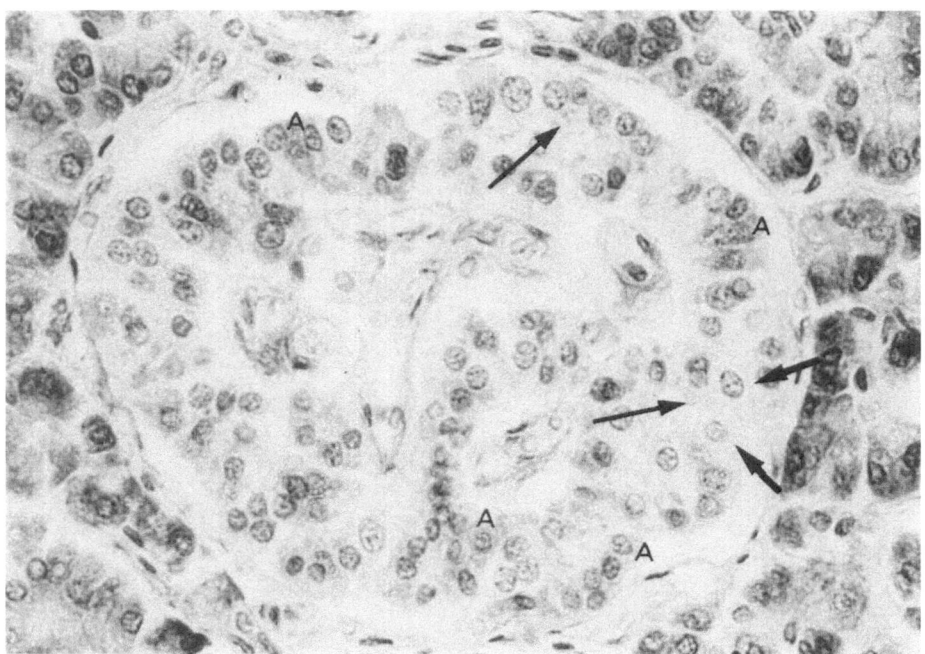

Figure 3. Recent-onset juvenile diabetic. High magnification of an apparently hyperactive islet. The darker cells are A cells (A). The lighter cells are B cells; they have enlarged nuclei (arrows) and show "Körnchen" (long arrows) in their cytoplasm. Gomori's chromium hematoxylin–phloxine. ×560. Reproduced at 105%.

Hydropic Changes   In some juvenile diabetics, mainly in those with an acute type of disease, part of the B cells have a hydropic appearance: Their cytoplasm looks empty, apparently containing neither granules nor any other organelles visible with the light microscope (Fig. 4). Much disagreement exists in the literature about the exact frequency of this lesion. Weichselbaum[14] reported it in over 50% of the diabetics, but Warren *et al.*[9] noticed it in only 36 of their 1376 cases. No straightforward explanation is available for these discrepant observations, except that Weichselbaum had only untreated cases.

Much importance was attached to this lesion by the older pathologists, who considered it to be of degenerative nature and a forerunner of the atrophy of the islet cells, a striking feature of the pancreas of juvenile diabetics. However, this interpretation became unlikely after the demonstration by Toreson,[15] that the empty appearance of the cytoplasm is due to glycogen deposits. Hydropic change due to glycogen deposition is characteristically seen in many forms of experimental diabetes,[16–20] including that due to glucose overload. It is thus associated with hyperglycemia, without permanent damage to the B cell, and is reversible. Recently, Pictet and Imagawa[20a] have shown that it can be produced in the B cells of cultured rat islets by varying the concentration of glucose in the medium. Since, even under these conditions, the hydropic change is reversible, we disagree with the term "deleterious" as used by these authors. In dogs made diabetic with growth hormone, Volk and Lazarus[21] observed, in addition to glycogen infiltration of the islet cells, another lesion, of truly degenerative nature, characterized by cytoplasmic vacuolization and nuclear pyknosis. They called this lesion "ballooning degeneration." Typical examples are difficult to find in the pancreas of human diabetics, although in some cases the hydropic change is associated with nuclear hypertrophy and hyperchromatism.

Nuclear Changes   Hypertrophy of the nuclei has been mentioned before, but in some cases of juvenile diabetes, irregularity and hyperchromatism, and even pyknosis, are particularly striking[8,9] (Fig. 4 and 5). To judge from the work of Ehrie and Swartz[22] on normal pancreas, these large nuclei are probably polyploid. Despite their intense hyperactivity, the B cells of acute juvenile diabetics rarely show mitoses,[8] whereas in nondiabetics and in elderly diabetics mitoses may appear in large numbers in certain pathological conditions, such as liver injury from various causes.[23,24]

Insulitis   It should be noted at the outset that this subject and its implications have recently been discussed in two excellent reviews[25,26] and two symposia,[27,28] to which the interested reader is referred for more detailed information.

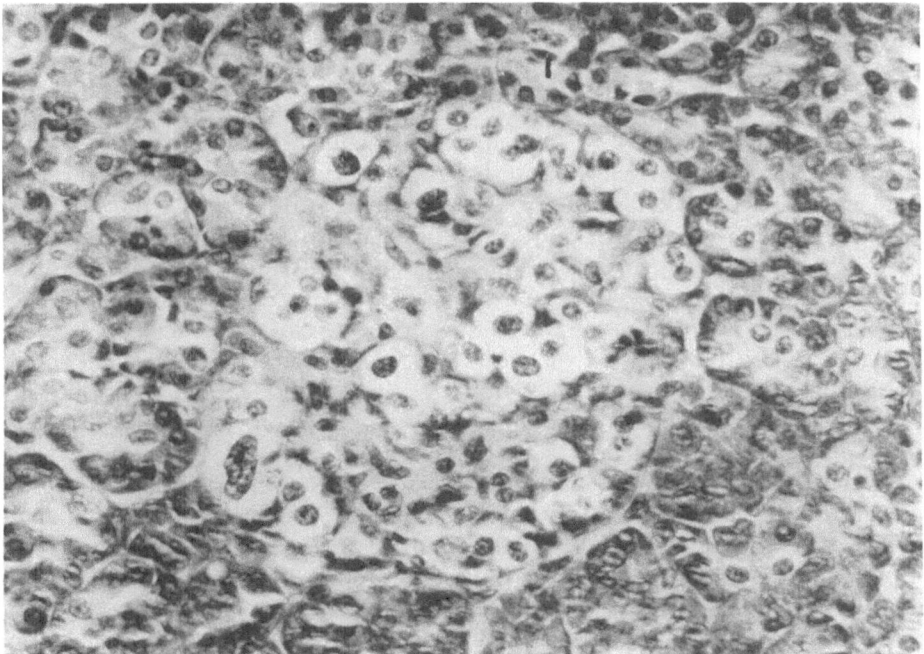

Figure 4. Recent-onset juvenile diabetic. Islet with hydropic change (clear cytoplasm) of the B cells. Note enlarged and sometimes irregular nuclei. Hemalum erythroxin saffron. ×420. Reproduced at 110%.

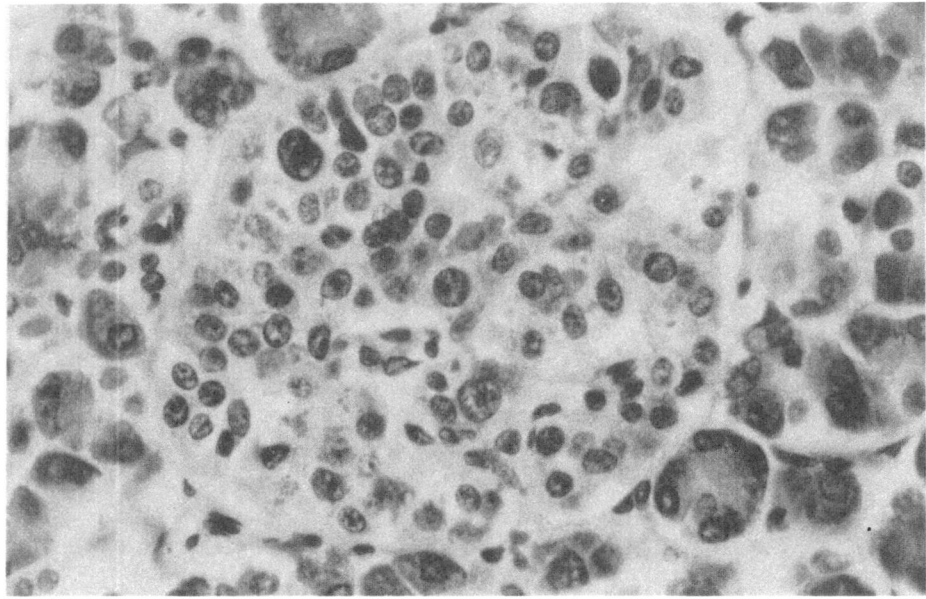

Figure 5. Recent-onset juvenile diabetic. Further example of enlarged, hyperchromatic, probably polyploid nuclei. Gomori's chromium hematoxylin–phloxine. ×600. Reproduced at 105%.

Lymphocytic infiltration of the islands of Langerhans (a process named "insulitis" by von Meyenburg[29]) and recognized for many years as a rare occurrence in the diabetic pancreas, has usually been regarded as a curiosity of little significance. Recently, with the phenomenal burgeoning of immunology, with the realization that lymphocytes are the basis of immune reactions, and with new evidence suggesting the possibility of viral etiology of some cases of diabetes (see Chapter 19) there has been a renewal of interest in "insulitis."

Lymphocytes infiltrating the islets were noted many years ago by early students of the pancreas in diabetes.[14,30–34] The lesion was described in the masterly review by Kraus[5] in 1929, but he apparently attached little significance to it. The early reports of Warren *et al.*[35–37] established the lesion as characteristic of early juvenile diabetes. Later, LeCompte[38] reported four cases, all in young diabetics of recent onset, and suggested that the rarity of the lesion might be more apparent than real. This impression was seemingly confirmed by Gepts,[8] who found it in 15 of 22 young diabetics who had died within 6 months of the first symptoms of the disease. However, it was not seen in those who had survived for more than a year.

Insulitis has been recognized mainly in case reports,[39–43] but the actual frequency of occurrence is not known. In one case it was associated with cytomegalic viral disease,[44] and a recent case report records the presence of insulitis accompanied by structures suggestive of virus particles.[44a] Ogilvie[45] regarded it as rare, and Doniach and Morgan[10] did not find it at all in a series of

13 acute juvenile diabetics. On the other hand, Junker *et al.*[46] noticed it in 6 of 11 acute juvenile diabetics dying within 1 year after onset and suggested that the failure of Doniach and Morgan to find the lesion may have been due to the scarcity of young children in their series. Thus, its frequency in human disease is uncertain. Only two cases have been reported in adults with long-standing diabetes.[47] It has been described in spontaneous diabetes in animals.[48-50] Perhaps the most remarkable example of spontaneous diabetes with insulitis in animals is that recently reported in a strain of rats by Nakhooda *et al.*[51] (See Chapter 17.)

Insulitis characteristically appears as an infiltration of some (usually not all) of the islets in a given pancreas by fairly small lymphocytes with scanty cytoplasm (Fig. 6). Occasionally a few large cells, apparently macrophages, are present. Rarely a few eosinophils or plasma cells may be seen. A few cases are reported in which the cellular infiltrate consisted predominantly of polymorphonuclear leukocytes.[37,38] It should be emphasized that the cellular infiltrate is, with rare exceptions, confined to the islets, although occasionally there are a few lymphocytes in the interstitial tissue or around ducts.

As noted above, the process is not uniform. Many islets may be involved, or only a few. Sometimes the infiltrated islet is large, on occasion even larger than normal (Fig. 7), and some of the nuclei of the B cells may be enlarged and hyperchromatic, suggesting polyploidy.[22] More often the infiltrated islets are

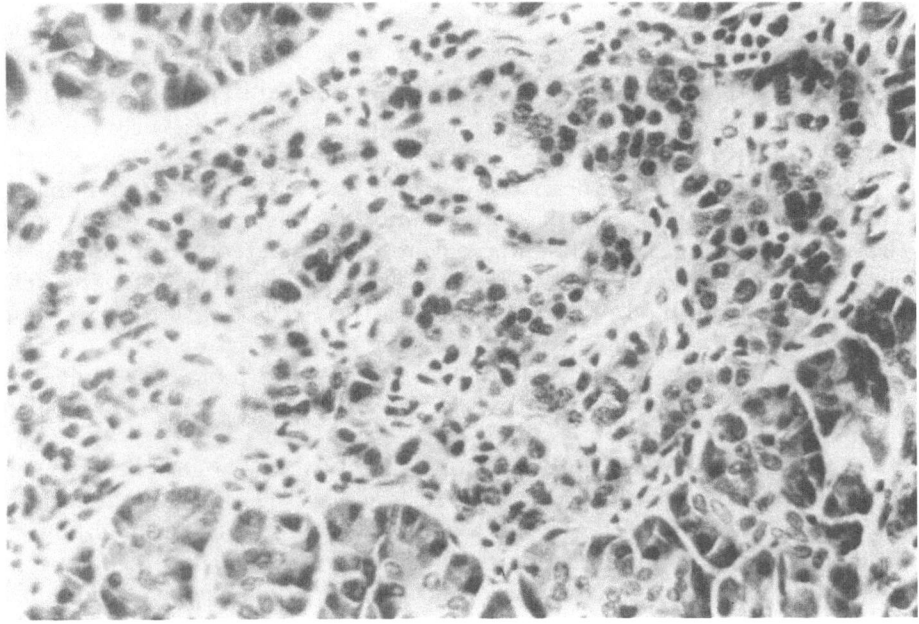

Figure 6. Recent-onset juvenile diabetic. Heavy lymphocytic infiltration (insulitis) in a fairly large islet, showing apparent hyperplasia and hyperactivity in the middle and atrophy on the left. ×560. Reproduced at 75%.

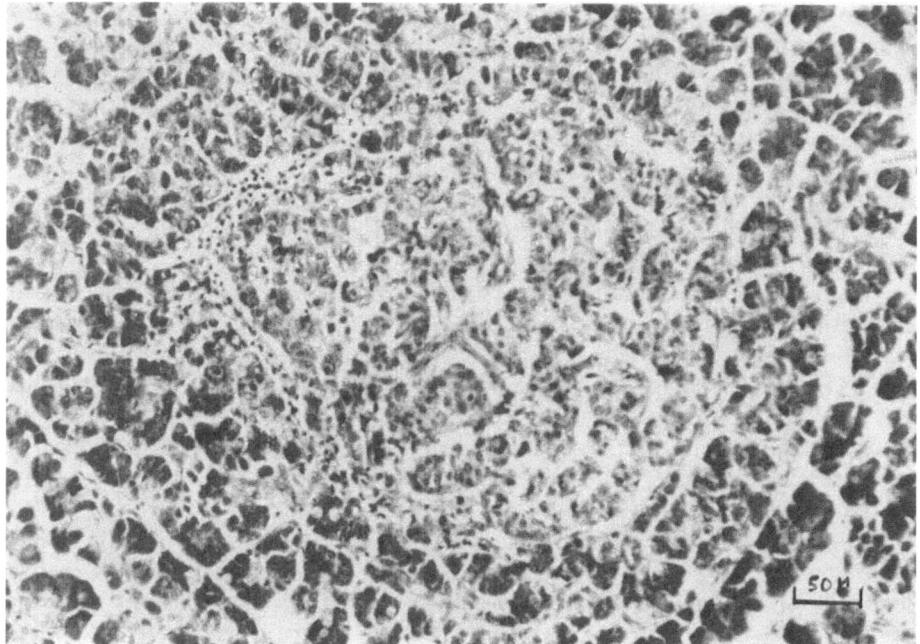

Figure 7. Recent-onset juvenile diabetic. Insulitis in a hypertrophic islet. The infiltration is more marked on the left side. Gomori's chromium hematoxylin–phloxine. ×160. Reproduced at 110%.

beginning to show the pattern of cords of small cells so characteristic of late juvenile diabetes (Figs. 8 and 9). In some such islets there is fairly advanced fibrosis.

The appearance just described of islets in various stages of apparent hyperplasia, infiltration (and presumed injury) by lymphocytes, atrophy, and fibrosis, suggests stages in an immunologic reaction in the course of which the B cells are eliminated and the islet is left consisting of apparently atrophic cells. However, with immunocytochemical methods, these cells appear to be secreting different types of pancreatic hormones as described below.

A special form of insulitis is the intense accumulation of eosinophil leukocytes sometimes seen around the hyperplastic islets in infants of diabetic mothers.[9,52]

Experimental Insulitis   Inflammation of the islets of Langerhans in experimental animals has been produced in several ways: (1) active immunization against homologous or heterologous insulin, (2) passive injection of antiinsulin serum, (3) injection of islet-rich pancreatic homogenates or pure islet tissue, (4) viruses, (5) the drug streptozotocin, in small doses. These will be considered in order.

1. Active immunization against insulin.   The first observation of experimental insulitis was accidental. Renold *et al.*[53] had injected cows with crystalline bovine and porcine insulin in Freund's adjuvant, for the purpose of studying the antibody response. Antibodies to both types of insulin were produced. Six

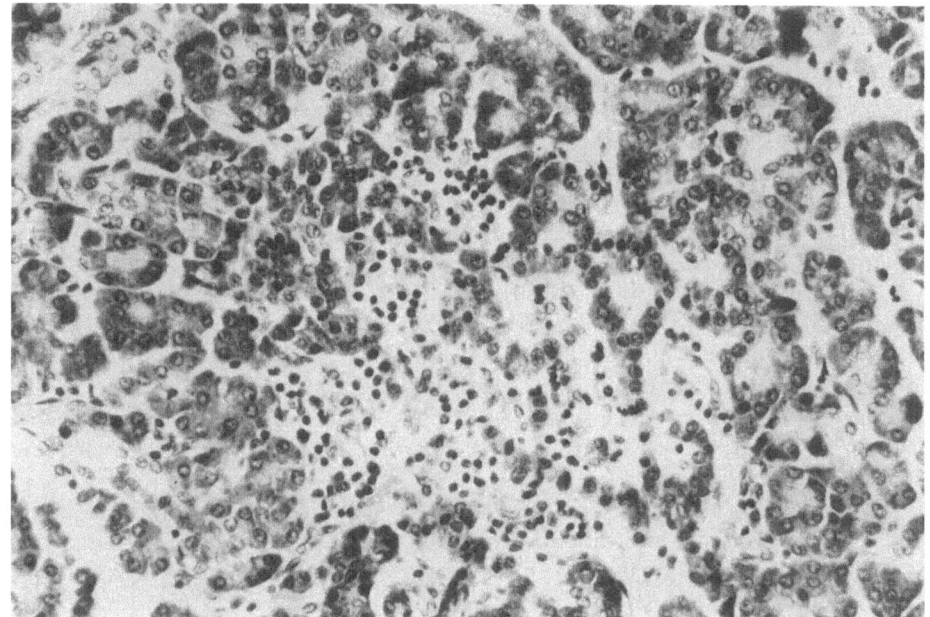

Figure 8. Recent-onset juvenile diabetic. Insulitis in an apparently atrophic islet, with narrow cords of islet cells and abundant mononuclear infiltrate. Gomori's chromium hematoxylin–phloxine. ×300. Reproduced at 110%.

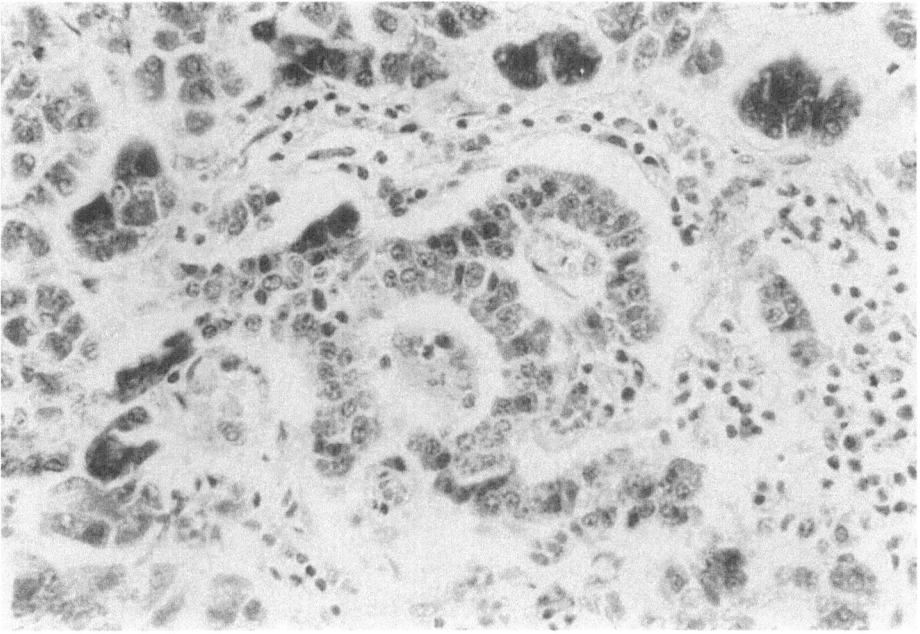

Figure 9. Recent-onset juvenile diabetic. Fairly advanced fibrosis in an islet also showing insulitis and apparent atrophy. B cells are essentially absent, and many of the remaining cells stain like A cells. Hematoxylin and eosin. Approximately ×400. Reproduced at 80%.

months after beginning injections of bovine insulin in adjuvant, one of the heifers died accidently of strangulation when her halter was caught in the superstructure of the stall. Examination of the pancreas revealed striking infiltration of the islets by lymphocytes. Thereafter, the other animals were studied carefully at autopsy. They showed varying degrees of insulitis.[54] Beside the heifer just mentioned, one other that had been given only homologous (bovine) insulin showed an extensive involvement of practically every islet by heavy infiltration of lymphocytes (Fig. 10). Although there was obvious loss of B cells and fibrosis in this as well as other animals (Fig. 11), none of them became demonstrably diabetic. Interestingly, the surviving B cells in affected islets often showed striking enlargement and evidence of hyperactivity in the form of a prominent Golgi apparatus (Fig. 12 and 13). Such evidence of stimulation is also commonly observed in the islets of juvenile diabetics of recent onset (Fig. 3).

Shortly after the work of Renold *et al.*,[53] Toreson *et al.*[55] noted insulitis as well as hyperglycemia in a rabbit immunized with crystalline beef insulin. Later experiments of similar nature in rabbits[56,57] led to further descriptions of experimental insulitis, with ultrastructural studies suggesting that the infiltrating cells could be classified as lymphocytes and immunoblasts, and that these cells were often in close relationship to B cells, sometimes inserting pseudopods

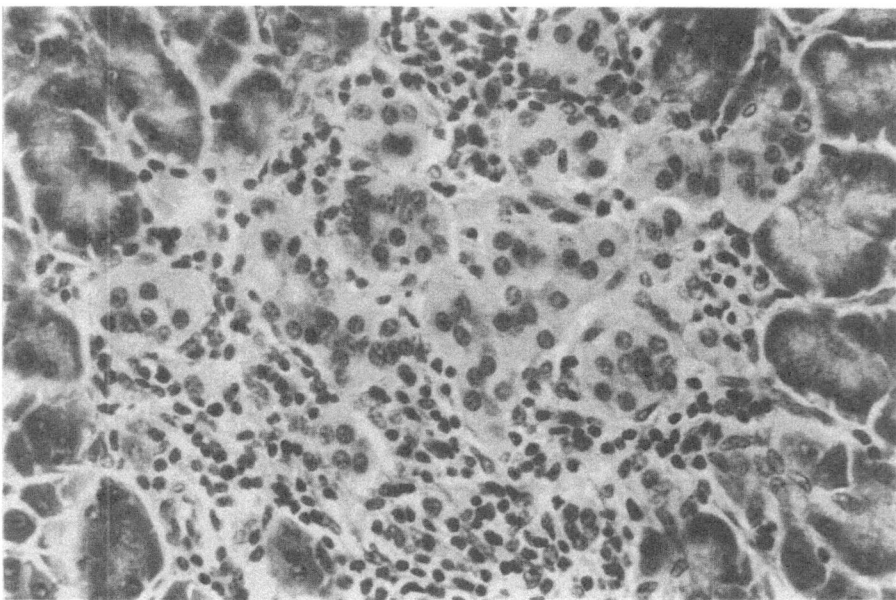

Figure 10. Severe insulitis with partial destruction of the islet in a cow injected repeatedly with homologous (bovine) insulin in Freund's adjuvant. Hematoxylin and eosin. Approximately ×500. Reproduced at 75%.

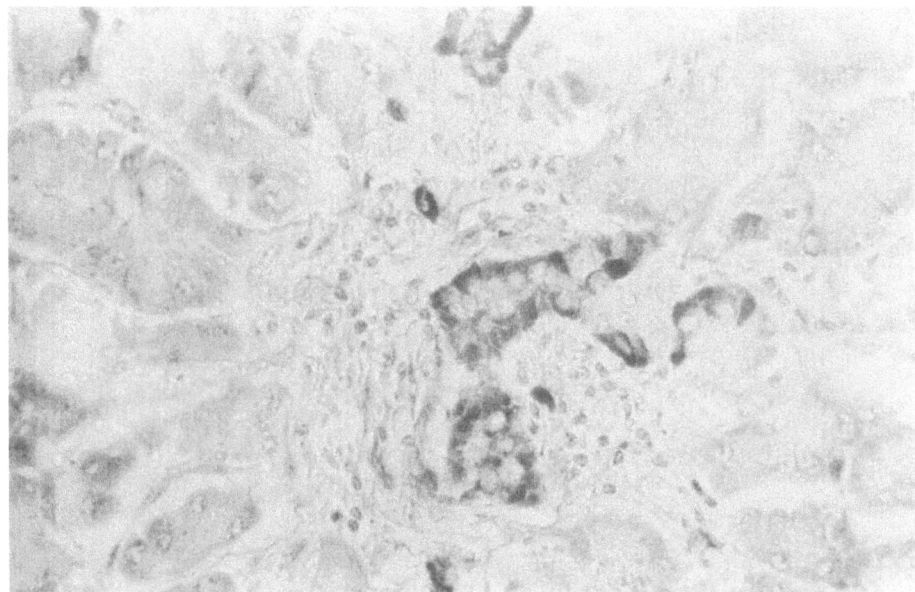

Figure 11. Islet of same animal as shown in Fig. 10 stained for B cell granules. The B cells (dark cytoplasm) are greatly reduced in number, and small groups of them are surrounded by fibrous tissue infiltrated by a few lymphocytes. Aldehyde-thionin ponceau-fuchsin. Approximately ×500. Reproduced at 75%.

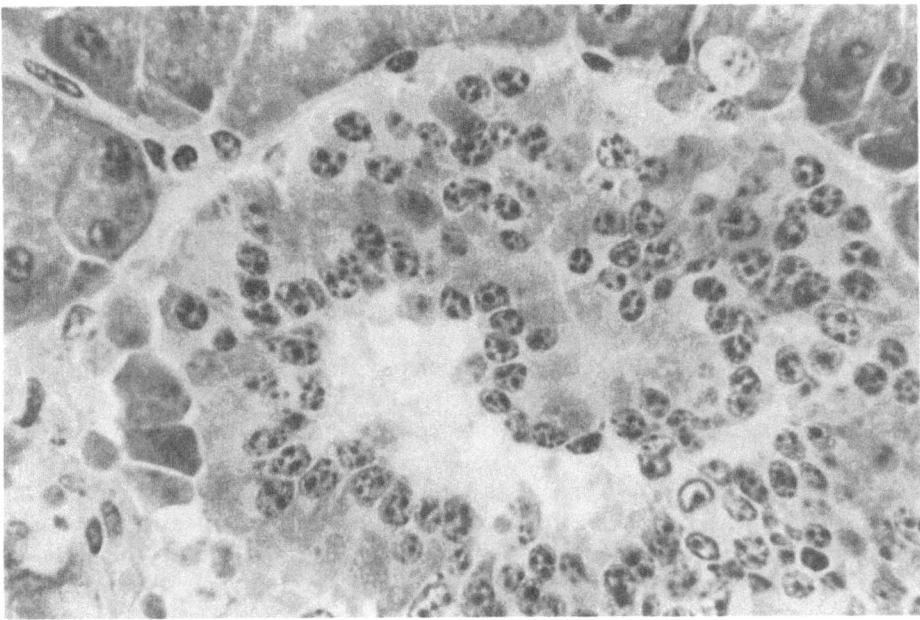

Figure 12. Islet of normal, uninjected cow (for comparison with Fig. 13, following page). Aldehyde-thionin trichrome. Approximately ×900. Reproduced at 75%.

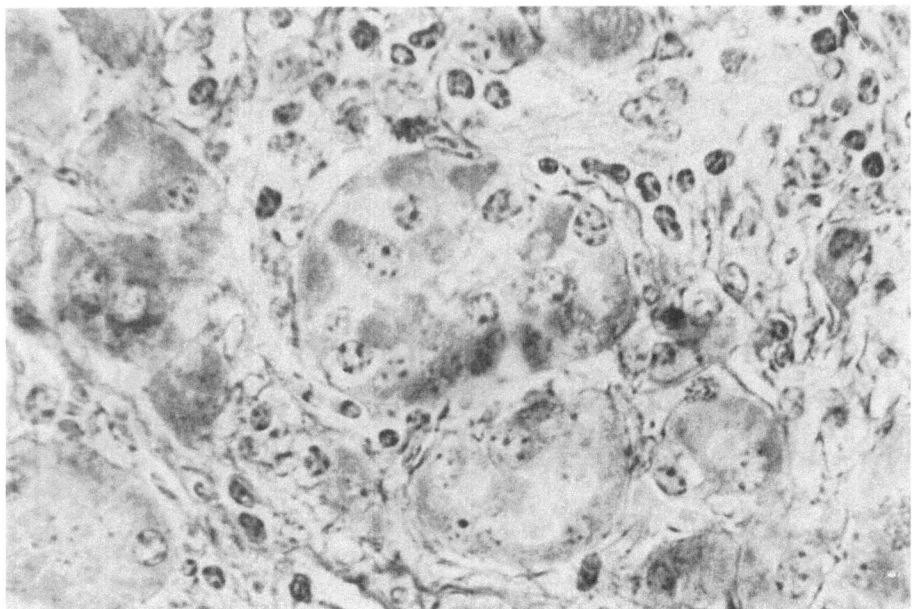

Figure 13. Islet of cow injected repeatedly with homologous (bovine) insulin in Freund's adjuvant (same animal as Fig. 10). Same magnification as Fig. 12, preceding page, to show enlarged cells with large nuclei and prominent Golgi areas. Note insulitis and beginning fibrosis at upper right and lower left. Aldehyde-thionin trichrome. Approximately ×900. Reproduced at 75%.

into them, with occasional lysis of the B cell membrane and release of its cytoplasmic contents. It thus appeared that the B cells were actually destroyed by a cell-mediated immunologic process of the type seen in delayed hypersensitivity. In general, the severity of the insulitis is correlated with high levels of circulating antibody to insulin, but this is not always true.[58]

Similar experimental results were obtained in sheep.[59,60] However, it appears that insulitis of this autoimmune type has not been produced in any animal species other than cattle, rabbits, and sheep, even though humoral antibodies to insulin (which can be associated with delayed hypersensitivity) have been produced in all species so far studied.[25]

Another unanswered question concerns the variable antigenicity of different forms of insulin and in particular the mechanism by which a homologous insulin becomes antigenic for the same species. This problem was noted by Renold *et al.*[53] who suggested that their results indicated a difference between endogenous circulating insulin and pancreatic insulin. Among the possible answers to this still unanswered question are the following: (a) molecular changes occurring during the extraction of insulin, perhaps more likely differences in the tertiary structure than the amino acid sequence[61]; (b) the concept that endogenous insulin is associated with other plasma proteins leading to a covering or modification of an antigenic site; and (c) the uncovering of an antigenic site during the extraction procedure.

2. Passive injection of antiinsulin serum. This may lead acutely to a form of insulitis characterized by an exudate of eosinophilic and neutrophilic leukocytes surrounding islets and ductules and appearing within a few hours after injection. Lacy and Wright[62] observed an exudate in the pancreatic tissue, not confined to the islets, after intraperitoneal injection of rats with guinea pig antiinsulin serum, but they noted involvement of islets only after intravenous injection. Their results have been confirmed by others.[63,64] The lesion is readily produced in mice as well as in rats. A single intravenous injection of 0.02 ml of antiinsulin (antibovine or antiporcine) guinea pig serum leads to a pure granulocytic (eosinophilic and neutrophilic) infiltration around the islets, reaching its maximum after 3 to 6 hr. The electron microscope reveals cloudy, electron-dense material (presumably antigen–antibody complex) being phagocytosed by leukocytes in the vicinity of B cells. A temporary hyperglycemia develops, and hyperactivity of B cells (enlargement of Golgi complex, increase in microvesicles and pregranules) can be recognized. Continuation of daily injections leads to hyaline thrombi in the islets and eventually, in a matter of weeks, to hyperplasia of islets and to an alteration in the cellular infiltrate, which now consists of mononuclear cells (immunoblasts sometimes acting as macrophages, lymphocytes, and a few plasma cells).[25]

As noted by Freytag and Klöppel,[25] the prompt (within 90 min) appearance of antigen–antibody precipitates and an exudate of eosinophil and neutrophil leukocytes suggest a sensitivity reaction of the immediate type, perhaps analogous to the Arthus phenomenon. This kind of cellular reaction would seem comparable in the human to the eosinophilic infiltrate in infants of diabetic mothers, rather than to the insulitis of the juvenile diabetic. It is of interest, however, that prolonged injections of antiinsulin serum can, as noted above, lead to a more chronic form of insulitis, presumably from superimposition of a reaction of delayed hypersensitivity.

3. Injection of pancreatic tissue. This has been carried out mainly by Nerup and associates,[65] the general method being to inject intracutaneously saline suspensions of heterologous or homologous pancreatic tissue in Freund's adjuvant. The tissue has usually been chosen to be rich in islets (fetal calf pancreas at 16 to 20 weeks gestation, or isolated mouse islets). Insulitis consisting of mononuclear cells, presumably lymphocytes, was found, associated with evidence of injury to B cells. Cellular sensitization was demonstrated *in vitro* by the leukocyte migration test, as had been previously done in human diabetics by the same group of workers.[66,67] Heydinger and Lacy[68] isolated rat islets by the collagenase method and injected them subcutaneously in rats which, on sacrifice some months later, showed fibrosis of the islets (Fig. 14). Rare lymphocytes were seen, but with no insulitis worthy of the name. However, the shortest period in their series was 2 months, and it is possible that an insulitis might have disappeared in that time.

4. Viruses. Craighead[69] was the first to show that insulitis, comparable to that sometimes seen in human juvenile diabetes, could be produced experimentally by infection of mice with a virus of the encephalomyocarditis group. His findings were soon confirmed by others.[70-74] Müntefering *et al.*[70,74] note that in their experiments the insulitis was transitory, usually appearing from the

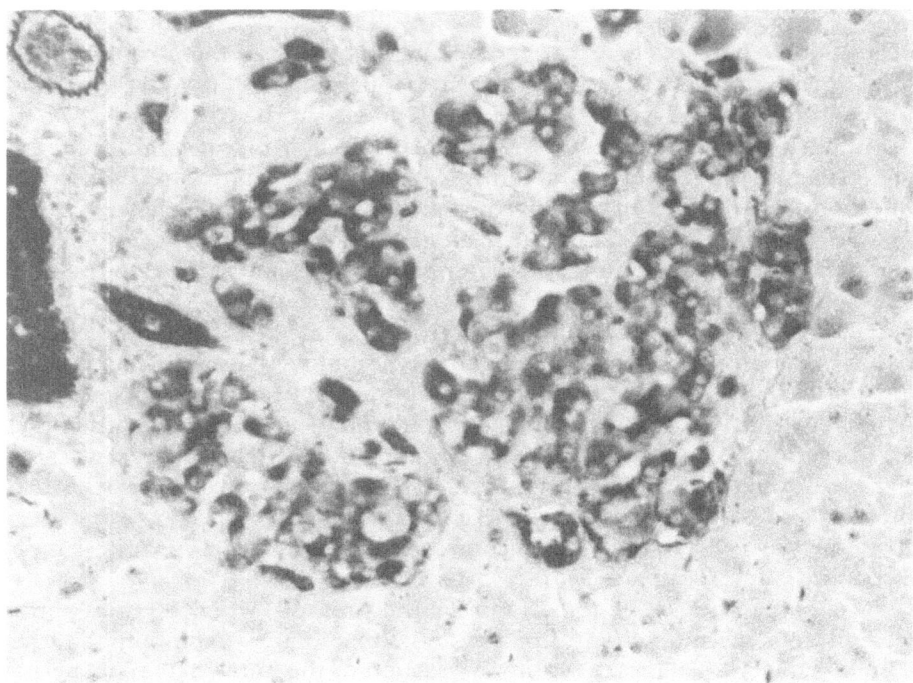

Figure 14. Fibrosis of islet of rat injected with homogenized rat islets. Surviving islet cells contain dark granules. Courtesy of Dr. Paul E. Lacy. From Heydinger and Lacy.[68] Aldehyde fuchsin. Approximately ×300.

seventh to the twelfth day, and imply that this finding might conceivably throw light on the supposed rarity of the lesion in human juvenile diabetes. Since the viral lesions are fully covered by Craighead in Chapter 19, they will not be discussed further here.

5. Streptozotocin. While giving small doses of streptozotocin to mice for another purpose, Like and Rossini[75] accidentally discovered that insulitis (Figs. 15 and 16) was a constant feature in their animals. Further investigation revealed that insulitis first appeared on the sixth and fifth days after the last injection in mice that received two or three daily injections, respectively (40 mg/kg, i.p.). Inflammation was more pronounced after three injections, and these animals also showed mild hyperglycemia (mean plasma glucose 214 mg/100 ml) on the seventh postinjection day. Another unexpected and most striking finding was the presence, in addition to the lymphocytes and macrophages, of numerous C-type virus particles in the B cells (not in A or D cells). The genome of the C-type viruses, which are responsible for murine leukemia,[76] is known to be present in many strains of wild and laboratory mice, as well as in many other species, including primates,[77,78] and similar particles have been seen in the B cells of mice.[78]

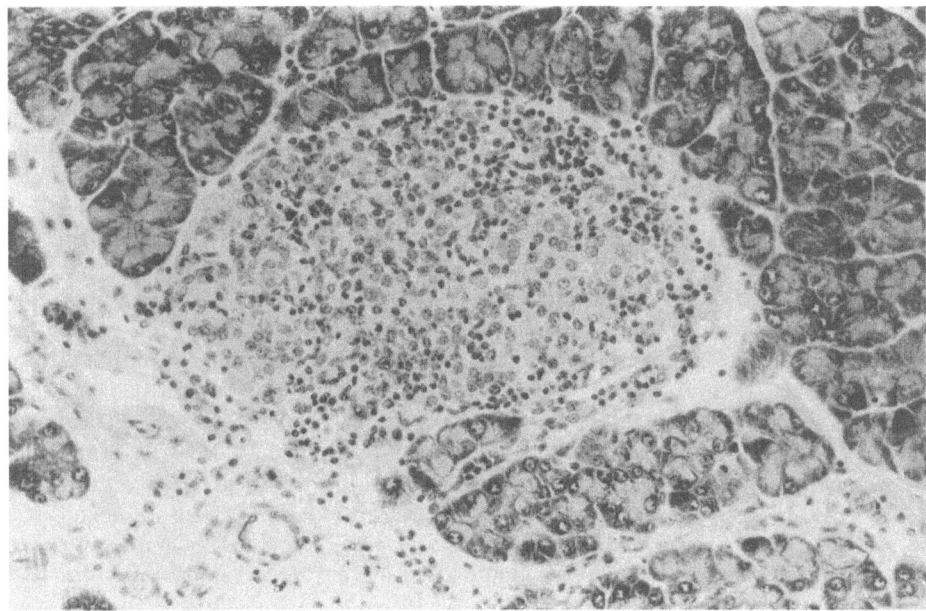

Figure 15. Inflamed islet from mouse sacrificed 6 days after receiving five injections of streptozotocin (40 mg/kg). The interior and periphery of the islet are permeated with large numbers of mononuclear cells, identified as lymphocytes and macrophages by electron microscopy. Courtesy of Dr. Arthur Like. From Like and Rossini.[75] Hematoxylin and eosin. Approximately ×250.

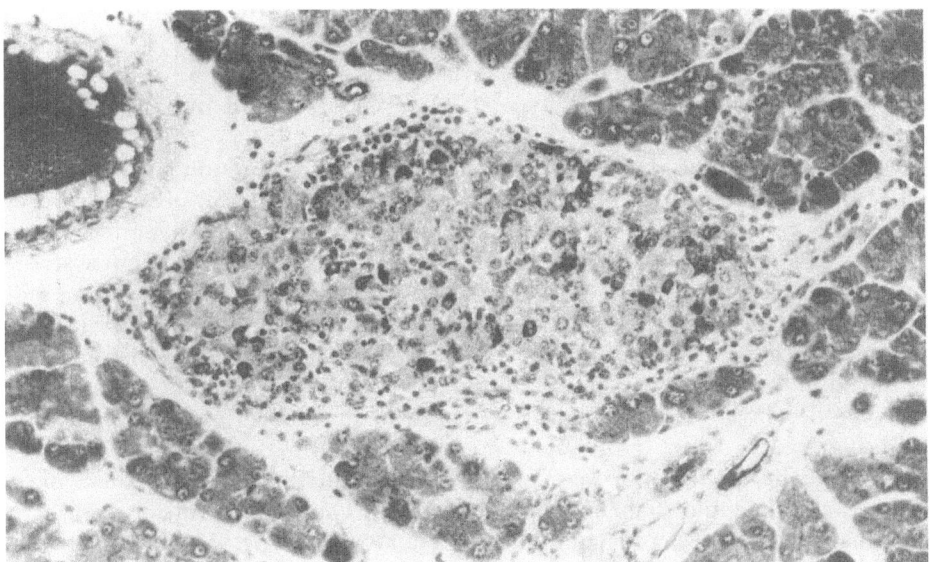

Figure 16. Islet of mouse treated like that in Fig. 15. Stained for B cell granules (black). In addition to insulitis there is marked degranulation of B cells, consistent with the presence of hyperglycemia. Courtesy of Dr. Arthur Like. Aldehyde fuchsin. Approximately ×160.

Further studies of this fascinating experimental model by the same authors have shown that there is genetic variation in the susceptibility of different strains of mice to the procedure[78a], also that prior treatment of susceptible mice with 3-*O*-methyl-D-glucose or anti-mouse-lymphocyte serum causes attenuation of the diabetic syndrome, and that both agents together prevent it. The authors suggest[78b] that a triad of factors: (1) direct B cell cytotoxicity, (2) virus induction within B cells, and (3) a cell-mediated autoimmune reaction, acting separately or in concert, appear to induce the destructive insulitis and severe diabetes.

Islet Hyalinosis   With the light microscope, insular hyalinosis appears as a deposit of acellular hyaline material between the islet cells and the capillaries. Many authors[79-83] have demonstrated that islet hyaline shares many staining characteristics with amyloid. It also has the same ultrastructural appearance.[84,85] However, tryptophane, a typical constituent of amyloid, cannot be demonstrated histochemically, either in islet hyaline,[85] or in the hyaline deposits which are commonly present in insulinomas.[86] The latter authors have therefore denied the identity of insulinoma hyaline with amyloid and have suggested that it consists of C-chains of the proinsulin molecule. Lacy[87] was unable to detect insulin in islet hyaline, but Westermark,[88] by treating crystalline insulin with dilute acid, according to the method of Bourke and Rougvie,[89] made a gel which showed tinctorial reactions of amyloid.

Although islet hyalinosis was first described by Opie[30] in the pancreas of a diabetic girl of 17, all authors agree that it is rare in young diabetics and occurs much more frequently in maturity-onset diabetics. Bell[90] found no example of hyalinosis in diabetics under 20 years of age; in his material it occurred in only 10% of the diabetes between 20 and 40 years, whereas it was present in 45.7% of diabetics over 60 years of age. Warren *et al.*[9] rarely observed islet hyalinosis in diabetics under age 40. In the material studied by one of the authors of this chapter,[8] only one, not entirely typical, example was found among 54 juvenile diabetics (Fig. 17).

The question as to why hyaline deposits are so common in the islets of older diabetics and so rare in those of younger patients has not been answered as yet. Recent observations by Westermark[88] suggest that islet hyalinosis is not an expression of so-called senile amyloidosis and that it differs from systemic immune amyloidosis. One could speculate that there is something wrong with the mechanism of insulin secretion in the B cells of older diabetics (and in tumoral B cells), leading to extracellular deposition of some cellular material involved in the secretory process. In juvenile diabetes, on the other hand, the B cells are destroyed by an unknown mechanism, and therefore hyaline deposits do not appear.

Islet Fibrosis   Islet fibrosis (Fig. 18) has been mentioned in all studies of the pancreas of juvenile diabetics. It is a frequent change in acute as well as in chronic cases.[8,9,91] It is present mainly in the atrophic type of islets. It could be partly due to islet inflammation and to a collapse of the framework of the islet after the disappearance of the B cells (Fig. 19). Heydinger and Lacy[68] produced fibrosis with rare lymphocytic infiltration in the islets of rats by repeated injections of isolated islets from the same species (Fig. 14). In cases of chronic juvenile diabetes, islet fibrosis is usually associated with a diffuse interlobular and interacinar fibrosis, as well as with severe vascular sclerosis.

Islet Hypertrophy and Islet Regeneration Abnormally large islets with a diameter exceeding 400 μm occur in the pancreas of juvenile diabetics who have died after a disease of short duration.[8,9,92] Maclean and Ogilvie[92] suggested that this hypertrophy might result from an excessive stimulation by an extra-pancreatic factor of unknown nature. Compensation for the atrophy of the majority of the other islets is another likely explanation.

The question as to when islet hypertrophy starts to appear remains unsettled, because of the lack of information concerning the appearance of the islets before the onset of diabetes. One of us (P.M.L.) has had the opportunity to review the autopsy findings in a boy of 14, genetically prediabetic, since both his parents were diabetic.[93] This boy died of cardiomyopathy, after a terminal episode of low blood pressure while in a respirator. His pancreas showed islet hyperplasia and hypertrophy (Fig. 20) with mitoses and nuclear pyknosis (Fig. 21). However, the relationship between these changes and the hypothetical development of diabetes later on cannot be ascertained, because other pathological factors may have been involved in their production.

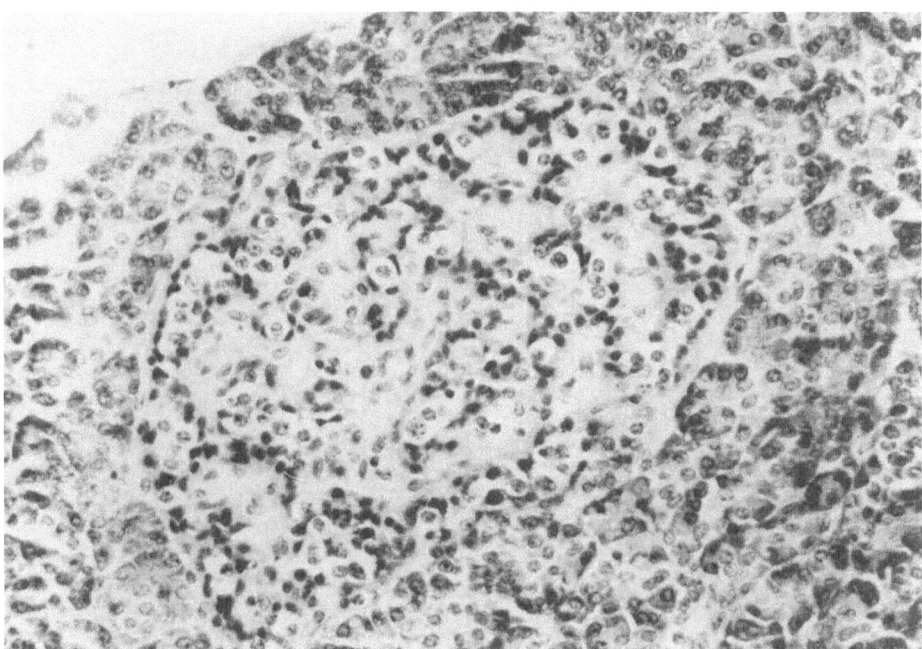

Figure 17. Amorphous hyaline deposits between the cells in an islet of a recent-onset juvenile diabetic. Hemalum erythrosin saffron. ×260. Reproduced at 110%.

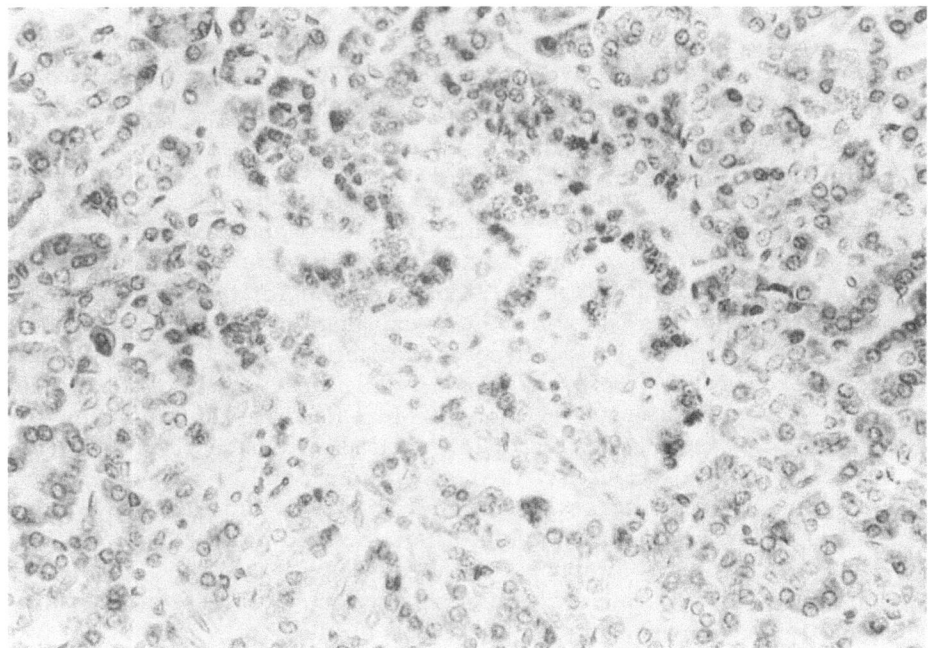

Figure 18. Acute juvenile diabetic. Marked fibrosis with thin cords of atrophic (?) islet cells and discrete lymphocytic infiltration. Gomori's chromium hematoxylin–phloxine. ×260. Reproduced at 105%.

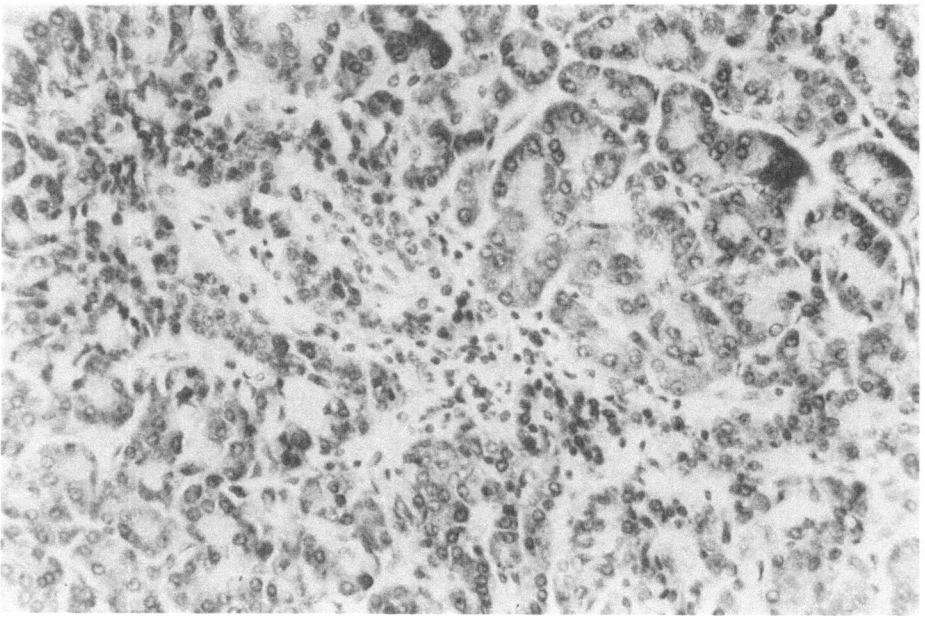

Figure 19. Recent-onset juvenile diabetic. Collapse of an islet, associated with insulitis. Gomori's chromium hematoxylin–phloxine. ×260. Reproduced at 105%.

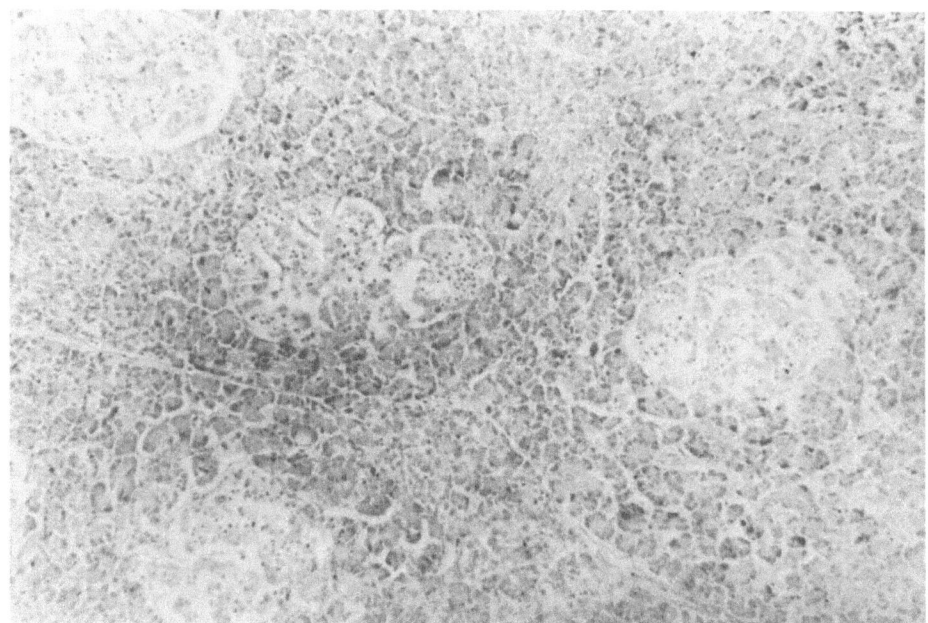

Figure 20. Hyperplasia and hypertrophy of islets in the pancreas of a 14-year-old boy who had two diabetic parents. Pyknotic nuclei are seen among large, active-looking cells. ×160. Reproduced at 80%.

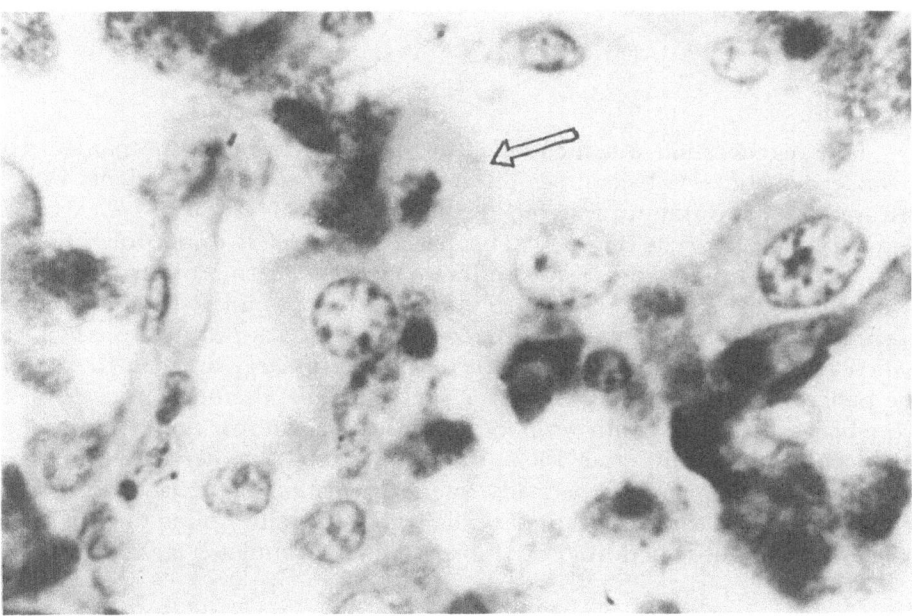

Figure 21. High magnification of cells in an islet of the case shown in Fig. 20, stained for B granules. The pyknotic cells contain B granules (black). The large cells with large nuclei and occasional mitotic figures (arrow) do not contain granules stainable with the usual methods. Aldehyde-thionin trichrome. ×1300. Reproduced at 75%.

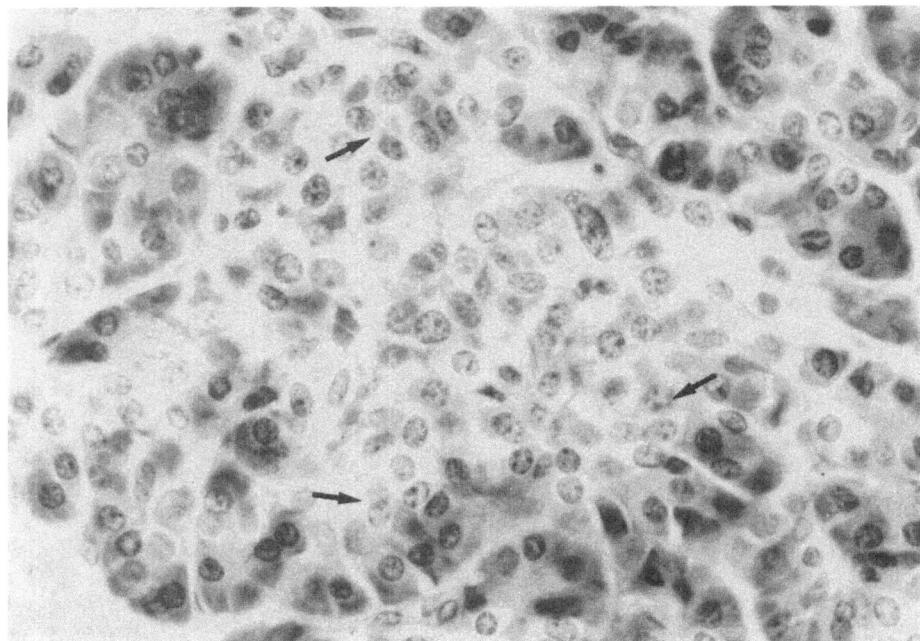

Figure 22. Recent-onset juvenile diabetic. Neoformation of an islet from centroacinar cells (arrows). Gomori's chromium hematoxylin-phloxine. ×600. Reproduced at 75%.

Islet regeneration was mentioned in the early studies of the pancreas of juvenile diabetics.[14,94] It assumes different aspects. In young patients with a disease of short duration, it is represented by a proliferation of centroacinar (Fig. 22) and duct cells (Fig. 23). This proliferation leads to the formation of islets composed of large cells, with a clear cytoplasm, often containing "Körnchen" (Fig. 24), and occasionally a few B or A granules. The distribution of these newly formed islets is quite irregular; they may appear in crops in a few pancreatic lobules, and may be completely absent in large areas of the rest of the pancreas (Figs. 25 and 26). In one such example, the newly formed islets were heavily infiltrated with lymphocytes (insulitis), whereas no such infiltrates could be found in the other islets. In chronic cases, regeneration assumes a more atypical appearance; it leads to the formation of islets consisting of irregular, sinuous cords of columnar cells, with a centrally located nucleus and a pale cytoplasm, usually devoid of visible secretion granules (Fig. 27).*

*In studying regeneration in tissue cultures of islets of primates (monkeys) Like and Chick (*Amer. J. Pathol.* 75:329, 1974) concluded that B cells seemed to be derived from preexisting B cells, not duct or acinar cells. We feel that these findings are not necessarily applicable to the human diabetic pancreas, where regeneration of B cells as well as other cell types seems to occur from duct cells and centroacinar cells, especially in the juvenile.

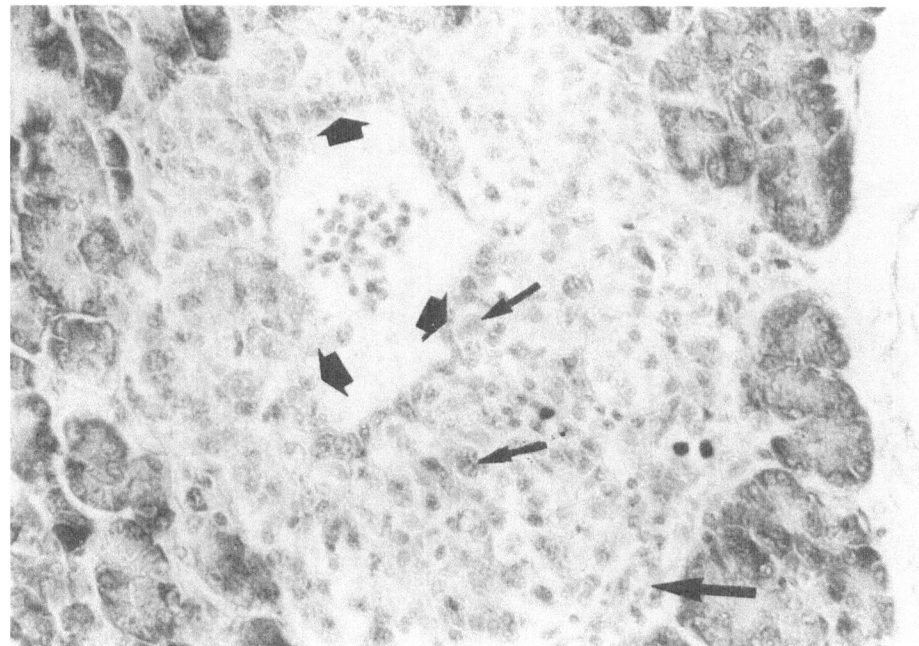

Figure 23. Recent-onset juvenile diabetic. Neoformation of an islet from duct epithelium (large arrows). Also note hypertrophic and irregular nuclei (short arrows) and discrete lymphocytic infiltration (insulitis) (long arrow). ×350. Reproduced at 105%.

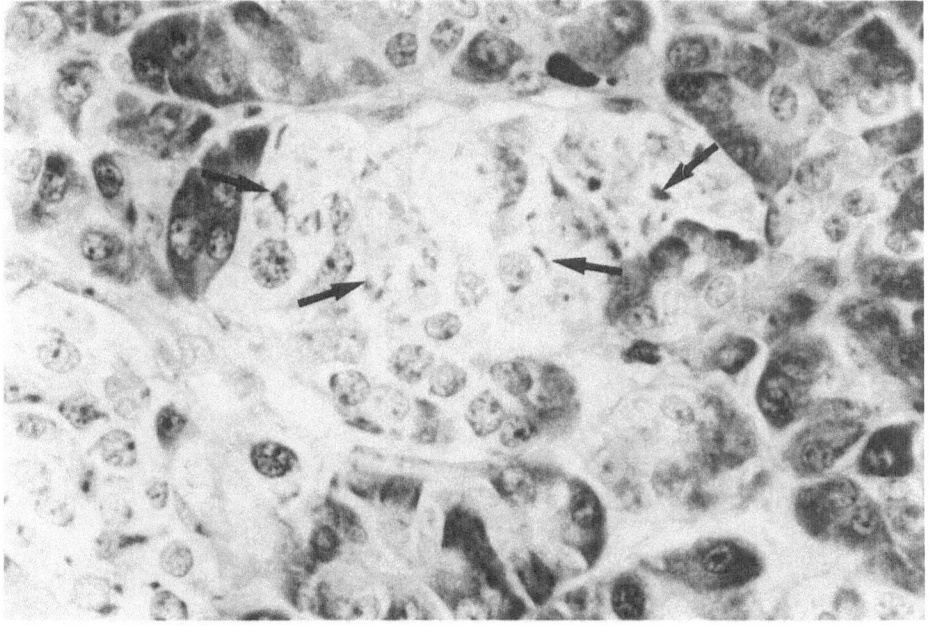

Figure 24. Recent-onset juvenile diabetic. Small, newly formed islets with cells having large nuclei and "Körnchen" (arrows). Gomori's chromium hematoxylin–phloxine. ×600. Reproduced at 105%.

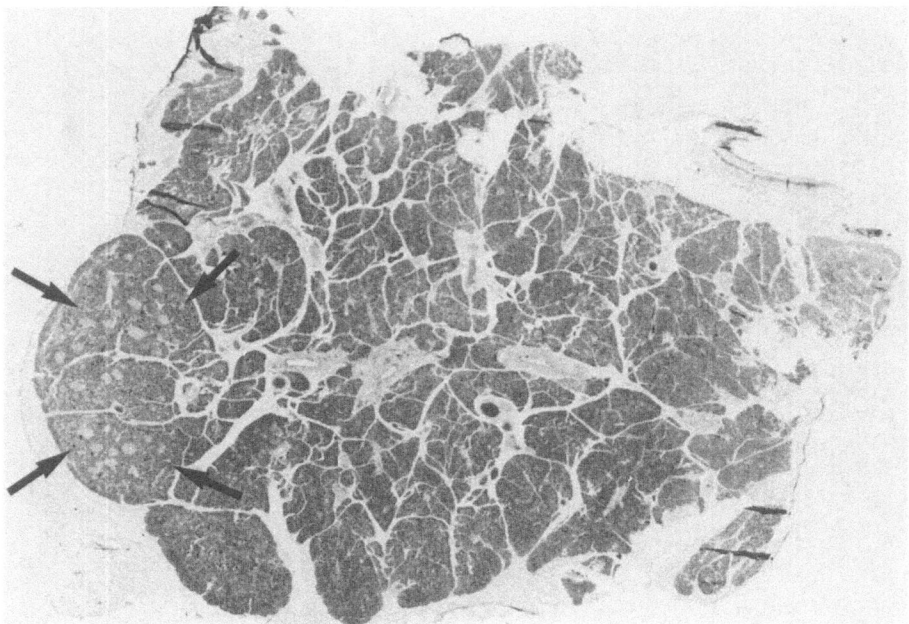

Figure 25. Recent-onset juvenile diabetic. Very active neoformation of islets in a few pancreatic lobules at left (arrows). Islets scarcely visible in remainder of section. Gomori's chromium hematoxylin-phloxine. ×12. Reproduced at 75%.

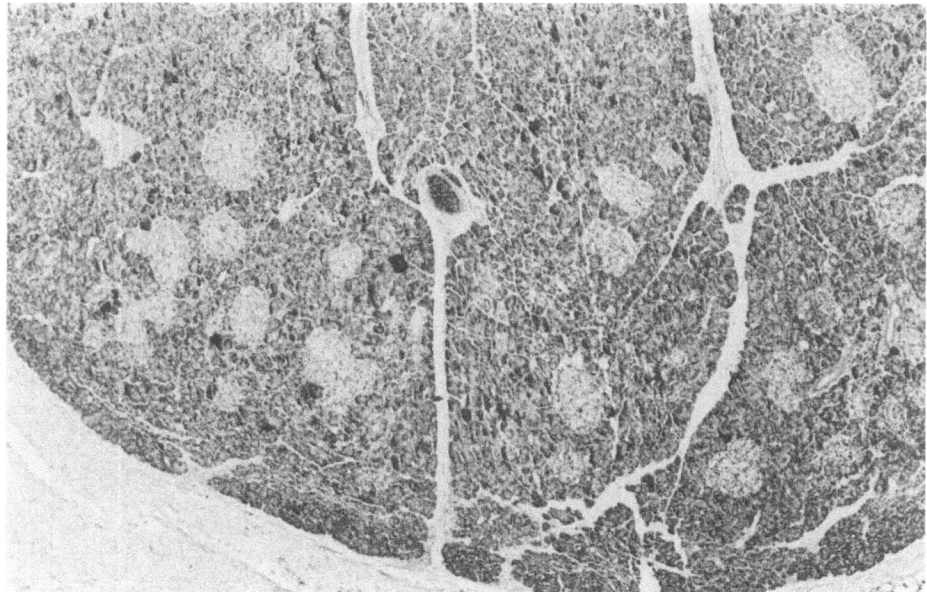

Figure 26. Higher magnification of area shown in Fig. 25, showing numerous newly formed islets (same case in Fig. 23). Gomori's chromium hematoxylin–phloxine. ×60. Reproduced at 75%.

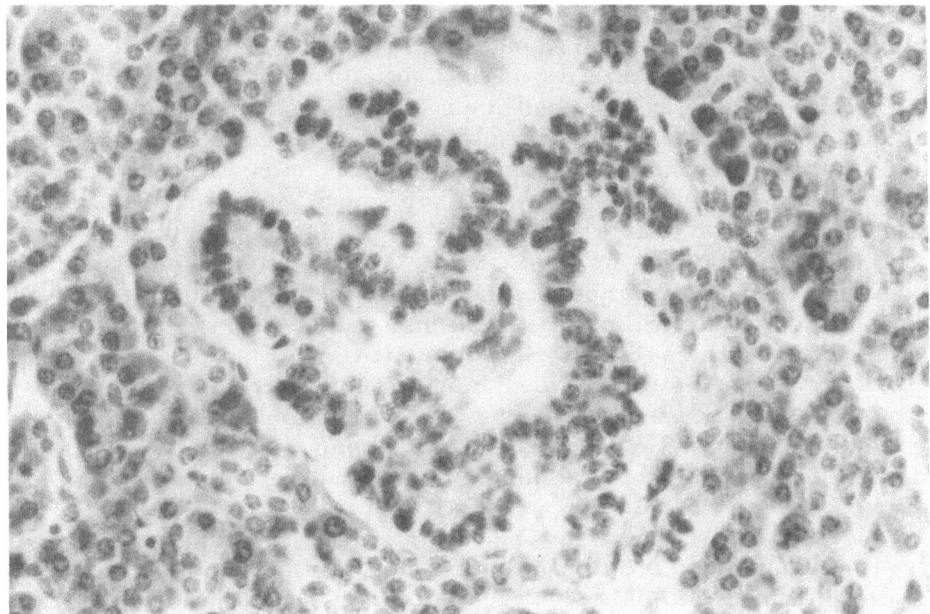

Figure 27. Regenerating islet consisting of ribbonlike cords of columnar cells. This pattern often represents hyperplasia of cells producing pancreatic polypeptide (see Fig. 32). Gomori's chromium hematoxylin–phloxine. ×350. Reproduced at 105%.

Quantitative Changes

The dispersion of the endocrine tissue of the pancreas in the form of small islets within a much larger exocrine gland greatly complicates quantitative studies. Moreover, in juvenile diabetics the irregular distribution of the islet lesions and the difficult identification of the islet cells constitute supplementary difficulties. However, the quantitative changes which are present in the pancreas of juvenile diabetics are so marked that they can be demonstrated even with very crude methods. Furthermore, new immunohistochemical methods have been introduced, which now allow a better insight into the changes in the cytological composition of the islets.

Size and Number of Islets   At the beginning of this century, studies of the diabetic pancreas revealed the fact that the number and the size of the islets are often reduced, especially in young patients. Actually, the islets may be so scarce and small in these diabetics, that it requires a prolonged search to find them. Such cases have induced a few authors to postulate a congenital hypoplasia of the pancreatic islets as a possible cause of juvenile diabetes.[5,95] This suggestion appears unlikely, because nearly complete absence of islets would result in diabetes from birth on. To our knowledge, the only convincing recorded case of congenital absence of islets is that of Laurence and Dodge.[96] In this case, the infant had a blood glucose of 800 mg/100ml at 36 hr of age and died shortly afterwards. This infant had a sibling who had died at 48 hr, but no histological examination of the pancreas was performed. The authors were led to suggest a previously undescribed X-linked inherited condition.

In cases of juvenile diabetes, in which the numerical reduction of the islets is less evident, it is easily confirmed by quantitative studies, which usually consist of counting the islets in a given area of pancreatic tissue. From such studies it appears that the pancreases of diabetics contain fewer islets than those of nondiabetics, that this change is more pronounced in young than in older patients,[5,14,32,97] and that within the juvenile group the reduction is more marked in chronic than in acute cases.[8,92] As already mentioned under the qualitative changes, the majority of the islets of juvenile diabetics are small and atrophic in appearance, but islets of medium and of large size are present in young diabetics with a disease of short duration.

Amount of Islet Tissue   As could be expected from the reduced number of islets, their small size, and, in the case of chronic juvenile diabetics, the reduction of the weight of the pancreas, the total amount of islet tissue is markedly decreased. Again, this change is more profound in cases with a disease of long duration than in acute cases.[8,92]

Changes in the Cytologic Composition of the Islets   A detailed study of the cytologic composition of the pancreatic islets of juvenile diabetics meets with several difficulties, including scarceness of the islets, especially in chronic cases, atrophy and degranulation of the islet cells, and lack of reliable methods to demonstrate all the known cell types in autopsy material.

These difficulties probably explain why so few cytologic studies of the islets of juvenile diabetics have been attempted. Maclean and Ogilvie[92] performed differential counts of A and B cells in 6 juvenile diabetics, among whom were 3 acute and 3 chronic cases. In the acute cases the A:B ratio proved to be approximately 1 to 2.7, in the chronic cases 1 to 1.1. In the material studied by Gepts,[8] such cell counts proved difficult to perform, because in the majority of cases the non-B cells were small and poorly stained. Furthermore, the routine methods for staining the islet cells do not distinguish between glucagon cells and other cell types, now known to be present in the pancreatic islets. Only the B cells remained recognizable in spite of their almost complete degranulation. Taking advantage of this fact, it was calculated that shortly after the clinical onset of the disease, the pancreas of juvenile diabetics contains less than 10% of the normal number of B cells. In 13 among 17 cases who had survived the initial diagnosis for longer than 1 year, B cells were no longer identifiable. In the remaining 4 cases, they were present in a small number in 2, in a moderate number in 1 and in a relatively large number in the last 1.[8]

In a more recent study, Doniach and Morgan[10] found a gross reduction of the islets already at the clinical onset of diabetes. In the acute cases, they observed granulated B cells in 10, and none in 3 others. In treated chronic cases with a duration of diabetes between 6 and 38 years, B cells were present in very low numbers in 7 cases, whereas none could be found in 6 others. In spite of minor discrepancies, this study led to the same conclusion as that of Maclean and Ogilvie[92] and that of Gepts.[8] B cells are still present, but in a markedly reduced number, when juvenile diabetes breaks out clinically; they tend to disappear with a prolonged evolution of the disease.

The situation is much less clear for the non-B cells of the pancreatic islets. It is true that the number and the function of these cells have not been completely clarifed as yet. After the description by Lane[98] of A and B cells, a third cell type, the D cell, was identified by Bloom.[99] The introduction of silver techniques then created a very confused situation because the methods applied by different authors apparently did not demonstrate the same type of cells. Moreover, the correspondence between the silver-impregnated cells and those differentiated by other staining methods remained somewhat controversial. Whereas some silver techniques (Gros–Schultze, Bodian, Holmes) impregnate all non-B cells and probably a small number of B cells as well,[100,101] the Davenport silver technique, modified by Hellerström and Hellman,[102] stains only part of the A cells, more particularly those which these authors called A_1 cells. Fujita[103,104] defended the opinion that A_1 and D cells are identical, a conclusion which the Swedish authors are reluctant to admit.[105]

From a number of elegant experiments (for a review see Hellman and Täljedal[106]), Hellman and Hellerström concluded that the A_2 cells, i.e., those that do not take up silver with their method, secrete glucagon. They were unable to propose a function for the A_1 cells, but they produced evidence that these cells secrete a factor which inhibits the release of insulin from B cells.[128] Some workers[107,108] have claimed to demonstrate gastrin in the A_1 or D cell; others[109,110] have failed to do so. However, Erlandsen *et al.*[110a] maintain that D cells contain both gastrin and somatostatin.

Another silver technique which has become widely applied is the one developed by Grimelius.[111] According to this author, it is almost specific for the glucagon-secreting A_2 cells. However, it seems to stain also the D_1 cells[111a] as well as the PP cells (which may be identical; see page 350).

Studies with the electron microscope at first added to the confusion, because divergent opinions were expressed by different authors, and also because of the application of a different nomenclature (for a review, see Lacy and Greider[112]). In the laboratory of one of us (W.G.) four types of cells were identified in the islets: A and B cells, and two other cell types which were provisionally called type III and type IV. Another very rare endocrine cell type, called type V, was observed among the acinar cells of the pancreas of adults.[113] Like and Orci,[115] studying human fetuses, described several cell types (A,B, and D cells and "other endocrine cells tentatively identified as serotonin, gastrin, epinephrine, and norepinephrine cells"). In 1973, a group of morphologists[116] met in Bologna and agreed on four islet cell types: A, B, D (corresponding to the type III of Deconinck *et al.*[113,114]) and D_1 (corresponding to the type IV of the same authors). The classification of the endocrine cells of the pancreas and the gut was discussed again at the International Symposium on the Gastro-entero-pancreatic System.[117]

An important step forward was made when it was demonstrated that cells with the ultrastructural characteristics of D cells secrete somatostatin,[118,119] a tetradecapeptide, first isolated from the hypothalamus by Vale *et al.*[120] and by Brazeau *et al.*[121] which later on was shown to be present in the pancreatic islets and in the gastric and duodenal mucosa as well.[110a,122–125] Since it was also demonstrated that somatostatin not only inhibits the release of growth hormone, but also that of insulin and glucagon, as well as that of several other hormones, the interesting possibility emerged that D cells may play a part in the local regulation of an integrated islet function,[126,127] but this provocative hypothesis must await confirmation. On the other hand, it became retrospectively clear that the factor which Hellman and Lernmark[128] had extracted from the A_1 cells and which was shown to inhibit insulin release is somatostatin.

The function of the D_1 cells remains unknown as yet.[113,114,128a] Buffa *et al.*[128b,c] have suggested that these cells secrete vasoactive intestinal peptide (VIP), a peptide which was first isolated from the intestinal mucosa, but also extracted from the pancreas later on.[128d] Another candidate for secretion by the D_1 cells, the "pancreatic polypeptide" was recently proposed by Heitz *et al.*[128e,f] Pancreatic polypeptide (PP) is a 36-amino acid peptide which was detected as a contaminant of chicken insulin by Kimmel *et al.*[129,130] Later on, Lin and Chance[131-134] isolated a similar factor from the bovine (BPP) and porcine as well as from the human (HPP) pancreas. The physiological functions of this polypeptide are poorly known as yet, but evidence has been proposed that it acts as a hormone.[135,136a,b,c] Cells secreting HPP are present in the pancreas of man.[111b,137,138a,b,c,d] In the normal human pancreas, most of them are located at the periphery of the islets, but some are found in the acinar tissue or in the epithelium of ducts, either isolated or in clusters. The ultrastructural identification of the PP cells is still controversial. As mentioned above, Heitz *et al.*[128d,e] have expressed the opinion that they are identical to the D_1 cells, but this suggestion was criticized by Sundler and Håkanson.[138e] Larsson *et al.*[111b] favor the type V cells of Deconinck *et al.*[113,114] for the origin of PP. The fact that the PP cells are numerous in the uncinate process of the dog pancreas induced Baetens *et al.*[138f] and Buffa *et al.*,[128c] as well as Forssmann *et al.*[138g], to suggest that these cells correspond to the F (or X) cells, described in that species by Bencosme and Liepa,[139] by Munger *et al.*,[140] and by Lazarus and Shapiro[141]. Cells with the ultrastructural characteristics of the F (or X) cells of the dog cannot be found in the pancreas of man.

Only recently have immunocytochemical techniques become available which allow a more precise identification of the islet cells. In Geneva, Orci *et al.*[142] applied these methods, as well as electron microscopy, to the pancreas of two chronic juvenile diabetics who for some time had been kept artificially alive after a road accident. In the perfectly fixed specimens of pancreatic tissue, they were able to show that two-thirds of the cells of the islets were composed of glucagon cells, and the remaining third of somatostatin cells. They were unable to find B cells. Results in seven cases of juvenile diabetes, recent-onset and chronic, have recently been reported by one of us.[138c] They were later on confirmed by more cases (unpublished observations). In recent-onset cases, cells secreting insulin (Fig. 28), glucagon (Fig. 29), somatostatin (Fig. 30), and human pancreatic polypeptide (Fig. 31) could be demonstrated. The B cells, which with the Gomori techniques appeared almost completely degranulated, still contained appreciable amounts of insulin; however, they appeared strongly reduced in number. The glucagon and the somatostatin cells were clearly visible and appeared increased in number, but in view of the markedly reduced amount of islet tissue, this increase was probably relative and also resulted from a decrease in the number of B cells. In cases with a disease of many years

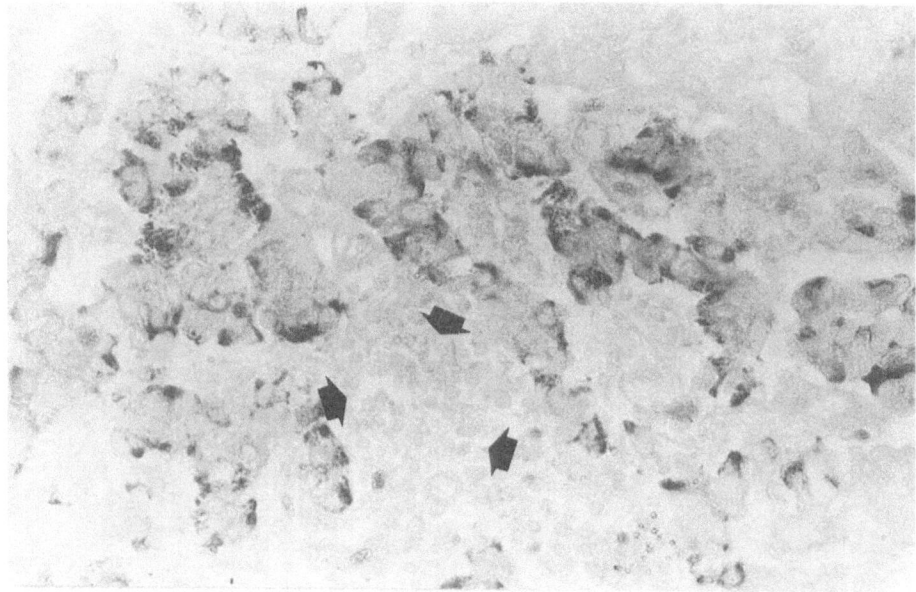

Figure 28. Recent-onset juvenile diabetic. Partly degranulated (dark) B cells demonstrated with a peroxidase-conjugated antibody to insulin. Also note insulitis (arrows). ×350.

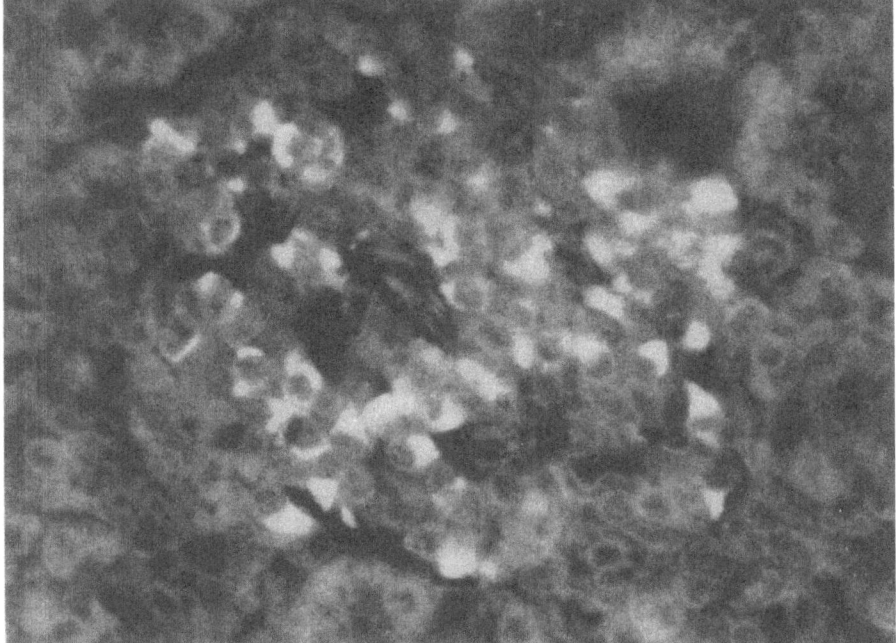

Figure 29. Numerous glucagon cells demonstrated with the indirect fluorescent antibody technique in an islet of recent-onset juvenile diabetic (same case as Fig. 28). ×350.

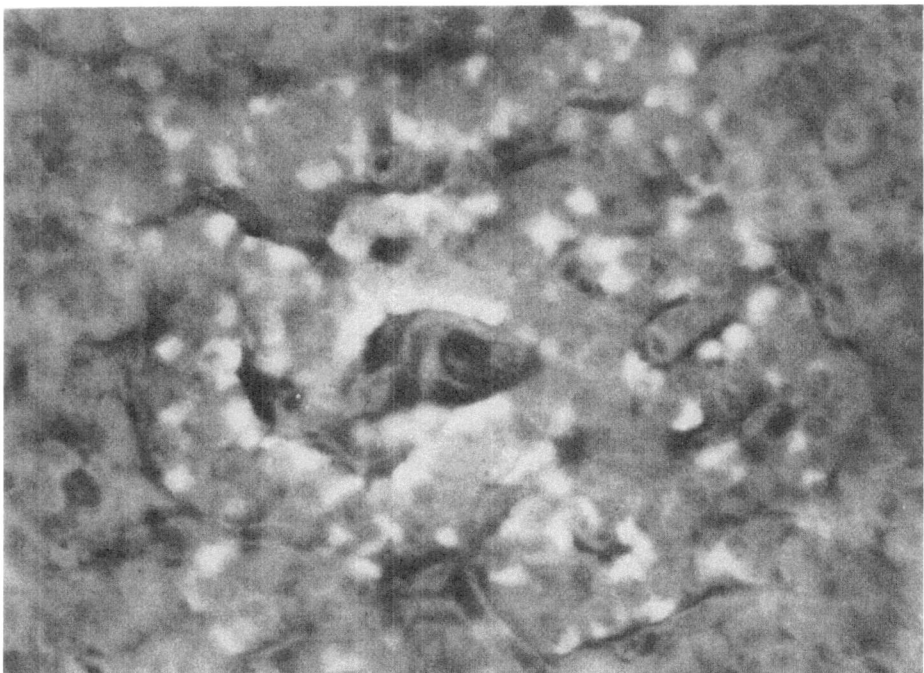

Figure 30. Numerous somatostatin cells demonstrated with the indirect fluorescent antibody technique in an islet of a recent-onset juvenile diabetic (same case as Figs. 28 and 29). ×350. Reproduced at 105%.

duration, many of the islets were predominantly composed of cells containing pancreatic polypeptide, whereas others contained glucagon and somatostatin cells. B cells could no longer be found.

These important findings confirm the progressive disappearance of B cells from the islets of juvenile diabetics. Moreover, they also reveal that the small non-B cells which compose these islets are neither undifferentiated nor inactive, but are actively engaged in the production of pancreatic hormones other than insulin. The physiological signification of the hyperplasia of the pancreatic polypeptide cells remains to be defined.

Changes in the Exocrine Tissue   In the pancreas of acute juvenile diabetics, foci of acute pancreatitis are not rare. They seem to represent terminal events, induced by dehydration and circulatory failure. In chronic juvenile diabetics, the acinar tissue surrounding the islets may itself appear atrophic. This finding may be explained by the observation of Malaisse-Lagae *et al.*[144] that the activity of the periinsular acini is governed by hormones emerging from the islets. It is conceivable that the reduced weight of the pancreas in chronic juvenile diabetics may be explained partly by this phenomenon.

Interlobular and interacinar fibrosis, as well as vascular sclerosis, commonly seen in the pancreas of chronic juvenile diabetics, may also contribute to the pancreatic atrophy.

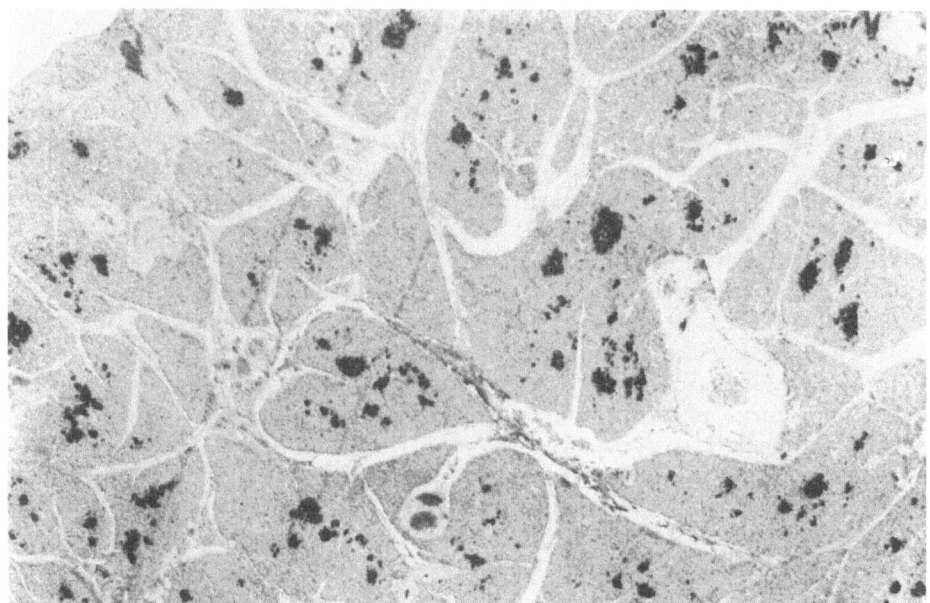

Figure 31. Pancreatic tissue of a juvenile diabetic showing numerous islets entirely composed of "pancreatic polypeptide" cells. Unlabeled antibody enzyme method of Sternberger using horseradish-peroxidase–anti-horseradish-peroxidase. ×22. Reproduced at 105%.

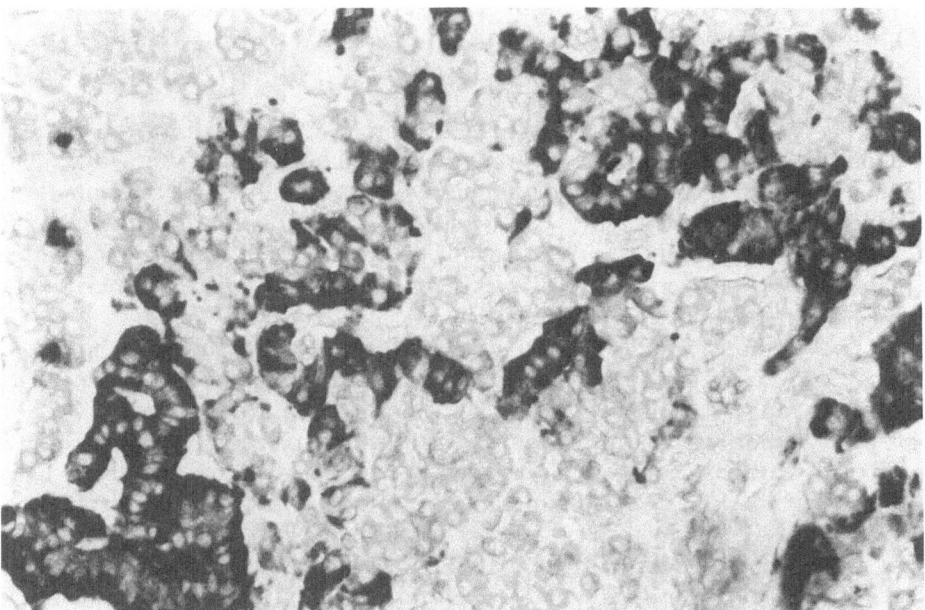

Figure 32. Higher magnification of Fig. 31, showing the islets composed of pancreatic polypeptide cells. The outlines of the islets are very irregular, and there are many reactive cells among the acinar cells. Notice also the centrally located nuclei of many pancreatic polypeptide cells and compare with the ribbonlike islets of Fig. 27. Unlabeled antibody enzyme method of Sternberger using horseradish-peroxidase–anti-horseradish-peroxidase. ×340. Reproduced at 105%.

Etiology and Pathogenesis of Juvenile Diabetes

We shall now consider what light the pathological changes described above may throw on the difficult questions of etiology and pathogenesis of the growth-onset form of diabetes. Any conclusions will necessarily be speculative.

To summarize the findings: The accumulated evidence suggests that, in the usual juvenile diabetic, some islets are probably large and hyperactive *before* the onset of clinical diabetes; that at some time during this preclinical phase an injury of some sort occurs, directed specifically at the B cells; that this injury may or may not be accompanied by a mononuclear cell infiltrate suggestive of an immunologic reaction; and that the end result is the apparently atrophic islet with some fibrosis, consisting essentially of non-insulin-producing cells, the B cells having been destroyed.

The large, active islets seen at the onset of diabetes in these young people are unexplained, but they might conceivably be the result of an increase in circulating growth hormone, which some investigators regard as frequent and perhaps significant in young diabetics,[145,146] or they may be a reaction to metabolic demands occurring around the time of puberty. Craighead[147] found that the hyperplastic islets induced in mice by gold thioglucose were more susceptible to the encephalomyocarditis virus in that they showed a more prominent mononuclear infiltrate and more necrosis than the islets of infected controls not given the drug.

The large, hyperchromatic nuclei often seen in the islets in early-onset diabetes of man are consistent with hyperactivity[23,148] and with polyploidy. Ehrie and Swartz[22] have made the interesting observation that only the B cells exhibit polyploidy.

The lymphocytic infiltrate or insulitis, found in two-thirds of the cases by Gepts[8] and in half of the cases by Junker *et al.*[46] although not observed at all by Doniach and Morgan,[10] is strongly suggestive of an immunologic reaction of the delayed hypersensitivity type. The transitory nature of the infiltrate in some forms of experimental insulitis (especially viral) suggests a possible explanation for failure to find it in all early cases. Ultrastructural studies of experimental models suggest that cytotoxic damage to B cells occurs.[57,70–72,74,149,150]

The demonstration of antibodies to pancreatic tissue in young diabetics[66,67,151–158] is suggestive of an autoimmune reaction, although autoantibodies are no longer considered necessarily a criterion of autoimmune disease.[159] Also, the experimental production of insulitis by injections of insulin or of pancreatic extracts, as noted above, suggests the possibility of an analogy with the human disease.[160] Perhaps of greater pertinence is the demonstration of cellular hypersensitivity to islet antigens other than insulin,[65,66] and a suggestion that the responsiveness of diabetic lymphocytes is altered.[161] One group of investigators[162] has observed a decreased number of T-lymphocytes in juvenile diabetics, another has not.[163]

Presumably, the appearance of an autoimmune disease requires some mechanism for the breakdown of immunologic tolerance for self. The disruption of this tolerance can occur in several ways, which are discussed by Heremans.[164] Among them is the action of a virus which might alter the B cell membrane in such a way as to make an antigen that the body's cells would recognize as "foreign." The injury to the B cell would then result from the immunologic cytoxic reaction rather than the direct effect of the virus. Of particular interest in this connection is the finding of Like and Rossini,[75] noted above, that a drug may apparently activate a latent virus in the B cell and lead to an insulitis. (For description of.experimental viral insulitis and for evidence that human diabetes may be associated with virus infections, see Chapter 19.)

Further evidence for an autoimmune basis for juvenile diabetes is the well-known association of diabetes with other supposed autoimmune diseases[163,174] and the presence of organ-specific antibodies to other endocrine glands.[166,168,171–182] Such an association has led to the question of whether certain individuals have a genetic predisposition to autoimmune disease[183] or to virus infections.[184] In the past few years there has been intensive study of the histocompatibility (HLA) antigens in diabetics, with the result that several groups of investigators have agreed that there is an increased prevalence of HLA-B8 (formerly HL-A8) and HLA-BW15 (formerly HL-W15*) in insulin-dependent nonobese diabetics.[185–195] Nerup *et al.*[196] noted that the frequency of HL-A8 (HLA-B8) was also reported to be increased in Addison's disease, suggesting that this genetic configuration might be a common denominator for the development of endocrine autoimmunity. The same group of workers[196a] have shown that evidence of antipancreatic autoimmunity (islet cell antibodies and/or cell-mediated autoimmunity) could be demonstrated in 73% of a series of 37 juvenile diabetics and predominantly in those who were HLA-B8 positive (89%), thus linking antipancreatic autoimmunity with a genetic marker of juvenile diabetes. Several authors have suggested that the possession of these antigens predisposes to diabetes because of a defective immune response to certain viral infections, a hypothesis which is possibly supported by a recent report of insulitis in a 10-month-old diabetic infant with Down's syndrome.[43]

An additional antigen (HLA-CW3) has also been reported as increased, along with the two mentioned above, in juvenile diabetics and their relatives with glucose intolerance under the age of 35 years, the association thus being dependent on age at onset of the disease.[199] In addition, the same group of workers conclude, from their own data combined with those of others, that there is a highly significant decrease in frequency of HLA-B7 in juvenile diabetics and their relatives, as compared with controls, this factor being found in only 10 of 68 blood relatives of patients.[200] They found particularly striking their failure to find HLA-B7 in any relative with glucose intolerance under the age of 35. They suggest that HLA-B7 is possibly a marker associated with a protective gene for juvenile diabetes.

The recent burgeoning of interest in the HLA system and its relation to disease, the appreciation of the association of diabetes with other recognized autoimmune diseases, the development of better methods for detecting islet cell antibodies, and the increasing evidence that viruses are probably involved in the etiology of some cases of insulin-dependent diabetes (see Chapter 19),

---

*The nomenclature of the factors of the HLA system has recently been revised by an international committee.[197,198]

have led to a wealth of new information and an active, sometimes disputatious literature.[201–206c] On the basis of such data, classifications are proposed, varying from relatively simple ones[206a,206b] to the more intricate one of Irvine[206c] which takes into account genetics, HLA factors, islet cell antibodies, viruses, and association with other recognized autoimmune states. Further data and more evidence will be required to establish hypotheses of this nature.

In summary, one may speculate that, in the usual case of juvenile diabetes, both genetic and environmental influences are involved; that there is probably early stimulation of the islets by some unknown mechanism; and that these stimulated islets are susceptible to an injurious agent such as a virus (exogenously acquired or "latent"), which then causes a breakdown of self-tolerance (possibly by modifying surface antigens), leading to an autoimmune reaction directed against the B cells and mediated by lymphocytes and macrophages, with destruction of B cells, ending in atrophy and fibrosis of islets, with permanent insulin-dependent diabetes.

The problem of the permanence of juvenile diabetes is unsolved as yet. In many tissues, injury is followed by regeneration. Indeed, islet regeneration is a prominent feature of the pancreas of juvenile diabetics and may explain the well-known "honeymoon period," which often follows the clinical outbreak of the disease. In the early clinical phases this regeneration tends to reproduce normal islets, with active B cells. As time goes by, this type of regeneration becomes rarer and is replaced by the development of atypical ribbonlike islets, in which B cells are difficult to demonstrate. These observations suggest that the capacity of the pancreatic tissue to produce normal new islets, and particularly new B cells, is not unlimited. Experimental studies confirm this view, although there are well-known species differences in this regard. In rats, subtotal pancreatectomy is followed by an intense islet regeneration, but this decreases as time goes on, and after 1 or 2 months permanent diabetes appears.[207] Logothetopoulos[208,209] has pointed out that the B cells are only capable of a limited number of mitotic divisions. Increased mitotic activity of the B cells, proliferation of the ductular epithelium, and marked islet hyperplasia were observed by Volk et al. in steroid-treated rabbits.[18,210] On the other hand, in dogs and cats the regenerative capacity appears to be much more limited, and in these species subtotal pancreatectomy rapidly leads to permanent diabetes.[16,17] In humans, the capability of the islet tissue to regenerate is not known; it is conceivable that it also may depend on genetic factors.

An important new observation is that the islets of chronic juvenile diabetics, which have always been described as atrophic, have now been shown to be composed of cells producing glucagon, somatostatin, and "human pancreatic polypeptide."[138d,142] The absence of B cells accounts for the unresponsiveness of these patients to factors which in normal individuals raise the insulin level in the blood. On the other hand, Unger et al.[143,211–213] have demonstrated high levels of glucagon in the blood of juvenile diabetics. It remains a matter of controversy[212,218] whether this glucagon originates in the A cells of the pancreatic islets or comes from extrapancreatic sources which have been shown to exist at least in the human and in the dog.[219–221] The role of somatostatin and of the other pancreatic hormones, such as the recently isolated "pancreatic polypeptide," in the physiopathology of juvenile diabetes requires further investigation. Of great interest in this connection are the findings of Floyd *et al.*[222] that plasma HPP was increased in 83% of a series of juvenile diabetics.

Acknowledgments

The authors express their gratitude to Dr. P. E. Lacy for Fig. 14, and to Dr. A. Like for Figs. 15 and 16. One of us (W.G.) thanks the following persons for the gifts of antisera: Dr. M. P. Dubois (Institut National de la Recherche Agronomique, Nouzelly, France) for antisomatostatin serum; Dr. P. Lefebvre (Université de Liège) for antiglucagon serum; Dr. A. E. Lambert for anti-insulin serum, and Dr. R. E. Chance (Lilly Research Laboratories, Indianapolis, Indiana) for sera against human and bovine "pancreatic polypeptide."

The authors also thank Mrs. Judith Brandt, who made most of the histologic preparations on which this work was based, and Mrs. Eveline Willems for typing the manuscript.

References

1. Danowski, T. S.: *Diabetes Mellitus, With Emphasis on Children and Young Adults.* Williams & Wilkins, Baltimore, 1957, p. 121.
2. Forsham, P. H.: In: *Diabetes Mellitus; Theory and Practice.* Edited by M. Ellenberg and H. Rifkin, McGraw-Hill, New York, 1970, p. 694.
3. Traisman, H. S.: In: *Diabetes Mellitus.* Edited by K. E. Sussman and R. J. S. Metz. American Diabetes Assoc., New York, 1975, p. 103.
4. Tattersall, R. B., and Fajans, S. S.: *Diabetes,* **24**:44, 1975.
5. Kraus, E. J.: In: *Handbuch der speziellen Pathologischen Anatomie und Histologie.* Edited by F. Henke and O. Lubarsch. Julius Springer, Berlin, Vol. 2, 1929, p. 662.
6. Vartiainen, I.: *Acta Med. Scand.,* **118**:538, 1974.
7. Terbrüggen, A.: *Virchows Arch.,* **315**:407, 1948.
8. Gepts, W.: *Diabetes,* **14**:619, 1965.
9. Warren, S., LeCompte, P. M., and Legg, M. A.: *The Pathology of Diabetes Mellitus.* Lea & Febiger, Philadelphia, 1966.
10. Doniach, I., and Morgan, A. G.: *Clin. Endocrinol.,* **2**:233, 1973.
11. Dourov, N., and Buyl-Strouvens, M. L.: *Arch. Fr. Pediat.,* **26**:641, 1969.
12. Ghon, A. and Roman, B.: *Präg. Med. Wochenschr.,* **38**:524, 1913.
13. Duschl, L.: *Münch. med Wochenschr.,* **70**:1388, 1923.
14. Weichselbaum, A.: *Sitzungsber. Akad. Wissensch. Math.-Naturwiss. Kl.,* **119**:73, 1910.
15. Toreson, W. E.: *Amer. J. Pathol,* **27**:327, 1951.
16. Homans, J.: *J. Med. Res.,* **33**:1, 1915.
17. Allen, F. M.: *J. Metab. Res.,* **1**:5, 1922.
18. Lazarus, S. S., and Volk, B. W.: *Arch. Pathol.,* **67**:4, 1959.
19. Dohan, F. C., and Lukens, F. D. W.: *Science,* **105**:183, 1947.
20. Dohan, F. C., and Lukens, F. D. W.: *Endocrinology,* **42**:244, 1948.
20a. Pictet, R., and Imagawa, W.: *Diabetes (Suppl. 1)* **25**:381, 1976.
21. Volk, B. W., and Lazarus, S. S.: *Diabetes,* **11**:426, 1962.

22. Ehrie, M. G., and Swartz, F. J.: *Diabetes*, **23**:583, 1974.
23. LeCompte, P. M., and Merriam, Jr., J. C.: *Diabetes*, **11**:35, 1962.
24. Potvliege, P. R., Carpent, G., and Gepts, W.: *Beitr. Pathol. Anat.*, **128**:335, 1963.
25. Freytag, G., and Klöppel, G.: *Curr. Top. Pathol.* **58**:49, 1973.
26. MacCuish, A. C., and Irvine, W. J.: In: *Clinics in Endocrinology and Metabolism. Autoimmunity in Endocrine Diseases.* Edited by W. J. Irvine. W. B. Saunders, London, 1975, p. 435.
27. Bastenie, P. A., and Gepts, W.: *Immunity and Autoimmunity in Diabetes Mellitus.* Excerpta Medica, Amsterdam, 1974.
28. Kobenhain Symposium on "Immunological Aspects of Diabetes Mellitus," *Acta Endocrinol. Suppl.*, 205, 1976.
29. Von Meyenburg, H.: *Schweiz. med. Wochenschr.*, **70**:247, 1940.
30. Opie, E.L.: *J. Exp. Med.*, **5**:527, 1900–01.
31. Schmidt, M. B.: *Münch. med. Wochenschr.*, **49**:51, 1902.
32. Cecil, R. L.: *J. Exp. Med.*, **11**:266, 1909.
33. Fischer, B.: *Frankf. Ztschr. Pathol.* **17**:218, 1915.
34. Heiberg, K. A.: *Arch. Kinderheilk.*, **56**:403, 1911.
35. Warren, S. and Root, H. F.: *Amer. J. Pathol.*, **1**:415, 1925.
36. Warren, S.: *JAMA*, **88**:99, 1927.
37. Stansfield, O. H., and Warren, S.: *N. Engl. J. Med.*, **198**:686, 1928.
38. LeCompte, P. M.: *Arch. Pathol.*, **66**:450, 1958.
39. Nagler, W. and Taylor, H.: *JAMA*, **184**:723, 1963.
40. Crome, L., Erdohazi, M., and Rivers, R. P. A.: *Arch. Dis. Child.*, **42**:677, 1967.
41. Steiner, H.: *Klin. Wochenschr.*, **46**:417, 1968.
42. Warne, G. L.: *Med. J. Australia*, **2**:934, 1973.
43. Gladisch, R., Bayer, H. P., Lipinski, C., and Stenzel, M. L.: *Kinderheilk.*, **119**:5, 1975.
44. Hultquist, G., Nordvall, S., and Lundström, C.: *Upsal. J. Med. Sci.*, **78**:139, 1973.
44a. Goldman, H., Bolande, R., Colle, E., and Marks, M.: *Diabetes* (Suppl. 1) **25**:365, 1976.
45. Ogilvie, R. F.: In: *The Aetiology of Diabetes and its Complications. Ciba Colloquia on Endocrinology.* Vol. 15. Edited by M. P. Cameron and M. O'Connor. Churchill, London, 1964, p. 49.
46. Junker, K., Egeberg, J., Kromann, H., and Nerup, J.: 1977 (in press).
47. LeCompte, P. M., and Legg, M.: *Diabetes*, **21**:762, 1972.
48. Christensen, N. O., and Schambye, P.: *Nord. Vet. Med.*, **2**:863, 1950.
49. Barboni, E., and Manocchio, I.: *Arch. Vet. Ital.*, **13**:477, 1962.
50. Gepts, W., and Toussaint, D.: *Diabetologia*, **3**:249, 1967.
51. Nakhooda, A. F., Like, A. A., Chappel, C. I., and Marliss, E. B.: *Diabetes* **26**:100, 1977.
52. Silverman, J. C.: *Diabetes*, **12**:528, 1963.
53. Renold, A. E., Soeldner, J. S., and Steinke, J.: In: *The Aetiology of Diabetes and its Complications. Ciba Colloquia on Endocrinology.* Vol. 15. Edited by M. P. Cameron and M. O'Connor. Churchill, London, 1964, p. 122.
54. LeCompte, P. M., Steinke, J., Soeldner, J. S., and Renold, A. E.: *Diabetes*, **15**:586, 1966.
55. Toreson, W. E., Feldman, R., Lee, J. C., and Grodsky, G. M.: *Amer. J. Clin. Pathol.*, **42**:531, 1964.
56. Toreson, W. E., Lee, J. C., and Grodsky, G. M.: *Amer. J. Pathol.*, **52**:1099, 1968.
57. Lee, J. C., Grodsky, G. M., Caplan, C. J., and Craw, L.: *Amer. J. Pathol.*, **57**:597, 1969.
58. Jansen, F. K., and Freytag, G.: *Diabetologia*, **9**:191, 1973.
59. Federlin, K., Renold, A. E., and Pfeiffer, E. F.: In: *Immunopathology.* Vol. 1. Edited by P. A. Miescher and P. Grabar, Schwabe, Stuttgart, 1968, p. 107.
60. Renold, A. E., Gonet, A. E., and Vecchio, D.: In: *Textbook of Immunopathology.* Vol. 2. Edited by P. A. Miescher and H. J. Müller-Eberhard. Grune & Stratton, New York, 1969, p. 595.
61. Berson, S. A., and Yalow, R. S.: *Nature (London)*, **191**:1392, 1961.
62. Lacy, P. E., and Wright, P. H.: *Diabetes*, **14**:634, 1965.
63. Logothetopoulos, J., and Bell, E. G.: *Diabetes*, **15**:205, 1966.
64. Freytag, G. and Klöppel, G.: *Beitr. Pathol. Anat.*, **139**:138, 1969.
65. Nerup, J., Andersen, O. O., Bendixen, G., Egeberg, J., Poulsen, J. E., Vilien, M., and Westrup, M.: *Acta Allerg.*, **28**:231, 1973.

66. Nerup, J., Andersen, O. O., Bendixen, G., Egeberg, J., and Poulsen, J. E.: *Diabetes,* **20**:424, 1971.
67. Nerup, J., Andersen, O. O., Bendixen, G., Egeberg, J., and Poulsen, J. E. *Acta Allerg.,* **28**:223, 1973.
68. Heydinger, D. K., and Lacy, P. E.: *Diabetes,* **23**:579, 1974.
69. Craighead, J. E.: *Amer. J. Pathol.,* **48**:375, 1966.
70. Müntefering, H., Schmidt, W. A. K., and Körber, W.: *Dtsch. Med. Wochenschr.,* **96**:693, 1971.
71. Wellmann, K. F., Amsterdam, D., Brancato, P., and Volk, B. W.: *Diabetologia,* **8**:349, 1972.
72. Volk, B. W., Wellmann, K. F., Brancato, P., and Amsterdam, D.: *Diabetes,* **21**:338, 1972.
73. Boucher, O. W., and Notkins, A. L.: *J. Exp. Med.,* **137**:1226, 1973.
74. Müntefering, H.: *Virchows Arch., A,* **356**:207, 1972.
75. Like, A. A. and Rossini, A. A.: *Science,* **193**:415, 1976.
76. Gross, L.: *N. Engl. J. Med.,* **294**:724, 1976.
77. Todaro, G. Y.: *Amer. J. Pathol.* **81**:590, 1975.
78. Like, A. A., and Chick, W. L.: *Diabetologia,* **6**:216, 1970.
78*a.* Like, A., Appel, M. C., Gazdar, A. F., and Rossini, A. A.: *Diabetes,* 1977 (in press).
78*b.* Rossini, A. A., Like A. A., Chick, W. L., Appel, M. C., and Cahill, G. F., Jr.: *Proc. Natl. Acad. Sci.,* 1977 (in press).
79. Gellerstedt, N.: *Beitr. Path. Anat.,* **101**:1, 1938.
80. Van Beek, C.: *Ned. T. Geneesk.,* **83**:646, 1939.
81. Arey, B.: *Arch. Pathol.* **36**:32, 1943.
82. Ahronheim, J. H.: *Amer. J. Pathol.,* **19**:873, 1943.
83. Ehrlich, J. C., and Ratner, J. M.: *Amer. J. Pathol.* **38**:49, 1961.
84. Lacy, P. E.: In: *The Aetiology of Diabetes and its Complications. Ciba Colloquia on Endocrinology.* Vol. 15. Edited by M. P. Cameron and M. O'Connor. Churchhill, London, 1964, p. 84.
85. Westermark, P.: *Virchows Arch., A,* **359**:1, 1973.
86. Pearse, A. G. E., Ewen, S. W. B., and Polak, J. M.: *Virchows Arch., B,* **10**:93, 1972.
87. Lacy, P. E.: In *Pathogenesis of Diabetes Mellitus.* Edited by E. Cerasi and R. Luft. Almqvist & Wiksel, Sweden. 1970, p. 109.
88. Westermark, P.: *Histochemistry,* **38**:27, 1974.
88*a.* Westermark, P.: *Virchows Arch. A,* **373**:161, 1977.
89. Bourke, M. S., and Rougvie, M. A.: *Biochemistry,* **11**:2435, 1972.
90. Bell, E. T.: *Diabetes,* **1**:341, 1952.
91. Lazarus, S. S., and Volk, B. W.: *The Pancreas in Human and Experimental Diabetes.* Grune & Stratton, New York, 1962.
92. Maclean, N., and Ogilvie, R. F.: *Diabetes,* **8**:83, 1959.
93. Case records of the Massachusetts General Hospital, No. 29. *N. Engl. J. Med.,* **273**:41, 1965.
94. Cecil, R. L.: *J. Exp. Med.,* **14**:500, 1911.
95. Moore, R. A.: *Amer. J. Dis. Child.,* **52**:627, 1936.
96. Laurence, K. M., and Dodge, J. A.: *Arch. Dis. Child.,* **50**:663, 1975.
97. Martius, K.: *Frankf. Z. Pathol.,* **17**:276, 1915.
98. Lane, M. A.: *Amer. J. Anat.,* **7**:409, 1907.
99. Bloom, W.: *Anat. Rec.,* **49**:363, 1931.
100. Creutzfeldt, W.: *Beitr. Pathol. Anat.,* **133**:113, 1953.
101. Gepts, W.: *Ann. Soc. Roy. Sci. Med. Nat.,* **10**:1, 1957.
102. Hellerström, C., and Hellman, B.: *Acta Endocrinol.,* **35**:418, 1960.
103. Fujita, T.: *Arch. Histol. Jap.,* **25**:189, 1964.
104. Fujita, T.: *Arch. Histol. Jap.,* **29**:1, 1968.
105. Bjorkman, N., Hellerström, C., Hellman, B., and Petersson, B.: *Z. Zellforsch.,* **72**:425, 1966.
106. Hellman, B., and Täljedal, J. B.: In: *Handbook of Physiology.* Sect. 7, *Endocrinology.* Edited by D. Steiner and N. Freinkel. Amer. Physiol. Soc., Washington, 1972, p. 91.
107. Lomsky, R., Länger, F., and Vortel, V.: *Nature, (London),* **223**:618, 1969.
108. Greider, M. H., and McGuigan, J. E.: *Diabetes,* **20**:389, 1971.
109. Lotstra, F., Vanderloo, W., and Gepts, W.: *Diabetologia,* **10**:291, 1974.

110. Creutzfeldt, W., Arnold, R., Creutzfeldt, C., Feurle, G., and Ketterer, H.: *Europ. J. Clin. Invest.,* **1**:461, 1971.
110*a*. Erlandsen, S. L., Hegre, O. D., Parsons, J. A., McEvoy, R. C., and Elde, R. P.: *J. Histochem. Cytochem.,* **24**:883, 1976.
111. Grimelius, L.: *Acta Soc. Med. Upsal.,* **73**:243, 1968.
111*a*. Solcia, E., Cappella, C., Vassallo, G., and Buffa, R.: *Internat. Rev. Cytol.* **42**:223, 1976.
111*b*. Larsson, L. I., Sundler, F., and Håkanson, R.: *Diabetologia* **12**:211, 1976.
112. Lacy, P. E., and Greider, M. H.: In: *Handbook of Physiology.* Sect. 7, *Endocrinology.* Edited by D. Steiner and N. Freinkel. Amer. Physiol. Soc., Washington, 1972, p. 77.
113. Deconinck, J., Potvliege, P. R., and Gepts, W.: *Diabetologia,* **7**:266, 1971.
114. Deconinck, J., Van Assche, F., Potvliege, P. R., and Gepts, W.: *Diabetologia,* **8**:326, 1972.
115. Like, A. A., and Orci, L.: *Diabetes,* (Suppl. 2), **21**:511, 1972.
116. Solcia, E., Pearse, A. G. E., Grube, D., Kobayashi, S., Bussolati, G., Creutzfeldt, W., and Gepts, W.: *Rend. Gastroenterol.,* **5**:13, 1973.
117. Fujita, T. (ed.): *Proceedings of the International Symposium on the Gastroenteropancreatic Endocrine System, Kyoto, 1975.* Excerpta Medica, Amsterdam, 1976.
118. Orci, L., Baetens, D., Dubois, M. P., and Rufener, C.: *Horm. Metab. Res.,* **7**:400, 1975.
119. Rufener, C., Amherdt, M., Dubois, M. P. and Orci, L.: *J. Histochem. Cytochem.,* **23**:866, 1975.
120. Vale, W., Brazeau, G., Grant, A., Nussey, R., Burgus, J., Rivier, N., Ling, N., and Guillemin, R.: *C. R. Acad. Sci. (Paris),* **275**:2913, 1972.
121. Brazeau, P., Vale, W., Burgus, R., Ling, N., Butcher, M., Rivier, J. and Guillemin, R.: *Science,* **179**:77, 1973.
122. Luft, R., Efendic, S., Hökfelt, T., Johansson, O., and Arimura, A.: *Med. Biol.,* **52**:428, 1974.
123. Dubois, M. P.: *Proc. Nat. Acad. Sci.,* **72**:1340, 1975.
124. Polak, J. M., Pearse, A. G. E., Grimelius, L., Bloom, S. R., and Arimura, A.: *Lancet,* **1**:1220, 1975.
125. Hökfelt, T., Efendic, S., Hellerström, C., Johansson, O., Luft, R., and Arimura, A.: *Acta Endocrinol. Suppl.,* 200, 1975.
126. Orci, L., Unger, R. H., and Renold, A. E.: *Experientia,* **29**:1015, 1973.
127. Orci, L., and Unger, R. H.: *Diabetes,* **26**:241, 1977.
128. Hellman, B., and Lernmark, A.: *Endocrinology,* **84**:1484, 1969.
128*a*. Creutzfeldt, W.: *Isr. J. Med. Sci.,* **11**:762, 1975.
128*b*. Buffa, R., Capella, C., Fontana, P., Trinci, and Said, S. J.: *Rendic. Gastroenterol.,* **8**:73, 1976.
128*c*. Buffa, R., Capella, C., Solcia, E., Frigerio, B., and Said, S. J.: *Histochemistry,* **50**:217, 1977.
128*d*. Said, S. I., and Faloona, G. R.: *New Engl. J. Med.,* **293**:155, 1975.
128*e*. Heitz, Ph., Polak, J. M., Bloom, S. R., and Pearse, A. G. E., *Gut,* **17**:755, 1976.
128*f*. Heitz, Ph., Polak, J. M., Bloom, S. R., Adrian, T. E., and Pearse, A. G. E.: *Virchows Arch. B. Cell Path.,* **21**:259, 1976.
129. Kimmel, J. R., Pollock, H. G., and Hazelwood, R. L.: *Endocrinology,* **83**:1323, 1968.
130. Kimmel, J. R., Pollock, H. G., and Hazelwood, R. L.: *Fed. Proc.,* **30**:1318 (Abst.), 1971.
131. Lin, T. M. and Chance, R. E.: *Gastroenterology,* **62**:852 (Abst.), 1972.
132. Lin, T. M., Chance, R. E. and Evans, D. C.: *Gastroenterology,* **64**:865, 1973.
133. Lin, T. M., Evans, D. C. and Chance, R. E.: *Gastroenterology,* **66**:852, 1974.
134. Lin, T. M., and Chance, R. E.: In: *Endocrinology of the Gut.* Edited by W. Y. Chey and F. P. Brooks. C. B. Slack, Thorofare, New Jersey, 1974, p. 143.
135. Langslow, P. R., Kimmel, J. R., and Pollick, H. G.: *Endocrinology,* **95**:558, 1973.
136. Hazelwood, R. L., Turner, S. D., Kimmel, J. R., and Pollock, H. G.: *Gen. Comp. Endocrinol.,* **21**:485, 1973.
136*a*. Schwartz, T. W., Rehfeld, J. F., Stadil, F., Larsson, L.-I., Chance, R. E., and Moon, N.: *Lancet,* **1**:1102, 1976.
136*b*. Adrian, T. E., Bloom, S. R., Besterman, H. S., Barnes, A. J., Cooke, T. J. C., Russel, R. C. G., and Faber, F. G.: *Lancet,* **1**:161, 1977.
136*c*. Schwartz, T. W. and Rehfeld, J. J.: *Lancet,* **1**:698, 1977.
137. Larsson, L.-I., Sundler, F., Håkanson, R., Pollock, H. G., and Kimmel, J. R.: *Histochemistry,* **42**:377, 1974.

138. Larsson, L.-I., Sundler, F., and Håkanson, R.: *Cell. Tiss. Res.,* **156**:167, 1975.
138a. Larsson, L.-I.: *Lancet,* **2**:149. 1976.
138b. Gersell, D. J., Greider, M. H., and Gingerich, R. I.: *Diabetes,* (Suppl. 1), **25**:364, 1976.
138c. Pelletier, G., and Leclerc, R.: *Gastroenterol.,* **72**:569, 1977.
138d. Gepts, W., De Mey, J., and Pipeleers-Marichal, M.: *Diabetologia,* **13**:27, 1977.
138e. Sundler, F., and Håkanson, R.: *Lancet,* **2**:1300. 1976.
138f. Baetens, D., Rufener, C., and Orci, L.: *Experientia,* **32**:785A, 1976.
138g. Forssmann, W. G., Helmstaedter, V., Metz, J., Greenberg, J., and Chance, R. E.: *Histochemistry,* **50**:281, 1977.
139. Bencosme, S. A., and Liepa, E.: *Endocrinology,* **57**:588, 1955.
140. Munger, B. L., Caramia, J., and Lacy, P. E.: *Z. Zellforsch.,* **67**:776, 1965.
141. Lazarus, S. S. and Shapiro, S. H.: *Anat. Rec.,* **169**:487, 1971.
142. Orci, L., Baetens, D., Rufener, C., Amherdt, M., Ravazzola, M., Studer, P., Malaisse-Lagae, F., and Unger, R. H.: *Proc. Natl. Acad. Sci.,* **73**:1338, 1976.
143. Unger, R. H.: *Diabetes,* **25**:136, 1976.
144. Malaisse-Lagae, F., Ravazzola, M., Robberechts, P., Vandemeers, A., Malaisse, W. J., and Orci, L.: *Science,* **190**:795, 1975.
145. Hansen, A. P.: *Dan. Med. Bull.,* (Suppl. 1), **19**:3, 1972.
146. Johansen, K., Soeldner, J. S., Gleason, R. E., Gottlieb, M. S., Park, B. N., Kaufman, R. L., and Tan, M. H.: *N. Engl. J. Med.,* **293**:57, 1975.
147. Craighead, J. E.: In: *Immunity and Autoimmunity in Diabetes Mellitus.* Edited by P. A. Bastenie and W. Gepts. Excerpta Medica, Amsterdam, 1974, p. 227.
148. Kiefer, G., and Sandritter, W.: *Beitr. Path.,* **158**:332, 1976.
149. Klöppel, G., Altenähr, E., and Freytag, G.: *Virchows Arch., A,* **356**:1, 1972.
150. Klöppel, G., Altenähr, E., and Freytag, G., and Jansen, F. K.: *Virchows Arch., A,* **364**:333,1974.
151. Mancini, A. M., Zampa, G. A., Vecchi, A., and Costanzi, G.: *Lancet,* **1**:1189, 1965.
152. Botazzo, C. F., Christensen, A. F., and Doniach, D.: *Lancet,* **2**:1279, 1974.
153. MacCuish, A. C., Jordan, J., Campbell, C. J., Duncan, L. J. P., and Irvine, W. J.: *Diabetes,* **23**: 693,1974.
154. MacCuish, A. C., Irvine, W. J., Barnes, E. W., and Duncan, L. J. P.: *Lancet,* **2**:1529, 1974.
155. MacCuish, A. C., Jordan, J., Campbell, C. J., Duncan, L. J. P., and Irvine, W. J.: *Diabetes,* **23**:695, 1974.
156. MacCuish, A. C., Urbaniach, S. L., Campbell, C. J., Duncan, L. J. P., and Irvine, W. J.: *Diabetes,* **23**:708, 1974.
157. Lendrum, R., Walker, G., and Gamble, D. R.: *Lancet,* **1**:880, 1975.
158. MacLaren, N. K., and Huang, S. W.: *Lancet,* **1**:997, 1975.
159. Stiller, C. R., Russell, A. S., and Dosseter, J. B.: *Ann. Int. Med.,* **82**:405, 1975.
160. Schalch, D. S.: In: *Immunological Diseases.* Edited by M. Samter. Little, Brown, Boston, 1971, p. 125.
161. Delespesse, G., Duchateau, J., Kennes, B., Lauvaux, J. P., Bastenie, P. P., and Govaerts, A.: In: *Immunity and Autoimmunity in Diabetes Mellitus.* Edited by P. A. Bastenie and W. Gepts. Excerpta Medica, Amsterdam, 1974, p. 83.
162. Cattaneo, R., Saibene, V., and Pozza, G.: *Diabetes,* **25**:223, 1976.
163. Hann, S., Kaye, R., and Falkner, B.: *Diabetes,* **25**:101, 1976.
164. Heremans, J. F.: In: *Immunity and Autoimmunity in Diabetes Mellitus.* Edited by P. A. Bastenie, and W. Gepts. Excerpta Medica, Amsterdam, 1974, p. 3.
165. Crooke, A. C., and Russell, D. S.: *J. Pathol. Bacteriol.,* **40**:255, 1935.
166. Solomon, J. L., and Blizzard, P. M.: *J. Pediat.,* **63**:1021, 1963.
167. Carpenter, C. C., Solomon, N., Silverberg, S. G., Bledsoe, T., Northcut, R. C., Klinenberg, J. R., Bennett, Jr., J. L., and Harvey, A. M.: *Medicine,* **43**:153, 1964.
168. Ungar, B., Stocks, A. E., Martin, F. I. R., Wittingham, S., and MacKay, I. R.: *Lancet,* **2**:415, 1968.
169. Gharib, H., and Gastineau, C. F.: *Mayo Clin. Proc.,* **44**:217, 1969.
170. Hung, W.: *Med. Ann. D. C.,* **39**:487, 1970.
171. Irvine, W. J., Clarke, B. F., Scarth, L., Cullen, D. R., and Duncan, L. J. P.: *Lancet,* **2**:163, 1970.

172. Goldstein, D. C., Drash, A., Gibbs, J., and Blizzard, R. M.: *J. Pediat.,* **77**:304, 1970.
173. Yoo, J., and Kozak, G. P.: *Postgrad. Med.,* **55**:62, 1974.
174. Nerup, J.: In: *Immunity and Autoimmunity in Diabetes Mellitus.* Edited by P. A. Bastenie and W. Gepts. Excerpta Medica, Amsterdam, 1974, p. 149.
175. Pettit, M. D., Landing, B. H., and Guest, G. M.: *J. Clin. Endocrinol. Metab.,* **21**:209, 1961.
176. Landing, B. H., Pettit, M. D., Wiens, R. L., Knowles, H., and Guest, G. M.: *J. Clin. Endocrinol. Metab.,* **23**:119, 1963.
177. Moore, J. M., and Neilson, J.: *Lancet,* **1**:645, 1963.
178. Deckert, T.: *Acta Med. Scand. Suppl.,* **476**:29, 1967.
179. Deckert, T.: In: *Immunity and Autoimmunity in Diabetes Mellitus.* Edited by P. A. Bastenie and W. Gepts. Excerpta Medica, Amsterdam, 1974, p. 277.
180. Bastenie, P. A.: In: *Immunity and Autoimmunity in Diabetes Mellitus.* Edited by P. A. Bastenie and W. Gepts. Excerpta Medica, Amsterdam, 1974, p. 164.
181. Nerup, J., and Binder, C.: *Acta Endocrinol.,* **72**:279, 1973.
182. Moulias, R., Goust, J. M., Croisier, B., Attali, A., and Berthaux, P.: In: *Immunity and Autoimmunity in Diabetes Mellitus.* Edited by P. A. Bastenie and W. Gepts. Excerpta Medica, Amsterdam, 1974, p. 140.
183. Fudenberg, H. H.: *Amer. J. Med.,* **51**:295, 1971.
184. Notkins, A. L.: *Viral Immunology and Immunopathology.* Academic Press, New York, 1975.
185. Singal, D. P., and Blagchman, M.: *Diabetes,* **22**:429, 1973.
186. Nerup, J., Platz, P., Andersen, O. O., Christy, M., Lingsoe, J., Poulsen, S. E., Ryder, L. P., Thomson, M., Nielsen, L. S., and Svejgaard, A.: *Lancet,* **2**:864, 1974.
187. Nerup, J., Andersen, O. O., Christy, M., Platz, P., Ryder, L., Thomson, M., and Svejgaard, A.: In: Kobenhain Symposium on "Immunological Aspects of Diabetes Mellitus. *Acta Endocrinol. Suppl.,* 205, 1976.
188. Menser, M. A., Forrest, J. M., and Honeyman, M.: *Lancet,* **2**:1508, 1974.
189. Cudworth, A. G., and Woodrow, J. C.: *Lancet,* **2**:1153, 1974.
190. Cudworth, A. G., and Woodrow, J. C.: *Diabetes,* **24**:345, 1975.
191. Cudworth, A. G., Woodrow, J. C., and Gamble, D. R.: *Lancet,* **2**:29, 1975.
192. Cudworth, A. G., and Woodrow, J. C.: *Brit. Med. J.,* **3**:133, 1975.
193. Löw, B., Schersten, B., Sartor, G., Thielen, T., and Mitelman, F.: *Lancet,* **1**:695, 1975.
194. Nelson, P. G., Pyke, D. A., Cudworth, A. G., Woodrow, J. C., and Batchelvi, J. R.: *Lancet,* **2**:193, 1975.
195. Ludwig, H., Mayer, W. R., and Schernthaner, G.: *Lancet,* **2**:1152, 1975.
196. Nerup, J., Andersen, O. O., Bendixen, G., Egeberg, J., and Poulsen, J. E.: In: *Immunity and Autoimmunity in Diabetes Mellitus.* Edited by P. A. Bastenie and W. Gepts. Excerpta Medica, Amsterdam, 1974, p. 107.
196a. Christy, M., Nerup, J., Bottazzo, G. F., Doniach, D., Platz, P., Svejgaard, A., Ryder, L. P., and Thomsen, M.: *Lancet,* **2**:142, 1976.
197. WHO-IUIS Terminology Committee. *Europ. J. Immunol.,* **5**:889, 1975.
198. Carpenter, C. B.: *N. Engl. J. Med.,* **294**:1005, 1976.
199. Schernthaner, G., Mayr, W. R., and Pacher, M.: *Horm. Metab. Res.,* **7**:521, 1975.
200. Ludwig, H., Schernthaner, G., and Mayr, W. R.: *N. Engl. J. Med.,* **294**:1066, 1976.
201. Lendrum, R., Walker, G., Cudworth, A. G., Woodrow, J. C., and Gamble, D. R.: *Brit. Med. J.,* **1**:1565, 1976.
202. Lendrum, R., Walker, G., Cudworth, A. G., Theophanides, C., Pyke, D. A., Bloom, A., and Gamble, D. R.: *Lancet,* **2**:1273, 1976.
203. Cudworth, A. G., Gamble, D. R., White, G. B. B., Lendrum, R., Woodrow, J. C., and Bloom, A.: *Lancet,* **1**:385, 1977.
204. Irvine, W. J., Gray, R. S., and McCallum, C. J.: *Lancet,* **2**:1097, 1976.
205. Irvine, W. J.: *Lancet,* **1**:189, 1977.
206. Irvine, W. J., McCallum, C. J., Gray, R. S., Campbell, C. J., Duncan, L. J. P., Farquhar, J. W., Vaughan, H., and Morris, P. J.: *Diabetes,* **26**:138, 1977.
206a. Bottazzo, G. F., and Doniach, D.: *Lancet,* **2**:800, 1976.

206*b*. Cudworth, A. G.: *Brit. J. Hosp. Med.,* **16**:207, 1976.

206*c*. Irvine, W. J.: *Lancet,* **1**:638, 1977.

207. Marx, M., Schmidt, W., and Goberna, R,: *Z. Zellforsch. Mikrosk. Anat.,* **110**:569, 1970.

208. Logothetopoulos, J., Brosky, G., and Kern, H.: In: *The Structure and Metabolism of the Pancreatic Islets.* Edited by S. Falkmer, B. Hellman, and I. Täljedal. Pergamon Press, Oxford, 1970, p. 15.

209. Logothetopoulos, J.: In: Handbook of Physiology. Sect. 7, *Endocrinology.* Edited by D. Steiner and N. Freinkel. Amer. Physiol. Soc., Washington, 1972, p. 67.

210. Volk, B. W., and Lazarus, S. S.: *Amer. J. Pathol.* **34**:21, 1958.

211. Unger, R. H.: *Amer. J. Med. Sci.,* **260**:79, 1970.

212. Unger, R. H.: *Adv. Int. Med.,* **7**:265, 1972.

213. Unger, R. H., and Orci, L.: *Lancet,* **1**:14, 1975.

214. Mashiter, K., Harding, P., Chere, M., Mashiter, G., Stout, J., Diamond, D., and Field, J.: *Endocrinology,* **96**:678, 1975.

215. Sasaki, H., Rubacalva, B., Baetens, D., Blasquez, E., Strikland, C., Orci, L., and Unger, R. H.: *J. Clin. Invest.,* **56**:135, 1975.

216. Dobbs, R., Sakurai, H., Sasaki, H., Falcona, G., Valverde, I., Baetens, D., Orci, L., and Unger, R. H.: *Science,* **187**:544, 1975.

217. Gerich, J. E., Karam, J. H., and Lorenzi, M.: *Lancet,* **1**:855, 1976.

218. Bloom, A. J., and Barnes, S. R.: *Lancet,* **1**:219, 1976.

219. Larsson, L.-I., Holst, J., Hakanson, R., and Sundler, J.: *Histochemistry,* **44**:281, 1975.

220. Baetens, D., Rufener, C., Unger, R., Renold, A. and Orci, L.: *C. R. Acad. Sci.,* **282**:196, 1976.

221. Grimelius, L., Capella, C., Buffa, R., Polak, J. M., Pearse, A. G. E., and Solicia, E.: *Virchows Arch., B,* **20**:217, 1976.

222. Floyd, J. C., Jr., Fajans, S. S., Pek, S., and Chance, R. E.: *Recent Progr. Hormone Res.,* **33**:519, 1977.

Chapter 16

The Islets of Infants of Diabetic Mothers

Klaus F. Wellmann and Bruno W. Volk

Ever since Dubreuil and Anderodias[1] observed, in 1920, the occurrence of pancreatic islet hypertrophy in a newborn infant and attributed this change to the hyperglycemic state of its diabetic mother, the relationship between a disturbed maternal carbohydrate metabolism and various pathologic alterations in the pancreas and in other tissues of the fetus or neonate has been the subject of a large number of reports in the medical literature. These include review articles concerned with the clinical[2-17] or with the morphologic aspects[4-7,11,18-30] of this relationship as well as pertinent reports of single[1,16-18,31-47] or multiple cases.[6,17,19,20,30,48-73] In the present chapter, the literature on quantitative, qualitative, and functional islet cell changes in neonates of diabetic mothers will be reviewed. To be discussed also are findings pertaining to the pancreas as a whole, some experimental data, questions related to the pathogenesis of the described alterations, and the problem of the development of permanent diabetes in infants born to diabetic mothers.

Quantitative Islet Cell Changes

The islets of Langerhans in newborn infants of diabetic mothers are characterized primarily by a conspicuous increase in their size (macronesia). The augmented islet diameter derives from an increase in both the size (hypertrophy) and the number (hyperplasia) of the constituent islet cells. Most authors[5,10,11,13,14,16,17,21,25,28,33,34,43,46,47,50-55,60-62,67-77] simply recorded the increased islet size in their cases without evaluating it quantitatively, although some appended qualifying terms such as "tremendous,"[30] "enormous,"[53,54] or "gigantic"[46] in characterizing these islets. Many others, however, did supply quantitative data which will now be reviewed.

In the pancreas of the neonate of a diabetic mother, Angyal[31] measured a mean islet diameter of 172 by 154 μm; the average of the means of 8 control

Klaus F. Wellmann and Bruno W. Volk • Isaac Albert Research Institute of the Kingsbrook Jewish Medical Center, and Downstate Medical Center, State University of New York, Brooklyn, New York. Present address of K.F.W.: Beekman Downtown Hospital, New York, New York. Present address of B.W.V.: University of California, Irvine, California.

cases was calculated to be 94 by 71 μm. In Bauer and Royster's case[18] the mean islet diameter was 135 by 109 μm, and in that of Bayer[32] it amounted to 254 μm, while some islets measured as much as 704 μm. In 245 control infants less than 3 days old, Borchard and Müntefering[19] found the mean for the medium islet diameters to be 85.6 $\pm$ 10.7 μm and that for the maximum diameters to be 209 $\pm$ 60.4 μm; the corresponding values in the 9 newborn infants of diabetic mothers were 120.5 $\pm$ 21.5 and 369.8 $\pm$ 124.3 μm, respectively. These authors concluded that a medium islet diameter of more than 100 μm or a maximum diameter in excess of 300 μm are highly suggestive of maternal diabetes. The average diameter in 38 control cases analyzed by Cardell[20] amounted to 124 by 99 μm, and that in 18 infants born to diabetic mothers was 157 by 130 μm; the largest islet in this series measured 761 by 486 μm. In the first case on record, that of Dubreuil and Anderodias,[1] the mean islet diameter was 290 by 212 μm, as compared to 116 by 100 μm in a control infant. Ehrich[35] encountered islets measuring 500 to 600 μm in size and more, while Feldmann[36] registered a two- to fourfold increase in islet diameter in another infant born to a diabetic mother. The average diameter in Gray and Feemster's[37] case amounted to 213 by 182 μm, whereas 6 controls yielded a mean figure of 116 by 102 μm. Heiberg[55] registered a mean diameter of 150 μm in the head and 195 μm in the tail portion of the pancreas in an infant of a diabetic mother and 137 μm in that of a control; the same case was also reported by Nothmann and Hermstein.[41] From Helwig's[56] figures on 9 infants with diabetic mothers and 9 normal neonates, one can calculate an average medium diameter of 229 by 187 μm for the first and 131 by 108 μm for the second group; largest maximum diameters for any islet were 693 and 654 μm, respectively.

The average islet diameter in 4 neonates of diabetic mothers observed by Hultquist *et al.*[57] was 172 by 134 μm, and that in 3 control infants was 85 by 63 μm. In Jacobsen's[39] case, the recorded diameters ranged from 64 to 280 μm. Kloos,[23] in 4 pertinent instances, found a mean diameter of 145 μm as compared with 66 μm in 3 controls. The average islet size in Mellgren's case[40] was 240 μm $\pm$ 6.7%. In a series of overweight neonate and stillborn infants of diabetic mothers, Naeye[63] recorded mean islet diameters that were 30% above those of controls; later, Naeye *et al.*[64] reported the following mean diameters: 182.4 μm in 21 infants of overtly diabetic mothers and 184.5 μm in 9 neonates or stillborn infants of latently diabetic mothers, compared with 109.2 μm in 42 offspring of healthy mothers. A fair number of islets measuring more than 200 μm in size was seen in 3 cases by Okkels and Brandstrup,[65] and islets with diameters of 250 to 400 μm were noted in 2 examples by Potter *et al.*[26] Rascoff *et al.*[66] found islets that had four to six times the normal size, while Seifert[27] recorded diameters in excess of 400 μm and up to 800 μm, and Smyth and Olney[44] observed that "entire lobules appeared as adenomatous formation of island tissue"; outside of the adenomatous formations, these authors saw discrete islets with an average diameter of 242 by 190 μm (largest islet: 880 by 560 μm), whereas the mean diameter in 10 control infants was 114 by 112 μm (largest islet: 225 by 192 μm). In von Bakay's case,[45] most islets measured between 300 and 400 μm although some had a maximum diameter of 700 or

800 μm; in the infant of a metabolically intact mother, the islet diameters varied between 120 and 180 μm, with an occasional value as high as 220 μm. In 23 infants of diabetic mothers observed by Warren *et al.*[30] most islets exceeded 250 μm in size.

Islet enlargement in infants of diabetic mothers is apparently most pronounced in the tail portion of the pancreas and is least conspicuous in the organ's head[38,41]; in control infants, on the other hand, Cardell[20] found no such topographical differences in islet size. The degree of macronesia correlates positively with the neonate's birth weight,[5,10,11,21,50,56,69,75] but there is no correlation with the severity of the mother's diabetes[23,25,26,50] or the degree to which this is controlled,[25,26] the presence or absence of maternal complications,[50] the use of exogenous estrogens or insulin,[50] or the level of the infant's blood sugar.[26]

Macronesia has been found in as early as the 4th month of gestation, in twin fetuses of a diabetic mother.[51] While Sudan[14] has stated that islet hyperplasia regresses within 4 to 5 days after the infant's delivery, persisting enlargement of islets has been observed in individual cases 2 weeks to 3 months after birth.[14,43]

While macronesia is usually present in the neonate of the diabetic mother, this is not invariably so. In the series of Driscoll *et al.*,[50] 46 of 57 (81%) such infants had appreciably enlarged islets; a similarly high percentage has been recorded by Pedersen[10] and van Assche.[77] Given *et al.*[52] found macronesia in 7 of 13 cases (54%), Miller and Wilson[75] in 10 of 18 (56%), Silverman[69] in 25 of 35 (71%), Warren *et al.*[30] in 23 of 27 (85%), and White and Hunt[17] in only 5 of 15 (33%) of their cases. Also, macronesia is not a specific indicator of maternal diabetes, since it has frequently been found in erythroblastosis fetalis; thus, Miller and colleagues[74] encountered it in 8 of 12 such infants (75%) and van Assche[77] in 4 of 15 cases (27%). While Potter[25] is "inclined to think that islet hyperplasia in children of normal women is rare," pertinent examples have, in fact, been recorded[19,72]; van Assche[77] encountered macropolynesia in 2 of 37 (5.4%) normal pregnancies.

Of particular interest is the observation that islet enlargement occurs not only in the offspring of mothers with overt diabetes but also in infants of prediabetic and latently diabetic mothers, as first proposed by van Beek.[16,70,71] Miller[62] observed islet hyperplasia in 2 such infants; it was only later that their mothers became diabetic. Naeye *et al.*[64] recorded similar findings in 17 stillborn or newborn infants whose mothers were not known to be diabetic at the time of delivery; on follow-up, 9 of these women revealed a disturbance of their carbohydrate metabolism. Macropolynesia was noted by van Assche[77] in 4 of 25 infants of women with "slightly reduced" carbohydrate tolerance.

In addition to their increased size (macronesia), the islets of infants born to diabetic mothers are frequently more numerous than normally seen (polynesia). Several authors[6,30,33,38,41,53,63,65,66] have recorded this observation without supplying quantitative data. In his case, Benner[33] termed the increase in size and number of islets "tremendous," and Driscoll *et al.*[21,50] found poly- and macronesia in 46 of 57 (81%) such infants. A doubling in the number of islets was reported by Ehrich.[35] In a review of the literature up to 1969, Borchard and Müntefering[19] found figures ranging from 136 to 1100 islets/cm² of pancreatic tissue for infants of diabetic mothers and from 19 to 1105 for those of metabolically normal mothers; in their own material, they counted a mean of 719.0 ± 99.1 islets/cm² in the diabetic and 593.9 ± 163.6 islets/cm² in the nondiabetic group of neonates less than 3 days old. Cardell[20] calculated an average number of 115 islets/50 mm² in 18 infants of diabetic mothers, compared with 72 islets/50 mm² in a control group; in the latter, the head portions of the organs showed the lowest mean, with 67 islets/50 mm², and the tails showed the greatest, with 78 islets/50 mm². Gray and Feemster[37] counted 184 islets/50 mm² in the infant of a diabetic mother, while the average value in 6 controls was 64. In the case of Jacobsen,[39] 289 islets were counted within 50 mm², and in that of Smyth and Olney,[44] 196 islets/50 mm²; these latter authors found a mean of 62 islets/50 mm² in 10 neonates of healthy mothers. Some observers, on the other hand, failed to see an increase in islet number,[1,32] and Angyal[31] actually registered a decrease to 133 islets/50 mm² in his case, since the average in 8 infants born to metabolically normal mothers amounted to 248/50 mm²; however, this decrease in number per square unit was more than offset by an increase in islet size. In 5 infants and fetuses of diabetic mothers, Kloos[23] counted an average of 270 islets/50 mm², whereas the average for 3 controls was 394. Klein and Fischer[6] summarized the situation by stating that polynesia is less important in such cases than is macronesia, and Borchard and Müntefering[19] concluded that the number of islets (they calculated a "critical figure" of 900 islets/cm²) was of little practical importance as an indicator for maternal diabetes or prediabetes.

Another way of looking at the problem is to determine the proportion of pancreatic tissue occupied by islets, expressed either as a percentage of a square unit as seen in histologic sections, or in terms of volume or weight. In sections from 245 normal neonates less than 3 days old, Borchard and Müntefering[19] found that the islet tissue took up a mean of 3.74 ± 1.46% of the organ, while in 9 infants of diabetic mothers the figure was 9.69 ± 3.78%; the critical upper limit of normal was deemed to be around 6%. In Cardell's[20,48] material, the area of islet tissue in 18 infants of diabetic mothers ranged from 1.8 to 9.9% (mean: 4.35 ± 2.27%), and that in 38 neonates of healthy mothers ranged from 0.7 to 2.6% (mean: 1.5 ± 0.45%); 13 of the 18 diabetic cases (72%) were considered to show an increase in islet tissue by area. Gordon[39] stated that in some microscopic fields the islets occupied up to 50% of the pancreatic tissue. Jackson and Woolf[59] recorded the following mean islet areas in a total of 8 stillborn infants: controls, 1.3%; infants with diabetic mothers, 6.5%; infants with prediabetic mothers (length of prediabetic period: 0–30 years), 7.5%; erythroblastosis cases, 7.1%. In 5 infants and fetuses of diabetic mothers, Kloos[23] found islet areas ranging from 1.44 to 13.0% (mean: 9.33%); in three controls, the range was 1.97 to 3.5%, with a mean of 2.66%. Van Assche[29] recorded islet areas in 40 normal neonates (5.1 ± 1.6%), 9 infants with mothers showing a slightly reduced carbohydrate tolerance (9.8 ± 5.6%), 10 neonates born to diabetic mothers (12.9 ± 8.9%), and 10 cases of erythroblastosis fetalis (9.0 ± 4.5%). In

88 unselected cases of stillbirth and neonatal death, Woolf and Jackson[72] measured islet areas ranging from 0.5 to 7.9% (mean: 2.13%); in 18 cases selected because of known macronesia, the proportion of islet tissue ranged from 4.1 to 13.6%. The mothers of 12 of the infants with islet hypertrophy were investigated, and 10 of them displayed impaired glucose tolerance.

Several authors have estimated the volume of islet tissue present in their cases of infants born to diabetic mothers and found it to be twice,[58] 4 times,[78] 14 times,[32] or even 20 to 30 times normal.[1,37,44] In five infants of diabetic mothers, D'Agostino and Bahn[49] recorded a mean islet weight of 202 mg and a mean islet mass amounting to 8.5 ± 0.7% of the whole pancreas; the corresponding figures for 9 controls were 68 mg and 3.2 ± 0.2%. In a study comprising 30 neonates (including stillborns) of diabetic mothers and 14 controls, Naeye[63] demonstrated that the islet mass is positively related to body weight; thus, the endocrine tissue constituted 10.8% of the pancreas in overweight infants, 5.4% in underweight infants (both of diabetic mothers), and only 3.5% in normal controls. Seifert[27] found that the relative islet mass (weight) increases from a normal value around 2% (of the whole pancreas) to 3.5% and more in infants of diabetic mothers, whereas Poursines and Cerati[42] reported that the islets in their case constituted as much as 21.7% of the pancreatic tissue mass.

Many authors have recorded cytological alterations of a quantitative nature in the pancreatic islets of infants born to diabetic mothers. In his case, Angyal[31] found most longitudinal diameters of the islet cells increased by 5 to 10 μm (maximum: 16 μm), from a normal range of 3 to 6 μm (maximum: 8 μm); Mellgren[40] also observed nuclei measuring between 5 and 15 μm in size. Other investigators[27,33,45,60] simply reported the occurrence of enlarged (and usually also pleomorphic and hyperchromatic) nuclei in such islets. While Hultquist and co-workers[58] stated that these changes normalize after 4 to 6 weeks, Schretter and Nevinny[43] still noted pleomorphic giant nuclei in the islets of a 32-day-old child. Large B cells were described by Driscoll *et al.*[21,50] and by Potter.[25]

A common finding in islets of infants born to diabetic mothers is a change in the ratio of A to B cells, in favor of the latter. Farquhar[78] remarked that in such cases the B cells increase in proportion to more than their normal share of about 50%. In the 4-month-old twin fetuses of a diabetic mother, Geyer and Staeffen[51] recorded a decrease of A cells from a normal 50% to 18%, with an increase in B cells to 55%; the remaining cells were termed "cellules intermediaires." Silver-positive cells amounted to 26 to 36% of all islet cells in 4 fetuses of diabetic mothers examined by Hultquist *et al.*[57]; in 3 controls, 46 to 52% of all cells were silver positive. In Kloos' series,[23] the proportion of B cells in 5 fetuses and infants of diabetic women ranged from 29.7 to 74.8%, and that in 3 controls ranged from 20.5 to 32.1%; in both groups, the larger islets tended to show the greatest number of B cells. McKay *et al.*[61] reported a numerical B cell increase coupled with an A cell decrease in such cases; they observed the B cells in all parts of the islets and not, as normally seen, clustered in their centers. A proliferation of B cells was also noted by Rascoff *et al.*[66] By using the means of values recorded by 12 different authors, Seifert[27] calculated an A:B ratio of

1:1–2 for infants of metabolically normal mothers and one of 1:3–5 for those of diabetic women. Van Assche[29] recorded the following average proportions for B cells: in 40 normal neonates, 40.0 ± 7.5%; in 9 infants of mothers with slightly reduced carbohydrate tolerance, 54.8 ± 12.3%; in 10 children born to diabetic women, 63.3 ± 8.9%; and in 10 cases of erythroblastosis fetalis, 40.0 ± 8.0%. Van Assche's earlier contention[28] that there is also an increase of silver-positive islet cells in the offspring of mothers with slightly or frankly reduced carbohydrate tolerance is not borne out by the figures contained in his most recent report[29]; thus, for the four groups (listed above), the percentages of silver-positive cells were: 40.5 ± 8.6%; 36.5 ± 6.2%; 31.0 ± 8.4%; and 31.0 ± 9.5%, respectively. With slightly reduced maternal glucose tolerance, fetal B cell hyperplasia occurred in 5 of 10 cases.[77] Van Assche[29,77] concluded, as did Gryaznova *et al.,*[55] that the increase in the percentage of B cells in the fetal or neonatal islets is a more nearly specific indicator of reduced maternal carbohydrate tolerance than is macro- or polynesia, since it occurs more frequently; furthermore, it is not encountered in erythroblastosis fetalis.

Qualitative Islet Cell Changes

In addition to the various quantitative alterations reviewed above (macro- and polynesia; increase in area, volume, and weight of islet tissue; reduction of A:B ratio), certain qualitative changes have been recorded in the islets of infants born to diabetic mothers. Nuclear pleomorphism and hyperchromasia[27,30,33,40,43,45,58,60,76] have already been mentioned and appear to affect primarily the B cells.[6,49,50] Occasionally blurring of the cell outlines,[43] increase in the mitotic index,[76] degranulation of B cells,[27] edema of the islets[36,45] or hydropic swelling of the islet cells,[36] an arrangement of islet cells in the form of ribbons,[61] foci of degeneration and fibrosis[25] or necrosis,[27,76] the alleged formation of islets from small ducts[30] or from acini,[27] and the appearance of wide and prominent capillaries within the islets[45,49] have been observed. Von Bakay[45] emphasized the presence of thick connective tissue capsules, especially around the larger islets, while Hultquist and Olding[79] recently recorded significant pancreatic islet fibrosis in 6 of 10 infants (aged 11 to 142 days) born to diabetic mothers; fibrosis covered an islet area of 5 to 10% in 3 cases, 10 to 20% in 2 cases, and more than 20% in the remaining case. The 3 infants with the most pronounced islet fibrosis were heavier than normal at birth. The pathogenesis of the islet fibrosis in these cases remained undetermined.

Infiltrates of eosinophilic leukocytes (and other cells) are very commonly seen in the pancreases of infants born to diabetic mothers. While these infiltrates can and do extend into the islets proper,[21,50,56,61,66] they are much more often confined to the periinsular interstitial tissue of the organ. Therefore, they will be discussed below, in the section dealing with extrainsular pancreatic changes.

Functional Islet Cell Changes

Enzymatic studies on islets in offspring of diabetic mothers have been conducted by only one group of researchers.[28,80,81] Gepts *et al.*[80] found a statistically significant increase in activity only for isocitric dehydrogenase, but the fact that this change was limited to the islets suggests that it can be related to an increase in their functional activity. It was observed in 12 cases (6 with slightly reduced maternal glucose tolerance and 6 with overt maternal diabetes) investigated by van Assche[81] that the enzymatic spectrum (various hydrolases, dehydrogenases, and diaphorases) in the fetal islets "differs in some way from the normal baby, but this divergence is very small and not constant"; 60 control cases were studied. Specifically, these minor differences constituted a slightly increased activity of 5'-nucleotidase, adenosine triphosphatase, acid phosphatase, and butyric dehydrogenase in newborn infants of diabetic mothers.[28]

Van Assche[29] also determined the insulin content in microdissected pancreatic islets of neonates. The mean concentration in 6 normal infants was 715.5 ± 182 μU/μg dry weight; in an infant born to a diabetic mother the concentration was 1326 μU/μg, in 2 infants of women with slightly impaired glucose tolerance, concentrations were 708 and 902 μU/μg, respectively, while in 3 cases of erythroblastosis fetalis the average value was 644 μU/μg. In 8 neonates with maternal diabetes, Gepts *et al.*[80] found a pancreatic insulin content ranging from 460 to 1326 μU/μg; the mean in normal controls was 700 μU/μg. These authors, and their co-workers,[28,82] explained the augmented insulin values by the larger proportion of islet tissue in these pancreases rather than by an increased insulin concentration of the individual B cell. A high pancreatic insulin content was found by Rose[67] in 3 of 4 infants of diabetic mothers. Steinke and Driscoll[83] determined the extractable insulin of pancreases from fetuses and infants. In 15 control cases with gestational ages between 20 and 32 weeks, the values ranged from 2 to 15 U/g (mean: 6.3 ± 1.1 U/g); somewhat lower figures have been found by Wellmann *et al.*[84] in 5 fetuses aged 16 to 20 gestational weeks (range: 1.16 to 7.31 U/g; mean: 3.27 U/g). In 13 older controls (34 weeks to term) examined by Steinke and Driscoll,[83] the range was 4 to 26 U/g and the mean was 12.7 ± 3.2 U/g, while in 9 infants (34 weeks to term) of diabetic mothers, the mean insulin concentration was increased to 21.1 ± 5.2 U/g (range: 4 to 50 U/g). These authors found the insulin values and the islet cell histology in their cases to correspond well with one another.

Several investigators[28,29,85–90] determined the serum or plasma insulin levels in such cases. In Baird and Farquhar's study,[85] the mean plasma insulin-like activity in 8 normal infants amounted to 200 μU/ml in the fasting state and 72 μU/ml 5 min after a glucose injection; in 6 neonates of diabetic mothers, the mean value rose from 149 μU/ml in the fasting state to as much as 700 μU/ml following glucose administration. Cole *et al.*[86] found the mean serum insulin level at birth significantly higher in 9 infants of diabetic women (24.1 ± 5.27 μU/ml) than that of 12 controls (10.0 ± 1.47 μU/ml). Isles and colleagues[87] determined that in 14 normal infants the mean plasma insulin level rose from

49 μU/ml before glucose loading to 139 μU/ml after 2 min; the level then fell but climbed again to reach 229 μU/ml after 1 hr. In contrast, the mean for a group of 6 neonates of non-insulin-treated diabetic mothers rose from a value of 34 prior to loading to one of 208 μU/ml 2 min after loading; there was, however, no second peak. In 7 normal neonates investigated by Stimmler *et al.*[89] the average plasma insulin level was 69 μU/ml in the umbilical vein and 74 μU/ml in heel stick blood; in 5 infants born to diabetic mothers, the averages read 477 and 355 μU/ml, respectively. Thomas *et al.*[90] found that the normal infant at birth has a low insulin level which is nearly equal in the umbilical vein (mean of 14 cases: 5.6 ± 0.7 μU/ml) and artery (mean: 6.6 ± 0.7 μU/ml). In 6 heavy infants born to untreated, latently diabetic mothers, the insulin levels were significantly higher than in the controls, and those in the umbilical vein (in three cases: 38, 42, and 12 μU/mg) were different from those measured in the artery (in the same three cases: 17, 34.5, and 18.5 μU/ml, respectively). These results are at variance with those obtained by Klink and Estrich,[88] who noted either a decrement or increment across the placenta in their nondiabetic rather than overtly or latently diabetic cases. Van Assche[28] also reported augmented insulin levels in the cord blood of neonates with maternal diabetes. The means as recorded in his latest compilation of data[29] are as follows: in 40 controls, 10.2 ± 2.5 μU/ml; in 9 infants of women with slightly impaired glucose tolerance, 19.5 ± 8.8 μU/ml; in 10 infants of diabetic mothers, 32.7 ± 8.8 μU/ml; and in 10 erythroblastosis cases, 17.0 ± 5.0 μU/ml. Jørgensen and colleagues[91] investigated the plasma insulin concentrations in the umbilical cord blood of 13 normal neonates and of 15 infants of diabetic mothers. At birth, the mean value for the controls was 15 μU/ml and that for the diabetic group was 144 μU/ml; these values rose to 41 and 243 μU/ml, respectively, 5 min after glucose injection, and to 72 and 167 μU/ml, respectively, 30 min after injection. In the normal infants, none of the obtained figures was higher than 128 μU/ml, while among the infants of diabetic women many were in excess of 500 μU/ml.

Several authors have recorded blood glucose concentrations in newborn infants of metabolically intact mothers and in those of diabetic women. In 185 mature, healthy neonates, Crawford[92] found values between 35 and 130 mg/100 ml in umbilical vein blood and between 25 and 130 mg/100 ml in umbilical artery blood; the correlation coefficients between the concentrations in maternal, umbilical vein, and umbilical artery blood were very high in almost all cases. In 19 neonates of normal mothers, Pedersen *et al.*[93] obtained a mean blood glucose concentration of 66 mg/100 ml on the first postpartem day; the mean in 27 infants of diabetic women was 63 mg/100 ml. These authors stated that during the first 24 hr of life in both groups, the infants' mean blood sugar figures were negatively correlated with the maternal blood sugar during the later months of pregnancy and positively with the maternal blood sugar at delivery. The mean glucose values obtained by Cole *et al.*[86] at the time of birth revealed no significant differences between the infants of gestational diabetic mothers and the normal controls. On the other hand, in heel stick blood of 5 neonates with maternal diabetes, 1 hr after birth, Stimmler and colleagues[89] found an average glucose concentration of only 19 mg/100 ml, while the average in 12 controls was 61 mg/100 ml. Rose[67] also stated that the initial postpartum drop in blood sugar is comparatively more pronounced in the offspring of the diabetic mother; symptomatic hypoglycemia occurs in 10 to 20% of these cases.[12]

Infants of diabetic mothers dispose of an intravenous glucose load much more rapidly than infants of metabolically normal women.[85] Isles *et al.*[87] determined the glucose tolerance as expressed by the "total index" *(Kt),* that is, the percentage of glucose disappearance from the plasma in 1 min. The *Kt* value of 14 infants of normal women (0.44 to 2.31, with a mean of 1.16) during the first hour after a glucose load differed little from that of infants of non-insulin-treated diabetic mothers (0.51 to 1.93, with a mean of 1.31). The *Kt* of both groups, however, differed significantly from that of infants of insulin-treated diabetic mothers whose range was from 0.83 to 5.78, with a mean of 3.30. In Persson's study,[94] the mean *Kt* values 1 to 6 hr after birth were as follows: in control infants, 0.80 ± 0.23; in infants of gestational diabetic mothers, 1.17 ± 0.42; and in the offspring of insulin-treated diabetic women, 1.27 ± 0.47.

Insulin antibodies, transferred from the mother, have been demonstrated in infants of insulin-treated diabetics[91]; they have a mean half-life of 25 days.[95] More recently, significantly elevated levels of C-peptide immunoreactivity have been found in umbilical cord blood of infants of insulin-requiring diabetics[12]; C-peptide is the connecting segment of the insulin molecule. While the presence of such antibodies may falsify the results of insulin immunoassay procedures,[12,88] their clinical significance is still poorly understood.[11]

Cole *et al.*[86] found no difference in the mean growth hormone values between infants of diabetic and nondiabetic mothers recorded at birth. However, after an oral glucose tolerance test, they were significantly higher in the diabetic group at 1 hr (61.9 ± 6.13 vs. 39.1 ± 5.00 ng/ml) and at 2 hr (57.8 ± 5.35 vs. 31.1 ± 3.83 ng/ml).

Extrainsular Pancreatic Alterations

The generalized macrosomia that characterizes many infants of diabetic mothers[8,19,21,48,50] is often shared by the pancreas. In some cases, increased pancreatic weights (up to three times normal) have been recorded.[31,38,41,43] In 21 overweight neonates of diabetic women, Naeye[63] found the mean pancreatic weight to be a modest 110% of normal; in 4 underweight infants with maternal diabetes, it was only 48% of normal.

Many authors have described the presence of eosinophilic infiltrates in the pancreases of infants born to diabetic mothers. In some cases, the infiltrates extend into the islets,[21,50,56,61,66] but much more often they are confined to the periinsular interstitial tissue of the organ.[6,10,14,19,27,28,30,33,48,49,52,53,63,69,96] Frequently, other cellular elements, including neutrophilic leukocytes, lymphocytes, histiocytes, and macrophages (some of them with hemosiderin granules), have been encountered along with the eosinophilic cells.[10,21,33,50,63] Fibrosis[10,21,49,50,63] and Charcot–Leyden crystals may also be present.[6,10,19,21,30,49,50,61] Eosinophilic infiltrates were found by Silverman[69] in 12 of 35 (34.3%) infants born to diabetic mothers; they were moderately prominent in 9 and very extensive in 3 cases. In Pedersen's review,[10] the incidence of eosinophilic infiltrates is stated to lie between 34 and 65%. Eosinophilic infiltrates may occur in occasional infants of nondiabetic mothers; Silverman[69] encountered them in 5.2% of his controls. Sudan[14] found that eosinophilic infiltrates tend to disappear within 4 to 5 days after birth.

In a clinicopathologic study, Silverman[69] concluded that stromal pancreatic eosinophilia was not related to the clinical grade of maternal diabetes, the number of previous pregnancies, or the administration of insulin to the mother. A statistically significant negative correlation existed between stromal eosinophilia and birth weight, length of gestation, and hours of postpartal life. No consistent change in stromal eosinophilia was noted between the first and second infants of six diabetic mothers who gave birth to more than one child included in this study.

The eosinophilic leukocytes display a distinct peroxidase activity.[6] The Charcot–Leyden crystals associated with them stain black with Heidenhain's iron hematoxylin, purple with phosphotungstic acid hematoxylin, red with acid fuchsin, blue with phloxine-methylene blue, and red with Prussian blue.[61] The eosinophilic infiltrates have been interpreted as allergic reactions related to excessive insulin production.[27] However, since insulin, when injected, fails to elicit local eosinophilia, McKay *et al.*[61] concluded that some unknown substance, possibly related to insulin, diffuses into the connective tissue around the islets. This material, which may be rich in sulfhydril groups, then attracts eosinophilic leukocytes and induces the observed periinsular inflammation. With breakdown of eosinophils, Charcot–Leyden crystals appear. The suggestion that the periinsular eosinophilic infiltrates merely represent persisting foci of extramedullary hematopoiesis[23] has been rejected,[6,96] since myeloid precursors are lacking in these cell nests. More recently, Gibb[96] proposed that the eosinophilic infiltrates are the morphologic expression of a localized organ-specific antigen–antibody reaction between the secreted fetal insulin and maternal antiinsulin antibodies transmitted via the placenta.

Morphologic changes other than those already mentioned are rarely encountered in the exocrine portion of the pancreas in infants of diabetic mothers. A dilatation of the pancreatic ducts and acute pancreatitis were recorded in two cases each by Given *et al.*[52]

Experimental Data

Data similar to those derived from infants of diabetic mothers have been obtained in experimental animals. Macrosomia and other alterations characteristic of the diabetic state have been observed in the offspring of rats rendered diabetic by alloxan[97,98] or by subtotal[99] or total pancreatectomy.[98,100] In neonates of alloxan-diabetic rats, Angervall[101] found poorly delineated islets with hydropic degeneration as well as an elevated mitotic index of the B cells, while the A cells appeared intact. In a similar group of animals of the same species, Baranov *et al.*[102] recorded an increase in the amount of insular tissue, an enhanced mitotic activity, and hyperplasia of the B cells; the severity of these changes paralleled the degree of the maternal diabetes. In sections from rat fetuses investigated by Frye,[103] the proportion of the pancreas occupied by islet tissue amounted to 6.23 ± 0.34% in the controls, to 11.56 ± 0.52% (or 185.5% of normal) in the offspring of nontreated alloxan-diabetic animals, and to 5.14 ± 0.35% (or 82.5% of normal) in those of insulin-treated diabetic mother animals. The average number of islets per unit area was between 2.2 and 2.6 in rats of all three groups. This author also found progressive hydropic and degranulative changes in the islets, beginning with day 18 of pregnancy. He saw no evidence of a *de novo* origination of islets in these animals. In the offspring of alloxan-diabetic rats, Hultquist[100] observed hydropic degeneration of islet cells and poor delineation of islets. In 14 control cases, the mean islet volume amounted to 0.040 mm³/g of body weight; in 13 young of diabetic animals it was 0.051 mm³/g, but in those with marked generalized macrosomia, the average islet volume was still higher (0.055 mm³/g). This latter observation agrees with the data obtained in 284 rats by Tejning,[104] who found a positive correlation between the total volume of the islands of Langerhans and body weight, body surface, and body length. Degranulation and occasional vacuolization of B cells were noted by Kim[105] in fetal rats from alloxan-diabetic mothers. In the infants of pancreatectomized rats, Kozma-de Bokay *et al.*[106] described hypertrophy and irregular delineation of islets as well as degranulation, enlargement, and hydrops of the B cells. Lazarow *et al.*[107] made similar observations in neonates of alloxan-diabetic rats; following delivery, it took 3 to 10 days for the B cells to become completely regranulated and for the glycogen to disappear. Nerenberg[108] found that maternal diabetes mildly inhibits the development of β granulation in fetal rats, but that the latter remained unaffected by the exogenous administration of glucose, insulin, or cortisone, or by starvation. Nikitin[109] recorded that the severity of the islet cell changes (increased mitotic activity, nuclear enlargement, degranulation, hyperplasia) in fetuses of alloxan-diabetic and alloxan-subdiabetic rats paralleled the degree of insulin deficiency.

Species other than the rat have rarely been utilized for such studies. In the young of severely ketoacidotic, diabetic Chinese hamsters, Carpenter *et al.*[110] found slightly enhanced islet volumes as well as glycogen infiltration and degranulation of B cells as long as 15 days after birth. Wellmann *et al.*[111] encountered predominantly pale secretory granules and prominent arrays of endoplasmic reticulum, both interpreted as indicating hyperfunction, in the B cells of the offspring of 9 alloxan-diabetic rabbits.

A few authors recorded the results of pancreatic insulin determinations in animals. Employing the epididymal fat pad method in the offspring of alloxan-diabetic rats, Dixit and colleagues[112] found that their microdissected islets contained only 7 to 19% of the insulin amounts present in those of normal fetuses; with the acid alcohol extract procedure, 5.3 U of insulin/g of tissue (one-third of normal) were detected in the fetuses of diabetic animals on the last day of gestation. Golob[113] failed to detect a significant difference in pancreatic insulin concentration between fetuses and neonates of normal and of streptozotocin-diabetic rats; however, the pancreatic insulin content of the latter was reduced, since their pancreases weighed less than those of the controls. In a study conducted by Wellmann *et al.*,[111] the pancreatic insulin concentrations in the offspring of 8 normal rabbits averaged 0.56 U/g of wet tissue, while the figure was somewhat higher (0.73 U/g) in the young of 9 alloxan-diabetic animals. Elevated plasma insulin levels have been measured by Carpenter *et al.*[110] in 15-day-old weanlings of severely diabetic Chinese hamsters.

The injection of labeled hormone into pregnant rats on the 21st day of gestation by Goodner and Freinkel[114] has shown that, in this species at least, no significant transplacental passage of insulin takes place, and that the placenta may be the major target site for maternal insulin within the conceptus. Asplund[115] determined the response of fetal pancreatic tissue to intermittent glucose infusions in pregnant rats during the last 5 days of gestation. While the pancreatic insulin content and the serum glucose levels of the fetuses, when killed, did not show any significant difference between the glucose-infused and control groups, the pancreatic islets of fetuses of glucose-infused mothers responded to a high glucose concentration *in vitro* with a considerably enhanced rate of insulin release. These findings suggest that the development of the B cell function before birth may be influenced even by minor, short-term increases in the maternal blood glucose levels. When pancreatic explants of fetal and neonatal rats were kept in a high glucose medium (500 mg/100 ml), Kaung *et al.*[116] detected 80 to 160% more insulin than was produced in a standard medium with 150 mg of glucose in 100 ml; these authors also concluded that the maturation of responsiveness to glucose appears to be inherent in the pancreas and is not dependent on other organ systems. In the offspring of streptozotocin-diabetic rhesus monkeys, Mintz and co-workers[117] noted a prompt two- to fivefold increase in fetal plasma insulin levels in response to glucose and amino acid infusions; these findings contrast with the unresponsiveness of the fetal insulin-releasing mechanism in normal primates. The fetal plasma growth hormone concentrations were unaltered.

Eosinophilic infiltrates located in the exocrine portions of the pancreas and resembling those in newborn infants of diabetic mothers were induced by Lacy *et al.*[118,119] in albino rats injected intraperitoneally with guinea pig antiinsulin serum. The infiltrates in some cases were associated with edema, focal necrosis, and hemorrhage, and occasionally extended into the islets. Their appearance was not related to the severity of the induced diabetes, and their nature suggested that they were allergic in origin.

Pathogenesis of Pancreatic Changes

A number of hypotheses have been advanced in an effort to explain the pathogenesis of the morphologic and functional changes seen in the fetus and newborn infant of the diabetic mother, including, in particular, those occurring in the pancreatic islets. Most authors subscribe to the concept that maternal hyperglycemia, per se, is primarily or exclusively responsible for the striking alterations that appear in the offspring of diabetic women.[1,4,5,8,11,14,15,18,23,31, 32,35,53,54,65,66,78,83,120] The hypothesis that "glucose poisoning"[15] induces fetal islet hyperplasia which, in turn, leads to hyperinsulinism with all its sequelae was first expounded by Dubreuil and Anderodias[1] in 1920 and has found its most ardent champion in Pedersen.[11,120] The results of animal experiments also favor this concept.[101, 117,121,122] For instance, Horii *et al.*[122] were able to reduce the incidence of diabetes-induced fetal malformations in the offspring of alloxanized mice from 28% (14 of 50 animals) to 0.2% (1 of 492) by abolishing hyperglycemia through insulin treatment.

On the surface, the hyperglycemia hypothesis appears to be incompatible with the fact that women who develop diabetes only at a later date often give birth to infants with the stigmata of diabetic fetopathy.[5,16,19,48,62,70-72,123] In fact, ever since Cornelia van Beek's pioneering observations,[16,70,71] beginning in 1939, the presence of macronesia, especially in conjunction with macrosomia, in the neonate has been utilized as a reliable indicator of maternal prediabetes.[5,15,19,48,59,62,72,123-125] It has therefore been suggested that such decreased glucose tolerance as prediabetic women may have in pregnancy can be balanced by the increased fetal use of glucose.[78] Thus, the maternal level may never rise to the renal threshold, while the fetus would still be subjected to an increased glucose load. The feasibility of this hypothesis has been shown by Hagen who, in a thesis quoted by Pedersen and Osler,[120] was able to ascertain that mothers of large babies have a higher blood sugar level outside and inside pregnancy, in the fasting state as well as at any time during glucose tolerance tests. Additional support for this hypothesis derives from animal experiments, such as that of Asplund discussed above[115] and similar ones reviewed by Farquhar.[78]

Among alternative modes of explanation, "maternal dyshormonosis"[22] of one type or another has enjoyed a certain measure of popularity. An overproduction of pituitary growth hormone in the mother has been postulated to be the decisive stimulant for diabetic fetopathy, especially by Cardell,[20,48] and also by Miller,[62,123] but it has been pointed out that there is no islet hyperplasia in infants of acromegalic women.[72,120] In a similar vein, hyperfunction of the maternal adrenal cortex is not likely to be responsible for the abnormalities observed in neonates of diabetic mothers, since in the few cases in which women with active Cushing's disease became pregnant, the stigmata of diabetic fetopathy were not evident.[120]

Yet another theory has been advanced by Vallance-Owen.[126,127] He found that the increased antagonism associated with the plasma albumin fraction of prediabetics can be transmitted to the fetus, and surmised that it is this antagonism to insulin that is instrumental in inducing "the characteristic hypertrophy of the islets and the fat, flabby appearance of the stillborn fetus of the prediabetic mother." The validity of this concept is yet to be confirmed.

The Development of Diabetes in Infants of Diabetic Mothers

In 1939, Cornelia van Beek[16] proposed that the prenatally affected islets of infants of diabetic mothers become insufficient through the stress of postnatal life, so that such children are more likely than their healthy peers to develop permanent diabetes. In order for this hypothesis to be valid, the observed incidence of diabetes in persons with diabetic mothers should exceed that to be expected on the basis of heredity alone. The available data are still limited, but they are compatible with the described proposition. Thus, Farquhar[128] reviewed 329 consecutive deliveries in diabetic women; fetal mortality was 20.9%. The incidence thus far of clinical juvenile diabetes among the survivors if 0.77% (2 cases), which is already 22 times greater than that of the general population under 16 years of age. Scheibenreiter and Thalhammer[125] compared the birth weights (as the only retrospectively demonstrable sign of diabetogenic fetopathy) of 336 full-term children of diabetic mothers with those of 336 infants of nondiabetic women; the birth weights of 1000 neonates and normal values recorded in the literature were used as controls. It was shown that a birth weight in excess of 4000 g is significantly more frequent in children of diabetic mothers than in those of the control group, and that birth weights above the 90th percentile of normal American newborns occurred in 26.6% of children of diabetic mothers, an incidence 2.5 times higher than predicted. However, it is still to be demonstrated through long-term studies that these children become diabetic more often than expected. Diabetic stigmata, such as macrosomia, polyuria, and impaired glucose tolerance, may persist in the offspring of alloxan-diabetic rats[129] for as long as 1 or 2 years[107] and may even manifest themselves again in subsequent generations.[97]

References

1. Dubreuil, G., and Anderodias: *C. R. Soc. Biol.,* **83**:1490, 1920.
2. Anonymous: *Lancet,* **1**:669, 1975.
3. Grenet, P., de Paillerets, F., Badoual, J., Galiet, J. P., Babinet, J. M., and Tichet, J.: *Arch. Franç. Pédiatr.,* **29**:925, 1972.
4. Hoet, J. P.: *Bull. Acad. Roy. Méd. Belg.,* Series 7, **7**:85, 1967.
5. Hoet, J. P. and Hoet, J. J., Jr.: In: *Handbuch des Diabetes Mellitus.* Edited by E. F. Pfeiffer. J. F. Lehmann, Munich, Vol. 2, 1971, p. 537.
6. Klein, H. J., and Fischer, R.: *Med. Welt,* p. 2621, 1968.
7. Kloos, K., and Vogel, M.: *Pathologie der Perinatalperiode.* G. Thieme, Stuttgart, 1974, pp. 182 & 306.
8. Mayer, J. B., and Camara, J. J. R.: *Dtsch. Med. Wochenschr.* **89**:974, 1964.
9. Morais, T., and Demers, P. P.: *Laval Méd.,* **38**:337, 1967.
10. Pedersen, J.: *The Pregnant Diabetic and Her Newborn: Problems and Management.* E. Munksgaard, Copenhagen, 1967, p. 71.
11. Pedersen, J.: In: *Handbuch des Diabetes Mellitus.* Edited by E. F. Pfeiffer. J. F. Lehmann, Munich, Vol. 2, 1971, p. 511.
12. Pildes, R. S.: *N. Engl. J. Med.,* **289**:902, 1973.
13. Skipper, E.: *Quart J. Med.,* **2**:353, 1933.
14. Sudan, J. P.: *Rév. Franç. Gynécol. Obstét.,* **64**:529, 1969.
15. Thalhammer, O.: *Pränatale Erkrankungen des Menschen.* G. Thieme, Stuttgart, 1967, p. 341.
16. van Beek, C.: *Ned. T. Geneesk.,* **83**:5973, 1939.
17. White, P., and Hunt, H.: *J. Clin. Endocrinol.,* **3**:500, 1943.
18. Bauer, J. T., and Royster, H. A., Jr.: *Bull. Ayer Clin. Lab. Penns. Hosp.,* **3**:109, 1937.
19. Borchard, F., and Müntefering, H.: *Virchows Arch. Path. Anat. A,* **346**:178, 1969.
20. Cardell, B. S.: *J. Pathol. Bacteriol.,* **66**:335, 1953.
21. Driscoll, S. G.: *Med. Clin. N. Amer.,* **49**:1053, 1965.
22. Kloos, K.: *Klin. Wochenschr.,* **29**:557, 1951.
23. Kloos, K.: *Virchows Arch. Pathol. Anat.,* **321**:177, 1952.
24. Lazarus, S. S., and Volk, B. W.: *The Pancreas in Human and Experimental Diabetes.* Grune & Stratton, New York, 1962, p. 234.
25. Potter, E. L.: *Pathology of the Fetus and Infant.* Year Book Medical, Chicago, 1961, p. 334.
26. Potter, E. L., Seckel, H. P. G., and Stryker, W. A.: *Arch. Pathol.,* **31**:467, 1941.
27. Seifert, G.: *Verh. Dtsch. Ges. Pathol.* **42**:50, 1959.
28. van Assche, F. A.: Thesis: The Fetal Endocrine Pancreas: A Quantitative Morphological Approach. Belgium, Catholic University of Leuven, 1970, p. 62.
29. van Assche, F. A.: In: *Carbohydrate Metabolism in Pregnancy and the Newborn.* Edited by H. W. Sutherland, and J. M. Stowers. Churchill Livingstone, Edinburgh, 1975, p. 68.

30. Warren, S., LeCompte, P. M., and Legg, M. A.: *The Pathology of Diabetes Mellitus.* Lea & Febiger, Philadelphia, 1966, p. 406.
31. Angyal, F.: *Centralbl. Allg. Path. Path. Anat.,* **66**:209, 1936.
32. Bayer, J.: *Virchows Arch. Pathol. Anat.,* **308**:659, 1942.
33. Benner, M. C.: *Arch. Pathol.* **32**:818, 1941.
34. Duncan, G. G., and Fetter, F.: In: *Diseases of Metabolism.* Edited by G. G. Duncan. W. B. Saunders, Philadelphia, 1947, p. 861.
35. Ehrich, W.: *Klin. Wochenschr.,* **13**:584, 1934.
36. Feldmann, I.: *Centralbl. All. Path. Path. Anat.,* **42**:435, 1928.
37. Gray, S. H. and Feemster, L. C.: *Arch. Path. Lab. Med.,* **1**:348, 1926.
38. Heiberg, K. A.: *Virchows Arch. Path. Anat.,* **287**:629, 1933.
39. Jacobsen, N. S.: *Ugeskr. Laeger,* **96**:347, 1934.
40. Mellgren, J. A.: *Nord. Med.,* **19**:1301, 1943.
41. Nothmann, M., and Hermstein, A.: *Arch. Gynäk.,* **150**:287, 1932.
42. Poursines, Y., and Cerati, P.: *Ann. Anat. Path.,* **16**:673, 1939.
43. Schretter, G., and Nevinny, H.: *Arch. Gynäk.,* **143**:465, 1930.
44. Smyth, F. S., and Olney, M. B.: *J. Pediatr.,* **13**:772, 1938.
45. Von Bakay, L., Jr.: *Virchows Arch. Path. Anat.,* **310**:291, 1943.
46. Wenig, K.: *Frankf. Z. Pathol.* **55**:188, 1941.
47. Wiener, H. J.: *Amer. J. Obstet. Gynecol.,* **7**:710, 1924.
48. Cardell, B. S.: *J. Obstet. Gynecol. Brit. Emp.,* **60**:834, 1953.
49. D'Agostino, A. N., and Bahn, R. C.: *Diabetes,* **12**:327, 1963.
50. Driscoll, S. G., Benirschke, K., and Curtis, G. W.: *Amer. J. Dis. Child.,* **100**:818, 1960.
51. Geyer, A., and Staeffen, J.: *Presse Méd.,* **65**:1079, 1957.
52. Given, W. P., Douglas, R. G., and Tolstoi, E.: *Amer. J. Obstet. Gynecol.,* **59**:729, 1950.
53. Gordon, W. H.: *J. Mich. St. Med. Soc.,* **34**:167, 1935.
54. Gordon, W. H.: *Ohio St. Med. J.,* **32**:540, 1936.
55. Gryaznova, I. M., Bolkhovotinova, L. M., and Vtorova, V. G.: *Vopr. Ohkr. Materin. Det.,* Vol. 17, No. 11, p. 22, 1972.
56. Helwig, E. B.: *Arch. Int. Med.,* **65**:221, 1940.
57. Hultquist, G. T., Lindgren, I., and Dalgaard, J. B.: *Nord. Med.,* **31**:1841, 1946.
58. Hultquist, G. T., Olding, L., and Larsson, Y. A. A.: *Fifth Congress of the International Diabetes Federation,* Excerpta Medica Int. Congr. Series No. 74; Abstract No. 129, 1964, p. 67.
59. Jackson, W. P. U., and Woolf, N.: *Diabetes,* **7**:446, 1958.
60. Liebegott, G.: *Beitr. Path. Anat. Allg. Pathol.,* **101**:319, 1938.
61. McKay, D. G., Benirschke, K., and Curtis, G. W.: *Obstet. Gynecol.,* **2**:133, 1953.
62. Miller, H. C.: *Amer. J. Med. Sci.,* **209**:447, 1945.
63. Naeye, R. L.: *Pediatrics,* **35**:980, 1965.
64. Naeye, R. L., Sims, E. A. H., Welsh, III, G. W., and Gray, M. J.: *Arch. Pathol.,* **81**:552, 1966.
65. Okkels, H., and Brandstrup, E.: *Acta Pathol. Microbiol. Scand.,* **15**:268, 1938.
66. Rascoff, H., Beilly, J. S., and Jacobi, M.: *Amer. J. Dis. Child.,* **55**:330, 1938.
67. Rose, V.: *Canad. Med. Assoc. J.,* **82**:306, 1960.
68. Rössle, R.: *Virchows Arch. Pathol. Anat.,* **308**:676, 1942.
69. Silverman, J. L.: *Diabetes,* **12**:528, 1963.
70. van Beek, C.: *Maandschr. Kindergen.,* **20**:84,129,141, 1952.
71. van Beek, C.: In: *Probleme der fetalen Endokrinologie.* Edited by H. Nowakowski. Springer Verlag, Berlin, 1956, p. 124.
72. Woolf, N. and Jackson, W. P. U.: *J. Pathol. Bacteriol.,* **74**:223, 1957.
73. Sisson, W. R., and White, P.: *Trans. Amer. Pediat. Soc.,* **48**:47, 1936.
74. Miller, H. C., Johnson, R. D., and Durlacher, S. H.: *J. Pediatr.,* **24**:603, 1944.
75. Miller, H. C., and Wilson, H. M.: *J. Pediatr.,* **23**:251, 1943.
76. Ringertz, N.: *Nord. Med.,* **19**:1302, 1943.
77. van Assche, F. A.: *Biol. Neonat.,* **12**:331, 1968.
78. Farquhar, J. W.: *Postgrad. Med. J.,* **38**:612, 1962.
79. Hultquist, G. T., and Olding, L. B.: *Lancet,* **2**:1015, 1975.
80. Gepts, W., Gregoire, F., van Assche, A., and de Gasparo, M.: In: *The Structure and Metabolism of the Pancreatic Islets.* Edited by S. Falkmer, B. Hellman, and I. B. Täljedal. Wenner-Gren International Symposium Series 16, Pergamon Press, Oxford, 1970, p. 283.

81. van Assche, F. A.: *Biol. Neonat.*, **14**:19, 1969.
82. de Gasparo, M., van Assche, A., Gepts, W., and Hoet, J. J.: *Rév. Franç. Étud. Clin. Biol.*, **14**:904, 1969.
83. Steinke, J., and Driscoll, S. G.: *Diabetes*, **14**:573, 1965.
84. Wellmann, K. F., Volk, B. W., and Brancato, P.: *Lab. Invest.*, **25**:97, 1971.
85. Baird, J. D., and Farquhar, J. W.: *Lancet*, **1**:71, 1962.
86. Cole, H. S., Bilder, J. H., Camerini-Davalos, R. A., and Grimaldi, R. D.: *Pediatrics*, **45**:394, 1970.
87. Isles, T. E., Dickson, M., and Farquhar, J. W.: *Pediatr. Res.*, **2**:198, 1968.
88. Klink, D. D., and Estrich, D.: *Lancet*, **1**:1393, 1964.
89. Stimmler, L., Brazie, J. W., and O'Brien, D.: *Lancet*, **1**:137, 1964.
90. Thomas, K., de Gasparo, M., and Hoet, J. J.: *Diabetologia*, **3**:299, 1967.
91. Jørgensen, K. R., Deckert, T., Mølsted-Pedersen, L., and Pedersen, J. *Acta Endocrinol.*, **52**:154, 1966.
92. Crawford, J. S.: *Biol. Neonat.*, **8**:222, 1965.
93. Pedersen, J., Bojsen-Møller, B., and Poulsen, H.: *Acta Endocrinol.*, **15**:33, 1954.
94. Persson, B.: In: *Carbohydrate Metabolism in Pregnancy and the Newborn.* Edited by H. W. Sutherland and J. M. Stowers. Churchill Livingstone, Edinburgh, 1975, p. 106.
95. Spellacy, W., and Goetz, F. C.: *Lancet*, **2**:222, 1963.
96. Gibb, G.: *Zbl. Allg. Path. Path. Anat.*, **104**:322, 1962.
97. Bartelheimer, H., and Kloos, K.: *Z. Ges. Exp. Med.*, **119**:246, 1952.
98. Kim, J. W., Runge, W., Wells, L. J., and Lazarow, A.: *Diabetes*, **9**:396, 1960.
99. Foglia, V. G.: In: *Early Diabetes.* Edited by R. A. Camerini-Davalos, and H. S. Cole. Academic Press, New York, 1970, p. 221.
100. Hultquist, G. T.: *Acta Pathol. Microbiol. Scand.*, **27**:695, 1950.
101. Angervall, L.: *Acta Endocrinol. Suppl.*, **44**:1, 1959.
102. Baranov, V. G., Nikitin, A. I., and Sokoloverova, I. M.: *Probl. Endokrinol.*, Vol. 17, No. 6, p. 96, 1971.
103. Frye, B. E.: *J. Morphol.*, **101**:325, 1957.
104. Tejning, S.: *Acta Med. Scand., Suppl.*, **198**:1, 1947.
105. Kim, J. N.: *Diabetes*, **14**:137, 1965.
106. Kozma-de Bokay, S., Jacquot, R., and Jost, A.: *J. Physiol.*, **53**:733, 1961.
107. Lazarow, A., and Heggestad, C. B.: In: *Early Diabetes.* Edited by R. A. Camerini-Davalos and H. S. Cole. Academic Press, New York, 1970, p. 229.
108. Nerenberg, S. T.: *Arch. Pathol.*, **58**:236, 1954.
109. Nikitin, A. I.: *Probl. Endocrinol.* Vol. 19, No. 4, p. 73, 1973.
110. Carpenter, A. M., Gerritsen, G. G., Dulin, W. E., and Lazarow, A.: *Diabetologia*, **6**:168, 1970.
111. Wellmann, K. F., Volk, B. W., Lazarus, S. S., and Brancato, P.: *Diabetes*, **18**:138, 1969.
112. Dixit, P. K., Lowe, I. P., Heggestad, C. B., and Lazarow, A.: *Diabetes*, **13**:71, 1964.
113. Golob, E.: *Z. Geburtsh. Gynäk.*, **171**:18, 1969.
114. Goodner, C. J., and Freinkel, N.: *Diabetes*, **10**:383, 1961.
115. Asplund, K.: *J. Endocrinol.*, **59**:285, 1973.
116. Kaung, H. L. C., Hegre, O. D., and Lazarow, A.: *Proc. Soc. Exp. Biol. Med.*, **148**:75, 1975.
117. Mintz, D. H., Chez, R. A., and Hutchinson, D. L.: *Clin. Res.*, **19**:68, 1971.
118. Lacy, P. E., and Wright, P. H.: *Diabetes*, **14**:634, 1965.
119. Lacy, P. E., Wright, P. H., and Silverman, J. L.: *Fed. Proc.*, **22**:604, 1963.
120. Pedersen, J., and Osler, M.: *Dan. Med. Bull.*, **8**:78, 1961.
121. Harding, P. G. R., Kinch, R. A. H., and Stevenson, J. A. F.: *Diabetes*, **11**:321, 1962.
122. Horii, K. I., Watanabe, G. I., and Ingalls, T. H.: *Diabetes*, **15**:194, 1966.
123. Miller, H. C.: *J. Pediatr.*, **29**:455, 1946.
124. Kriss, J. P., and Futcher, P. H.: *J. Clin. Endocrinol.*, **8**:380, 1948.
125. Scheibenreiter, S., and Thalhammer, O.: *Dtsch. Med. Wochenschr.* **91**:216, 1966.
126. Vallance-Owen, J.: *Adv. Metab. Dis.*, **1**:191, 1964.
127. Vallance-Owen, J., and Lilley, M. D.: *Lancet*, **1**:806, 1961.
128. Farquhar, J. W.: *Arch. Dis. Child.*, **44**:36, 1969.
129. Yamamoto, H.: *Endocrinol. Jap.*, **18**:375, 1971.

Chapter 17

Spontaneous Diabetes in Animals

Arthur A. Like

Although a large body of information has been gathered by physicians and scientists during the first half century of the insulin era, human diabetes mellitus is still a poorly understood disease. Most informed individuals agree that although the tendency to develop diabetes may be inherited, environmental factors are also involved in the etiology and the progression of the syndrome's symptom complex, of which hyperglycemia is the unifying phenomenon. The importance of heredity stems from the well-known familial incidence of diabetes. The importance of environmental factors rests upon evidence suggesting a viral etiology of juvenile-onset diabetes, and upon evidence linking the frequency of maturity-onset diabetes with the degree of nutritional (i.e., caloric) prosperity.

Given the widespread belief that both genetic and environmental factors contribute to and modify the pathogenesis of human diabetes, and given the obvious fact that it is impossible to control the genetic background, and almost impossible to control environmental conditions of human population groups, it is easy to understand why researchers have been interested in studying examples of spontaneous diabetes in laboratory animals wherein it would be more feasible to study and control both the genetics and environment.

In the 26 years that have elapsed since the report by Ingalls *et al.*[1] describing a new mutation in the mouse characterized by profound obesity, numerous articles have been published describing the physiology and pathology of a number of spontaneous diabetic syndromes occurring in laboratory rodents. These publications have been carefully summarized in three recent reviews[2-4] and have been augmented by the reports contained in three workshops[5-7] devoted to laboratory animal models of spontaneous diabetes mellitus. Rather than present a review of these superb reviews and workshops, this chapter will be devoted to an examination of these syndromes through the eyes of a histopathologist and from the unifying vantage point of the pancreatic islets. It is, after all, the structural and functional alterations within the pancreatic endocrine cells which determine to a large extent the progression and outcome of the diabetic syndrome.

Arthur A. Like • University of Massachusetts, Worcester, Massachusetts.

Lethal and Nonlethal Diabetic Syndromes

Table 1 illustrates a convenient, albeit simplified and possibly naïve classification of many, but not all of the frequently studied spontaneous diabetic animals. This classification groups the models into two categories: those which manifest *lethal* and *nonlethal* syndromes. In the lethal category are animal models in which the diabetic syndrome is severe and significantly reduces life expectancy. In contrast, the animals of the nonlethal group either experience a full life span with the disease, or may in fact eventually return to the normoglycemic state. The classification is based upon the hypothesis that it is the ability of the organism to produce new pancreatic β cells that determines whether the syndrome will or will not be lethal. The pancreatic islets of animals included in the lethal category reveal destruction of β cells with transient and/or inadequate replacement. The resulting decrease in β cell numbers is eventually associated with an absolutely decreased or inappropriately low level of circulating immunoreactive insulin (IRI). In the nonlethal group are animals which manifest significant β cell proliferation in response to diabetes, and the resulting increased number of functioning β cells is usually associated with elevated levels of circulating IRI. The assignment of sand rats and Chinese hamsters to both categories is in recognition of the variable severity of the disease in these animals. The frequency of lethal (ketotic) syndromes among sand rats is very low and in the author's own experience was essentially limited to one group of animals received in 1965.[5] Similarly, among Chinese hamsters, although examples of lethal (ketoacidotic) and nonlethal syndromes exist, the nonlethal predominate.[29] The hamsters and sand rats with nonlethal syndromes reveal an increased β cell mass together with elevated levels of circulating IRI, and the lethal examples evidence decreased β cell numbers, low levels of IRI, and more severe metabolic abnormalities.

It is therefore proposed that in the case of nonlethal syndromes, presently

Table 1. Spontaneous Diabetic Syndromes

Nonlethal	Lethal
C57Bl/6J-*ob/ob* (obese) [1,8–19]	C57Bl/KsJ-*db/db* (diabetes) [59–61]
KK (Japan and Toronto) [20–23]	Chinese hamster [c]
C3Hf X I F$_1$ (Wellesley) [24–27]	*Psammomys obesus* [d] [45]
Chinese hamster [a] [28–37]	*Acomys cahirinus* [e]
Psammomys obesus (sand "rat") [b] [38–44]	Bio Breeding Lab (BBL) rat [62–64]
Acomys cahirinus (spiny "mouse") [46–49]	

[a]Chinese hamsters with "mild" syndromes: animals with "trace" glycosuria, erratic syndrome, and spontaneous remission.
[b]Most sand rats studied have had a mild to moderate clinical course, without ketoacidosis.
[c]Chinese hamsters with severe syndromes, notably those with ketoacidosis, have shortened life expectancy.
[d]The first shipment of animals received (at Joslin Research Laboratory) in 1965 rapidly developed ketoacidosis. Subsequently, this has been observed only sporadically.
[e]Spiny mice with ketoacidosis have recently been observed only infrequently.
References in brackets.

unknown regulatory mechanisms respond to the metabolic abnormalities and/ or the reduction in β cell numbers by stimulating β cell replication and thereby enhancing the insulin synthetic capacity of the animals. This corrective process of β cell hyperplasia either does not occur or is of insufficient magnitude among the animals experiencing lethal syndromes, with the result that β cell loss exceeds replacement and insulin deficiency remains uncorrected. To illustrate and elaborate upon this approach to an understanding of the spontaneous diabetic animal models, physiologic and morphologic data will be presented on several of the more widely studied examples. These data will illustrate the features of lethality or nonlethality mentioned above, and will substantiate the validity of the classification.

Physiological Observations

Table 2 illustrates and compares selected physiological features of the major animal models studied.

Obesity. All of the nonlethal models except the Chinese hamster (remission) manifest obesity throughout their lifetime, with the degree of obesity most marked among the murine species. Abnormal subcutaneous fat deposits are first recognized during the 3rd to 5th weeks of life among C57Bl/6J-*ob/ob* (obese) and Toronto-KK mice. The accumulation of excess adipose tissue is more gradual and less abnormal in appearance among C3Hf X I hybrid mice, *Psammomys obesus* (sand "rats") and *Acomys cahirinus* (spiny "mice"). Among the lethal models, only spiny mice are apparently perpetually obese; the C57Bl/KsJ-*db/db* mice are markedly obese during most of their lifetime but lose weight in the several weeks prior to death; the Chinese hamsters and Bio Breeding Laboratory (BBL) rats are never obese.

Hyperglycemia. All of the animal models have elevated blood glucose (BG) levels at least during the early months of their lives. The nonlethal animals characteristically evidence less dramatic levels of hyperglycemia early in the syndromes and frequently demonstrate reductions in BG, often approaching or achieving normoglycemic status during the later periods of their existence. This tendency to normalize BG levels is not characteristic of the lethal animal models. On the contrary, BG remains elevated and often achieves its highest levels late in the syndrome (eg., ketotic Chinese hamsters, BBL rats, and *db/db* mice).

Circulating IRI. Perhaps the most accurate indicators of disease severity are the levels of plasma or serum immunoreactive insulin (IRI) recorded during the later periods of the syndromes, and the relationship of plasma IRI and BG levels. Among nonlethal models, plasma IRI is usually absolutely elevated throughout life and may return to or toward normal in association with the late achievement of normoglycemia. In contrast, plasma IRI of the lethal syndrome animals is usually only moderately and transiently elevated early in life, and declines in the later periods to levels that are either absolutely below normal or are inappropriately low in relation to the magnitude of hyperglycemia.

Table 2. *Physiological Features of Diabetic Syndromes*

Animals	Obesity		Hyperglycemia		Plasma IRI		Pancreatic IRI	Ketoacidosis	Genetics
	Early	Late	Early	Late	Early	Late			
Nonlethal									
C57B1/6J-*ob/ob*	++	+++	+	−[b]	↑	↔[b]	↕[d]	−	Autosomal recessive
Toronto—KK	++	+++	+	−[b]	↑	↕	↑	−	Polygenic
C3Hf X I (Wellesley)	+	++	+	−	↑	↕	↑	−	Hybrid
Chinese hamster (remission)	−	−	+	±	↕	↑	↕	−	Polygenic
Sand rat	+	++	+	−[b]	↑	↕	↑	−	Polygenic
Spiny mouse	++	++	±	+	↑	↑	↑	−	Polygenic
Lethal									
C57B1/KsJ-*db/db*	++	++[a]	++	+++	↑	↓	↓	−	Autosomal recessive
Chinese hamster (ketotic)	−	−	+++	+++	↑[c]	↓	↓	+	Polygenic
Sand rat (1965)	−	−	+++	+++	↑[c]	↓	↓	+	Polygenic
Spiny mouse	++	++	+	+	↑	↓	↓	+	Polygenic
Bio Breeding rat	−	−	+++	+++	↓	↓	↓	+[e]	?

[a] Preterminal weight loss.
[b] Decreases but may not always reach normal levels.
[c] Transient.
[d] Decreased early in syndrome but increases with regranulation of β cells.
[e] Most but not all rats studied.
(+) Present, (−) absent, (?) unknown, (↑) greater than normal, (↓) less than normal, (↔) normal levels.

Pancreatic Insulin. Data are available for all but one of the animal groups listed. The quantity of extractable IRI is elevated in all of the nonlethal models and absolutely decreased among all but one *(Acomys)* of the lethal diabetic animals. Hence, with the exception of the spiny mice, circulating and pancreatic insulin levels change in relationship with each other. The phenomenon of an early decrease followed by a later increase in extractable pancreatic insulin noted for the *ob/ob* mice is explained by the β cell degranulation which accompanies enhanced insulin secretory activity early in the syndrome. Later in life as the glycemic levels are normalized, β cell hyperplasia and secretory regranulation both occur and account for the increased pancreatic IRI.

Ketoacidosis. Only the most severely diabetic of the lethal animals experience ketoacidosis. These animals usually manifest the most dramatic reductions in circulating IRI and, except for the spiny mice, the most severe reduction in extractable pancreatic insulin.

Plasma and Pancreatic Glucagon. Data concerning the changing levels of plasma and pancreatic glucagon in these laboratory animals are at best fragmentary at this time, undoubtedly due to technical difficulties, lack of uniform expertise in performing the glucagon immunoassay, as well as problems with antibody specificity. It is for these reasons that the questionable and contradictory available data are omitted from Table 2.

Morphological Observations

Table 3 lists the major morphological phenomena of the animal models studied.

β Cell Hyperplasia. A key feature of the pancreatic islets which can be utilized to distinguish lethal and nonlethal diabetic animals is the presence of increased or decreased numbers of β cells in the fully established syndrome. The islets of all but one of the animal models evidencing lethal syndromes reveal not only an absence of β cell hyperplasia but an absolute decrease in β cell numbers. There is, therefore, a clear correlation between β cell numerical deficiency and insulinopenia on the one hand and diabetic severity on the other hand. The spiny "mouse" is the only known exception to this generalization (see below). The lethal diabetic animals also evidence β cell necrosis, usually at an early stage of the syndrome. This is associated with pronounced insulitis only in the recently described BBL rats. Islet inflammation, but of a focal and mild degree, has also been noted in C57Bl/KsJ-*db/db* mice.

β Cell Degranulation. The degranulation of β cells noted during the early hyperglycemic periods of the milder (nonlethal) animal models is followed later in life by regranulation, apparently a manifestation of decreased insulin release and increased storage in response to normalization of glycemic levels. β cell degranulation is observed during both the early and late stages of the lethal models and is ostensibly a result of maximum insulin release by the surviving β cells in response to unrelenting hyperglycemia. The eventual condition of absolute or relative deficiency of circulating and extractable IRI occurs, therefore, as a result of a reduction in the number of β cells available for IRI secretion.

Table 3. Morphologic Observations of Pancreatic Islets

Animals	β cells					α cells	
	Hyperplasia	Degranulation	Necrosis	Virus	Glycogen	Increased—late	Insulitis
Nonlethal							
C57B1/6J-ob/ob	4+	E	−	+	−	−	−
Toronto-KK mouse	4+	E	−	NS	−	−	−
C3Hf × I mouse	4+	E	−	+	−	NS	−
Chinese hamster[a]	+	+	−	−	−	NS	−
Sand rat	2+	E[c]	−	−	+	NS	−
Lethal							
Spiny mouse	3+	−	−	[d]	+	?	−
Chinese hamster	−[b]	E & L	+	−	+	+	−
Sand rat	−	E & L	+	−	+	NS	±
C57B1/KsJ-db/db	−[b]	E & L	+	+	−	+	±
Bio Breeding rat	−	E & L	+++	NS	NS	NS	3+[e]

[a]Chinese hamsters that experience spontaneous remission.
[b]Transient burst of islet cell mitoses early in syndrome.
[c]Variable late in syndrome.
[d]Viral particles observed in α cell.
[e]Minimal or absent at end stage.
(+) Present, (−) absent, (E) early in syndrome: cytoplasmic granulation increased later in syndrome, (L) late in syndrome, (NS) not studied.

Type C Viruses. These are observed within intact and otherwise normal β cells in several of the murine species and are presumably related to the acknowledged presence of this virus within the murine genome. The presence of increased numbers of C-type viruses within necrotic β cells of diabetic *(db)* mice is as yet unexplained.

β Cell Glycogen. Storage of β cell glycogen is an observation noted generally in non-mouse species (the spiny "mouse" is not a member of the murine species) and is not specifically related to syndrome lethality.

Pancreatic α and δ Cells. These cells have been reported[65] to be increased in number in the C57B1/KsJ-*db/db* but not in the C57B1/6J-*ob/ob* mice, and may be another manifestation of disease severity. α cells are also believed to be numerically increased in nonremission diabetic Chinese hamsters.[31] Evidence of α and δ cell numerical changes have not yet been fully confirmed by measurements of extractable hormone content in these animals.

Pancreatic Islets of Nonlethal Diabetic Syndromes

C57B1/6J-ob/ob (Obese) Mice

Perhaps the earliest recognized example of spontaneous genetic diabetes mellitus in a laboratory rodent, the *ob/ob* mice have certainly been the most thoroughly studied. For the purposes of this chapter, the morphology of their pancreatic islets will be used to illustrate the major features common to most of the nonlethal models of spontaneous diabetes.

Physiologically, the *ob/ob* mice are characterized by hyperphagia and early onset of obesity (3–5 weeks of age). Mild hyperglycemia [blood glucose (BG) levels usually not exceeding 250 mg/100ml] becomes manifest within the first month after weaning, with BG returning toward normal at 12–16 weeks of age. Elevation of circulating IRI is first noted immediately prior to the onset of hyperglycemia, and plasma IRI remains elevated during the greater portion of the animal's life, sometimes returning toward control levels late in the syndrome after normalization of BG.

Although the nature of the primary pathogenetic defect is not yet known with certainty, several summary observations are worth listing: (1) The possible etiologic significance of peripheral (skeletal and cardiac muscle, liver, adipose tissue) insulin resistance[15] and the role of hyperinsulinemia in the genesis and progression of the syndrome[18,19] have recently received more attention and have been placed on a more quantitative basis as a result of insulin receptor interaction studies based upon the availability of insulin receptor binding assays[66–68]; (2) many of the animals' metabolic abnormalities can be attributed to the combined effects of hyperglycemia, increased levels of physiologically active insulin, availability of other metabolic substrates, and peripheral insulin resistance; (3) the concept that a single gene *(ob)* defect is responsible for the complex characteristics of the syndrome has been modified by evidence that other (background) genetic factors may substantially alter the severity of the disease manifestations.[60,61]

Pancreatic Islet Morphology.   The appearance of the islets of Langerhans of *ob/ob* mice (Figs. 3–6) closely resembles that of other nonlethal animals and contrasts with the appearance of the pancreatic islets of nondiabetic mice (Figs. 1, 2, and 10). β cell degranulation is the earliest (4–6 weeks) recognizable alteration. β cell hyperplasia also occurs early in life so that islets of *ob/ob* mice at 10–12 weeks of age are both enlarged and degranulated (Fig. 3a). With normalization of glycemic levels (12–16 weeks) β cell regranulation occurs (Figs. 3b,c). In contrast with β cell hyperplasia, α cell numbers have not been

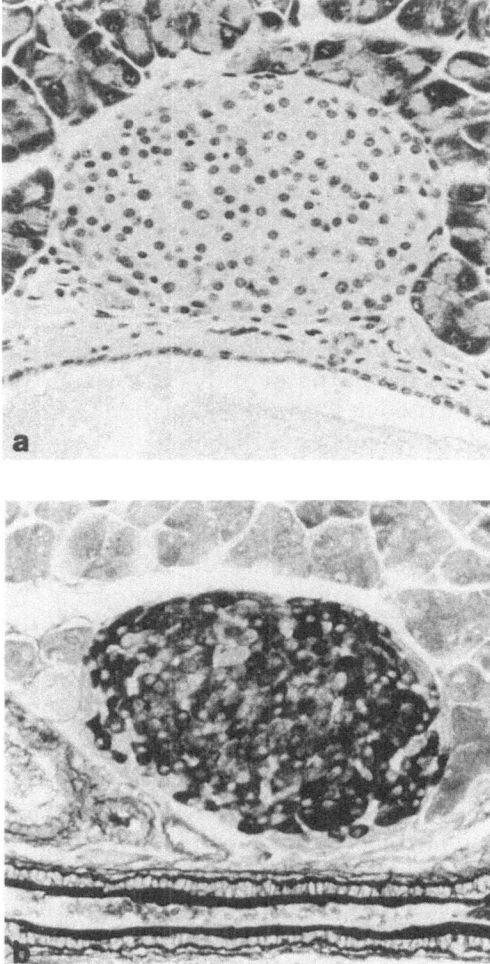

Figure 1. Pancreatic islets of normal mice. Tissue fixed in Bouin's solution. (a) The well-delineated islet is surrounded by acinar cells and is adjacent to an exocrine duct. Hematoxylin and eosin. ×256. (b) The deeply stained, well-granulated β cells (black in photograph) are characteristic of normoglycemic animals. Unstained alpha cells are located at periphery of islet. Aldehyde fuchsin. ×256.

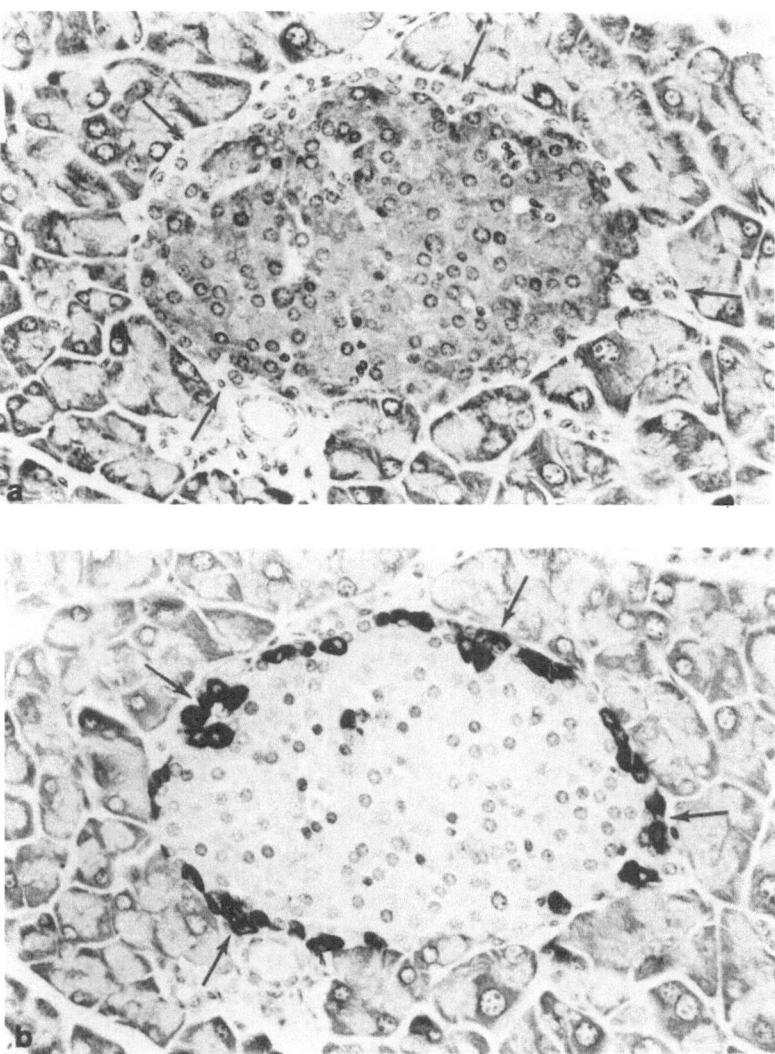

Figure 2. Pancreatic islets of normal mice. Tissue fixed in Bouin's solution. Immunohistochemical peroxidase-antiperoxidase technique (PAP) utilized for identification of insulin and glucagon. Parts a and b are adjacent sections. (a) Insulin-containing β cells stain deeply after reaction with guinea pig antiinsulin serum and PAP technique. Arrows indicate peripheral unstained α cells. ×300. (b) Peripheral glucagon-containing α cells (arrows) stain intensely after reaction with rabbit antipancreatic glucagon antiserum and PAP technique. Centrally located β cells are unstained. Compare with adjacent section in part a. ×300.

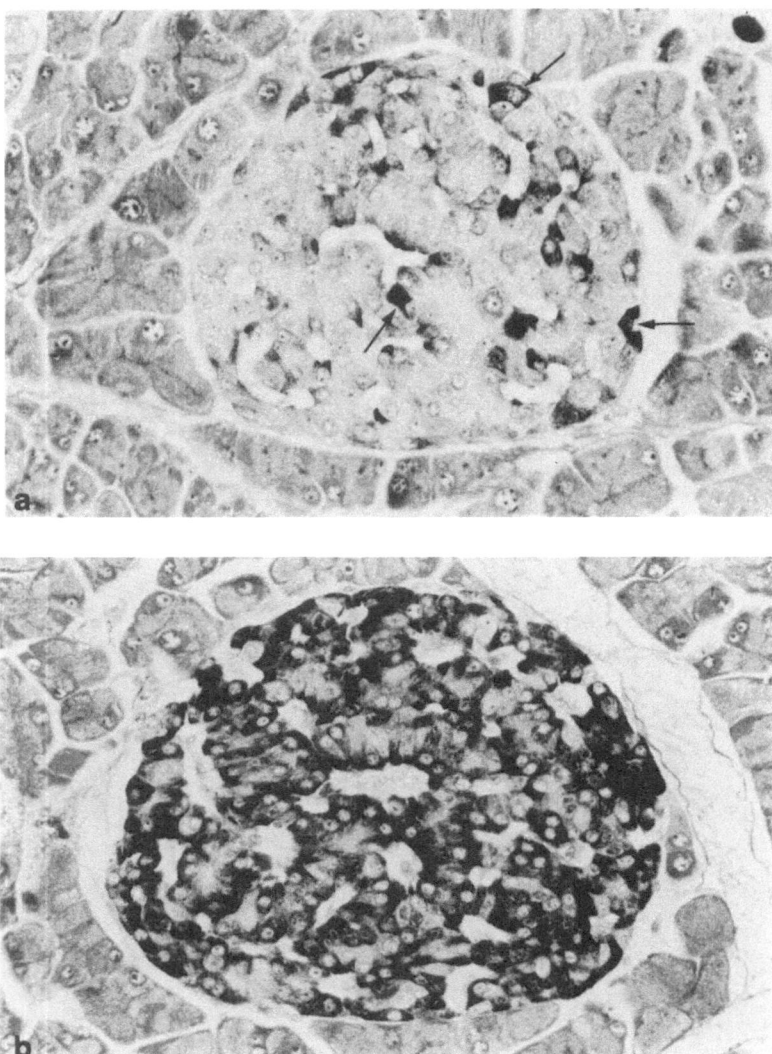

Figure 3. Pancreatic islets of C57Bl/6J-*ob/ob* mice. (a) The moderately enlarged islet of young *ob/ob* mouse reveals almost complete β cell degranulation. Arrows identify several β cells which are still granulated and are therefore aldehyde fuchsin positive. ×300. (b) Islet of an older *ob/ob* mouse with almost fully granulated β cells (black in photograph). Blood glucose (BG) of this mouse was approaching normal and pancreatic immunoreactive insulin (IRI) content was markedly elevated.

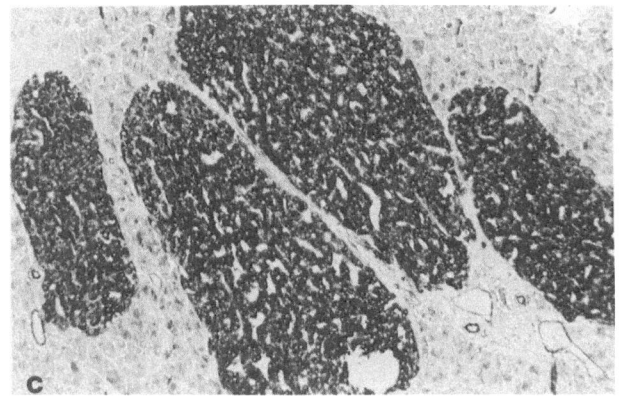

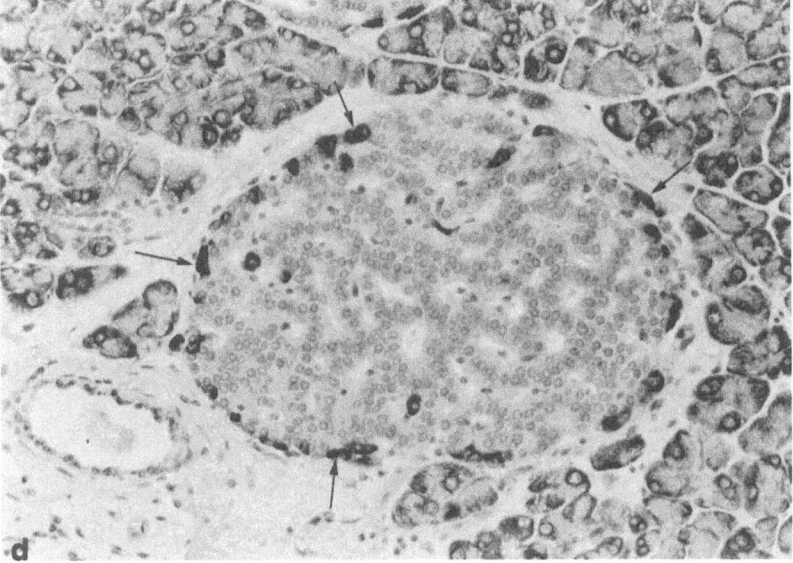

Aldehyde fuchsin. ×300. (c) Islets of older *ob/ob* mouse at low magnification to demonstrate the degree of β cell hyperplasia. The prominently enlarged islets are well granulated. Aldehyde fuchsin. ×72. (d) Islet of *ob/ob* mouse comparable in age with that of Fig. 3b, stained with the PAP technique after reaction with antipancreatic glucagon antiserum. α cells (arrows) are not increased in C57B1/6J-*ob/ob* mice.[65] ×212.

Figure 4. β cells in young *ob/ob* mouse. Secretory degranulation is prominent and associated with increased rough endoplasmic reticulum (RER) and enlarged Golgi structures (G). Arrow heads indicate remaining β granules. Compare with β cells of normoglycemic mice in Figs. 6 and 10. ×32,340.

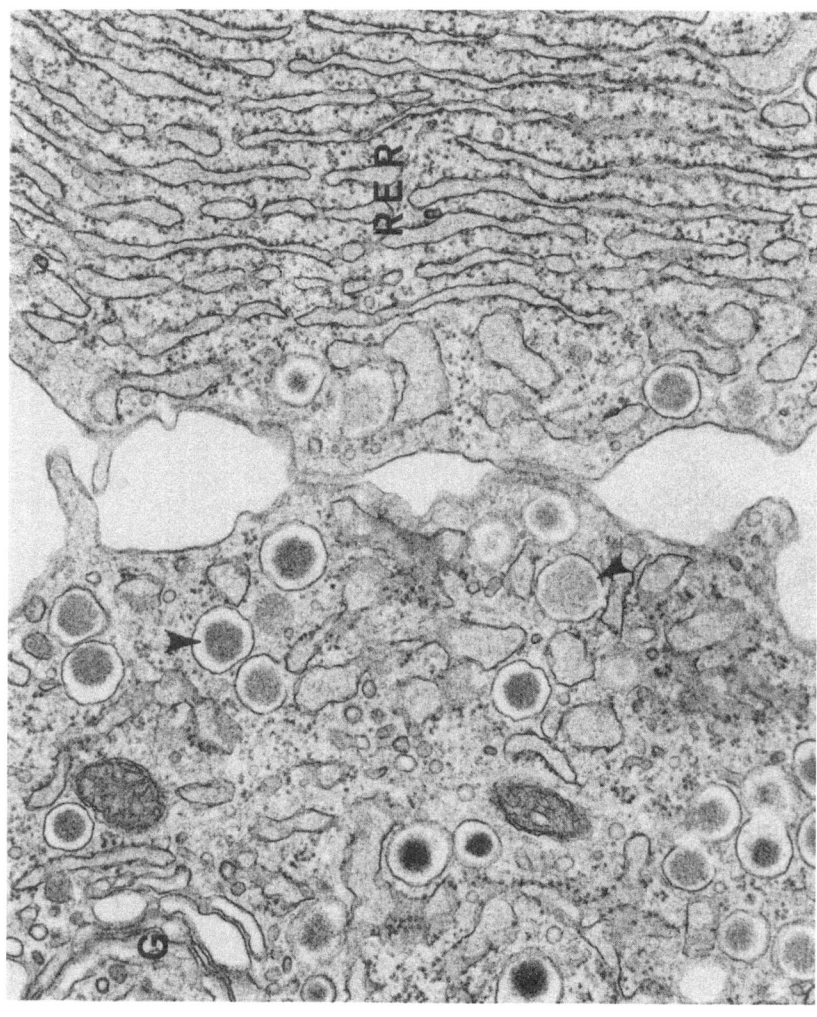

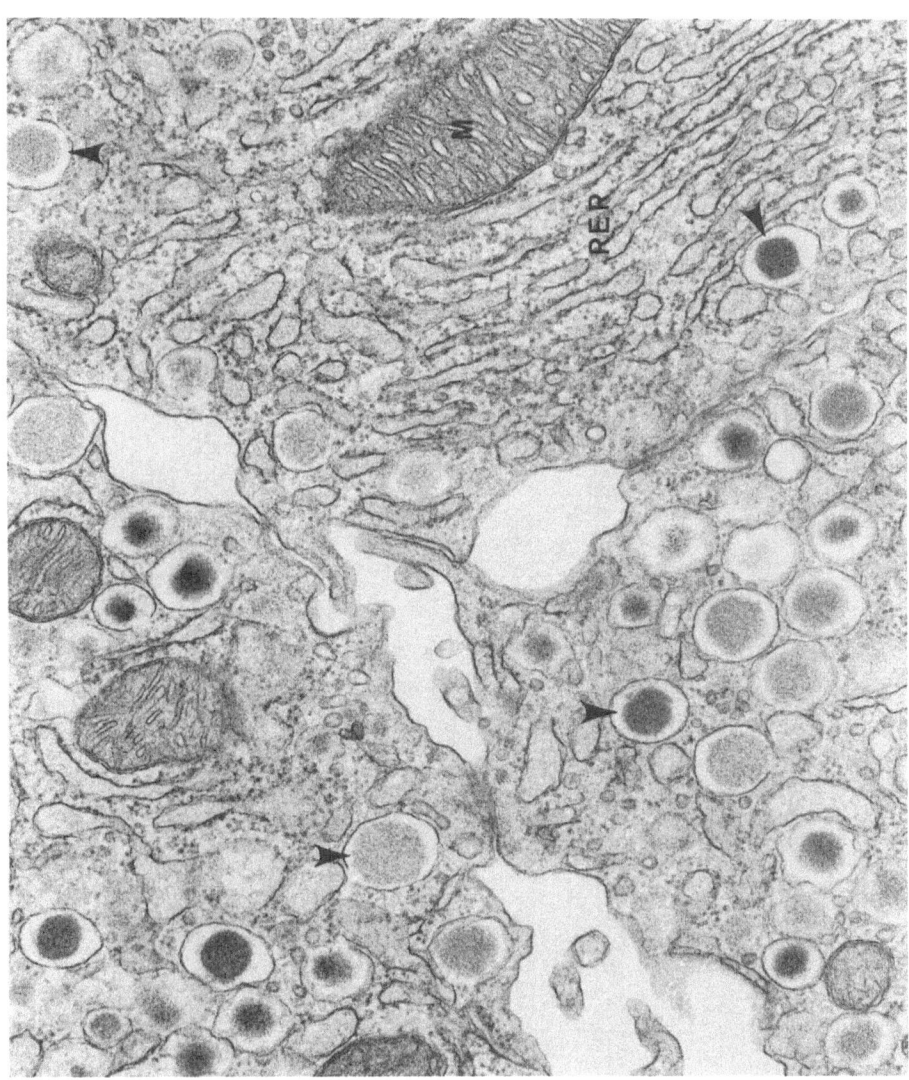

Figure 5. β cells in *ob/ob* mouse somewhat older than that of Fig. 4, with increased number of secretory granules (arrow heads). BG levels of this animal were somewhat lower. M, mitochondrion; RER, rough endoplasmic reticulum. ×32,340.

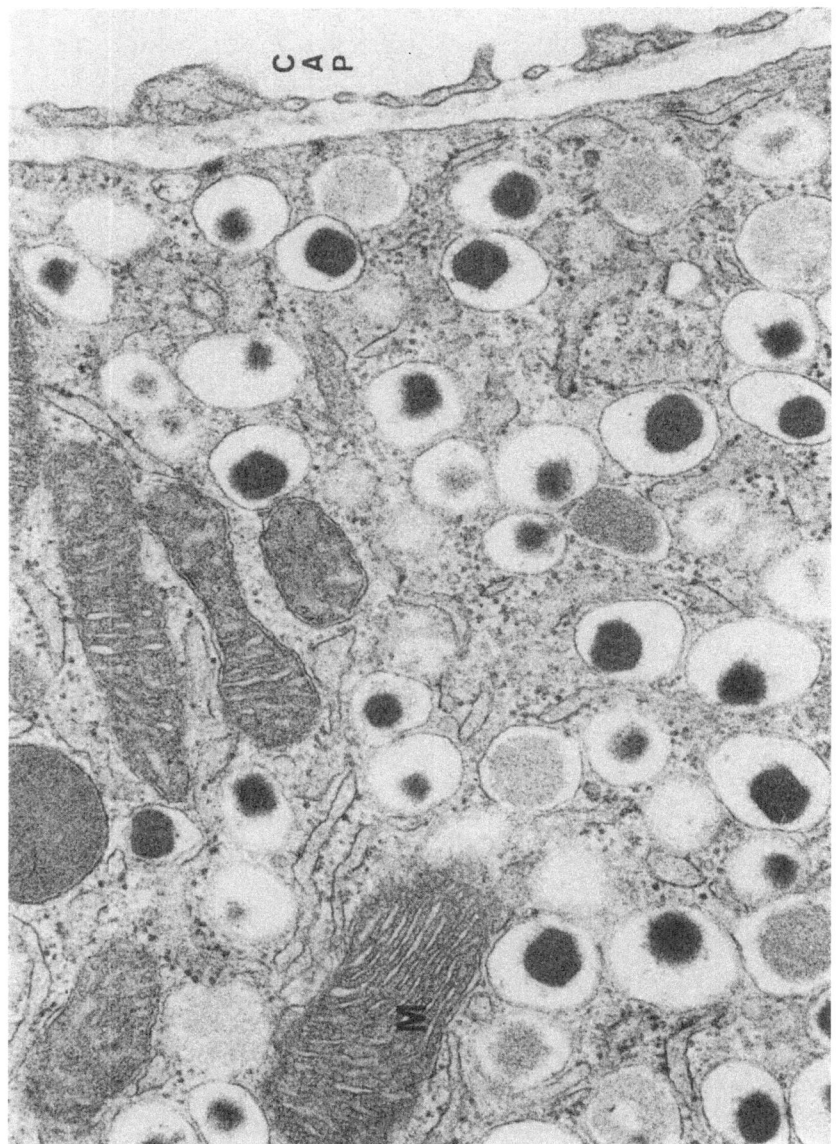

Figure 6. β cell and adjacent capillary (CAP) from an old, normoglycemic *ob/ob* mouse. Secretory granules are abundant and RER is inconspicuous. This cell is morphologically identical with β cells from normal mice. (See Fig. 10.) ×39,600.

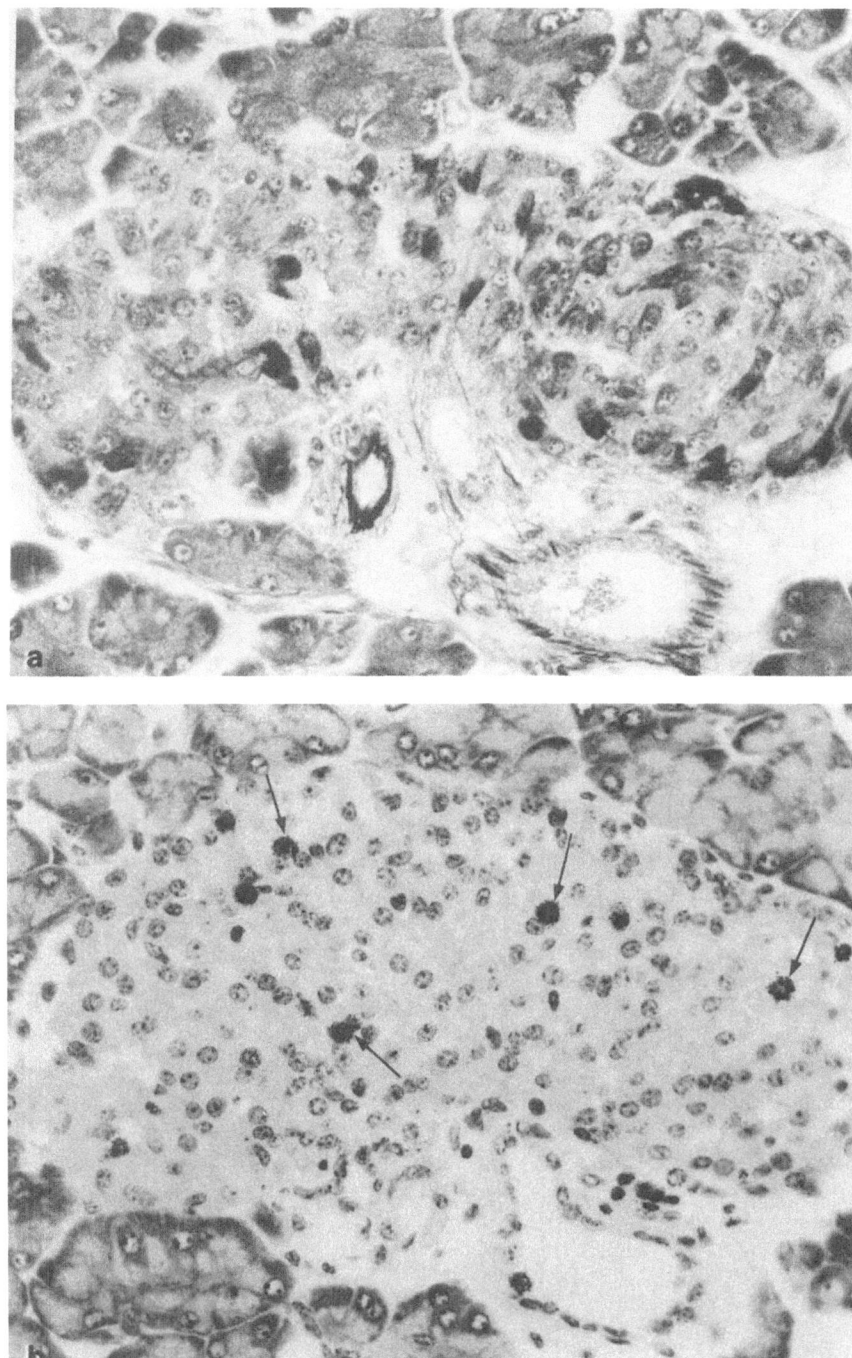

Figure 7. Pancreatic islets of diabetic (C57Bl/KsJ-*db/db*) mouse during early hyperglycemic period. Serum IRI levels were still elevated. (a) Aldehyde fuchsin stain revealing partial β cell degranulation. Islet configuration is intact. ×500. (b) Autoradiography (of adjacent section) after [³H]thymidine administration reveals labeling predominantly of islet cells (arrows). ×500.

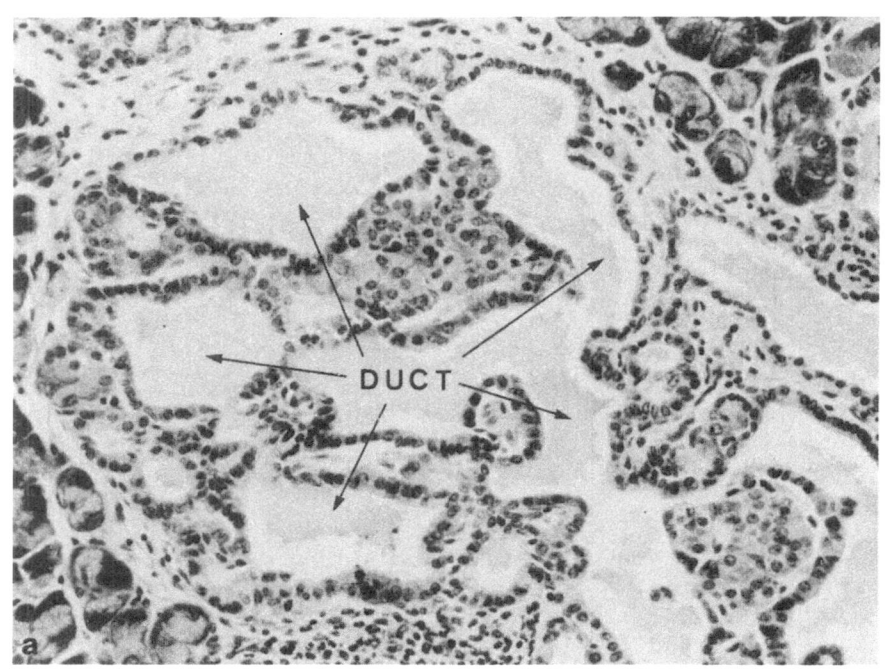

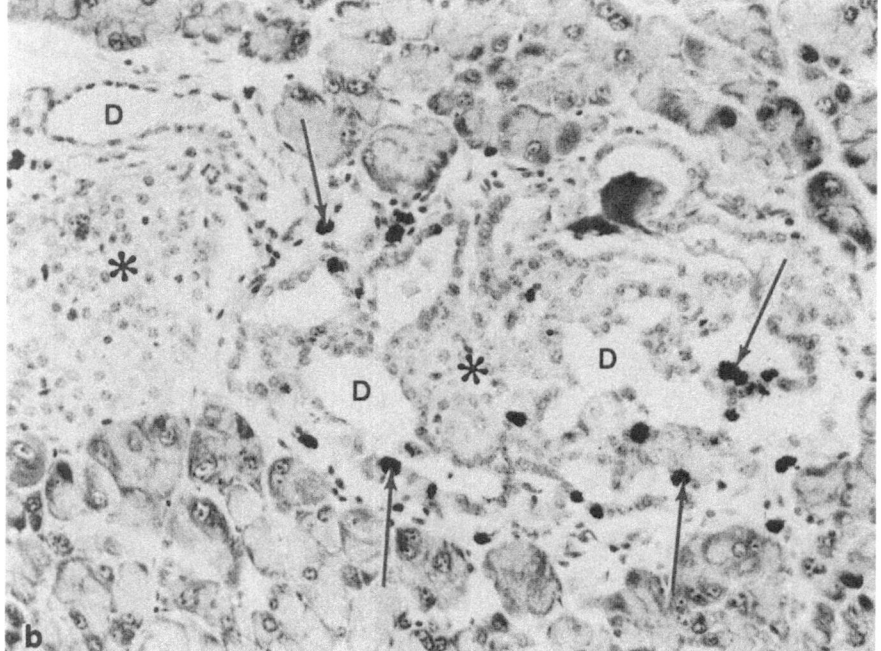

shown to be increased in the *ob/ob* mouse (Fig. 3d).[65] Ultrastructural studies confirm the light-microscopic findings and correlate well with available physiological data. Hence, β cells of *ob/ob* mice with hyperglycemia and increased plasma IRI reveal secretory degranulation with increased rough endoplasmic reticulum and enlarged Golgi structures (Fig. 4). Evidence of β cell necrosis is absent. With the gradual reduction of BG, β cell regranulation commences (Fig. 5) and is more complete with normalization of BG (Fig. 6). Individual fully granulated β cells (Fig. 6) cannot be differentiated from those of normal mice (Fig. 10); however, the enlarged islets, replete with fully granulated β cells (Fig. 3c), correlate well with the increased extractable pancreatic IRI and are characteristic of, and in fact cannot be distinguished from, the islets of the other nonlethal murine syndromes studied to date (Table 2).

β cell hyperplasia is also observed in spiny mice and sand rats with mild, nonketotic syndromes. The β cells of these animals can be differentiated from those of murine species because of the presence of β cell glycogen deposits and other subtle ultrastructural features. Although β cell hyperplasia and islet enlargement have been described in diabetic Chinese hamsters undergoing spontaneous remission (see below and Fig. 20b), the magnitude of the islet enlargement is not as pronounced as in the murine strains listed in Table 2.

Pancreatic Islets of Lethal Diabetic Syndromes

The unifying feature of the pancreatic islet morphology in the lethal models of diabetes is a reduction in β cell number with a concomitant decrease in available pancreatic and circulating IRI. The other species-specific morphologic features are illustrated below because of their unique and sometimes distinctive appearance and also because these features may shed light upon the presently illusive pathogenetic mechanisms responsible for the reduction in β cell mass.

C57Bl/KsJ-db/db (Mutation Diabetes) Mice

Following the first report by Hummel *et al.*[50] in 1966, the importance of this model of spontaneous diabetes literally exploded upon the scientific community, with many investigators researching various facets of this unique syndrome.[69] Physically and physiologically, the mice homozygous for the *db* and *ob* genes are virtually indistinguishable during the early weeks of life. Early

---

Figure 8. Pancreatic islets of diabetic *(db/db)* mice late in the syndrome. A network of ductal structures has infiltrated the islets with striking distortion of the usual configuration. Small clusters of residual islet cells (*) as well as inflammatory cells (bottom of part a) are visible. (a) Hematoxylin and eosin. ×256. (b) Autoradiography [³H]thymidine administration reveals uptake of label by proliferating ductal cells (arrows). Islet cells (*) are no longer labeled with any frequency late in the syndrome. ×256.

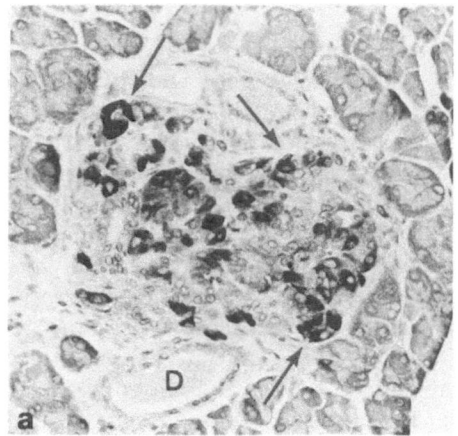

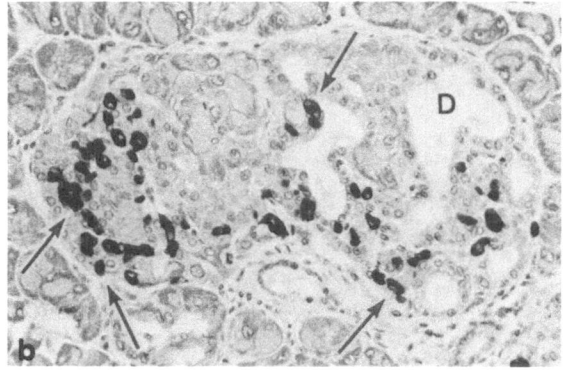

Figure 9. Pancreatic islets of diabetic *(db/db)* mice late in the syndrome, after immunohistochemical identification of insulin- (a) and glucagon- (b, c) containing cells by the PAP technique. (a) Arrows indicate residual β cells (black in photograph) haphazardly scattered among the ducts (D) and acinar cells which are located within the islet interior. ×190. (b) Arrows indicate α cells grouped in clusters and singly throughout the islet. Again, ducts (D) and acinar cells distort the islet structure. ×190.

hyperphagia, obesity, hyperinsulinemia, and hyperglycemia are present in both. The C57Bl/KsJ-*db/db* mice differ from the C57Bl/6J-*ob/ob* animals, and from the other nonlethal murine strains, in that the clinical course of the *db/db* mice is more rapidly progressive and more severe after the initial 8–10 weeks of life. Therefore, BG levels are considerably higher among *db/db* mice and increase further with advancing age rather than returning toward normal. Plasma IRI is only transiently elevated among *db/db* mice, rapidly returning toward or below normal levels after the first 8–10 weeks of age. Finally, life expectancy is significantly reduced among *db/db* mice with most animals dying usually between 5 and 7 months of age. As is true for the *ob/ob* mice, the

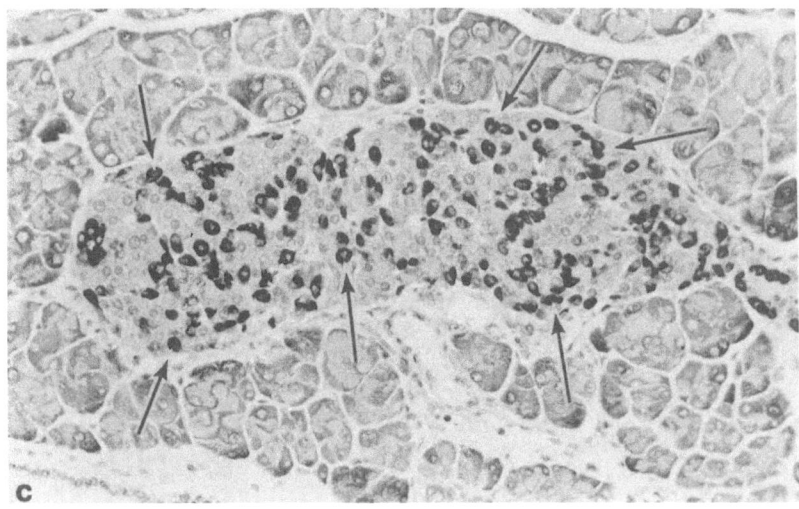

Figure 9(c) Another islet with increased number of glucagon-containing cells (arrows). α cells are believed to be significantly increased in old C57Bl/KsJ-*db/db* mice.[65] ×190.

primary pathogenetic defect(s) responsible for the *db/db* and the other murine syndromes is also not known. It is worth reemphasizing that the *db/db* and *ob/ob* mice share the following attributes, in addition to those listed above: (1) Peripheral insulin resistance, presumably based upon "insulin receptor interaction" defects. In the *db/db* mice, insulin resistance persists in older animals, even after circulating IRI levels have returned to normal or below. (2) Importance of genetic background upon syndrome severity. When the *db* gene is transferred from the original C57Bl/Ks to the related C57Bl/6 background, disease severity is considerably blunted, and the resulting pathophysiological pattern and islet morphology are essentially the same as in the C57Bl/6J-*ob/ob* mice. Parenthetically, it should be emphasized that when the *ob* gene is placed on the C57Bl/Ks background, disease severity is augmented and resembles that of the *diabetes mutation* (C57Bl/KsJ-*db/db*).[60,61]

Pancreatic Islet Morphology. The earliest histologic alteration in the *db/db* mice is partial β cell degranulation, sometimes noted in prehyperglycemic animals, but more uniformly observed and more prominent in degree within islets of mice with established hyperglycemia (Fig. 7a). This morphologic evidence of enhanced insulin secretory activity correlates well with increased levels of serum IRI and with autoradiographic evidence of increased β cell replication (Figs. 7b and 13). This early and transient evidence of β cell mitotic activity and the associated mild increase in islet size give way with time to a reduction in β cell number, a unique ingrowth of ductal structures and acinar cells (Figs. 8, 9, 16–18), and an end to the increased β cell incorporation of tritiated thymidine (Fig. 8b). Surviving β cells continue to be degranulated (Figs. 9a, 12, 16, and

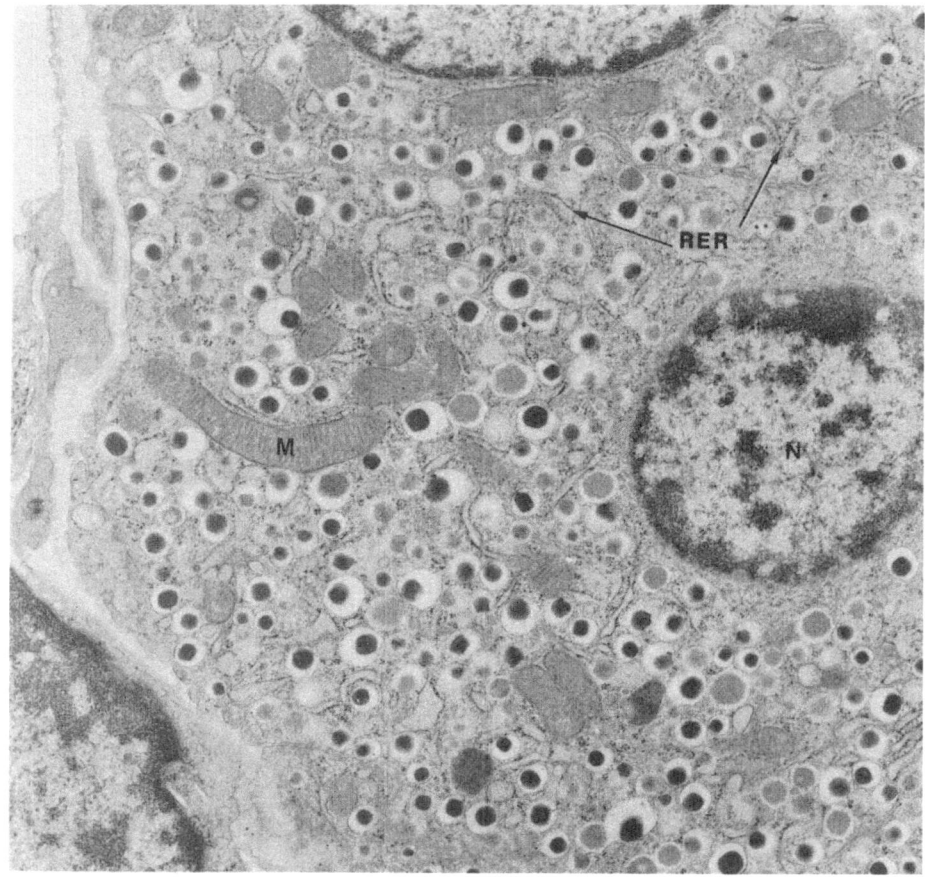

Figure 10. β cells from normal mouse (C57Bl/KsJ). Beta secretory granules are abundant and rough endoplasmic reticulum (RER) is inconspicuous. N, nucleus; M, mitochondrion. ×14,250. Reproduced at 85%.

17), however, well-granulated α cells appear to increase in number and are frequently located within the islet interior rather than at the islet periphery (Fig. 9c). Although there is considerable variability from islet to islet (compare Figs. 8 and 9), most islets reveal a decreased number of β cells, which correlates well with the reduction in serum and extractable pancreatic IRI.

Ultrastructurally, early β cell degranulation in *db/db* mice (Fig. 12) resembles that observed in the *ob/ob* mice. Evidence of β cells incorporating tritiated thymidine (Fig. 13) and undergoing mitotic division supports the optical microscopic data that a transient burst of β cell replication occurs early in the diabetic syndrome. As the animals progress into the later stages of the syndrome, the decrease in β cell number is accompanied by a reduction in the incorporation of

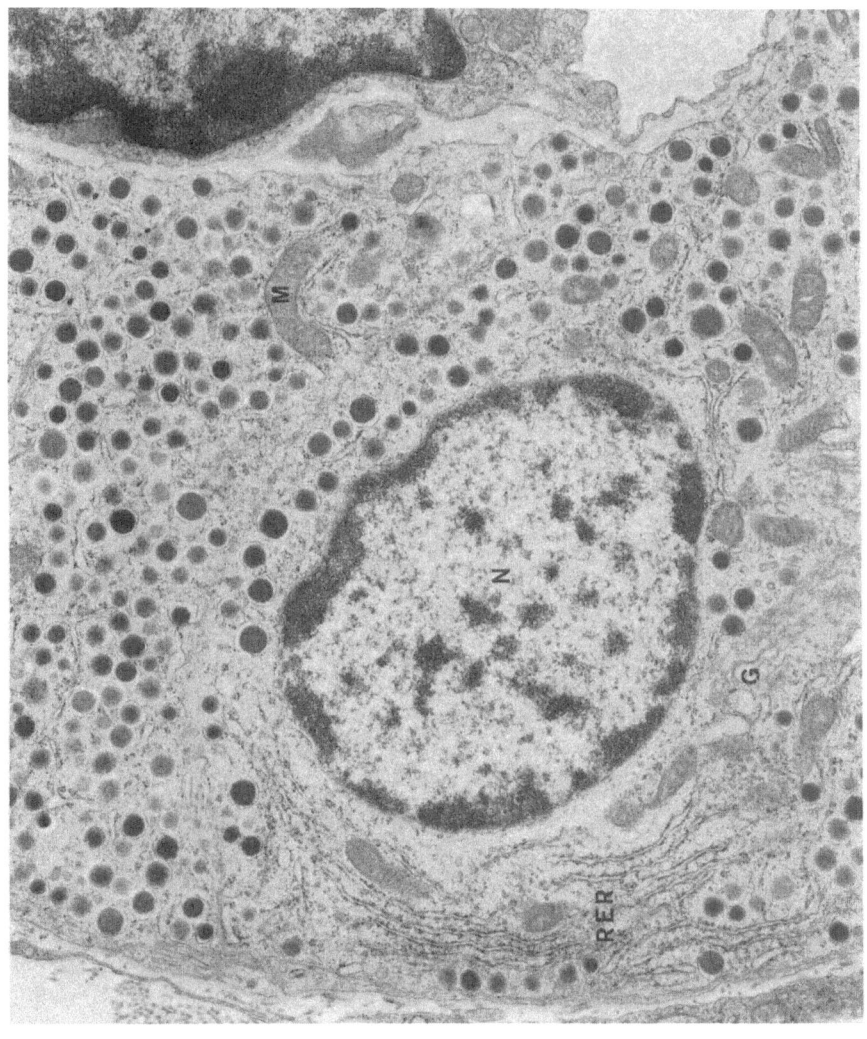

Figure 11. α cells from normal mouse (C57B1/KsJ). Abundant secretory granules are contained within tightly fitting sacs and are more electron dense than β granules. The RER and Golgi structures (G) are of normal size. ×14,250. Reproduced at 85%.

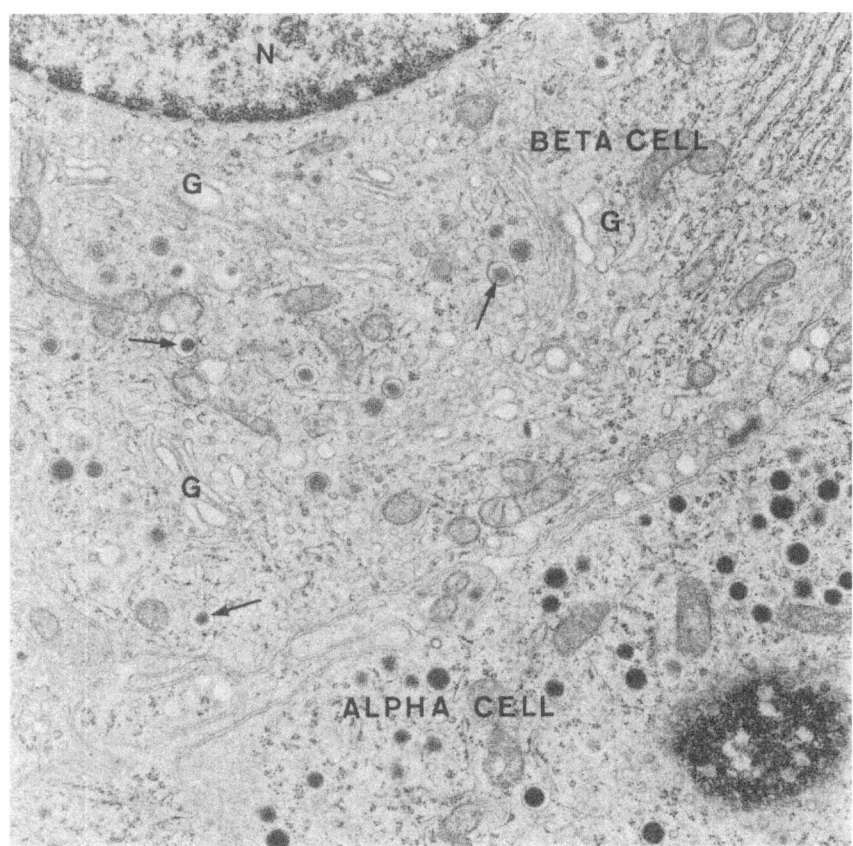

Figure 12. β and α cells of diabetic *(db/db)* mouse with early hyperglycemia. β secretory storage granules (arrows) are less numerous and smaller in size. Rough endoplasmic reticulum and Golgi structures (G) are prominent. α cell is unchanged. ×14,000.

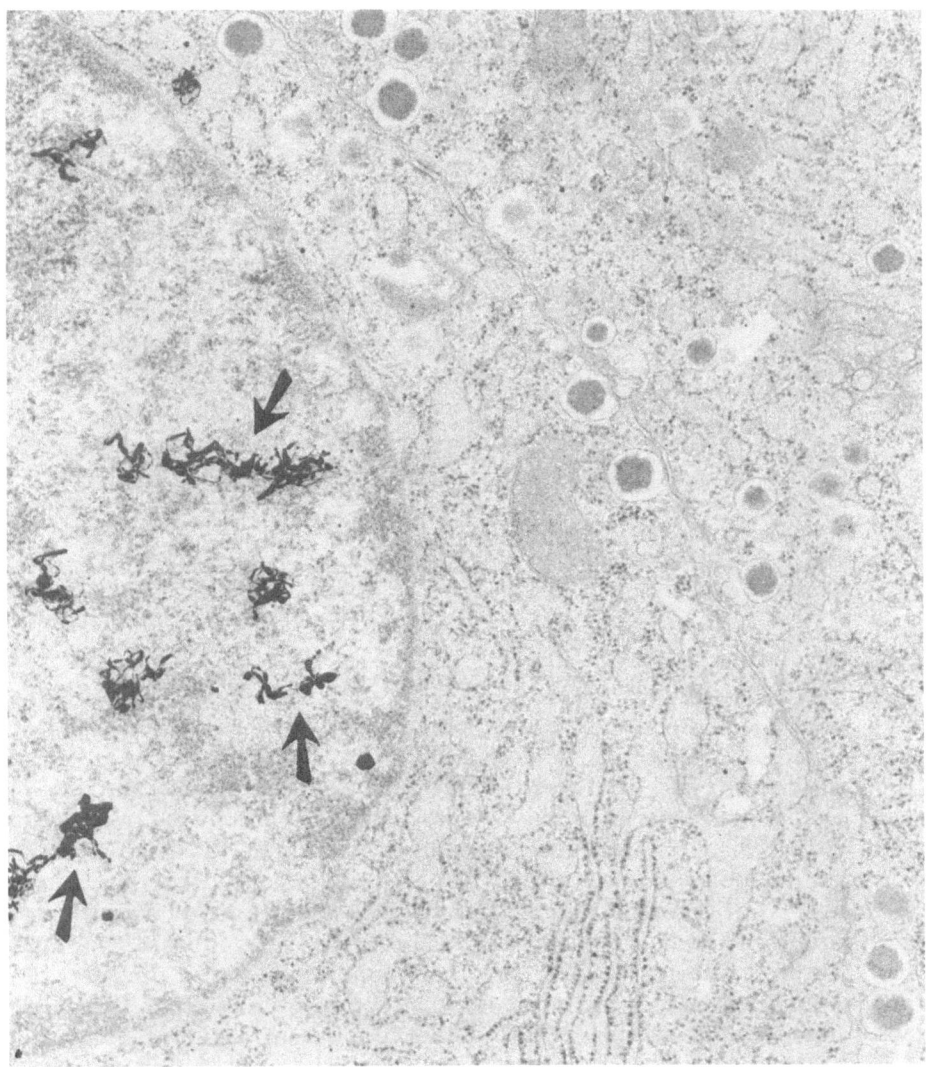

Figure 13. β cells of diabetic *(db/db)* mouse with early hyperglycemia. Electron-microscopic radioautography after [³H]thymidine administration reveals silver grains overlying nucleus, indicating path of exiting β particles. β secretory granules are reduced in number. ×22,000.

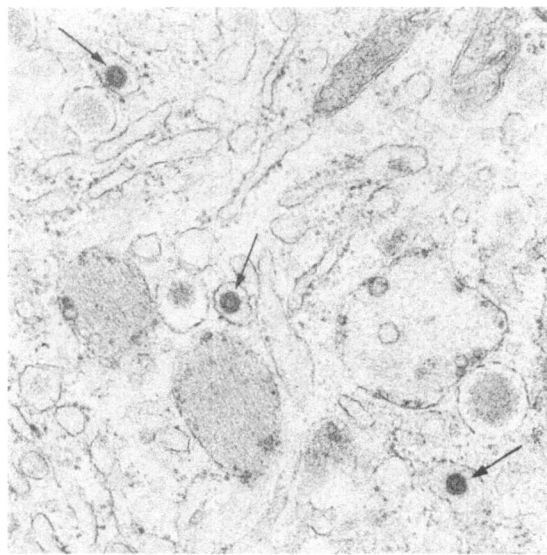

Figure 14. β cell of diabetic mouse (C57Bl/KsJ-*db/db*) revealing the presence of three immature type-C viruses (arrows). The murine leukemia virus is considered to be part of the genome of all mice. ×32,800.

[³H]thymidine and occurs in the presence of even more pronounced secretory degranulation. β cells of young *db/db* mice can frequently be distinguished from those of the *ob/ob* mice by the greater frequency of intracisternal and intravesicular type C virus particles in the *db/db* mice (Fig. 14) and by the presence of β cell necrosis (Fig. 15). More readily recognizable are the ductal structures and the differentiated acinar cells within the islet interior of older well established *db/db* mice. The ducts are frequently lined by cells containing characteristic zymogen granules of acinar cells (Figs. 16 and 17) or secretory granules of small intestinal Paneth or mucous cells (Fig. 18). The luminal surfaces of the latter often possess numerous microvilli. Most important, however, is the virtually complete absence of α and β cells along the lining or luminal surfaces of the ducts (Figs. 16–18), suggesting that in the adult *db/db* mouse, the proliferating ducts may not have the potential to differentiate into endocrine cells. They are apparently capable of giving rise to other ductal cells, Paneth (or mucous) and pancreatic acinar cells, and are presumably responsible for the unique presence of these cell types within the interior of these islets. The individual α cells of diabetic mice (Figs. 18 and 19) cannot be distinguished from those of normal animals (Fig. 11). The numerical increase and their frequent location within the islet interior rather than at the islet periphery are best appreciated by light microscopy (see Figs. 9b and 9c).

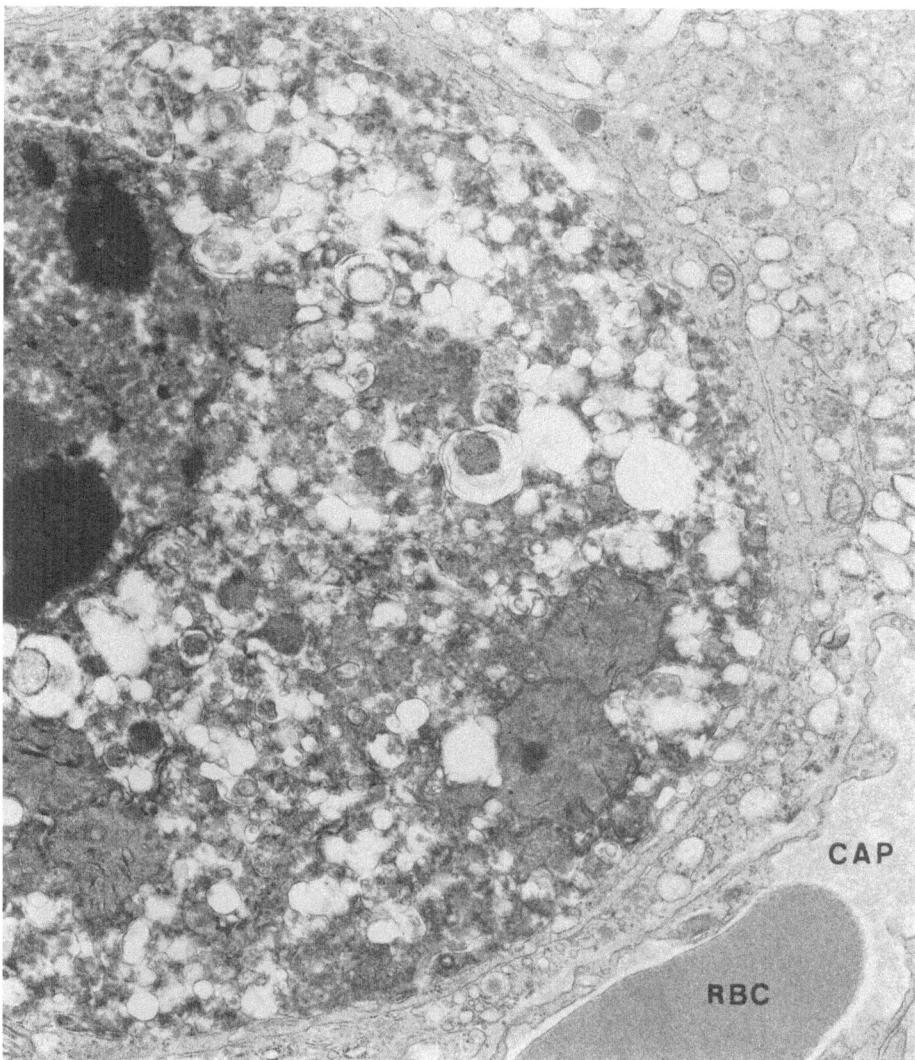

Figure 15. Portion of necrotic β cell in *db/db* mouse with established hyperglycemia. The nucleus is pyknotic and the cytoplasm is clumped and electron dense. CAP, capillary; RBC, red blood cell. ×14,250.

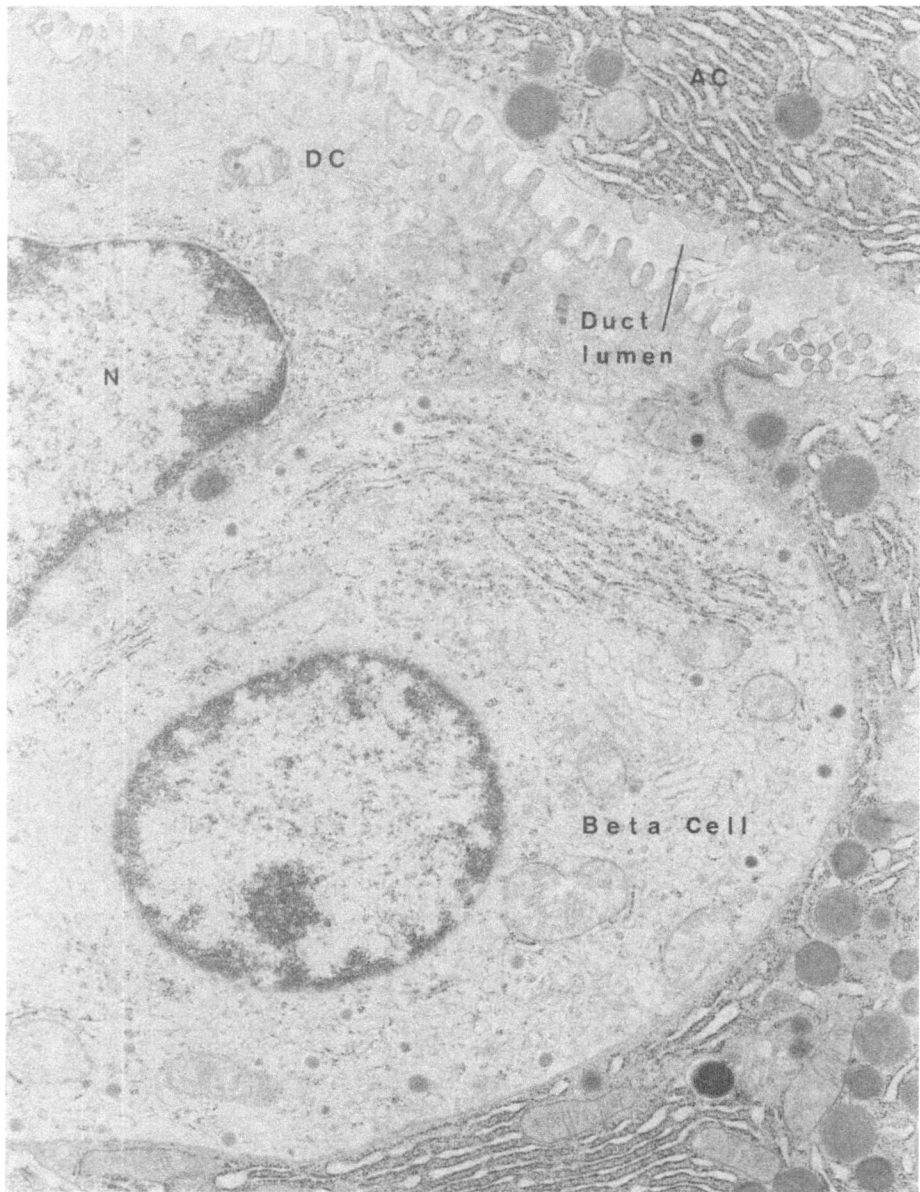

Figure 16. Diabetic *(db/db)* mouse. Portion of islet with infiltrating ductal structure lined by two acinar cells and a ductal cell (DC). The degranulated β cell is close to, but does not border on, the duct lumen. AC, acinar cell. × 14,250. Reproduced at 85%.

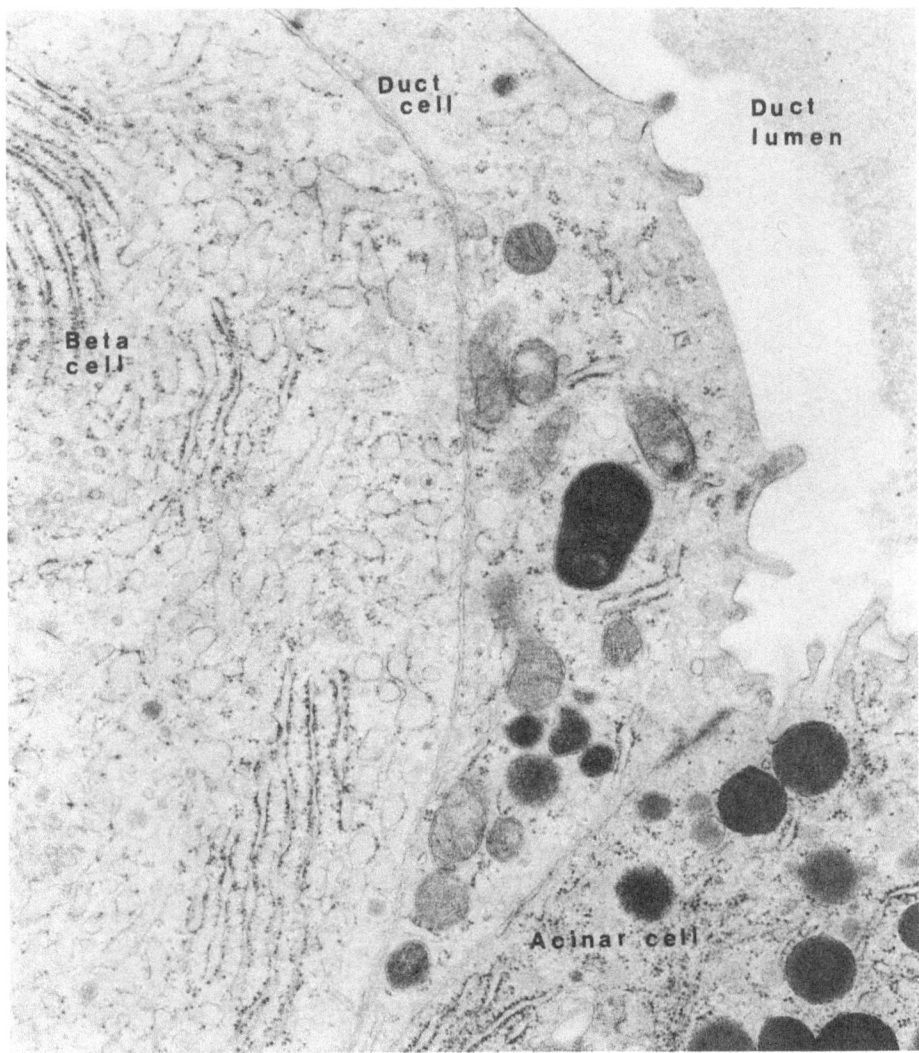

Figure 17. Diabetic *(db/db)* mouse. Another ductal structure lined by acinar and ductal epithelial cells with an adjacent degranulated β cell. The width of the ductal cell is too narrow to be resolved by light microscopy. ×22,000. Reproduced at 90%.

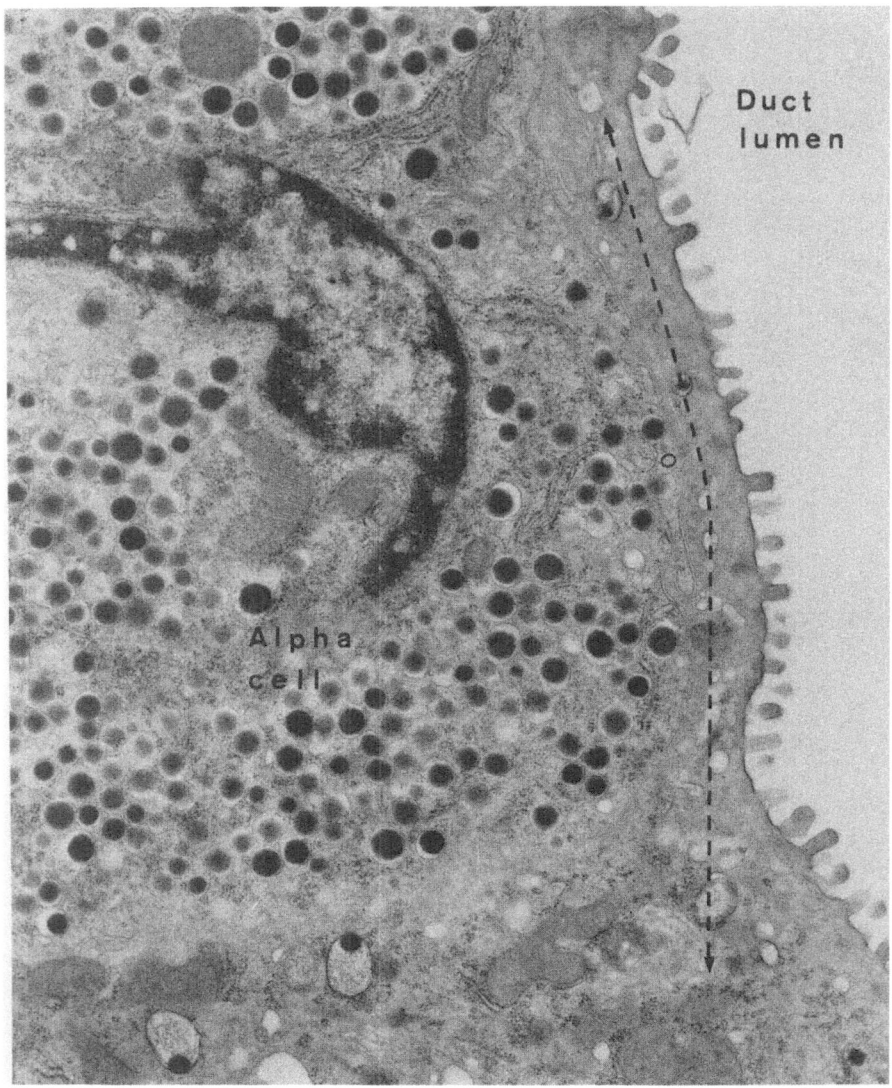

Figure 18. Diabetic *(db/db)* mouse. This micrograph illustrates a duct lumen with bordering ductal cell (interrupted arrow) separating the lumen from adjacent α cell. ×14,250.

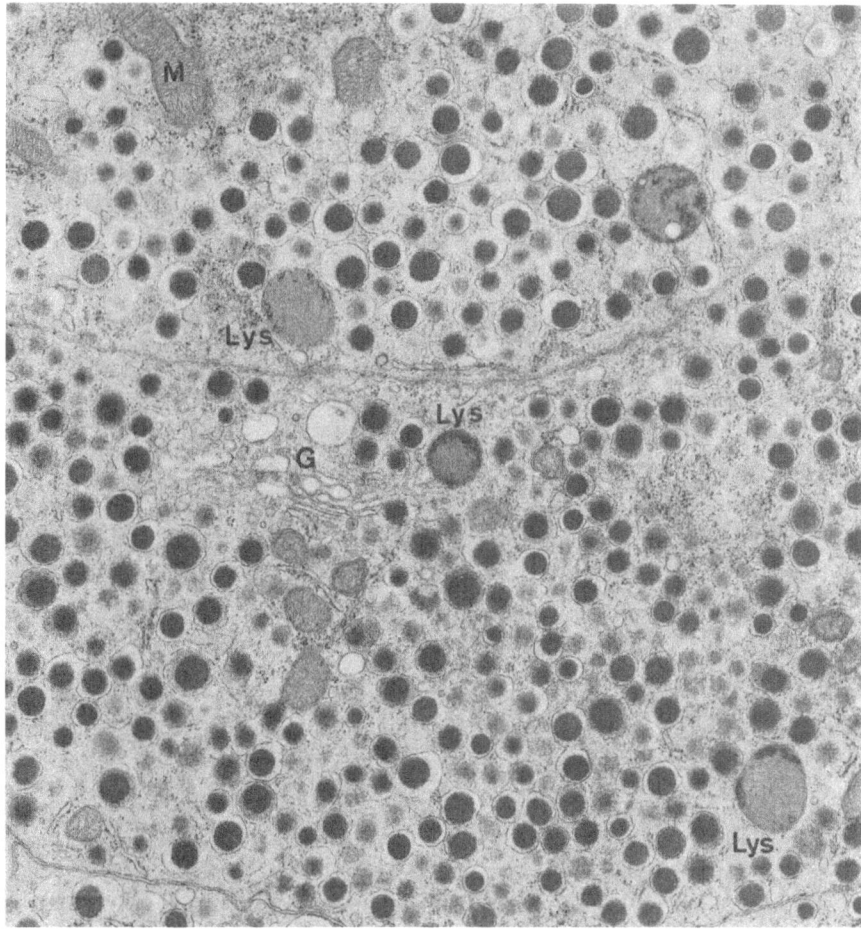

Figure 19. α cells of C57Bl/KsJ-*db/db* mouse. These cells cannot be distinguished from α cells of normal mice. The number of lysosomes (numerous in this micrograph) is quite variable among *db/db* mice. M, mitochondrion; Lys, lysosomes; G, Golgi structures. ×14,250.

Diabetic Chinese Hamsters

Meier and Yerganian first reported the presence of diabetes mellitus in a colony of Chinese hamsters.[28] In the original and subsequent publications,[29-35] the following characteristics were documented. The diabetic syndrome is considered to be the result of a polygenic inheritance with at least four genes involved; when any two genes are inherited, the animals become diabetic. The syndrome is characterized by early (preweaning) hyperphagia, variable onset of glycosuria and hyperglycemia, and the absence of obesity. Peripheral adipose tissue and skeletal muscle are normally responsive to insulin *in vitro*. Syndromes

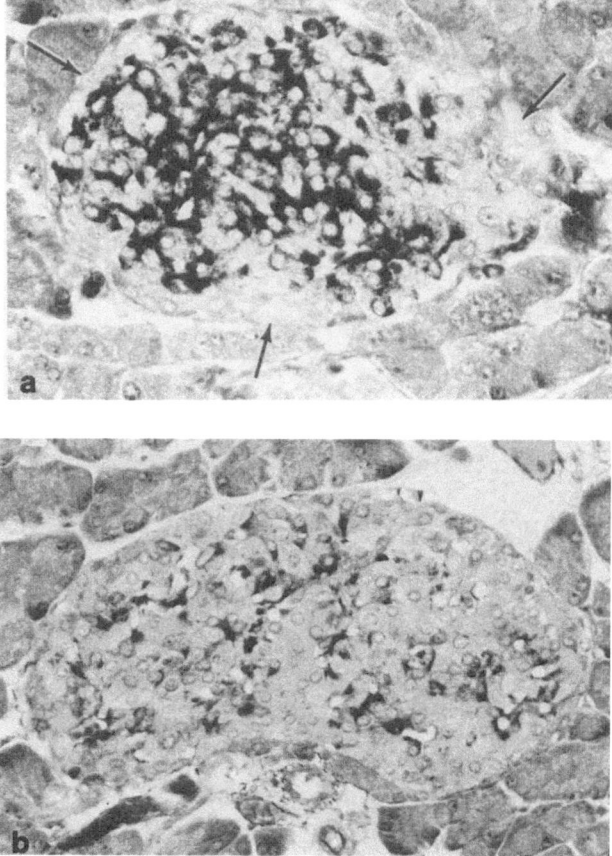

Figure 20. Pancreatic islets of Chinese hamster. (a) Normal hamster. The deeply staining, well-granulated β cells (black in photograph) are characteristic of animals with normal BG. Arrows indicate the peripheral α cells. Aldehyde fuchsin. ×380. (b) Hamster after spontaneous remission. BG normal and plasma IRI elevated. Islet is enlarged and composed of increased numbers of β cells, many of which are partially degranulated. Aldehyde fuchsin. ×288.

of variable severity have been described, including intermittent hyperglycemia (trace glycosuria), mild but persistent diabetes, moderately severe but nonketotic diabetes, and severe diabetic ketoacidosis. Recently, nonketotic diabetic hamsters undergoing spontaneous remission were reported.[36,37]

Pancreatic Islet Morphology. When one considers islet size and configuration, disposition of α and β cells, and the intensity of aldehyde fuchsin staining, the light- and electron-microscopic appearance of the islets of normal Chinese hamsters (Figs. 20a, 22, 23) cannot be distinguished from that of other nondiabetic rodents. Early after the onset of hyperglycemia, the islets are somewhat increased in size, contain partially degranulated β cells and increased numbers of

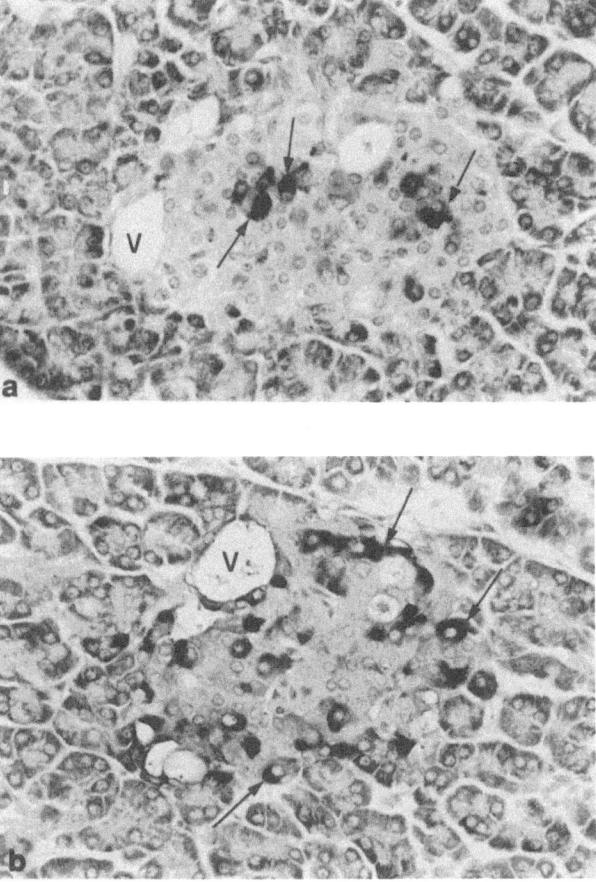

Figure 21. Islets of diabetic (ketotic) hamster after immunohistochemical identification of insulin and pancreatic glucagon by PAP technique. Islets are decreased in size and contain vacuolated, glycogen-filled β cells (V). (a) Insulin-containing β cells (arrows) are dramatically decreased in number and correlate well with pronounced hyperglycemia and decreased plasma IRI. ×300. (b) Glucagon-containing α cells (arrows) are numerous. ×300.

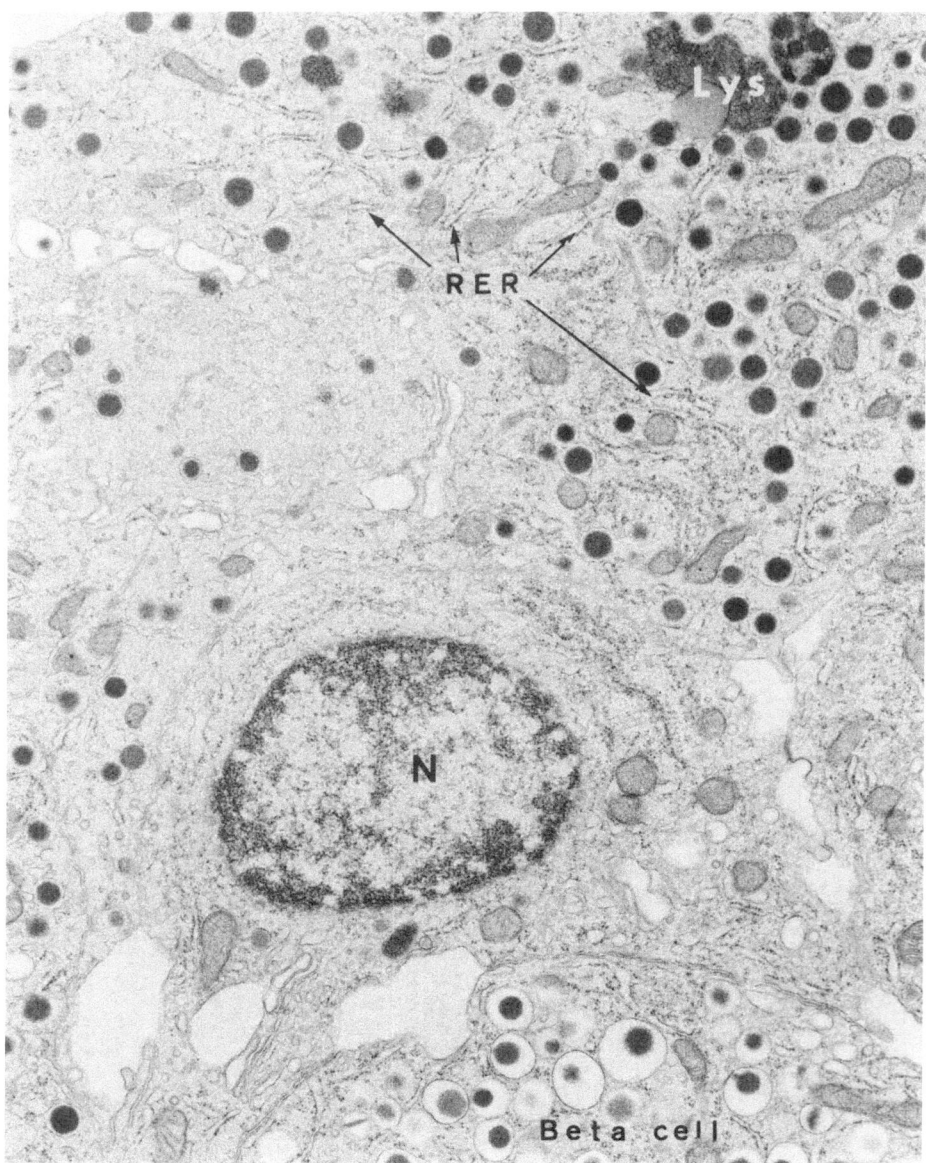

Figure 22. Peripheral portion of normal hamster islet. Several α cells and one β cell contain many secretory granules. The large lysosomal structure (Lys) is characteristic of hamster α cells. ×15,700.

cells synthesizing DNA in preparation for mitotic division. Plasma IRI is increased among Chinese hamsters with early-onset diabetes. With the progression of the diabetic syndrome, plasma IRI declines in the face of increasing or continued hyperglycemia, β cell numbers decrease, secretory degranulation is more pronounced, and cytoplasmic vacuolization due to glycogen storage is noteworthy (Fig. 21). The magnitude of the decrease in β cell numbers and in islet size is directly proportional to the severity of the diabetic syndrome and therefore is most pronounced among hamsters with ketoacidosis. It would appear that α cells are more numerous in animals with the ketotic diabetic syndrome (Fig. 21b). The pancreatic islets of diabetic hamsters that have experienced spontaneous remission are enlarged and contain increased numbers of pancreatic β cells (Fig. 20b).

Ultrastructurally, partial β cell degranulation in diabetic hamsters (Fig. 24) resembles that described in *ob/ob* and *db/db* mice. Furthermore, secretory degranulation is more pronounced in animals with greater elevations of BG (Figs. 25 and 27), and again it is not possible to differentiate among the intact β cells of the several diabetic rodents (Figs. 4, 12, and 25). All reveal an expanded rough endoplasmic reticulum, enlarged Golgi structures, secretory degranulation, and margination of the residual β granules. Unique among diabetic Chinese hamster islets, however, is the presence of necrotic β cells having a

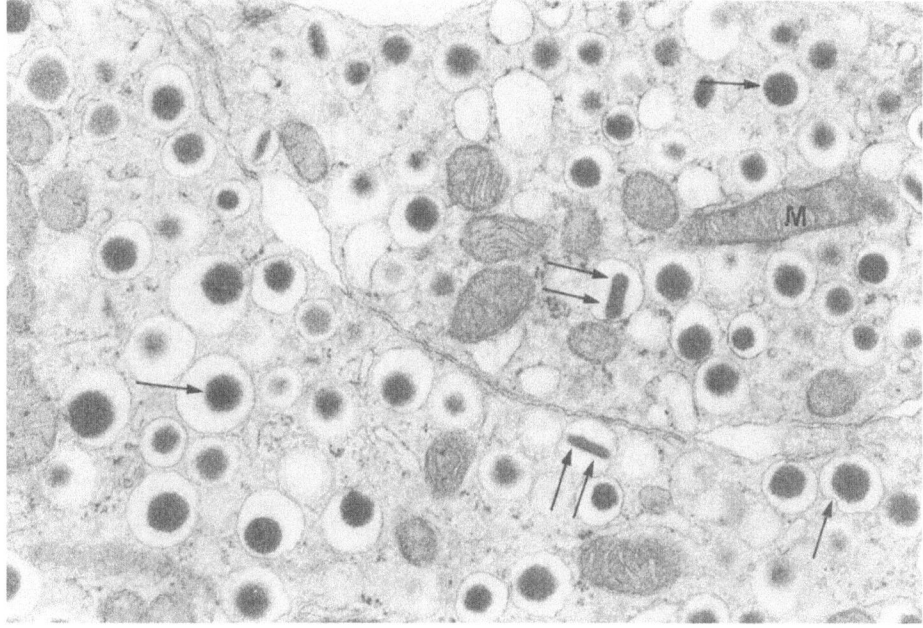

Figure 23. Normal hamster β cells under higher magnification, containing numerous characteristic spherical secretory granules (single arrows). Bar-shaped granules (double arrows) are found in β cells of many rodents. ×22,300.

characteristic ultrastructural configuration (Fig. 26). β cell cytoplasmic glycogen deposition is also a feature of the diabetic Chinese hamster islets and has been observed in the sand rat and spiny mouse (Table 2). α cells of normoglycemic and diabetic hamsters (Fig. 28) can be distinguished ultrastructurally from those of other laboratory animals. It has also been reported that the α cells of *ketotic* hamsters reveal lysosomal digestion of secretory granules, secretory degranulation, and dilated cisternae of the rough endoplasmic reticulum.[70] The islets of hamsters with diabetic syndromes of variable severity can be distinguished ultrastructurally from one another primarily by the frequency of β cell necrosis and the number of surviving β cells. These features most closely correlate with the degree of BG elevation and plasma IRI depression.

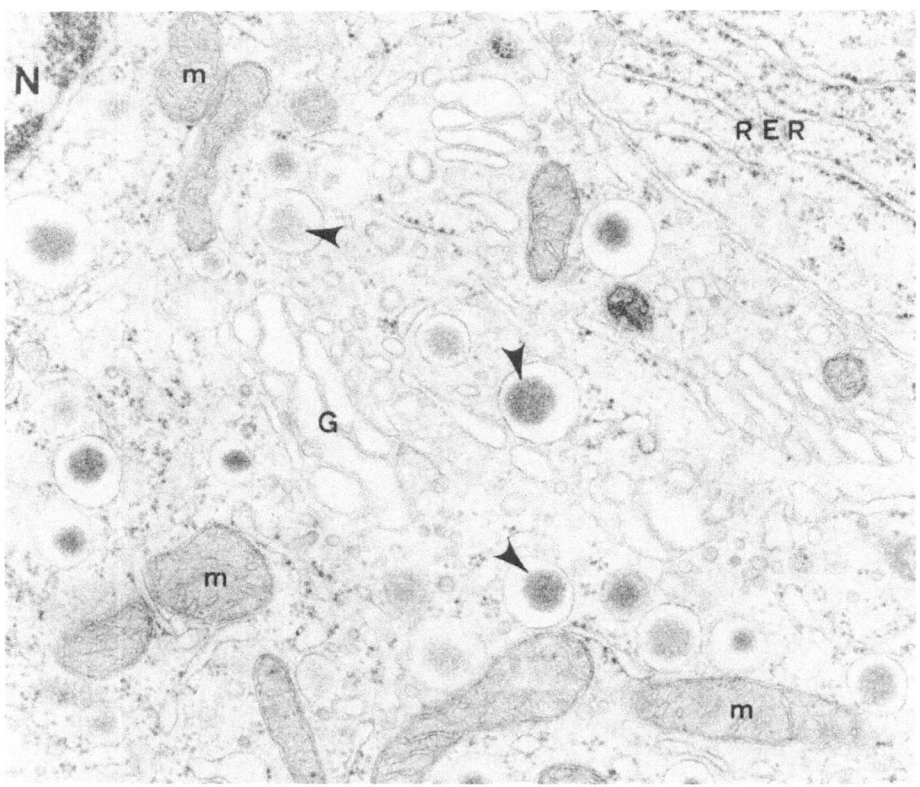

Figure 24. β cells of diabetic hamster. Secretory granule depletion is noteworthy, with remaining β granules (arrow heads) more variable in size and electron density than in normal hamsters (see Fig. 23). Rough endoplasmic reticulum (RER) and Golgi structures (G) are enlarged. ×25,500.

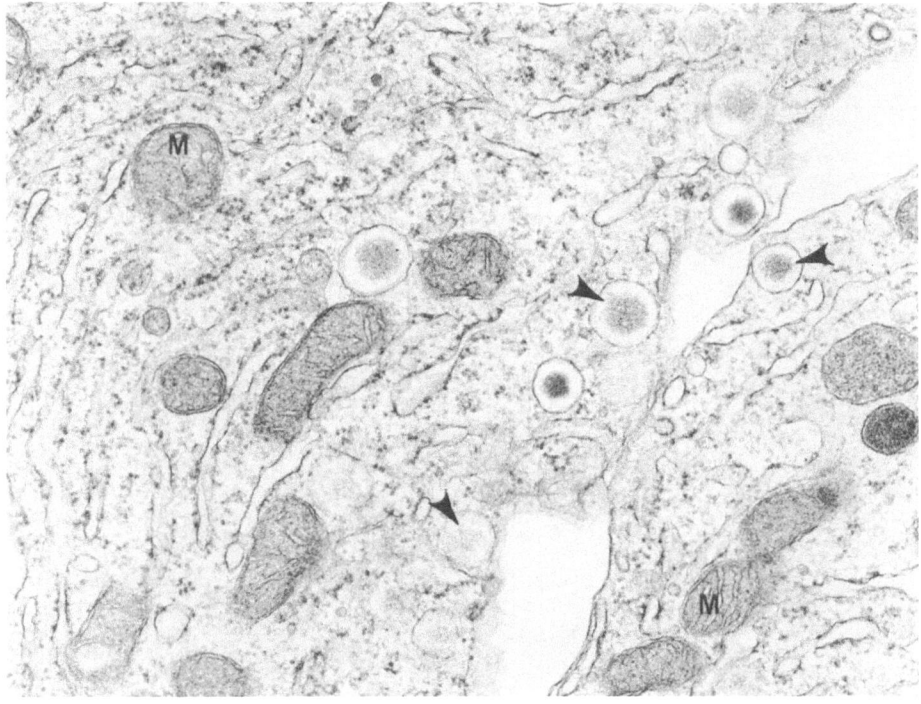

Figure 25. β cells of diabetic hamster. Secretory degranulation is prominent with margination of several of the remaining β granules (arrow heads) at the cell plasma membranes. ×33,000.

Bio Breeding Laboratory Rat

This most recently reported diabetic model was recognized in an outbred colony of Wistar rats by C. I. Chappel of the Bio Breeding Laboratories in Ottawa, Canada. It is characterized by early age of onset (48–120 days), variable degree of severity (hyperglycemia 250–730 mg/100 ml, hypoinsulinemia 0–1 ng/ml, hyperketonemia) and absence of obesity.[62,63,64] In the small number of animals studied, most have been moderately to severely ketotic and, if not treated with insulin, showed rapid weight loss, glycosuria, polyuria, dehydration, and death within 1–2 weeks. Animals with minimal ketonemia are stable and maintain their body weights, polyuria, and glycosuria for periods greater than 1 month. All rats reveal considerably reduced plasma and pancreatic IRI, elevated (relative or absolute) immunoreactive glucagon (IRG), and an exaggerated plasma IRG response to injected arginine.

Preliminary light-microscopic studies of pancreatic islets reveal a spectrum of lesions. Destructive inflammatory lesions are observed in a number of rats with mild elevation of BG (and, therefore, are possible examples of early-onset

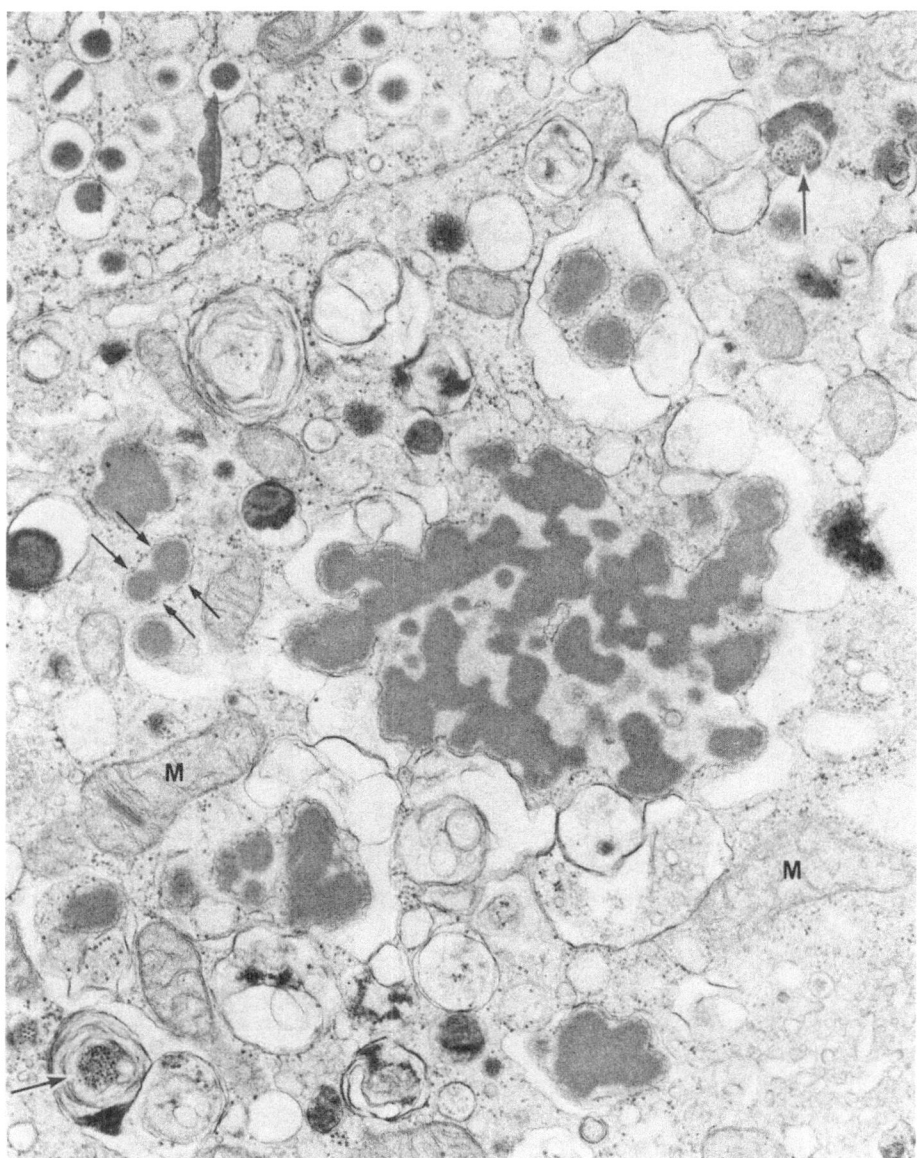

Figure 26. β cell of diabetic hamster with evidence of cytoplasmic degeneration. Varying sized aggregates of electron-dense material are present and frequently herald subsequent cell necrosis. Smaller aggregates of this material are clearly membrane enclosed (double arrows). Glycogen deposits (single arrows) are also visible. ×24,500. Reproduced at 90%.

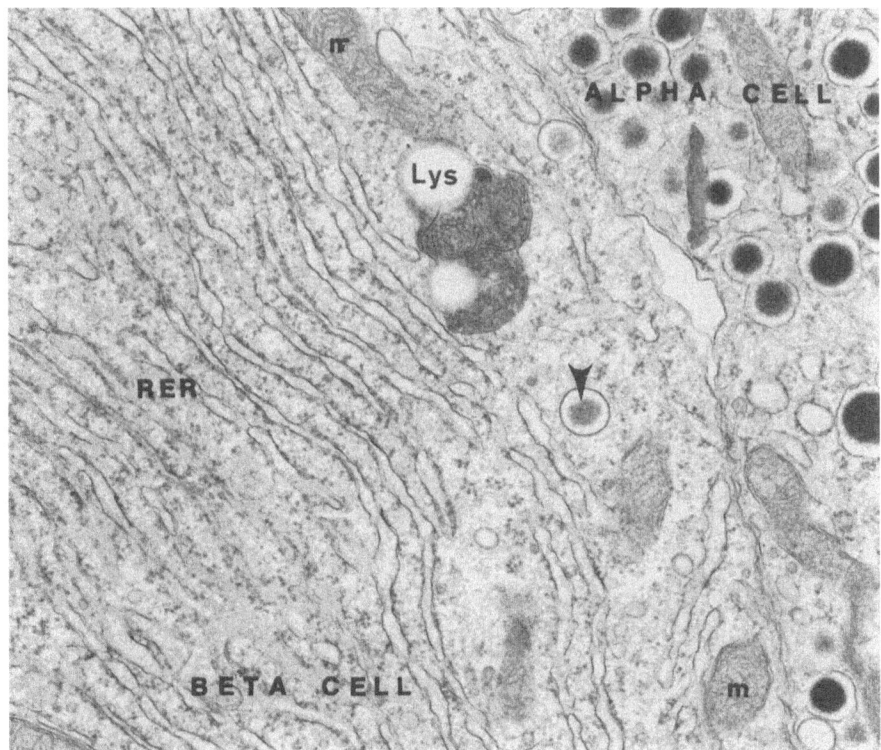

Figure 27. Diabetic hamster. Degranulated β cell and adjacent well-granulated α cell. Residual β granules are indicated (arrow heads), as is the expanded RER. Most α cells of diabetic hamsters cannot be distinguished from those of normal animals (see Figs. 22 and 28). Lys, lysosome. ×33,000.

disease) as well as in several normoglycemic littermates of animals with profound diabetic syndromes. These "early" lesions are characterized by an infiltration of mononuclear leukocytes within and around the islets, with the spreading apart and distortion of the cords or columns of endocrine cells (Figs. 29 and 30). The islets of rats succumbing after a fulminating syndrome, or of animals maintained with insulin replacement therapy are small, difficult to find in histologic sections, and composed virtually of non-β cells, with little or no evidence of inflammation (Fig. 31a). Although quantitative studies have not been reported, there is immunohistochemical evidence of abundant numbers of α cells within the inflamed and end-stage islets (Fig. 31b).

In spite of the fact that the number of animals investigated is small and the reported observations are very preliminary, this new model of spontaneous diabetes, without obesity, in which inflammatory islet lesions, β cell destruction, insulin deficiency, and ketoacidosis occur, is most reminiscent of the human juvenile-onset diabetic syndrome.[71] Inflammatory islet lesions have also been

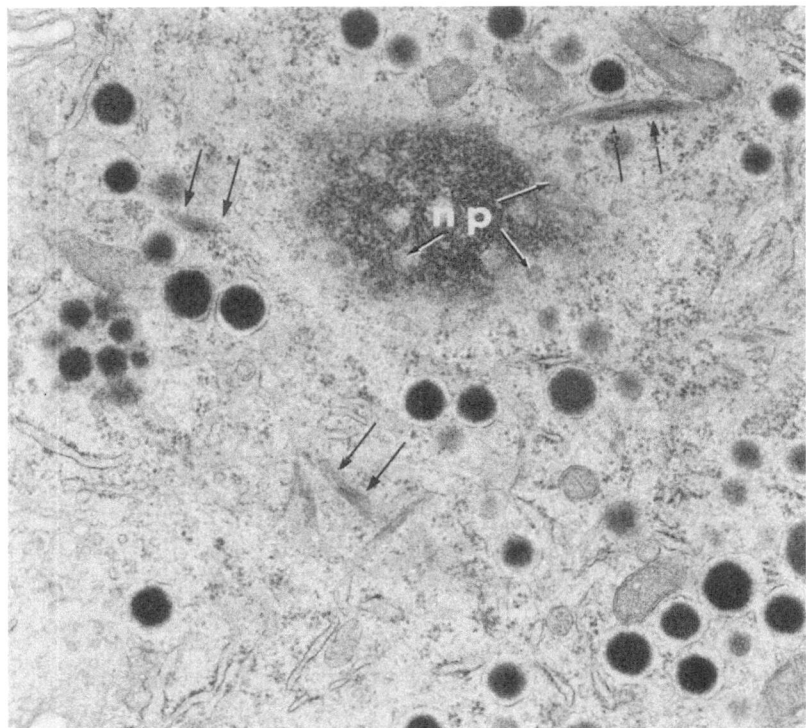

Figure 28. α cell from diabetic hamster. The perinuclear bundles of coarse microfilaments (paired arrows) are observed in both diabetic and nondiabetic animals. np, nuclear pores. ×27,600.

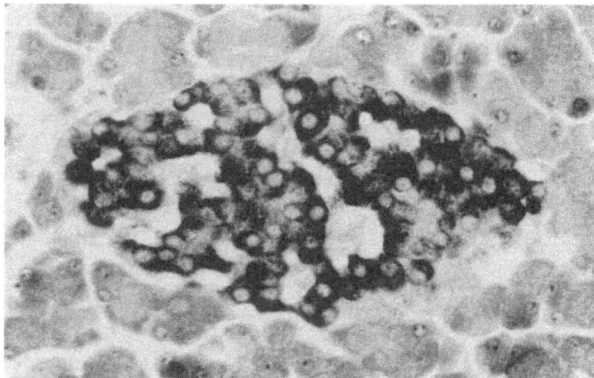

Figure 29. Pancreatic islet of normal Bio Breeding Laboratory (BBL) rat. There is no evidence of degranulation or of inflammation. Aldehyde fuchsin. ×300.

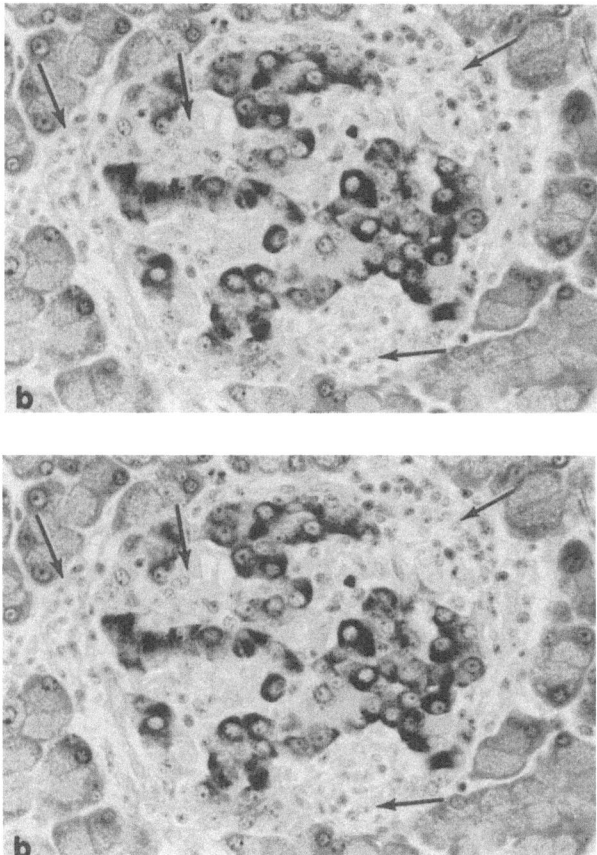

Figure 30. Pancreatic islets from BBL rat shortly after the onset of hyperglycemia. (a) Hematoxylin and eosin stained section demonstrating the mononuclear leukocytes (arrows) permeating and surrounding the pancreatic islet. ×192. (b) Aldehyde fuchsin stain. The usually compact cords of β cells are dispersed by the infiltrating inflammatory cells (arrows). Partial β cell degranulation is also present and correlates with the moderate hyperglycemia. ×300.

observed in experimental virus-induced diabetes,[72] after unsuccessful attempts to produce an immune-type diabetes,[73] and after multiple subdiabetogenic injections of streptozotocin.[74]

Concluding Remarks

It is the purpose of this chapter to: (1) survey, briefly, the major physiological and morphological characteristics of the most frequently studied laboratory

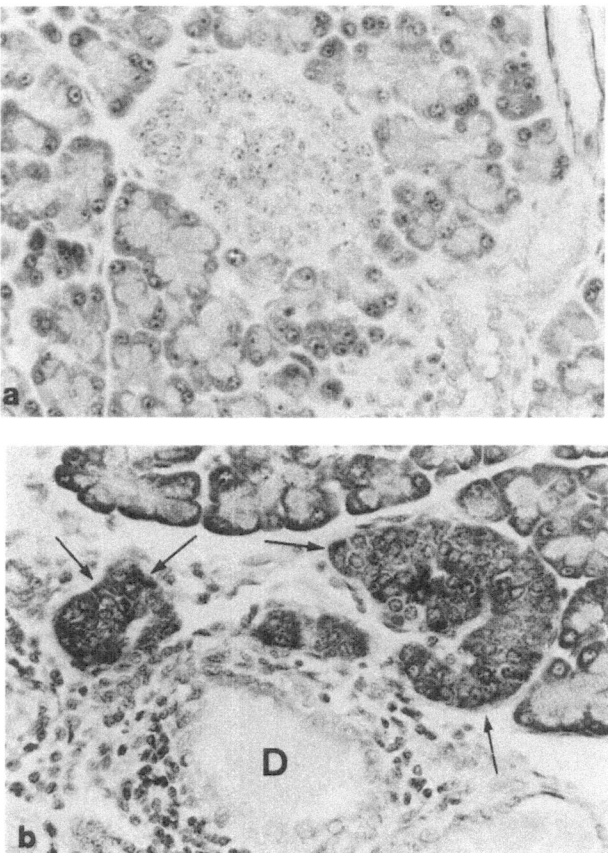

Figure 31. Pancreatic islets from BBL rat with advanced diabetes and ketoacidosis. (a) Very small islet consisting entirely of aldehyde fuchsin negative (presumably α and δ) cells. Residual inflammatory cells are infrequent (but see part b), and fibrosis is not observed. Aldehyde fuchsin. ×300. (b) Immunohistochemical stain for pancreatic glucagon, using the PAP technique, documents the presence of predominent α cells (arrows) within this small "end-stage" islet. Residual inflammatory cells surround the adjacent exocrine duct (D). ×300.

models of spontaneous diabetes; and (2) describe in detail the morphological features of the pancreatic islets of several of these animal models, selected to illustrate a conceptual approach to the pathogenetic evolution of these diabetic syndromes. According to the concept proposed, the severity of diabetes in each model studied is a function of the magnitude of insulin deficiency, which in turn (with the possible exception of the spiny "mouse") is directly related to the number of surviving and functioning β cells. Although the fundamental defect(s) which triggers the initiation of carbohydrate intolerance is still not known, there are no *morphologic data* to support the viewpoint that the primary event in these spontaneously diabetic rodents is an intrinsic β cell insensitivity to physiological secretory stimuli. On the contrary, it is difficult and probably not possible to differentiate morphologically between the *intact* β cells of the several lethal and nonlethal diabetic animals. In the presence of sustained hyperglycemia, all reveal ultrastructural evidence of enhanced protein synthesis and secretion. Although it is possible to identify ultrastructurally the degenerative and necrotic β cells of the *db/db* mouse, the Chinese hamster, and the sand rat, it would appear that it is the *fact* of necrosis, rather than the manner of cell destruction, that is of paramount importance to the outcome of the disease.

The morphologic and physiologic data presented are consistent with the conclusion that if β cell hyperplasia is sufficient to provide the physiologically necessary extra increment of IRI and/or to overcome a β cell loss brought about by known or unknown factors, then the supply of circulating IRI will be maintained, and a mild or nonlethal syndrome will occur. If, on the other hand, β cell numbers are reduced, and plasma IRI levels are significantly decreased, then insulin deficiency and a severe or lethal syndrome will be virtually inevitable.

Greater emphasis must therefore be directed towards the twin objectives of: (1) Deciphering the mechanism(s) for, and eventually the prevention of, β cell destruction; and (2) evaluating, and, in the future, manipulating, the factors (genetic and possibly environmental) which control β cell replication in the living organism.

Acknowledgments

This work was supported in part by an NIH PHS Research Grant AM-19155, and a grant from The Juvenile Diabetes Foundation.

The author is indebted to Ms. Claudia Berger, Ms. Serena Davis, and Ms. Paula Erlandson for expert and enthusiastic technical assistance; to Mr. Peter Healy for skillful photographic assistance; to Dr. M. C. Appel for invaluable instruction in the immunohistochemical techniques; to Dr. Roger Unger for the generous supply of antipancreatic glucagon antiserum; and to Dr. Peter Wright for the antiinsulin antiserum.

References

1. Ingalls, A. M., Dickie, M. M., and Snell, G. D.: *J. Hered.,* **41**:317, 1950.
2. Renold, A. E.: *Adv. Metab. Dis.,* **3**:49, 1968.
3. Stauffacher, W., Orci, L., Cameron, D. P., Burr, I. M., and Renold, A. E.: *Rec. Progr. Horm. Res.,* **27**:41, 1971.
4. Cameron, D. P., Stauffacher, W., and Renold, A. E.: In: Handbook of Physiology. Sec. 7, *Endocrinology.* Vol. 1, *Endocrine Pancreas.* Edited by R. O. Greep, E. B. Astwood, D. F. Steiner, N. Freinkel, and S. R. Geiger. Amer. Physiol. Soc., Washington, Chap. 39, 1972, p. 611.

5. First Brook Lodge Workshop on Spontaneous Diabetes in Laboratory Animals. *Diabetologia,* **3**:63, 1967.
6. Second Brook Lodge Workshop on Spontaneous Diabetes in Laboratory Animals. *Diabetologia,* **6**:12, 1970.
7. Third Brook Lodge Workshop on Spontaneous Diabetes in Laboratory Animals. *Diabetologia,* **10**:491, 1974.
8. Bleisch, V. R., Mayer, J., and Dickie, M. M.: *Amer. J. Pathol.,* **28**:369, 1952.
9. Wrenshall, G. A., Andrus, S. B., and Mayer, J.: *Endocrinology,* **56**:335, 1955.
10. Christophe, J., Dagenais, Y., and Mayer, J.: *Nature (London)* **184**:61, 1959.
11. Gepts, W., Christophe, J., and Mayer, J.: *Diabetes,* **9**:63, 1960.
12. Hellman, B., Brolin, S. E., Hellerström, C., and Hellman, K.: *Acta Endocrinol.,* **36**:609, 1961.
13. Solomon, J., and Mayer, J.: *Nature (London)* **193**:135, 1962.
14. Björkman, N., Hellerström, C., and Hellman, B.: *Z. Zellforsch.,* **58**:803, 1963.
15. Stauffacher, W., Crofford, O.B., Jeanrenaud, B. and Renold, A. E.: Ann. N.Y. Acad. Sci., **131**:528, 1965.
16. Stauffacher, W., Lambert, A. E., Vecchio, D., and Renold, A. E.: *Diabetologia,* **3**:230, 1967.
17. Westman, S.: *Acta Soc. Med. Upsal.,* **73**:81, 1968.
18. Mahler, R. J., Szabo, O., Adler, K., and Levine, R.: *Fed. Proc.,* **29**:380, 1970.
19. Mahler, R. J., and Szabo, O.: *Amer. J. Physiol.,* **221**:980, 1971.
20. Nakamura, M.: *Proc. Jap. Acad.,* **38**:348, 1962.
21. Nakamura, M., and Yamada, K.: *Diabetologia,* **3**:212, 1967.
22. Dulin, W. E., and Wyse, B. M.: *Diabetologia,* **6**:317, 1970.
23. Appel, M. C., Chang, A. Y., and Dulin, W. E.: *Diabetologia,* **10**:625, 1974.
24. Jones, E. E.: In: *Structure and Metabolism of the Pancreatic Islets.* Edited by S. E. Brolin, B. Hellman, and H. Knutson. Pergamon Press, Oxford, 1964, p. 189.
25. Like, A. A., Steinke, J., Jones, E. E., and Cahill, Jr., G. F.: *Amer. J. Pathol.* **46**:621, 1965.
26. Cahill, Jr., G. F., Jones, E. E., Lauris, V., Steinke, J., and Soeldner, J. S.: *Diabetologia,* **3**:171, 1967.
27. Gleason, R. E., Lauris, V., and Soeldner, J. S.: *Diabetologia,* **3**:175, 1967.
28. Meier, H., and Yerganian, G. A.: *Proc. Soc. Exp. Biol. Med.,* **100**:810, 1959.
29. Gerritsen, G. C., and Dulin, W. E.: *Diabetologia,* **3**:74, 1967.
30. Carpenter, A. M., Gerritsen, G. C., Dulin, W. E., and Lazarow, A.: *Diabetologia,* **3**:92, 1967.
31. Luse, S. A., Caramia, F., Gerritsen, G. C., and Dulin, W. E.: *Diabetologia,* **3**:97, 1967.
32. Butler, L.: *Diabetologia,* **3**:124, 1967.
33. Boquist, L.: *Acta Pathol. Microbiol. Scand.,* **75**:399, 1969.
34. Gerritsen, G. C., and Blanks, M. C.: *Diabetologia,* **6**:177, 1970.
35. Gerritsen, G. C., and Dulin, W. E.: *Acta Diabetol. Lat. (Suppl. I),* **9**:597, 1972.
36. Like, A. A., Gerritsen, G. C., Dulin, W. E., and Gaudreau, P.: *Diabetologia,* **10**:501, 1974.
37. Like, A. A., Gerritsen, G. C., Dulin, W. E., and Gaudreau, P.: *Diabetologia,* **10**:509, 1974.
38. Schmidt-Nielson, K., Haines, H. B., and Hackel, D. B.: *Science,* **143**:689, 1964.
39. Haines, H. B., Hackel, D. B., and Schmidt-Nielsen, K.: *Amer. J. Physiol.,* **208**:297, 1965.
40. Hackel, D. B., Schmidt-Nielsen, K., Haines, H. B., and Mikat, E.: *Lab. Invest.,* **14**:200, 1965.
41. Hackel, D. B., Frohman, L., Mikat, E., Lebovitz, H. E., Schmidt-Nielson, K., and Kinney, T. D.: *Diabetes,* **15**:105, 1966.
42. Miki, E., Like, A. A., Steinke, J., and Soeldner, J. S.: *Diabetologia,* **3**:135, 1967.
43. Like, A. A., and Miki, E.: *Diabetologia,* **3**:143, 1967.
44. Malaisse, W. J., Like, A. A., Malaisse-Lagae, F., Gleason, R. E., and Soeldner, J. S.: *Diabetes,* **17**:752, 1967.
45. Miki, E., Like, A. A., Soeldner, J. S., Steinke, J., and Cahill, Jr., G. F.: *Metabolism,* **15**:749, 1966.
46. Gonet, A. E., Stauffacher, W., Pictet, R., and Renold, A. E.: *Diabetologia,* **1**:162, 1965.
47. Stauffacher, W., Orci, L., Amherdt, M., Burr, I. M., Balant, L., Froesch, E. R., and Renold, A. E.: *Diabetologia,* **6**:330, 1970.
48. Cameron, D. P., Stauffacher, W., Orci, L., Amherdt, M., and Renold, A. E.: *Diabetes,* **21**:1060, 1972.

49. Malaisse-Lagae, F., Ravazzola, M., Amherdt, M., Gutzeit, A., Malaisse, W. J., and Orci, L.: *Diabetologia*, **11**:71, 1975.
50. Hummel, K. P., Dickie, M. M., and Coleman, D. L.: *Science*, **153**:1127, 1966.
51. Coleman, D. L., and Hummel, K. P.: *Diabetologia*, **3**:238, 1967.
52. Chick, W. L., and Like, A. A.: *Diabetologia*, **6**:243, 1970.
53. Coleman, D. L., and Hummel, K. P.: *Diabetologia*, **10**:607, 1974.
54. Like, A. A., and Chick, W. L.: *Science*, **163**:941, 1969.
55. Like, A. A., and Chick, W. L.: *Diabetologia*, **6**:207, 1970.
56. Like, A. A., and Chick, W. L.: *Diabetologia*, **6**:216, 1970.
57. Coleman, D. L., and Hummel, K. P.: *Amer. J. Physiol.*, **217**:1298, 1969.
58. Coleman, D. L.: *Diabetologia*, **9**:294, 1973.
59. Chick, W. L., and Like, A. A.: *Diabetologia*, **6**:252, 1970.
60. Hummel, K. P., Coleman, D. L., and Lane, P. W.: *Biochem. Genet.*, **7**:1, 1972.
61. Coleman, D. L., and Hummel, K. P.: *Diabetologia*, **9**:287, 1973.
62. Nakhooda, A. F., Like, A. A., Chappel, C. I., and Marliss, E. B.: *Clin. Res.*, **23**:638A, 1975.
63. Nakhooda, A. F., Like, A. A., Chappel, C. I., and Marliss, E. B.: *Diabetes (Suppl. 1)* **25**:378, 1976.
64. Nakhooda, A. F., Like, A. A., Chappel, C. I., Murray, F. T., and Marliss, E. B.: *Diabetes*, **26**:100, 1977.
65. Baetens, D., Coleman, D. L., and Orci, L.: *Diabetes (Suppl. 1)*, **25**:344, 1976.
66. Kahn, C. R., Neville, Jr., D. M., Gorden, P., Freychet, P. and Roth, J.: *Biochem. Biophys. Res. Commun.*, **48**:135, 1972.
67. DeMeyts, P., Roth, J., Neville, D. M., Jr., Gavin, J. R., III, and Lesniak, M.A.: *Biochem. Biophys. Commun.*, **55**:154, 1973.
68. Freychet, P., Laudat, M. H., Laudat, P., Rosselin, G., Kahn, C. R., Gorden, P., and Roth, J.: *FEBS Lett.*, **25**:339, 1972.
69. Staats, J.: *Diabetologia*, **11**:325, 1975.
70. Orci, L., Stauffacher, W., Dulin, W. E., Renold, A. E., and Rouiller, C.: *Diabetologia*, **6**:199, 1970.
71. Gepts, W.: *Diabetes*, **14**:619, 1965.
72. Craighead, J. E., and McLane, M. F.: *Science*, **162**:913, 1968.
73. Klöppel, G., Altenähr, E., and Freychet, P.: *Virchows Arch. Path. Anat.*, **356**:15, 1972.
74. Like, A. A., and Rossini, A. A.: *Science*, **193**:415, 1976.

Chapter 18

Chemically and Hormonally Induced Diabetes

W. E. Dulin and M. G. Soret

Any discussion concerning diabetogenic chemicals and hormones is immediately confronted with a need for a working definition of "diabetogenic." Since the definition of diabetes is confusing and not generally agreed upon by most researchers in the field, in this discussion we will define a diabetogenic agent as any which will cause "any temporary or permanent decrease in glucose metabolism, regardless of mechanism, which results either in an abnormal glucose tolerance or fasting hyperglycemia with or without glucosuria." It is recognized that this is a debatable definition, but the authors feel that it will suffice for this discussion.

One of the problems with a subject of this scope is that it becomes evident that considerable species differences exist in response to these agents, and this may cloud the entire issue. Consequently, we will consider a compound diabetogenic, even though it may be limited to a few or even to one species. Even with those compounds which are considered to be diabetogenic by most researchers, one finds some species that do not respond in a classical manner.

There are several recent reviews on this subject of chemically and hormonally induced diabetes[1-6] which cover the subject extensively. Therefore, we will attempt to restrict this discussion to the points the present authors consider most important. We will separate the presentation into a discussion of chemically induced and hormonally induced diabetes, even though it is recognized that hormones are chemicals.

Chemical Diabetogenic Agents

Introduction

The diabetogenic chemicals which are described can be separated into two general classes: those which produce a permanent diabetes by destruction of the β cells and with a result in insulin deficiency (streptozotocin, alloxan,

---

W. E. Dulin and M. G. Soret • The Upjohn Company, Kalamazoo, Michigan.

quinolines, and dithizone), and those which do not irreversibly destroy the β cells but which may cause a temporary decrease in available insulin and/or induce secondary effects which counteract the insulin actions (cyproheptadine, benzothiodiazines and closely related compounds, and asparaginase).

Streptozotocin

The diabetogenic property of streptozotocin was first reported in 1963.[7] Since this first report on streptozotocin several hundred publications have appeared. An extensive review covering essentially all the historical background was published in 1972.[8] An extensive review has also been published on the comparison of alloxan and streptozotocin.[9]

Streptozotocin was first reported as an antibacterial agent in 1959.[10,11] It was later found to exhibit also an inhibitory action on the growth of certain tumors[12] and an *in vitro* effect on cultured cells.[13] Streptozotocin was obtained from fermentation cultures of *Streptomyces achromogenes*,[14] but it has now been synthesized.[15,16] Synthetic streptozotocin has been shown to possess the same spectrum of biological activity as that produced by the fermentation product. The structure of streptozotocin has been determined[17] and its chemical name is 2-deoxy-2-(3-methyl-3-nitrosourea)1-*d*-glucopyranose ($\alpha + \beta$) (Fig. 1). It is commonly referred to as the *N*-nitroso-*N*-methylurea or 1-nitroso-1-methylurea derivative of 2-deoxyglucose.

Although considerable research has been reported on the mechanism of the antitumoral, tumorogenic, and antibacterial actions of streptozotocin,[8] this discussion will be confined to its effects on the α and β cells of the pancreas and its relationship to diabetes.

The chemical specificity of the diabetogenic effect of streptozotocin has received little attention; however, some analogs have been made but were found to be ineffective in producing diabetes.[18] Only one closely related compound has shown diabetogenic activity, and this was the ethyl urea derivative.[19] The *N*-nitroso-*N*-methylurea portion of the molecule exhibits diabetogenic activity when given at relatively high doses, and it produces the same direct effect on the islets as streptozotocin.[20,21]

Streptozotocin is diabetogenic in the rat,[7,12,22,23] dog,[7,24,25] monkey,[25-28] lamb,[29] Chinese hamster,[20,30-34,39] and normal mice.[19,21,35,36] An effect on the

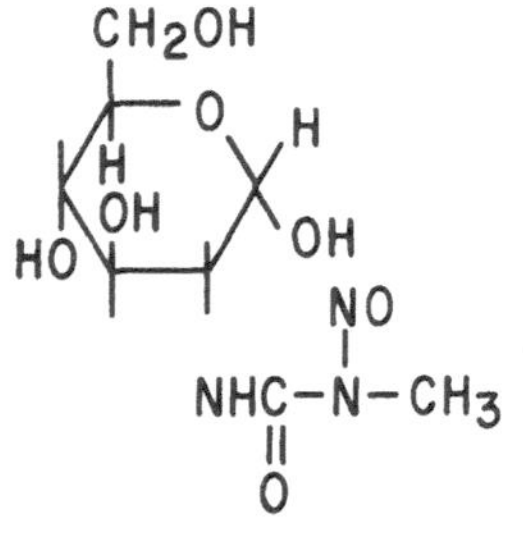

Figure 1. Structure of streptozotocin.

pancreatic β cells and induction of diabetes have been observed in the guinea pig[37] and rabbit,[32] but diabetes is produced with difficulty in these species.[38-41] Permanent diabetes is more easily produced in the guinea pig if drug injection is preceded by insulin-induced hypoglycemia.[40] Streptozotocin did not induce damage to the β cells in fish[42] (as evidenced by morphology of β cells, but with no blood sugar values), chicken,[43,44] cat,[45] diabetic KK mouse,[46] or diabetic spiny mice.[47] It should be pointed out that in the case of the chicken, diabetes might not be expected to appear with the destruction of β cells, since pancreatectomy has been shown to induce hypoglycemia rather than hyperglycemia in this species.[48] Studies in the *ob/ob* obese diabetic mouse have shown that there is no increase in the diabetic state when this mouse is treated with streptozotocin, although it will produce destruction of β cells, as evidenced by morphology and a decrease in pancreatic insulin.[49] However, it should be emphasized that in this particular animal, decreased plasma insulin may increase sensitivity to insulin and therefore improve the diabetic state.[49] In a very limited study with two animals, streptozotocin was shown to produce diabetes at 60 mg/kg in one miniature pig, but not in a second animal at a 40 mg/kg dose.[51]

A permanent or a relatively permanent hyperglycemia with streptozotocin generally occurs after approximately 24 hr; however, the overall response of streptozotocin is a triphasic one.[22,23,52] The triphasic blood sugar response after streptozotocin is characterized by initial hyperglycemia occurring 1–2 hr after the injection, followed by hypoglycemia from 6–12 hr and by permanent hyperglycemia at approximately 24 hr. The initial hyperglycemia is not associated with an increase in plasma insulin at 1 hr, even though blood sugar levels are increased.[22] There does not appear to be any decrease in tissue sensitivity to insulin.[53] Since there is no change in plasma insulin even though there is hyperglycemia, it is suggested that streptozotocin might inhibit insulin release. This has been shown to occur by studying insulin release from islets removed 60 min following streptozotocin injection[54] or by incubating islets for 60 and 120 min *in vitro* with streptozotocin.[55] These observations suggest that at least part of the early hyperglycemic response to streptozotocin may be a result of inhibition of insulin release.

The hypoglycemic phase is apparently due primarily to increased plasma insulin. It has been observed by several investigators in several species that there is a marked increase in plasma insulin during this phase,[22,23,52] but no decrease in pancreatic insulin.[22,23,52,56] The fact that the pancreatic insulin is not significantly decreased might be interpreted to mean that insulin synthesis can keep pace with release or that a slight decrease in the pancreatic insulin may be quantitatively sufficient to cause hyperinsulinemia without a significant change. The hyperglycemic phase which occurs by 24 hr results from a deficiency of insulin, since both the plasma and pancreatic insulin are markedly reduced at this time.[22,23,56]

It is generally accepted that the pancreatic effects of streptozotocin are primarily on the β cells, since morphological changes in the β cells have been extensively demonstrated. However, there have been some reports of toxic effects of streptozotocin on the α-2 cells, but this has been minimal and not correlated with measurement of glucagon.[20,34] It is of considerable interest that in the Chinese hamster streptozotocin is also toxic to the α cells as well as to the β cells.[41,77,78] These observations on α cell damage have been extended in our laboratories and reported below. Correlated with morphologically demonstrated damage to the α cell is a measurable decrease in glucagon content of the pancreas (Table 1). This decrease in glucagon is partially compensated for in the Chinese hamster by an increase in stomach glucagon levels (Table 1). The lower level of glucagon may account for the only moderately severe diabetes which results with streptozotocin in the Chinese hamster.

The observations that nicotinamide inhibited the diabetogenic activity of streptozotocin[57] as well as reversed its effect when given as long as 2 hr after streptozotocin injection[53] suggest that streptozotocin may act by decreasing β cell NAD levels. The earlier finding that nicotinic acid and nicotinamide inhibited the diabetogenic action of alloxan suggested that this might also occur with streptozotocin.[58] To substantiate the hypothesis that streptozotocin may be acting on the β cell by decreasing NAD content of the islets, NAD levels were determined in islets of streptozotocin-treated animals and found to be markedly decreased.[21,59–62] This decreased NAD level in the islets of streptozotocin-treated animals could be prevented by administration of nicotinamide.[60–62]

The mechanism by which streptozotocin decreases NAD levels of β cells may be by decreasing uptake of precursors and/or decreasing synthesis as well as increasing breakdown of preformed NAD. Evidence exists to indicate that all these mechanisms may be altered by streptozotocin. Decreased uptake of nicotinamide in islets and in the liver has been observed with streptozotocin.[60,63] It has also been found that streptozotocin treatment results in decreased NAD synthesis[60,63] and an increased breakdown of NAD.[61–63] NAD has been shown to be reduced to as little as 10% of normal by 2 hr following streptozotocin.[61]

The glucose portion of streptozotocin is not an absolute requirement for the diabetogenicity of this compound, since the N-nitroso-N-methylurea alone can produce β cell damage and diabetes as well as decrease islet NAD levels[20,21]; however, larger doses are required than for streptozotocin. It has been speculated that glucose may act as a carrier for the N-nitroso-N-methylurea portion, which is the cytotoxic agent. The observation that uptake of streptozotocin in β cells was 3.8 times that of N-nitroso-N-methylurea would support this hypothesis.[62]

Streptozotocin exists as an approximate 50–50 mixture of the α and β anomers at equilibrium.[64] Since it has been shown that the α anomer of glucose is a more effective stimulator of insulin secretion than the β anomer,[65,66] as well as a better protector of β cells against alloxan toxicity,[67] the specificity for toxicity of streptozotocin on β cells might be more related to the α anomer of the glucose moiety. Data were obtained on the relative diabetogenic activity of predominantly α or β anomers of streptozotocin in rats. It was found that a preparation of 90% α and 10% β streptozotocin was more potent as a diabetogenic agent than a preparation of 75% β and 25% α (Table 2).

A study of the inhibitors of streptozotocin diabetes is of great interest, since it may aid in defining some of its mechanism of action. As described above,

Table 1. *Plasma, Pancreatic, and Stomach Glucagon, and Plasma and Pancreatic Insulin of Chinese Hamsters at Various Times after Treatment with Streptozotocin (175 mg/kg i.p.)*

Treatment	Number	Time after treatment	Blood sugar (mg/100 ml)	Insulin		Glucagon		
				Plasma (µU/ml)	Pancreatic (U/ml)	Plasma (pg/ml)	Pancreatic (µg/g)	Stomach (ng/g)
Saline	6	3 hr	82 ± 4	74 ± 12	0.9 ± 0.1	23 ± 8	1.5 ± 0.2	4.0 ± 0.6
Streptozotocin	6	3 hr	129 ± 30	28 ± 9	0.8 ± 0.1	5 ± 3	1.3 ± 0.2	3.5 ± 0.4
Saline	6	6 hr	104 ± 5	105 ± 24	0.8 ± 0.1	20 ± 13	1.9 ± 0.2	4.3 ± 0.6
Streptozotocin	3	6 hr	293 ± 31	23 ± 19	0.7 ± 0.1	967 ± 536	1.8 ± 0.2	3.3 ± 0.7
Saline	6	6 hr	125 ± 6	55 ± 14	—	7.5 ± 5	—	—
Streptozotocin	6	6 hr	272 ± 43	27 ± 9	—	253 ± 38	—	—
Saline	5	12 hr	99 ± 3	67 ± 24	1.0 ± 0.1	3.4 ± 0.2	3.2 ± 0.6	11 ± 5
Streptozotocin	5	12 hr	322 ± 20	0	0.8 ± 0.1	47.8 ± 32	1.3 ± 0.3	10 ± 2
Saline	4	24 hr	91 ± 5	43 ± 26	1.0 ± 0.2	3.5 ± 1	2.6 ± 0.4	7.8 ± 3
Streptozotocin	4	24 hr	329 ± 39	0	0.02 ± 0.01	0.5 ± 0.5	0.05 ± 0.03	2.2 ± 0.2
Saline	5	2.5 weeks	91 ± 3	90 ± 14	1.4 ± 0.1	2.6 ± 2	2.7 ± 0.6	8.4 ± 3
Streptozotocin	5	2.5 weeks	369 ± 55	0	0.03 ± 0.02	26 ± 17	0.02 ± 0	62 ± 33
Saline	6	6 weeks	105 ± 3	110 ± 21	1.5 ± 0.1	0.3 ± 0.3	2.8 ± 0.4	6.7 ± 1
Streptozotocin	5	6 weeks	330 ± 11	0	0.02 ± 0	39 ± 19	0.3 ± 0.1	28 ± 7

Table 2. Comparative Diabetogenic Effects of Predominantly α or β Streptozotocin Anomers

Treatment	Anomer (%)	Number	Dose (mg/kg)	Blood sugar[a] (mg/100 ml)
Saline	—	5	—	108 ± 3.7
Streptozotocin	75 (β)[b]	5	40	121 ± 3.7
Streptozotocin	75 (β)	5	50	133 ± 9
Streptozotocin	90 (α)[c]	5	40	123 ± 3.7
Streptozotocin	90 (α)	5	50	244 ± 40
Saline	—	5	—	87 ± 1.2
Streptozotocin	75 (β)	5	50	144 ± 38
Streptozotocin	75 (β)	5	65	299 ± 15.4
Streptozotocin	90 (α)	5	50	281 ± 47
Streptozotocin	90 (α)	5	65	329 ± 20

[a]Nonfasting blood sugar 1 week after treatment.
[b]Lot No. 9681-GGS-118FI.
[c]Lot No. 11676-RCH-112.

nicotinamide but not nicotinic acid will inhibit the diabetogenic activity of streptozotocin.[53,57,75] Pyrazinamide, diphenylhydantoin and 2-deoxy-glucose have also been shown to inhibit the induction of diabetes with streptozotocin.[53,72,73] Glucose,[53] epinephrine,[53,73] NAD,[53] glucosamine,[53] glutamic acid, asparagine, cystein, tolbutamide, guanidoacetic acid, glutamic acid, glycine, glutathione, p-amino benzoic acid, and ethyl alcohol did not block streptozotocin diabetes.[53] Diazoxide was reported inactive by one investigator[53] but effective in blocking streptozotocin by another.[74]

One interesting aspect of the action of streptozotocin on the destruction of β cells is its potential for elimination of insulin-secreting tumors, which provides streptozotocin with a clinical utility. It has been found that many patients with untreatable hypoglycemia will respond favorably to streptozotocin treatment.[68–71] It is of considerable interest that none of these patients exhibit diabetes after extensive therapy with streptozotocin, which would suggest that the normal human β cell may be relatively resistant to this drug. It has been reported that only in one case has a reversible glucose intolerance occurred following streptozotocin treatment.[70]

Extensive studies have been done on the morphological changes caused by streptozotocin. The earliest pathologic changes of the β cell following streptozotocin treatment were observed at 1 hr in rats[22] and guinea pigs.[76] The changes were minimal and involved some hypertrophy of the Golgi apparatus in guinea pigs and occasional nuclear pyknosis in mice.

Earliest evidence of β cell damage in rabbits was found 2 hr after injection of streptozotocin. Electron microscopy of β cells showed some margination of nuclear chromatin, decrease of interchromatinic material, and compact nucleoli.[41] The capillary poles of some β cells showed cytoplasmic electron-lucent areas which contained ribosomes, vesicles, and ergastoplasmic strands.

Mitochondria were swollen, and the endoplasmic reticulum (ER) was often prominent in these cells.

At 3 hr after treatment of animals with streptozotocin, most β cells in guinea pigs showed vesiculation of the ER.[76] β cell pyknosis has been observed in Chinese hamsters 3 hr posttreatment.[34] Chromatin clumping and rarefaction of the interchromatinic material was marked in rabbits at 3 hr. Pyknotic nuclei devoid of nucleoli, swollen mitochondria, and irregularly distended ER cisternae were also observed.[41,77]

At 4.5 hr the distention of the ER was very pronounced in guinea pigs.[76] Rupture of β cell plasma membrane and loss of granules were also found at this time. By 6 hr the destruction of the ER was almost complete. Of interest was that storage granules, mitochondria, and nuclei remained intact at this time in guinea pigs.[76] β cell necrosis was observed in the Chinese hamster at 6 hr.[34]

By 18 hr after streptozotocin injection, the β cells were disintegrating, nuclear pyknosis was common, and almost complete loss of granules occurred in rabbits.[41,77] By 24 hr in most species the β cell destruction is essentially complete.[78]

There is little morphological change in the β cells of resistant species, such as the cod[42] and chicken.[43] Streptozotocin causes irreversible changes to the β cells of the islet of Langerhans, but the effect on α and D cells appears to be variable.

In most species the α and D cells are not significantly affected by streptozotocin. However, in the Chinese hamster, α and D cells may be destroyed.[78] In the rabbit, some α cells were affected and showed the early nuclear chromatin clumping and interchromatinic rarefaction, but the α cell secretory granules were intact, and D cells were unaffected.[41,77]

Long-term observations have shown a decrease in the number and size of islets in streptozotocin-treated animals. These islets were characterized by infrequent β cells and a large number of α cells.[24,25,37,40,49,79]

We have extended earlier observations on the effects of streptozotocin on the islet cells of the Chinese hamster. One hour after the intraperitoneal administration of 175 mg/kg of streptozotocin, many islet β cells showed some chromatin clumping and rarefaction of the interchromatinic substance (Fig. 2) as compared to islets from controls (Fig. 3). The cytoplasmic matrix of these cells appeared to be disintegrating, although all mitochondria, some secretory granules, and a few rough endoplasmic reticulum (RER) sacs were intact. α and D cells were difficult to locate 1 hr after treatment (Fig. 4), although these cells were easily found in all control islets.

At 3 hr, most islet cells were severely affected as described by earlier reports[41,47] in the rabbit and in the Chinese hamster.[34] Differentiation between α and β cells was generally difficult, although in some fields α cells (Fig. 5) and D cells (Fig. 6) were still identifiable. The damaging effects of streptozotocin was equally evident in all islet cell types. In most cells, the granular sacs were greatly distended (Figs. 7 and 8), the ER was distended (Figs. 6 and 8) or practically absent (Fig. 9), and nuclear pyknosis was well advanced (Figs. 5, 7,

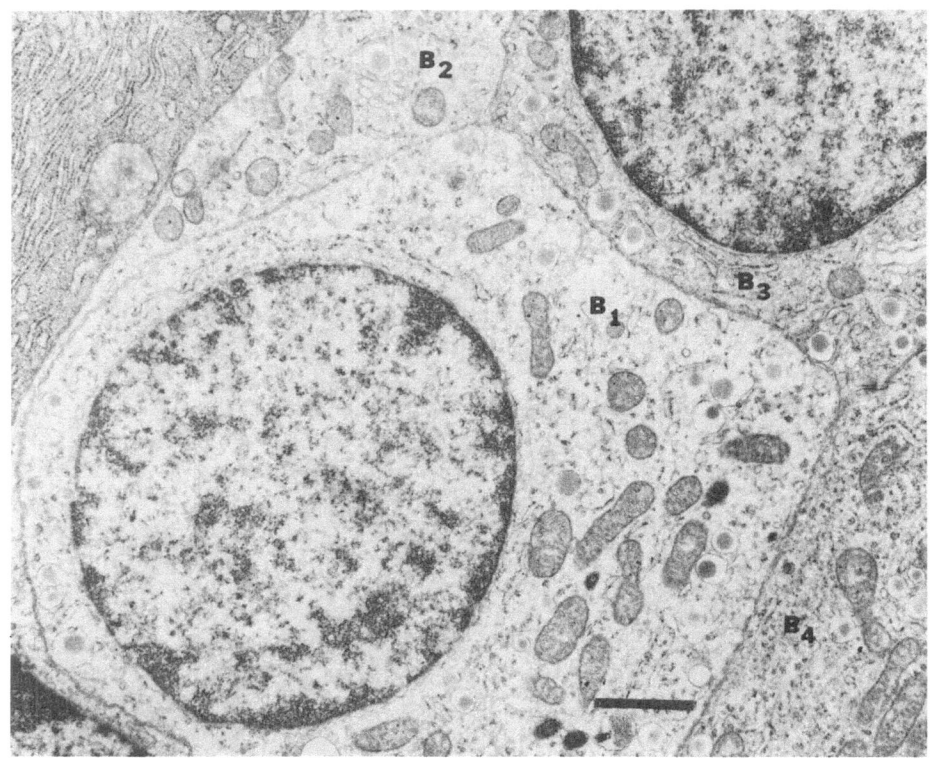

Figure 2. Pancreatic islet from a Chinese hamster 1 hr after intraperitoneal administration of streptozotocin. Two β cells (B_1 and B_2) show disintegration of the cytoplasmic matrix. The nucleus of B_1 shows some chromatin clumping, while the interchromatinic substance appears slightly rarefied. Other β cells (B_3 and B_4) are not visibly affected. Bar = 1 μm.

and 8). Mitochondrial changes varied from cell to cell. In some instances, they appeared swollen, while in adjacent cells they were rather compact (Fig. 8). Some cells presented a structureless cytoplasm in which a few granules and distended RER sacs could be observed (Fig. 9); other cells were still rich in organelles in the presence of heavily pyknotic nuclei (Fig. 8).

Damage to α cells was clearly demonstrable by the 6th hr posttreatment (Fig. 10). The most remarkable alteration was the dilation of the ER cicternae, including the formation of large vesicles from the nuclear sac. There was no change in pancreatic insulin or glucagon at this time (Table 1).

Total disintegration of the islet occurred by 24 hr. Only a few secretory granules and lysosomes could be recognized (Fig. 11). Islets from pancreases of three streptozotocin-treated Chinese hamsters were difficult to locate at this time. It should be emphasized that in the same area of pancreases of untreated animals, islets were easily and consistently found. The extensive morphological damage and extremely low insulin and glucagon levels in the pancreas (Table 1) shows that the islet destruction at 24 hr in these animals was complete. The small amount of plasma glucagon could arise from the stomach (Table 1).

Six weeks after streptozotocin treatment, five hamsters exhibited blood sugar levels ranging from 300 to 367 mg/100 ml. Only one islet was found after extensive search in each of two of these hamsters, and these were small and cell types were not easily identifiable (Fig. 12). Of the five cells observed in one of these islets, one was clearly a β cell, two were clearly D cells, and two were probably β cells as suggested by cytoplasmic glycogen deposition. These morphological findings are correlated with the extremely low levels of glucagon and insulin in the pancreas at this stage (Table 1). These observations indicate that streptozotocin destroys essentially all islet cells in the Chinese hamsters. It should also, however, be pointed out, that whereas plasma insulin was not

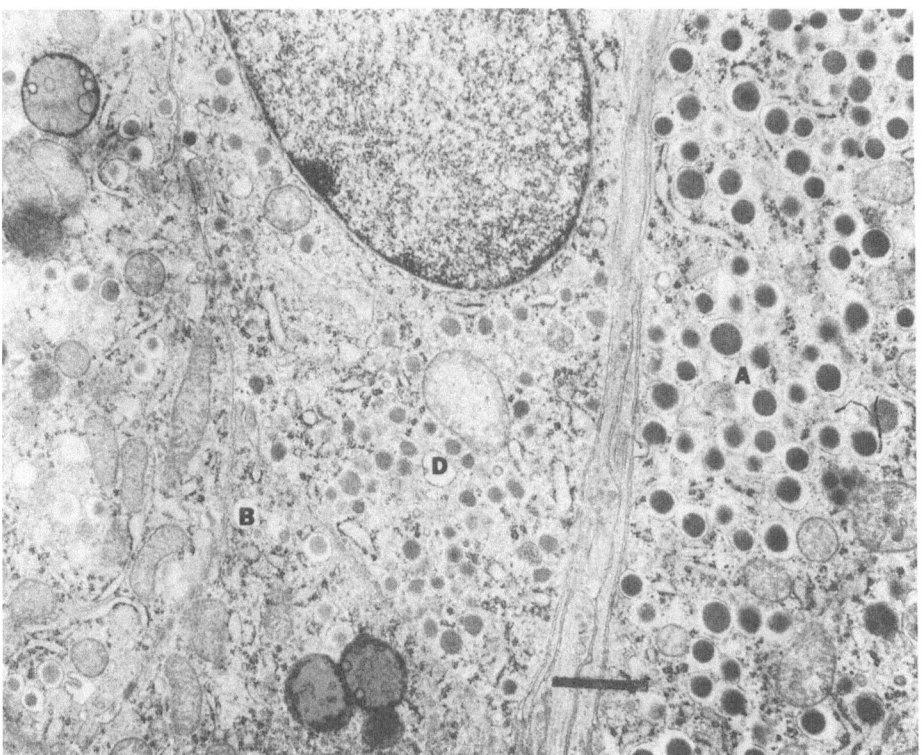

Figure 3. α (A), β (B), and D cells (D) from pancreatic islands of control Chinese hamsters are frequently found and easily identified. Bar = 1 μm.

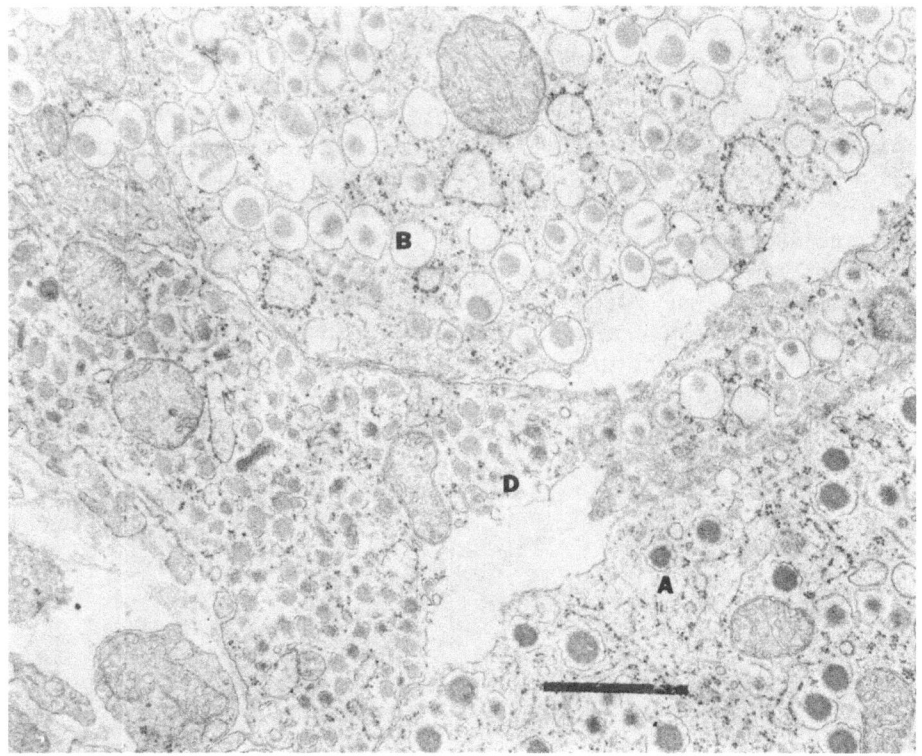

Figure 4. Pancreatic island from a Chinese hamster 1 hr after streptozotocin treatment. α (A) and D cells (D) are difficult to locate, but β cells (B) are easily found. Diminished electron density of the islet substance is common at this time. Bar = 1 μm.

measurable at 6 weeks, the plasma glucagon was slightly elevated, but this could probably originate from increased levels of stomach glucagon, since the pancreatic glucagon was extremely low at this stage.

Alloxan

The first indication that alloxan (Fig. 13) was capable of inducing a transient hyperglycemia was in 1937 in studies showing an early period of hyperglycemia followed by marked hypoglycemia and convulsions after injection of alloxan.[80] The first reports relating alloxan to a toxic effect on the β cells of the islets and a diabetogenic action were published in 1943.[81-86] Since that time, numerous studies have been reported and many reviews have been written concerning this effect of alloxan.[4,5,87-93]

Alloxan can produce diabetes in the rabbit, rat, dog, cat, sheep, monkey, turtle, pigeon, and mouse.[50,87] The guinea pig and chicken are the only species which have been reported to be resistant to alloxan.[43,94–96] The reason for the failure of alloxan to produce diabetes in the guinea pig and chicken is not known. In man, alloxan has been administered for relieving hypoglycemia resulting from tumors, and there is some evidence which indicates that it may cause a destruction of the normal pancreatic islets without any significant effect on the neoplastic tissues.[85,91]

Many compounds closely related to alloxan have been tested for their diabetogenic effects. Alloxan can be considered a pyrimidine, and it is closely related to uracil, thymidine, and cytosine. Some analogs of alloxan, such as methyl, ethyl, and propyl alloxan and dialuric acid, are diabetogenic.[87] Alloxan, however, has a very short half-life in blood of approximately 1 min and is not measurable by 2 min.[97,98]

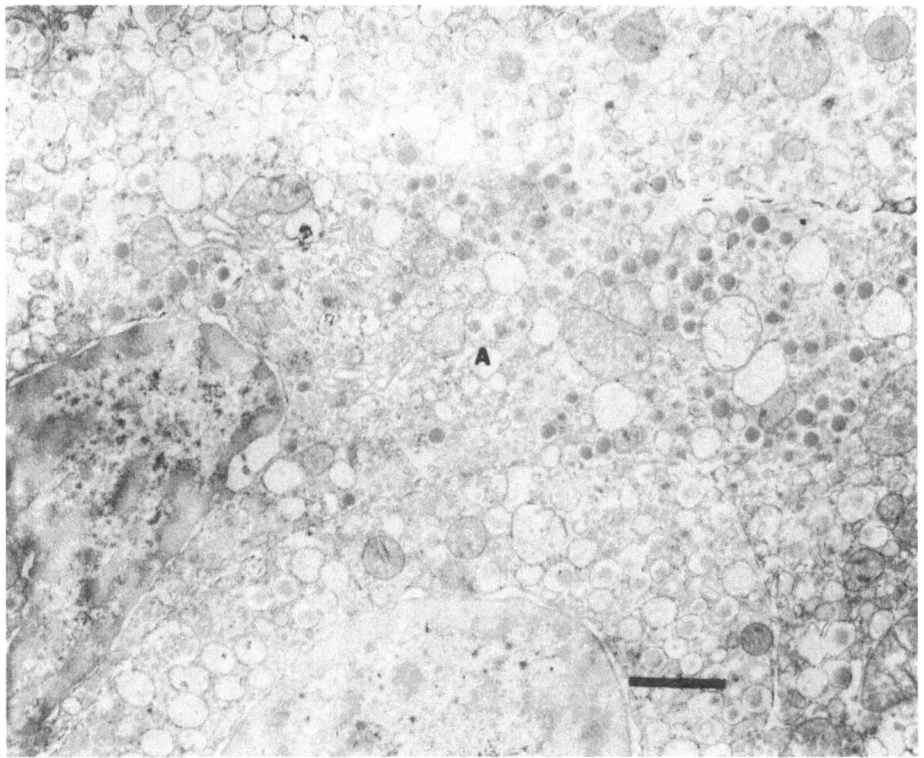

Figure 5. Pancreatic islet from Chinese hamster 3 hr after streptozotocin treatment. All islet cells are severely affected. An obviously damaged α cell (A) shows a pyknotic nucleus. Bar = 1 μm.

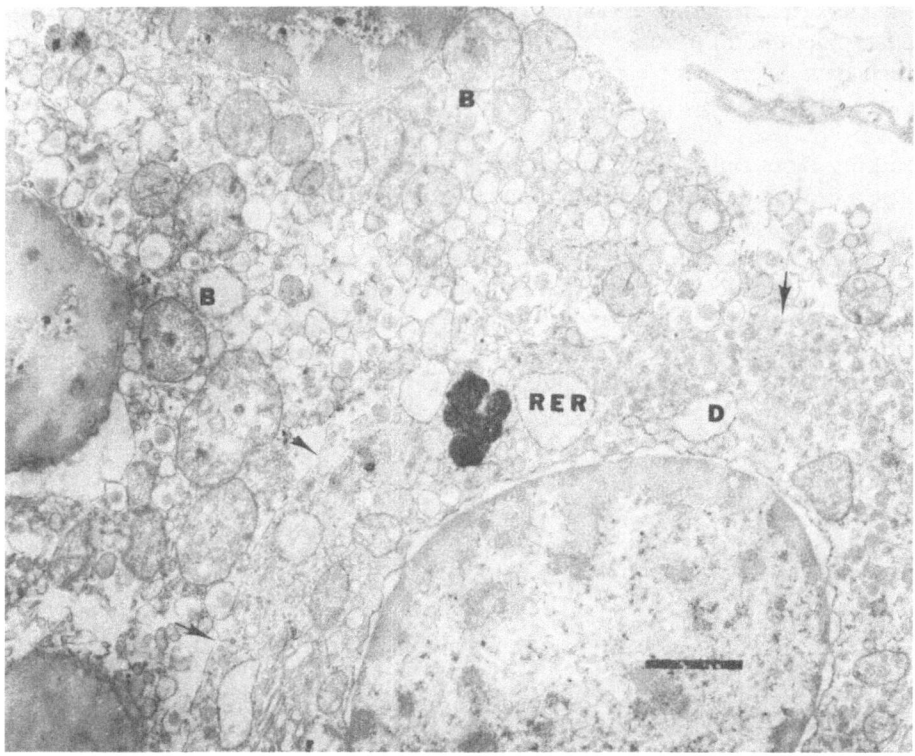

Figure 6. Damage to a D cell (D) from a Chinese hamster islet 3 hr after streptozotocin treatment. Notice the dilation of the RER, disintegration of plasma membrane, (→) and early nuclear pyknosis. Advanced nuclear pyknosis of two β cells (B). Bar = 1 μm.

Alloxan results in a triphasic blood sugar response with an initial elevation of blood sugar 2–4 hr after injection, a period of marked hypoglycemia which may induce convulsions from 6–12 hr, and finally a hyperglycemia at 24 hr.[80,87,99,102]

The mechanism of the early hyperglycemia is not clear, although there are several explanations that have been presented. However, since this phase is not understood and since it does not occur in fasted animals, whereas alloxan will still induce diabetes in the fasted animal,[100,101] these authors consider that whatever alloxan does to blood sugar during this early hyperglycemic phase is unimportant in relation to its diabetogenicity.

It is generally agreed that the hypoglycemic response is related to the release of a large amount of insulin from the β cells, with an increase in plasma insulin.[103,104] The final stage is explained by the destruction of β cells and an insulin deficiency, with a low level of plasma insulin.[103,104]

The mechanism by which alloxan kills the β cell is apparently an extracellular one, since the alloxan remains extracellular. It is distributed in pancreatic islet tissue in concentrations similar to that of D-mannitol, which remains in the extracellular space.[105,106] It has been shown that alloxan increases the permeability of islet cells since islets treated with alloxan become permeable to mannitol.[107] There is also some evidence that this change in permeability induced by alloxan is restricted to the islet cells. It has also been shown that the release of insulin by islets previously exposed to alloxan is reduced in response to high levels of glucose,[108] and this can also be interpreted as indicating a membrane effect of the compound. There is some evidence that the action of alloxan may be at the glucose receptor site on the β cell membrane. Evidence supporting this hypothesis is the observation that glucose can protect against the diabetogenic effects of alloxan,[109,110] and alloxan blocks glucose-stimulated insulin release.[108]

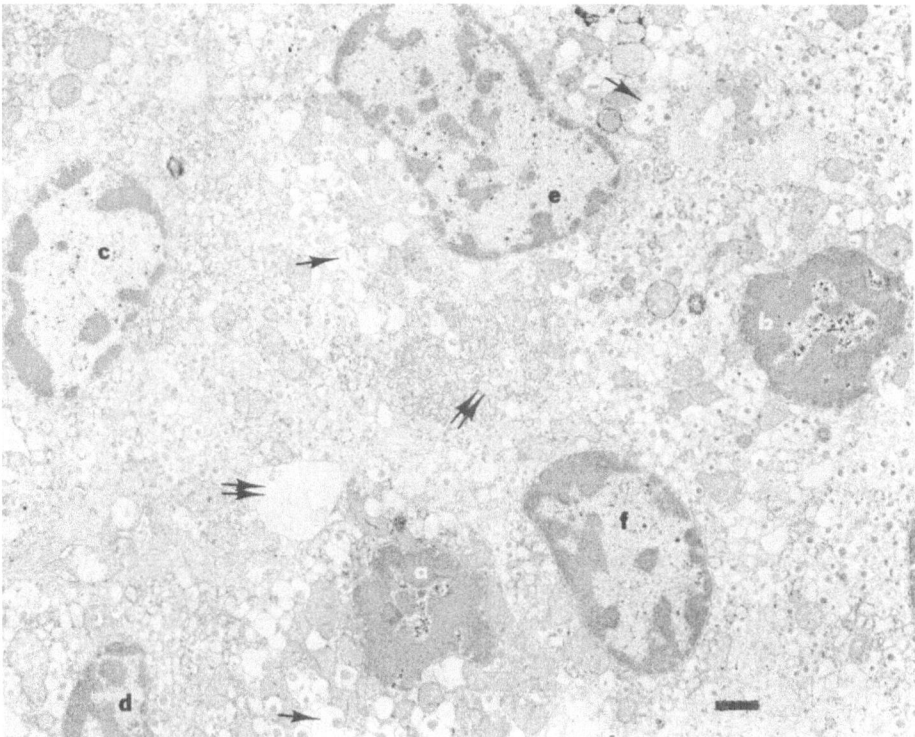

Figure 7. Pancreatic islet from a Chinese hamster 3 hr after streptozotocin treatment. All islet cells are affected. Some nuclei are clearly pyknotic (a, b), others show peripheral chromatin clumping and rarefaction (c, d) or some aggregation (e, f) of interchromatinic material. There is a distention of granular sacs (→) and of the endoplasmic reticulum cisternae (⇉). Bar = 1 μm.

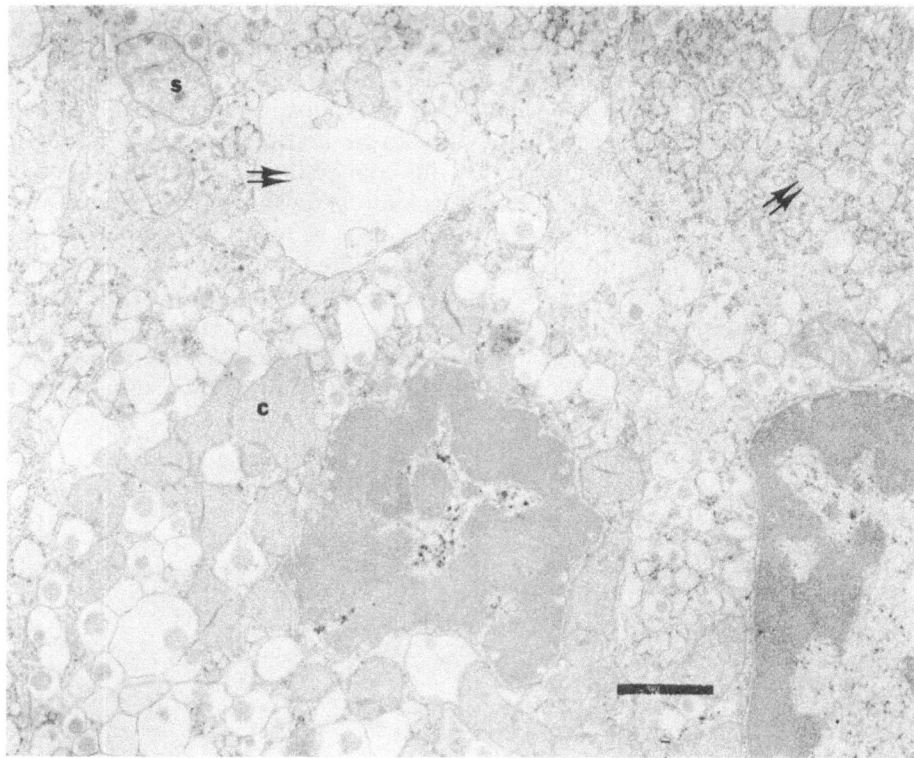

Figure 8. Detail of Fig. 7. Pyknotic nucleus, distended endoplasmic reticulum cisternae ($\rightrightarrows$), and swollen (s) and compact (c) mitochondria in adjacent cells. Bar = 1 μm.

Further evidence to support the hypothesis that alloxan acts at the membrane level and probably at the glucose receptor site is the observation that the α anomer of glucose is a more potent inhibitor of alloxan toxicity than the β anomer,[112] while there is no preferential metabolism of these anomers.[111] In addition, the α anomer is also a stronger stimulus of insulin secretion than the β anomer.[65,66] Also supporting the proposed membrane action of alloxan is the finding that the nonmetabolizable sugars, 2-deoxyglucose and 3-O-methylglucose, inhibit the diabetogenic action of alloxan but are not metabolized.[112] It is also of interest that the α anomer of 3-O-methylglucose is a better protector against the β cell toxicity of alloxan than the β anomer.[112] This stereospecificity further indicates a similarity of the glucose receptor and the alloxan-induced destruction of β cell membrane at the membrane site. However, it must be considered critical that additional proof will be required before the membrane site can be unequivocally accepted. Nevertheless, restriction of alloxan to the extracellular space of the islets, its interaction characteristics with glucose, and its extremely short half-life strongly support an extracellular site, probably at the membrane level. If this hypothesis is true, we will still be required to demonstrate the mechanism of the toxicity to the β cell since other agents that compete with glucose on insulin release are not β cell toxic agents.[113–115]

Histological changes in the islets of Langerhans of rats[116] and rabbits[117] were observed as soon as 5 min after administration of alloxan. The initial changes were loss of granules from β cells of both species. Fragmentation of the cytoplasm occurred in rats at 5 min. In rabbits, at 10–15 min, further degranulation occurred in centrally located cells presumed to be β cells. Peripheric α cells appeared normal. Rats killed at 15 min showed increased pericapillary spaces in the islets, probably owing to islet cell shrinkage.[116] The earliest time period after alloxan treatment when the islets were observed with the electron microscope was 15 min in rabbits. The changes which occurred at this time were clumping of chromatin and some aggregation of the interchromatinic material in most β cells.[77] Pericapillary cells of rat islets showed ragged disintegration 1.5 hr posttreatment.[118]

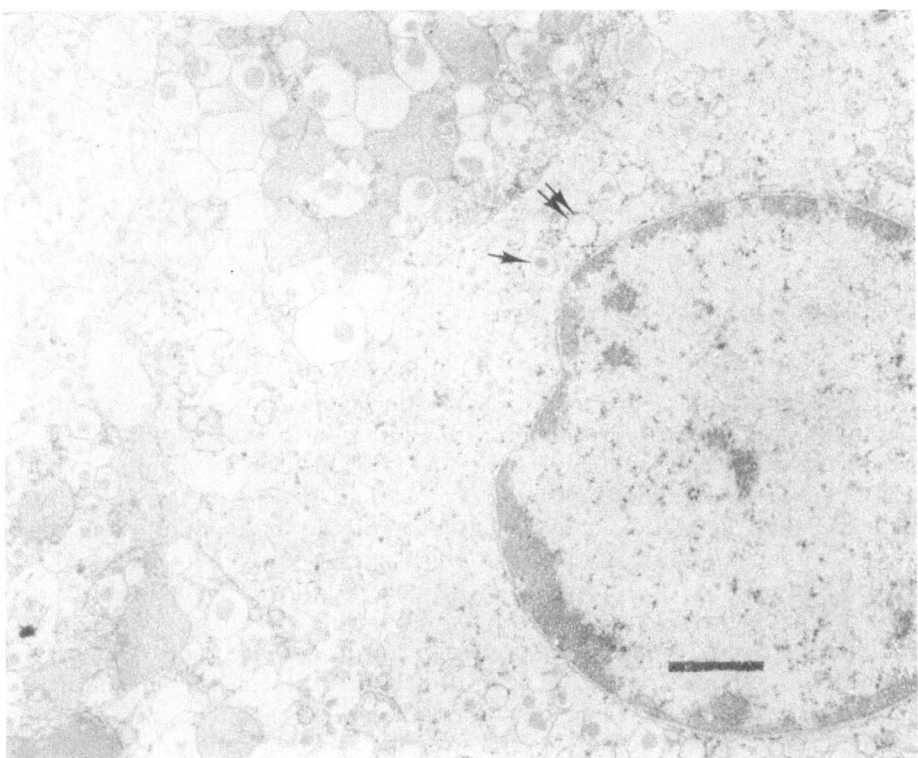

Figure 9. Pancreatic islet of a Chinese hamster 3 hr after streptozotocin treatment. Some cells show structureless cytoplasm in which a few granules (→) and RER sacs (⇉) can be found. Bar = 1 μm.

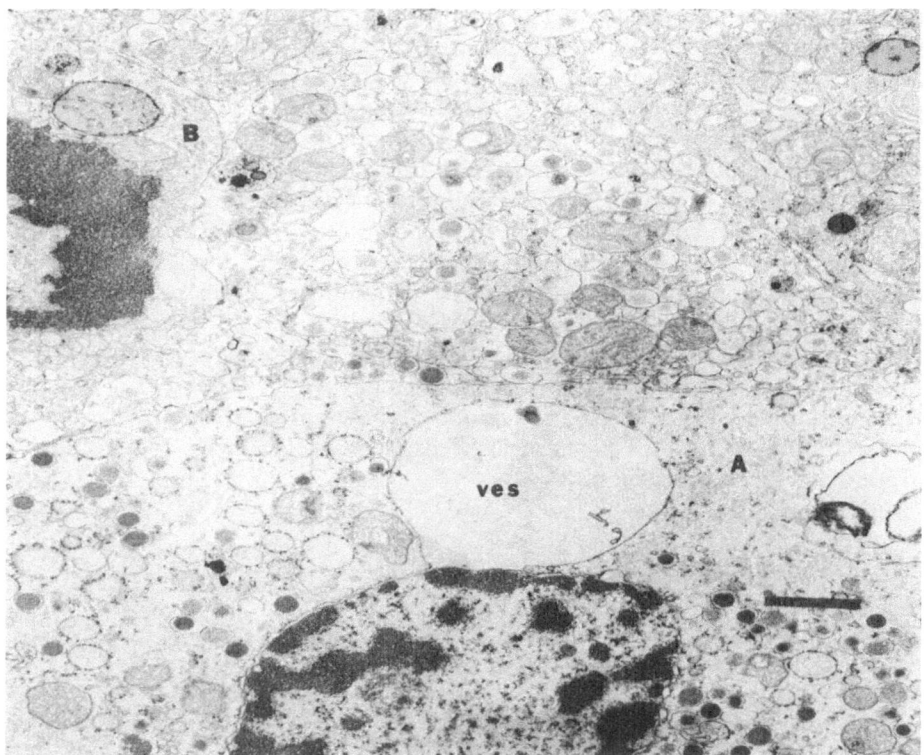

Figure 10. The pancreatic islet of a Chinese hamster 6 hr after streptozotocin treatment. A large vesiculation (ves) of the nuclear sac of a severely damaged α cell (A), marked nuclear pyknosis of a β cell (B), and loss of granules are evident. Bar = 1 μm.

Two hours after alloxan the pancreatic β cells showed large clumps of chromatin and marked aggregation of the interchromatinic material.[77] Distortion of the general architecture of the islet, as evidenced by shrunken central cells in collapsed islets, was observed at this time.[117] At 4 hr the β cell nuclei appeared shrunken, and further progression of chromatin clumps and coarse aggregates of interchromatinic material occurred.[77] At 5–7 hr coalescence of central islet cells and complete disintegration of other cells in the islets were observed in rabbits[117] and in rats. Loss of chromatin from necrotized β cells occurred between 18 and 24 hr posttreatment in rabbits,[77] and rabbits dying within 10 days showed decreased volume of islets which consisted primarily of α cells.[120] Two months following alloxan treatment one rabbit was observed, and revealed islets containing only α cells,[117] while in another rabbit no islet tissue was found at all at 3 months posttreatment.[116] Female rats after 1 year of alloxan-induced diabetes showed decreased sizes of islet tissue, decreased numbers of β cells, and decreased β to α cell ratios.[119] Response to alloxan treatment varies from species to species with regard to morphological changes in the pancreatic islets. Although most species exhibit islet cell damage with alloxan, the pancreatic islets of guinea pigs and birds are resistant to this drug.[43,121,122]

Comparison of Alloxan and Streptozotocin Diabetes

Examination of the information in the preceding sections indicates that streptozotocin and alloxan produce some similar effects, which might be interpreted to mean that they act the same way on the β cell. Since these are structurally different compounds, it was considered important to summarize the comparative actions of these two compounds. Since this has been done by several previous authors,[4,5,8,9] this discussion will highlight only the most significant points.

The principal similarities of streptozotocin and alloxan are that they both produce irreversible damage to the β cells in a variety of species and both produce a triphasic change in blood sugar. No reports have shown any effect of alloxan on α cells, while streptozotocin will destroy α cells in at least two species.

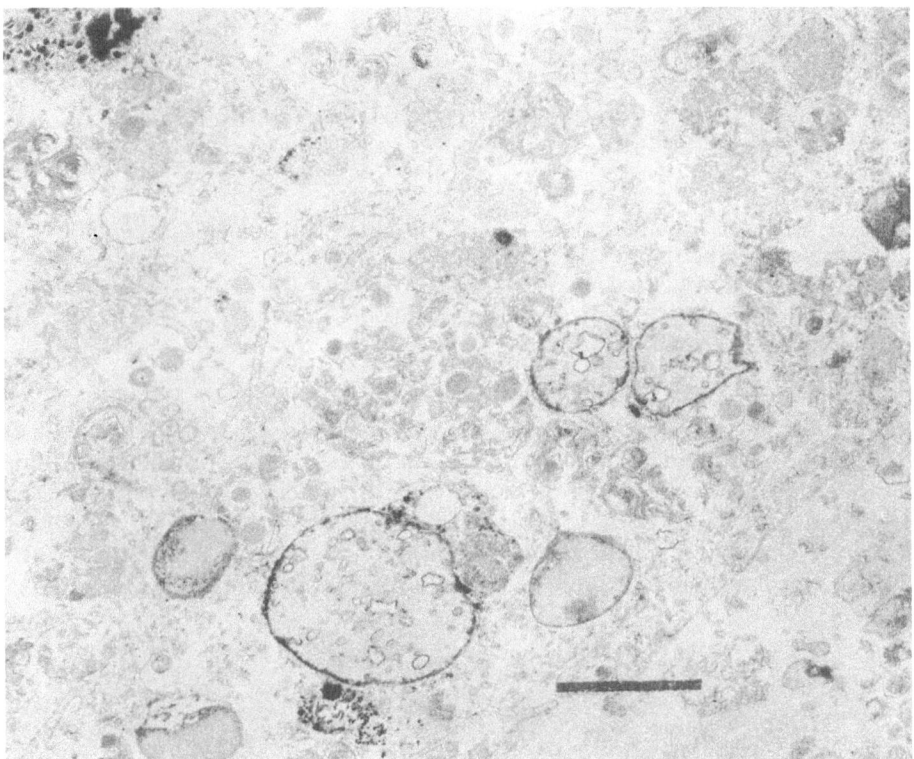

Figure 11. Pancreatic islet from a Chinese hamster 24 hr after streptozotocin treatment. Total disintegration of the islet. Bar = 1 μm.

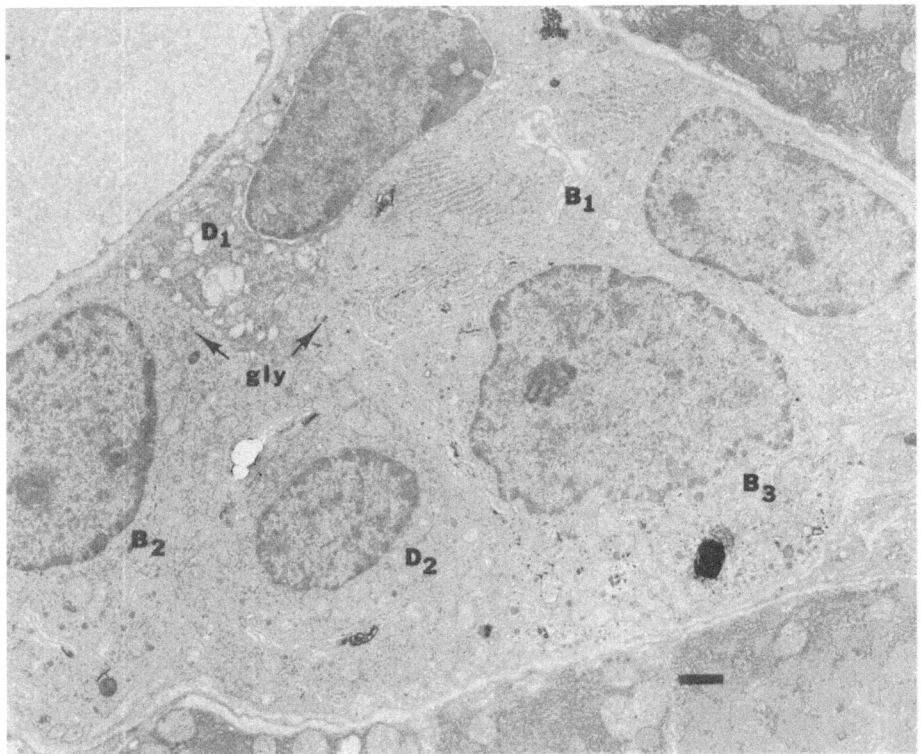

Figure 12. Pancreatic islet from Chinese hamster 6 weeks after streptozotocin treatment. Islets are extremely scarce and very small. One β cell (B₁) and two D cells (D₁ and D₂) were easily identified. Two other cells were considered β cells (B₂ and B₃) because of cytoplasmic deposition of glycogen (gly). Bar = 1 μm.

One of the most striking differences between these two chemicals is related to the ability of various compounds to inhibit their effects on the β cell. Glucose inhibits the action of alloxan but has little effect on streptozotocin-induced diabetes. Nicotinamide, but not nicotinic acid, protects against the effects of streptozotocin, while both will block the diabetogenic effect of alloxan. In addition, nicotinamide will protect against streptozotocin if administered as long as 2 hr later, while it must be given before or simultaneously with alloxan

Figure 13. Structure of alloxan.

in order to counteract the effects of that drug. Epinephrine blocks the effects of alloxan but not streptozotocin.

The half-life of alloxan is about 1 min and is completely gone from the blood in 2 min whereas streptozotocin has a half-life of approximately 10–15 min. The effects of alloxan are therefore very rapid, while those of streptozotocin require a longer time period.

It has been found that NAD levels of liver and islets are decreased with streptozotocin, while the liver NAD is not changed following alloxan treatment. Since liver NAD was not altered by alloxan, it suggests that islet NAD also may not be changed. This could be interpreted to mean that alloxan may not be toxic to the islets by decreasing NAD levels.

The available evidence supports the hypothesis that alloxan acts extracellularly on the β cell membrane, while streptozotocin probably acts intracellularly. It therefore seems reasonable to conclude that alloxan and streptozotocin damage the β cell through two different mechanisms.

Comparison of the sequence of the morphological events shows differences between streptozotocin and alloxan. The effects of alloxan are readily apparent within 5 min following administration. The earliest changes were loss of granules and cytoplasmic fragmentation. Damage to the nuclei of most β cells evidenced by chromatin clumping and aggregation of interchromatinic material have been observed within 15 min after treatment. With streptozotocin, no islet cell damage has been described prior to 1 hr after treatment. The initial changes were minimal and include occasional pyknotic β cells and hypertrophy of the β cell Golgi complex. In some species the first changes have been observed only after 2 hr posttreatment with streptozotocin, and these include chromatin clumping and some rarefaction of the interchromatinic material. The only similarity of the early change produced by alloxan and streptozotocin is the chromatin clumping which occurs later with streptozotocin. After 4.5 hr the nuclear and cytoplasmic β cell changes were similar with streptozotocin and alloxan. One important difference between alloxan and streptozotocin is that in the rabbits some of the α cells are affected by streptozotocin, and this has not been reported with alloxan. The chicken is resistant to both alloxan and streptozotocin, whereas the guinea pig is sensitive to streptozotocin but completely resistant to alloxan.

Benzothiodiazine Diuretics and Hypotensives

An extensive review of this subject matter has been made in a single volume of the *Annals of the New York Academy of Science.*[123] Therefore, this presentation will only summarize some of the pertinent information. Chlorothiazide was the first of this series reported to be an effective diuretic agent[124,140] and began a new era of diuretic drugs and later of antihypertensive drugs. Early clinical studies showed chlorothiazide caused hyperglycemia in some individuals[125–127] and deterioration of diabetes.[142] Following these reports, numerous studies were carried out to define the mechanism of the hyperglycemic action of this group of drugs. Diazoxide, a later benzothiodiazine, was found to be hypotensive without being diuretic.[128,129] The chemical structures of the major compounds in this series are shown in Fig. 14.

In contrast to some of the early benzothiodiazines, diazoxide causes sodium and water retention but still retains its ability to increase blood sugar.[129,130] Other compounds of this type which are also diabetogenic are furosemide, trichlorothiazide, and hydrochlorothiazide.[125,129,131,132] In this discussion we will assume that all of these compounds have the same basic mechanism of diabetogenic activity, and therefore they will be discussed as a class.

One of the major efforts on mechanism of action studies has been to correlate increased blood sugar with a decreased insulin secretion during glucose tolerance tests in man and experimental animals treated with these drugs.[133-139,141] The marked inhibition of insulin secretion has led to the use of these compounds in clinical situations of hypoglycemia.[143-145,155] The effect on insulin secretion was found to be a direct action of diazoxide on the islets, since

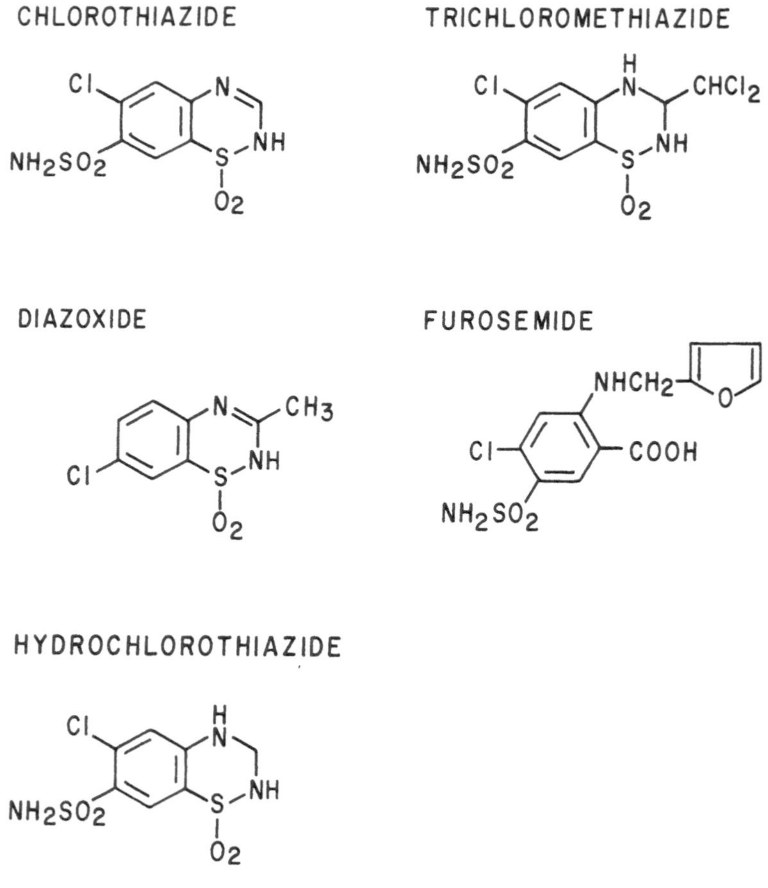

Figure 14. Structure of benzothiodiazines.

these drugs inhibited release of insulin.[115,146,147] It soon became apparent that increased blood sugar was caused by other mechanisms in addition to decreased insulin secretion. This conclusion was drawn from the observations that these compounds, when given to severely diabetic humans or animals,[129] caused a further increase in blood sugar.[2,129,130,148-151] Since these diabetics were deficient in insulin it was concluded that diazoxide had a peripheral effect on glucose utilization. The findings that adrenergic blockers reduced hyperglycemic activity of these drugs indicated that catecholamines may be involved in some way with this hyperglycemic effect.[130,152] Additional evidence implicating the catecholamines in hyperglycemic activity was the observation that an increase in plasma catecholamines occurred during benzothiodiazine treatment of animals and man.[153,154] These reports also showed that the diazoxide produced similar activities to those of epinephrine infusion, such as increased free fatty acid, tachycardia, and a widened pulse pressure. In conclusion, it can be stated that the benzothiodiazines increase blood sugar in man and in animals by direct inhibition of pancreatic insulin release, which results in elevated blood sugar, as well as by increasing epinephrine and other catecholamine secretions, which may also increase blood sugar.[130,151,155]

The diabetogenic effect of this group of drugs does not involve damage to the β cells, since the diabetes is reversible upon withdrawal of drug.[130] The only significant morphological change associated with the benzothiodiazines is accumulation of insulin in the pancreas and β cell granulosis.[163]

Quinolines, Dithizone, and Related Compounds

The first evidence that quinolines were diabetogenic was in a report without data involving a recall of previous experiments.[81] Styrylquinoline-90, which is 2-acetoacetylaminostyryl-6-dimethylaminoquinoline-methyl chloride, produced a minor and temporary blood sugar change in rabbits and rats.[81,156] The rationale for studies with these compounds was based on the demonstration that dithizone and oxine were useful for the histochemical detection of zinc in tissues, since these compounds have a marked affinity for zinc.[157,158] Since then a considerable number of studies have been done with these compounds, as well as with a large number of related chemicals. Most of the related chemicals, however, have been found to be inactive. All active quinolines require an 8-hydroxy group.[159-162] Of interest is the observation that the diabetogenicity of this type of compound is restricted to the rabbit. Rats, guinea pigs, cats, dogs, and hamsters are resistant to their diabetogenic effect.[162] Reviews which have included or discussed these compounds cover most of the early history as well as the majority of the references.[3] It is definitely not clear what the mechanism of activity of these compounds is, although they are strong chelating agents and bind zinc, which is found in association with the insulin in the β cells. However, it is not clear whether zinc chelation is the basic mechanism of action by which these compounds destroy the β cells, since many animal species containing zinc in the pancreas are resistant to these drugs, and not all chelating agents induce diabetes.[161]

It has been shown that oxine and dithizone produced a triphasic blood sugar response[159] similar to that produced by alloxan and streptozotocin. Hyperglycemia occurs 2–4 hr after treatment, followed by a hypoglycemia which may occur from 5–20 hr, and after approximately 24 hr there is a permanent hyperglycemia in a small number of treated animals.[159] The structure of oxine and dithizone, the basic compounds studied in this series of chemicals, are shown in Fig. 15.

The morphological changes produced with 8-hydroxyquinoline when given intravenously to rabbits were observed as early as 6 hr posttreatment and included nuclear pyknosis, degranulation, and some vacuolation of islet cells. From 18–35 hr after treatment there was progressive necrosis and disintegration of β cells. By 72 hr the islets were composed of 80–90% α cells, and in the permanent diabetic state the islets were reduced in size and in number.[159] Similar findings have been reported for a number of chemically different 8-hydroxyquinoline derivatives.[164] Dithizone diabetes in rabbits[159] was characterized by an early disappearance of β cell granules and final death of most β cells in all pancreatic islets. β cell degranulation was found within 2 hr after intravenous administration of the drug. Necrosis of β cells progressed from 8–24 hr at which time disintegration was observed. By 48 hr the islets were composed almost completely of α cells. Animals killed 5 and 8 days after treatment had islets which were reduced in number and size and were made up primarily of α cells.

Cyproheptadine

Cyproheptadine (Fig. 16) is an antiserotonin, antihistaminic compound[165] which is used clinically to stimulate weight gain in adults and children through

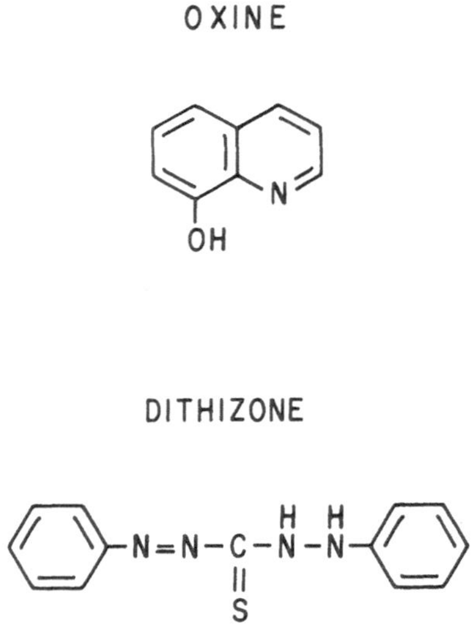

OXINE

DITHIZONE

Figure 15. Structure of quinoline (oxine) and dithizone.

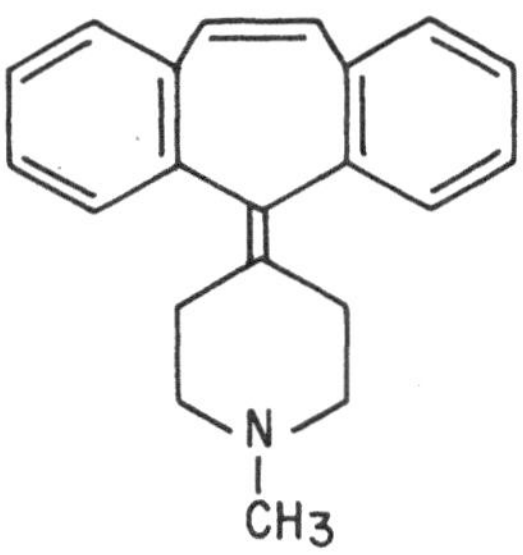

Figure 16. Structure of cyproheptadine.

the mechanism of increase in caloric intake.[166-169] Rats treated with cyproheptadine for 14 days may exhibit normal fasting blood sugars, but they may also show a decreased tolerance to glucose and a diminished insulin release with glucagon stimulation.[170] Others have found that fasting blood sugar levels of rats treated from 2–4 days with cyproheptadine are significantly elevated.[171] In man, cyproheptadine did not produce any alteration of glucose tolerance or plasma insulin levels during a glucose tolerance test.[167] Cyproheptadine added to perifusion medium in isolated rat islets completely abolished the increased insulin release induced by 300 mg/100ml of glucose but had no effect on the basal insulin release.[172] The data available do not allow one to determine the mechanism of action of cyproheptadine on the β cell nor the reason for its peculiar specificity for the rat.

Oral administration of cyproheptadine for 14 days to mice, rats, and hamsters produced no islet cell degeneration,[170] whereas rats showed marked vacuolation of the cytoplasm. Electron microscopy of the islets from orally treated rats[170,171] showed progressive degranulation of the β cells, dilation of the endoplasmic reticulum cisternae, and loss of ribosomes from the surface of the RER. Rats were given 1, 2, 4, 7, and 14 consecutive daily treatments and were killed 14–18 hr after the last dose. The β cell degranulation was observed after the first dose. Marked degranulation of the β cells and the formation of large vesicles by fusion of the RER dilated cisternae increased in severity after the fourth to the fourteenth dose. There were no changes in the α or D cells. Morphological recovery of the islets was completed 2 weeks after the seventh dose in rats.[171]

L-*Asparaginase*

L-Asparaginase, an enzyme isolated from *Escherichia coli*, has been used clinically for treatment of leukemia and other tumors. One of the reported side effects has been a temporary, nonketotic hyperglycemia in some of the patients.[173-176] It is difficult to evaluate the mechanism of action of this drug. Its hyperglycemic effect could not be associated with any specific action on the pancreas, although it has been reported to decrease plasma insulin levels.[174,175,177] Since insulin contains L-asparagine, it is possible that the enzyme might alter the structural integrity of insulin, but this was found not to be true, since incubation of insulin with L-asparaginase did not alter the hormone.[177] In rabbits, 2000 U/kg or more of L-asparaginase will induce a reversible diabetes often associated with an increased BUN (blood urea nitrogen) but no increase in alkaline phosphatase, SGOT, or serum amylase and with no significant influence on pancreatic morphology.[181] L-Asparaginase exerts its antitumor activity by decreasing the availability of L-asparagine to cells which, due to a deficiency of the enzyme L-asparagine synthetase, require an exogenous source of this amino acid.[178-180]

If L-asparaginase reduces plasma levels of L-asparagine, it may result in an inability of the β cell to synthesize insulin because of possible insufficient asparagine. Deficient insulin synthesis could then result in hyperglycemia. Based on the observed decreased plasma insulin, the inactivity of the enzyme on insulin structure, and the absence of general pancreatitis, it seems reasonable to conclude that the β cells may lack the enzyme L-asparagine synthetase and consequently must be provided with an exogenous source of L-asparagine. This hypothesis will have to be tested with studies on *in vitro* synthesis of insulin in the presence of this enzyme.

Hormonal Diabetogenic Agents

A number of hormones have been implicated as a contributory and/or a causative factor in diabetes mellitus. Those which are generally assumed to play an important role are glucocorticoids, adrenalin, sex hormones (particularly the oral contraceptives), glucagon, and some of the pituitary hormones. Although other hormones may play a role in the pathogenesis of diabetes, these authors consider the information on them to be inconclusive, and they will therefore not be discussed. Thyroid hormone and some of the specific anterior pituitary hormones, such as ACTH and prolactin, are considered to be members of this group. The most important hormone with recent information available is glucagon, and therefore it will be described in more detail.

Glucagon

There are a number of excellent and recent reviews concerning the role of glucagon in diabetes.[182-185] The purpose of this discussion is to emphasize the major developments in the elucidation of the glucagon role in diabetes and its possible mechanisms of action.

The first indication of the presence of a hyperglycemic factor in the pancreas was based on the finding that injection of pancreatic extracts which were proposed to be partially purified insulin caused a temporary increase in blood sugar.[186] A purified material was later isolated from pancreatic extracts and was shown to increase blood sugar. These findings indicated that the hyperglycemic action observed by the earlier researchers with pancreatic extracts was not due to an aberrant action of insulin.[187] This purified material was given the name glucagon.[187] The structure of glucagon has been determined,[188] and it has been shown to be a 29-amino acid polypeptide. The availability of pure glucagon made possible numerous studies concerning its mechanism of induction of hyperglycemia. The development of an immunoassay to measure concentrations in circulating blood aided in further defining the role of glucagon in diabetes.[189-191] Indirect evidence that glucagon may be diabetogenic in man is derived from studies on patients who had glucagon-producing tumors who exhibited high blood sugar levels and high levels of the hormone. Some of these patients were diabetic,[192] and one was reported to exhibit ketosis as well as fasting hyperglycemia.[192] Removal of the glucagon-producing tumors normalized one of these patients.[193] The fact that glucagon produces hyperglycemia in normal dogs,[194] rabbits,[195] and humans[182,196,197] suggests that it has a potential to induce diabetes. Nevertheless, it is difficult to induce diabetes in normal rats unless they are force fed[198,199] or simultaneously treated with cortisone.[200] In rabbits treated with 2 mg/kg per day of glucagon there was a transient hyperglycemia of varying degrees after each injection. Of nine of these rabbits treated for more than 3 months, two developed resistance to the hyperglycemic action of glucagon and seven showed a sustained increase in blood sugar. Diabetes persisted from 18–63 days following cessation of treatment. However, the rabbits did eventually revert to normal. Interestingly, there was an increase in the number of islets in resistant animals; they were seen to have a greater number than animals which exhibit hyperglycemia.[195] Since glucagon has also been shown to stimulate insulin secretion,[201,202] it is difficult to explain the sustained hyperglycemia in some of these animals, unless the glucagon at the dosage used was able to change the insulin:glucagon ratio to a point which would overcome an insulin action.

Recent data have shown that there is a normal level of fasting glucagon in maturity-onset and juvenile-type diabetic humans,[203] even with hyperglycemia, which would be expected to decrease the glucagon.[204] In addition, L-arginine infusions stimulate a larger than normal plasma level of glucagon in the diabetic.[205] These observations, when considered in conjunction with the hyperglycemic action of glucagon, provide further indirect evidence that elevated glucagon may play an important role in the pathogenesis of diabetes. However, more convincing proof would be that a reduction of glucagon in diabetics would ameliorate the disease. Evidence for this became available when it was discovered that somatostatin, a 14-amino acid polypeptide obtained from hypothalamus, was capable of reducing plasma levels of insulin and glucagon.[206] Since this discovery, investigators have found that suppression of glucagon by infusion of somatostatin reduces hyperglycemia in the diabetic[207] and hyperglycemia and ketosis in ketotic diabetics, even after withdrawal of insulin therapy.[208] These later observations clearly imply that elevated glucagon is a contributing factor in the hyperglycemia and ketosis of diabetes.

The mechanism by which glucagon induces hyperglycemia and elevated ketosis has been convincingly described. The increase in blood sugar arises from increased glycogenolysis and increased gluconeogenesis. Increased glycogenolysis is shown by rapid increase in arterial blood glucose following intraportal injection of glucagon[194] and breakdown of liver glycogen, with a concomitant rise of medium glucose from liver slices or perfused rat liver *in vitro.*[209-210] Evidence that glucagon increases gluconeogenesis has been obtained by showing increased nitrogen excretion[198,212] and increased blood sugar from alanine in normal postabsorptive man[213] as well as increased conversion of lactate to glucose by perfused livers.[214]

Another role of glucagon in diabetes is its effect on fat metabolism. It has been found that glucagon will increase lipolysis, which results in an increase in plasma-free fatty acids.[215,216] It also increases ketone bodies, which, when elevated to sufficiently high levels, results in increased levels of urine ketones. It also increases ketone bodies in insulin-dependent diabetics, further contributing to the metabolic problem of this type of diabetic.[217] This increase in ketones results from both increase in fatty acids as well as selectively increased oxidation of fatty acids to ketones, regardless of the free fatty acid levels.[218]

Although glucagon has been shown to play an important role in producing the undesirable metabolic problems in the diabetic, there is no evidence that it can cause permanent diabetes with a destruction of β cells. The observation that inhibition of glucagon levels in the diabetic with somatostatin reduces severity of diabetes indicates that if selective inhibition of glucagon can be accomplished in the early stages of diabetes, long-term beneficial effects might be expected. The ratio of glucagon to insulin may be the most significant aspect of glucagon control in diabetics, since many effects of glucagon and insulin are antagonistic.[219]

Morphologically it has been found that long-term glucagon treatment of rabbits will result in total loss of α cells and degranulation, hypertrophy, and hyperplasia of β cells.[220,221] Glycogen infiltration of β cells and of ductular cells have also been observed.[220] α cells were shown to recover slowly after withdrawal of treatment.[220] Dogs and force-fed rats, when treated for 7 days, showed degranulation of β cells.[198] The pancreatic islets of force-fed rats showed degranulation and hydropic degeneration of some β cells.[198] From these observations it can be concluded that glucagon apparently does not cause any long-term, permanent detrimental effects on the β cells.

Growth Hormone

The relationship of growth hormone to carbohydrate metabolism has been extensively reviewed.[222-227] The first evidence that the pituitary might have an influence on diabetes was that the severity of diabetes decreased after removal of that gland.[228] Further evidence of the diabetic role of the anterior pituitary was the observation that extracts of anterior pituitary produced hyperglycemia in intact dogs and partially depancreatized cats and increased the blood sugar in diabetics.[229-234] The assignment of the diabetogenic principle from the pituitary to growth hormone was shown by the observation that purified growth hormone produced diabetes in the dog and cat.[235-237] It was also shown that growth hormone could cause deterioration of diabetes in man.[239,240] Glucose tolerance has been found to decrease in many normal subjects after only several days of purified growth hormone injection, but it reaches a diabetic state in only a few.[241] Acromegalics exhibit diabetes at 10 times the rate of that in the general population. However, many acromegalic patients with high growth hormone levels are only mildly diabetic, and many are not diabetic at all.[242,243] It is of interest that in acromegalics with normal glucose tolerance curves the plasma insulin levels show an immediate and exaggerated rise[244] when challenged with glucose. In contrast, acromegalics with a diabetic type of glucose metabolism or decreased glucose tolerance show a delayed insulin response to a glucose challenge similar to that of nonacromegalic diabetics.[243] Although permanent diabetes has been produced in the dog and cat with purified growth hormone preparations, it is difficult to produce diabetes in the rat, guinea pig, or rabbit.[231] It should be emphasized that to date there is no evidence that permanent diabetes can be produced in normal human beings with growth hormone, although growth hormone will induce glucose intolerance in normal man.[241] In hypophysectomized women maintained on 0.7 mg/kg of cortisone per day, growth hormone at 0.3 mg/kg for 2 days has produced glucosuria.[239] The observation described above that active acromegalics with normal glucose tolerance tests had higher than normal plasma insulin, while those with a diabetic-like glucose tolerance had diabetic type of insulin response, suggests that the pancreatic reserve of insulin may be an important factor in growth-hormone-induced diabetes.

There is some evidence that pituitary hormones can act synergistically in the production of diabetes in rats. In intact rats transplanted with a tumor which produces 100- to 1000-fold increases of growth hormone, ACTH, and prolactin, there was no evidence that these animals became diabetic. Plasma insulin levels in these animals increased to approximately 200 μU/ml, indicating that they could compensate for a stressful situation in which more insulin was required. In 80% depancreatized rats, glucosuria resulted from transplantation of the growth-hormone-producing tumors. It was of interest that in the 80% depancreatized rats glucosuria was still evident 3 weeks after removal of the tumor.[245] Studies with pure hormones also showed that growth hormone or ACTH injected into 80% depancreatized rats induced glucosuria after 2–5 days of treatment, although rapid recovery occurred after treatment was stopped.[246]

The mechanism by which growth hormone produces a diabetes-like syndrome is complex and not understood. There is some indication that in the dog, growth hormone treatment results in insulin antagonism.[247,248] Further evidence for insulin antagonism has been obtained by studies *in vitro* with skeletal and heart muscle from rats which have been exposed to growth hormone.[249,250] Growth hormone also caused an increase in glucose release from the liver of normal or hypophysectomized dogs.[251] In the perfused human arm, it has been shown that glucose utilization by adipose and muscle tissue in active acromegalics is decreased. In normal people, growth hormone inhibited glucose uptake by both adipose and muscle tissue and inhibited the ability of insulin to increase glucose uptake.[238] It therefore seems logical to conclude that one effect of growth hormone is to increase insulin demand, which in situations of restricted reserve may cause diabetes.[239] However, to confuse the picture somewhat, it has been observed that growth hormone will increase plasma insulin and glucose turnover in the dog.[252] Therefore, the mechanism by which growth hormone induces diabetes remains questionable. Nevertheless, in some animals there is morphologic evidence of adverse effects and possibly permanent damage to β cells.

Morphologically, it has been shown that anterior pituitary extracts given in daily doses to dogs caused progressive degranulation, hydropic degeneration, and death of pancreatic β cells.[231,232] Treatment for 7 days caused only a temporary diabetes, and complete histological recovery was observed 4–5 days after cessation of treatment. However, with prolonged treatment a permanent diabetic state was induced in dogs, which was characterized by irreversible hydropic degeneration, decrease of β cells, decrease of insulin secretion, and scarcity of pancreatic islets.[230] Cats[234] as well as rodents[230] can only be made diabetic with anterior pituitary extracts after partial pancreatectomy. In cats, β cell degranulation and hydropic degeneration were reversible if the animals were treated with insulin during the first 3 months of diabetes. After 4 months, the hydropic degeneration was irreversible and resulted in atrophic islets and permanent diabetes.[234]

Glucocorticoids

In this discussion, ACTH and the adrenal glucocorticoids will be considered as producing identical effects, since the primary effect of ACTH is to stimulate production of adrenal glucocorticoids. Although ACTH has some extrapancreatic actions,[253] the authors of this review consider that this action is unlikely to contribute significantly to the production of diabetes.

The primary glococorticoids secreted by the adrenal glands which can be considered are corticosterone (compound B), hydrocortisone (compound F), and, to a lesser degree, cortisone (compound E). Although numerous synthetic derivatives of these compounds have been made, most of which are many times more potent than the naturally occurring compounds, we will consider these to be in the same class and, for all practical purposes, to produce the same physiological effects. The structures of the principal hormones are shown in Fig. 17.

Several reviews are available on the effects of glucocorticoids on carbohydrate metabolism.[254–256,314] The first indications that the adrenals may produce something that influences carbohydrate metabolism were the observations that their removal resulted in the reduction of the severity of diabetes in depancreatized animals and that the adrenal hormones could produce hyperglycemia in fasted adrenalectomized animals and in man.[257–261] Glucocorticoids were first shown to cause hyperglycemia and increased nitrogen excretion in normal and adrenalectomized animals.[262] It has been recognized by clinical investigators that many patients with Cushing's syndrome, which results from hypersecretion of glucocorticoids, would exhibit fasting hyperglycemia, glucosuria, or abnormal glucose tolerance. These findings led to the conclusion that the adrenals can produce hormones which will decrease carbohydrate tolerance.[254,263] Since hyperplasia and hypertrophy of the adrenal glands or Cushing's syndrome can

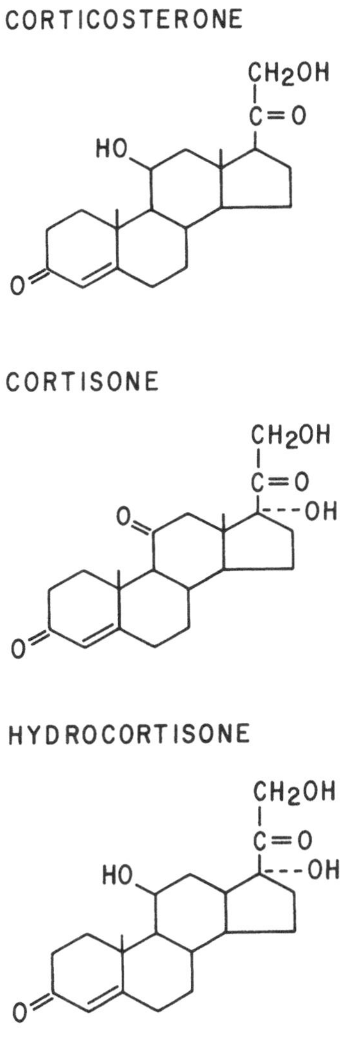

CORTICOSTERONE

CORTISONE

HYDROCORTISONE

Figure 17. Structure of glucocorticoids.

lead to excess production of hydrocortisone, and since the removal of the adrenal lesions restores carbohydrate metabolism to normal, this diabetes can be expected to be reversible.[264] In man and most laboratory animals, glucocorticoid treatment leads to abnormal glucose metabolism. This has been shown in the rabbit,[265,266,268,269,272] rat,[262,267,273] mouse,[262] cat,[258,268] guinea pig,[268,270,273] Chinese hamster,[271] and man,[263,277] but not in the dog.[268,273,274]

The mechanism by which glucocorticoids produce abnormal glucose tolerance has been studied in detail, and one may conclude that this abnormality results from several basic mechanisms. An increased gluconeogenesis was first proposed, based on an increased nitrogen excretion in animals[258,262,267] and man[276] as a result of glucocorticoid treatment. However, the increased nitrogen mobilization was not of sufficient magnitude to account for all of the increased glucose.[266,280,281] Other evidence supporting increased gluconeogenesis has been obtained by studies directly measuring glucose production. Using labeled glucose infusion, it has been shown that cortisone can cause a sevenfold increase in the rate of gluconeogenesis[278] *in vivo. In vitro* studies with liver slices have also demonstrated an increased conversion of alanine and pyruvate to glucose when glucocorticoids were added to the medium.[255,279,280] In addition to increased production of glucose, there is some evidence of a decreased glucose utilization following glucocorticoid treatment. Oxidation of [^{14}C]glucose is decreased in rats treated with the glucocorticoids,[281] and there is decreased glucose uptake by fat tissue removed from rats treated with these compounds.[282]

In contrast to these observations, clinical studies have provided no evidence of decreased insulin sensitivity in man, even though abnormal glucose metabolism was present.[283-285] These observations suggest that the principal mechanism whereby glucocorticoids increased blood sugar is increased production and decreased utilization of glucose in some species.

In all species reported on (rabbit, guinea pig, dog, and rat), adequate doses of corticosteroids induced β cell degranulation,[272,286-288,290] hypertrophy,[272,288,290] and hydropic degeneration[266,272,286,288,289] of β and ductular cells and transformation of ductular and acinar cells into β cells.[272,286,288,290] The diabetic state following corticosteroid therapy disappeared gradually after discontinuation of the corticoid treatment.[286] However, some of the morphological alterations probably remain for some time, such as hyperplasia and hypertrophy of the islets[286,288] and degeneration of β and ductule cells, which were affected with severe glycogen deposition.[272,286]

Adrenal Medullary Hormones—Epinephrine

Extensive reviews have been recently written on the influence of adrenal medullary hormones on carbohydrate metabolism.[291-294] One of the earliest indications that epinephrine or related monoamines could be involved in diabetes was the observation of patients with pheochromocytomas which were often diabetic or had a decreased glucose tolerance.[295-298] This decrease generally resulted from a tumor of the adrenal medulla, which produced significant elevations in levels of catecholamines, including epinephrine.[295] Removal of the tumor generally restored the carbohydrate metabolism to normal,[295-297] suggesting that adrenal-medullary-hormone-induced diabetes is reversible. Decreased insulin sensitivity has been observed in some patients with pheochromocytomas.[296,298] The structure of the principal hormone of adrenal medulla, epinephrine, is shown in Fig. 18.

Hyperglycemia has also been shown to occur *in vivo* as a result of infusion of epinephrine.[299-303] The mechanism of this hyperglycemia has been subjected to extensive investigations. In general, it is concluded that hyperglycemia from epinephrine results from a variety of metabolic actions of this hormone. It has been shown by many investigators that it will inhibit secretion of insulin *in vitro*. Addition of epinephrine to pieces of rabbit pancreas[304] or rat pancreatic

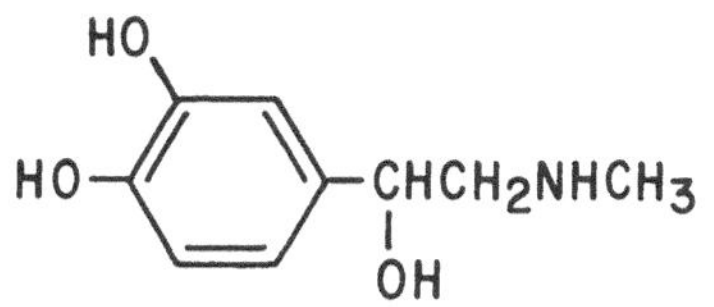

Figure 18. Structure of epinephrine.

tissue[114] will reduce insulin release. It has also been observed that in man the infusion of epinephrine reduces plasma insulin, even though the blood sugar is elevated.[305,306] In the dog, the peripheral infusion of epinephrine reduces the insulin release,[307] and the infusion of epinephrine into the gastroepiploic artery results in hyperglycemia, which can be explained by this reduction of insulin.[308]

In addition to reducing insulin levels, epinephrine also inhibits glucose utilization by muscle. Studies with intact or adrenal-demedullated dogs infused with uniformly labeled glucose have shown that epinephrine will decrease glucose utilization.[307,309] It has been shown that epinephrine inhibits *in vitro* glucose utilization by muscle tissue from rats that have been treated with epinephrine,[310,311] owing a direct inhibition of glucose uptake.[312] In addition to these effects of epinephrine, there is some evidence that epinephrine may cause insensitivity to insulin, since some patients with pheochromocytomas are less sensitive to insulin.[292,294] In some animal studies, injection of epinephrine resulted in decreased response to insulin.[313]

A more recently reported effect of epinephrine which may lead to decreased glucose tolerance is its ability to increase glucagon secretion.[315] Since glucagon may contribute to hyperglycemia and other undesirable effects observed in the diabetic, this increase in glucagon can be expected to modify glucose tolerance.[182,195,196] Infusion of epinephrine into juvenile diabetics or normal individuals results in increased blood sugar and glucagon levels.[315] Prevention of the glucagon increase resulted in a decrease of epinephrine-induced hyperglycemia by 40–50%.[315] The increased glucagon may contribute to epinephrine-induced hyperglycemia, although it cannot account for all epinephrine action on carbohydrate metabolism, since somatostatin-blocked epinephrine-induced glucagon release does not completely reverse epinephrine-induced hyperglycemia. These observations lend additional support to the multifaceted mechanisms of epinephrine-induced hyperglycemia.

There is little evidence that epinephrine can cause a permanent damage to the β cell with the resultant permanent diabetes. Although epinephrine increases blood sugar and causes glucosuria under severe conditions of stress or high doses, these generally revert to normal when epinephrine levels are reduced by removing the stress or withdrawing treatment. Also, in patients with epinephrine-producing tumors, hyperglycemia reverts to normal when the tumor is removed. There was only one report on the morphological changes induced by adrenalin on the pancreatic islet tissue, and this was in dogs infused continuously into the pancreaticoduodenal artery.[308] Biopsies of the pancreas from intact animals following 2, 4, and 6 hr of continuous infusion with adrenalin showed damage to the β cell membranes and cytoplasmic vascular poles of the β cells within 2 hr. By 4 hr, the β cells along the blood vessels had lost most of the membranes and part of the cytoplasm. By 6 hr it was impossible to distinguish the various types of cells in the islets, since the islets appeared as masses containing granules of insulin and a few pyknotic nuclei. Three of nine dogs which were partially pancreatectomized and perfused with adrenalin for 6 hr developed hyperglycemia from 2–6 days after infusion. The pancreases of the three hyperglycemic animals showed marked alterations of the pancreatic β cells. Although this damage appeared to be irreversible, the animals recovered spontaneously from the adrenalin treatment.

Sex Hormones

The recent widespread use of the oral contraceptives which have been indicated by some to precipitate glucose intolerance has renewed research activity on the relationship of these agents to diabetes.[316–322,327,328,330] However, many have observed no change in glucose tolerance following administration of these hormones.[316,323–326] Indications that sex hormones, particularly the female sex hormones, might be involved in a diabetes-like state were the observations that diabetes is frequently manifested during pregnancy at a time when sex hormones are elevated, and latent diabetes may become manifest during pregnancy.[275,329,331–334] One problem ascribing a diabetogenic effect to sex hormones is that there are numerous synthetic derivatives of the naturally-occurring sex hormones with a variety of physiological actions. These may be derived from estrogens, androgens, or progestins. The structures of the basic compounds are shown in Fig. 19. The contraceptive estrogens are generally derived from ethinyl estradiol, and the oral progestin-like compounds are derived from 17-α-ethinyl-19-norethisterone, 19-nortestosterone, or 17-ace-toxy-progesterone (Fig. 19).

One indication that some of these compounds affect glucose tolerance is a small increase in plasma insulin levels[329] which seems to be inconsistent with a diabetogenic action. Also, data from animal studies make the clinical observations difficult to interpret, since different effects of these compounds have been observed in animals. For example, an increased insulin release by isolated pancreas or pieces of tissue in vitro[339] occurred in tissue taken from animals previously treated with estrogen.

In 95% depancreatized animals, removal of the ovaries will increase the incidence and severity of diabetes, which indicates the ovarian hormones may be protective.[335] In ovariectomized, pancreatectomized rats, estrogen will decrease the incidence and severity of diabetes.[336] Diabetes has also been shown to be attenuated in animals with estrogen treatment, particularly in dogs[338] and monkeys.[340] Stilbesterol has been shown to be diabetogenic in force-fed rats or partially depancreatized rats,[337] or 95% depancreatized castrated female rats. In the 95% depancreatized rats only testosterone was found to be diabetogenic.[336] One study with chlormadione acetate (a progesterone-like compound) in dogs showed it produced diabetes in two animals within 1 year. These animals

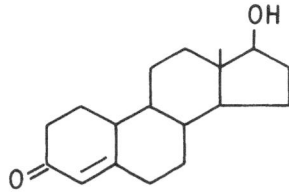

Figure 19. Structure of sex hormones.

remained diabetic, which indicated that a permanent diabetes could be produced in at least one species with this type of compound.[338] There was only one significant observation related to the morphological influence of the sex hormones on the pancreas.[338] Following 1 year of treatment with chlormadione acetate, only two dogs were diabetic, and histological abnormalities related to diabetes were found in the pancreas. These changes were a marked reduction in the number and size of the islets, and degranulated and some vacuolated β cells.[338]

It is obvious that the influence of sex hormones on diabetes is very complex, and insufficient data are available to make any generalized conclusion.

References

1. Jahnecke, J.: *Med. Klin.*, **68**:1046, 1973.
2. Malaisse, W., and Malaisse-Lagae, F.: *Nouv. Presse Med.*, **1**:473, 1972.
3. Okamoto, K.: In: *Diabetes Mellitus: Therapy and Practice*. Edited by M. Ellenberg and H. Rifkin. McGraw Hill, New York, 1970, p. 230.
4. Rerup, C. C.: *Pharmacol. Rev.*, **22**:485, 1970.
5. Fischer, L. J., and Rickert, D. E.: *Crit. Rev. Toxicol.*, **3**:231, 1975.
6. Lazarus, S. S., and Volk, B.: In: *The Pancreas in Human and Experimental Diabetes*. Grune & Stratton, New York, 1962, pp. 78, 82, 102, 141.
7. Rakieten, N., Rakieten, M. C., and Nadkarni, M. W.: *Cancer Chemother. Rep.*, **29**:91, 1963.
8. Rudas, B.: *Arzneimettel-Forschung (Drug Res.)*, **22**:830, 1972.
9. Hoftiezer, V.: A Comparison of Streptozotocin and Alloxan-Induced Diabetes in the rat. Univ. of Minnesota, Ph.D. Thesis, University Microfilms, Ann Arbor, 1970.
10. Vavra, J. J., DeBoer, C., Dietz, A., Hanka, L. J., and Sokolski, W. T.: *Antibiotics Annual*. Antibiotica, New York, 1959–1960, p. 230.
11. Lewis, C., and Barbiers, A. R.: *Antibiotics Annual*. Antibiotica, New York, 1959–1960, p. 247.
12. Evans, J. S., Gerritsen, G. C., Mann, K. M., and Owen, S. P.: *Cancer Chemother. Rep.*, **48**:1, 1965.
13. Bhuyan, B. K.: *Cancer Res.*, **30**:2017, 1970.
14. Herr, R. R., Eble, T. E., Bergy, M. E., and Jahnke, H. K.: *Antibiotics Annual*. Antibiotica, New York, 1959–1960, p. 236.
15. Hessler, E. J., and Jahnke, H. K.: *J. Org. Chem.*, **35**:245, 1970.
16. Burns, H. D., and Heindel, N. D.: *Org. Prep. Proced. Int.*, **6**:259, 1974.
17. Herr, R. R., Jahnke, H. K., and Argoudelis, A. D.: *J. Amer. Chem. Soc.*, **89**:4808, 1967.
18. Bannister, B.: *J. Antibiot.*, **25**:2677, 1972.
19. Anderson, T., McMenamin, M., and Schein, P. S.: *Biochem. Pharmacol.*, **24**:746, 1975.
20. Wilander, E.: Thesis: On the Development of Diabetes Mellitus in Chinese hamsters given streptozotocin and N-nitroso-methylurea. Institute of Pathol., Univ. of Uppsala and Umea, 1974.
21. Gunnarsson, R., Berne, C., and Hellerström, C.: *Biochem. J.*, **140**:487, 1974.
22. Junod, A., Lambert, A. E., Orci, L., Pictet, R., Gonet, A. E., and Renold, A. E.: *Proc. Soc. Exp. Biol. Med.*, **126**:201, 1967.
23. Junod, A., Lambert, A. E., Stauffacher, W., and Renold, A. E.: *J. Clin. Invest.*, **48**:2129, 1969.
24. Gans, J. H., and Cater, M. R.: *Life Sci.*, **10**:301, 1971.
25. Schein, P. S., Rakieten, N., Cooney, D. A., Davis, R., and Vernon, M. L.: *Proc. Soc. Exp. Biol. Med.*, **143**:514, 1973.
26. Mintz, D. H., Chez, R. A., and Hutchinson, D. L.: *J. Clin. Invest.*, **51**:837, 1972.
27. Pitkin, R. M., and Reynolds, W. A.: *Diabetes*, **19**:85, 1970.
28. Howard, C. F.: *Diabetes*, **21**:138, 1972.
29. Alexander, D. P., Britton, H. G., Cohen, N. M., Mashiter, K., Nixon, D. A., and Smith, F. G.: *Biol. Neonate*, **17**:381, 1971.
30. Sibay, T. M., Hausler, H. R., and Hayes, J. A.: *Ann. Ophthalmol.*, **3**:596, 1971.
31. Berman, L. D., Hayes, J. A., and Sibay, T. M.: *J. Nat. Cancer Inst.*, **51**:1287, 1973.
32. Richter, K. D., Loge, O., and Losert, W.: *Arzneimittel-Forschung*, **21**:1654, 1971.
33. Wilander, E.: *Horm. Metab. Res.*, **7**:15, 1975.
34. Wilander, E., and Boquist, L.: *Horm. Metab. Res.*, **4**:426, 1972.
35. Beloff-Chain, A., and Rookledge, K. A.: *Israeli J. Med. Sci.*, **8**:808, 1972.
36. Findlay, J. A., and Rookledge, K. A., Beloff-Chain, A., and Lever, J. D.: *J. Endocrinol.*, **56**:571, 1973.
37. Petersson, B., Hellerström, C., and Gunnarsson, R.: *Horm. Metab. Res.*, **2**:313, 1970.
38. Kushner, B., Lazar, M., Furman, M., Lieberman, T. W., and Leopold, I. H.: *Diabetes*, **18**:542, 1969.
39. Losert, W., Rilke, A., Loge, O., and Richter, K. D.: *Arzneimittel-Forschung (Drug Res.)*, **21**:1643, 1971.

40. Brosky, G., and Logothetopoulos, J.: *Diabetes,* **18**:606, 1969.
41. Lazarus, S. S., and Shapiro, S. H.: *Diabetes,* **21**:129, 1972.
42. Thomas, N. W.: *Horm. Metab. Res.,* **3**:21, 1971.
43. Langslow, D. R., Butler, E. J., Hales, C. N., and Pearson, A. W.: *J. Endocrinol.,* **46**:243, 1970.
44. Phillips, W. A., The Upjohn Company: Personal communication, 1969.
45. Weinstein, S., and Gertner, S. B.: *Pharmacology,* **6**:129, 1971.
46. Iwatsuka, H., Shino, A., and Taketomi, S.: *Diabetes,* **23**:856, 1974.
47. Orci, L., Junod, A., Renold, A. E., and Rouiller, A. E.: *4th Annual Meeting of the European Association for Study of Diabetes,* 1968.
48. Mikami, S., and Ono, K.: *Endocrinology,* **71**:464, 1962.
49. Batchelor, B. R., Stern, J. S., Johnson, P. R., and Mahler, R. J.: *Metabolism,* **24**:77, 1975.
50. Mahler, R. J., and Szabo, O.: *Amer. J. Physiol.,* **221**:980, 1971.
51. Marshall, M., Sprandel, U., and Zöllner, N.: *Res. Exp. Med.,* **165**:61, 1975.
52. Schein, P. S., and Bates, R. W.: *Diabetes,* **17**:760, 1968.
53. Dulin, W. E., and Wyse, B. M.: *Diabetes,* **18**:459, 1969.
54. Creutzfeldt, W., Frericks, H., and Creutzfeldt, C.: In: *Diabetes, Proc. of the 6th Congress of the International Diabetes Fed.* Edited by J. Ostman, and R. D. G., Milner. Excerpta Medica, Amsterdam, 1969, p. 110.
55. Golden, P., Baird, L., Malaisse, W. J., Malaisse-Lagae, F., and Walker, M. M.: *Diabetes* **20**:513, 1971.
56. Dixit, P. K., Tam, B. B., and Hernandez, R. E.: *Proc. Soc. Exp. Biol. Med.,* **140**:1418, 1972.
57. Schein, P. S., and Loftus, S.: *Cancer Res.,* **28**:1501, 1968.
58. Lazarow, A., Liambies, J., and Tausch, A. J.: *J. Lab. Clin. Med.,* **36**:249, 1950.
59. Schein, P. S., Cooney, D. A., McMenamin, M. G., and Anderson, T.: *Biochem. Pharmacol.,* **22**:2625, 1973.
60. Hinz, M., Katsilambros, N., Maier, V., Schatz, H., and Pfeiffer, E. F.: *FEBS Lett.,* **30**:225, 1973.
61. Ho, Chen-Kung, and Hashim, S. A.: *Diabetes,* **21**:789, 1972.
62. Anderson, T., Schein, P. S., McMenamin, M. G., and Cooney, D. A.: *J. Clin. Invest.,* **54**:672, 1974.
63. Chang, A. Y.: *Biochim. Biophys. Acta,* **261**:77, 1972.
64. Oles, P. J., The Upjohn Company: Personal communication, 1975.
65. Grodsky, G. M., Fanska, R., West, L., and Manning, M.: *Science,* **186**:536, 1974.
66. Niki, A., Niki, H., Miwa, I., and Okuda, J.: *Science,* **186**:150, 1974.
67. Rossini, A. A., Cahill, G. F., Jeanloz, D. A., and Jeanloz, R. W.: *Science,* **188**:70, 1975.
68. Schein, P. S.: *Cancer,* **30**:1616, 1972.
69. Broder, L. E., and Carter, S. K.: *Ann. Int. Med.,* **79**:108, 1973.
70. Schein, P. S., O'Connell, M. J., Blom, J., Hubbard, S., Magrath, I. T., Bergevin, P. H., Wiernik, P. H., Ziegler, J. L., and DeVita, V. T.: *Cancer,* **34**:993, 1974.
71. DuPriest, R. W., Huntington, M. C., Massey, W. H., Weiss, A. J., Wilson, W. L., and Fletcher, W. S.: *Cancer* **35**:358, 1975.
72. Philip, M., Ramani, L. N., and Zachariah, P.: *Curr. Sci.,* **43**:313, 1974.
73. Schimmel, R. J., and Graham, D.: *Horm. Metab. Res.,* **6**:475, 1974.
74. Culbert, S., Sharp, R., Rogers, M., Felts, P., and Burr, I. M.: *Diabetes,* **23**:282, 1974.
75. Stauffacher, W., Burr, I., Gutzeit, A., Beaven, D., Veleminsky, J., and Renold, A. E.: *Proc. Soc. Exp. Biol. Med.,* **133**:194, 1970.
76. Howell, S. L., and Whitfield, M.: *Horm. Metab. Res.,* **4**:349, 1972.
77. Lazarus, S. S., and Shapiro, S. H.: *Lab. Invest.,* **27**:174, 1972.
78. Wilander, E.: *Acta Pathol. Microbiol. Scand.,* **82**:767, 1974.
79. Shinkawa, Y., Kataoka, K., and Fujita, H.: *Hiroshima J. Med. Sci.,* **22**:447, 1973.
80. Jacobs, H. R.: *Proc. Soc. Exp. Biol.,* **37**:407, 1937.
81. Dunn, J. S., Sheehan, H. L., and McLetchie, N. G. B.: *Lancet,* **I**:484, 1943.
82. Dunn, J. S., and McLetchie, N. G. B.: *Lancet,* **II**:384, 1943.
83. Dunn, J. S., Kirkpatrick, J., McLetchie, N. G. B., and Telfer, S. V.: *J. Pathol. Bacteriol.,* **55**:245, 1943.
84. Bailey, C. C., and Bailey, O.: *JAMA,* **122**:1165, 1943.

85. Brunschwig, A., Goldner, M. G., Allen, J. G., and Gomori, G.: *JAMA,* **122**:966, 1943.
86. Goldner, M. G., and Gomori, G.: *Endocrinology,* **33**:297, 1943.
87. Lukens, F. D. W.: *Physiol. Rev.,* **28**:304, 1948.
88. Bailey, C. C.: *Vit. Horm.,* **7**:365, 1949.
89. Duff, G. L.: *Amer. J. Med. Sci.,* **210**:381, 1945.
90. Lazarow, A.: *Physiol. Rev.,* **29**:48, 1949.
91. Webb, J. L.: In: *Enzyme and Metabolic Inhibitors.* Edited by J. L. Webb. Academic Press, New York, 1966, p. 367.
92. Frericks, H., and Creutzfeldt, W.: In: *Handbook of Diabetes Mellitus.* Edited by E. F. Pfeiffer. Lehmann, Munich, 1969, p. 811.
93. Lazarus, S. S., and Volk, B. W.: In: *The Pancreas in Human and Experimental Diabetes.* Grune & Stratton, New York, 1962, p. 83.
94. Johnson, D. D.: *Endocrinology,* **46**:135, 1950.
95. Johnson, D. D.: *Endocrinology,* **47**:393, 1950.
96. West, E. S., and Highet, D. M.: *Proc. Soc. Exp. Biol. Med.,* **68**:60, 1948.
97. Leech, R. S., and Bailey, C. C.: *J. Biol. Chem.,* **157**:525, 1945.
98. Patterson, J. W., Lazarow, A., and Levey, S.: *J. Biol. Chem.,* **177**:197, 1949.
99. Bailey, C. C.: In: *The Treatment of Diabetes,* 8th Ed. Edited by H. F., Root, E. White, and A. Marble. Lee & Febiger, Philadelphia, 1974, p. 178.
100. Wrenshall, G. A., Collins-Williams, J., and Best, C. H.: *Amer. J. Physiol.,* **160**:228, 1950.
101. Kass, E. H., and Waisbren, B. A.: *Proc. Soc. Exp. Biol. Med.,* **60**:303, 1945.
102. Lazarow, A., and Palay, S. L.: *J. Lab. Clin. Med.,* **31**:1004, 1946.
103. Howell, S. L., and Taylor, K. W.: *J. Endocrinol.,* **37**:421, 1967.
104. Lundquist, I., and Rerup, C.: *Europ. J. Pharmacol.,* **2**:35, 1967.
105. Cooperstein, S. J., and Lazarow, A.: *Amer. J. Physiol.,* **207**:423, 1964.
106. Watkins, D., Cooperstein, S. J., and Lazarow, A.: *Amer. J. Physiol.,* **207**:431, 1964.
107. Watkins, D., Cooperstein, S. J., and Lazarow, A.: *Amer. J. Physiol.,* **207**:436, 1964.
108. Tomita, T., Lacy, P. E., Matschinsky, F. M., and McDaniel, M. L.: *Diabetes,* **23**:517, 1974.
109. Bhattacharya, G.: *Science,* **117**:230, 1953.
110. Zawalick, W. S., and Beidler, L. M.: *Amer. J. Physiol.,* **224**:963, 1973.
111. Bailey, J. M., Fishman, P. H., and Pentchev, P. G.: *J. Biol. Chem.,* **243**:4827, 1968.
112. Rossini, A. A., Arcangeli, M. A., and Cahill, G. F.: *Diabetes,* **24**:516, 1975.
113. Malaisse, W., Malaisse-Lagae, F., and Wright, P. H.: *Endocrinology,* **80**:99, 1967.
114. Malaisse, W., Malaisse-Lagae, F., Wright, P. H., and Ashmore, J.: *Endocrinology,* **80**:975, 1967.
115. Howell, S. L., and Taylor, K. W.: *Lancet* I:128, 1966.
116. Hughes, H., Ware, L. L., and Young, F. G.: *Lancet,* **246**:148, 1944.
117. Bailey, O. T., Bailey, C. C., and Hagan, W. H.: *Amer. J. Med. Sci.,* **203**:450, 1944.
118. Ridout, J. H., Ham, A. W., and Wrenshall, G. A.: *Science,* **100**:57, 1944.
119. Baranov, V. G., Sokoloverova, I. M., and Nikitin, A. I.: *Ark. Pathol.,* **34**:31, 1972.
120. Duffy, E., *J. Pathol. Bacteriol.,* **57**:199, 1945.
121. Goldner, M. G., and Gomori, G.: *Proc. Soc. Exp. Biol. Med.,* **58**:31, 1945.
122. Brosky, G., and Logothetopoulos, J.: *Fed. Proc.,* **27**:547, 1968.
123. *Annals New York Academy of Science.* Diazoxide and the treatment of hypoglycemia. Edited by H. Millard Smith, Vol. 150, pp. 193–467.
124. Ford, R. V., Moyer, J. H., and Spurr, C. L.: *Arch. Int. Med.,* **100**:582, 1957.
125. Wilkins, R. W.: *Ann. Int. Med.,* **50**:1, 1959.
126. Finnerty, F. A.: *Hypertension: The First Hahneman Symposium on Hypertensive Disease.* Edited by J. Moyer. Saunders, Philadelphia, 1955, p. 653.
127. Goldner, M. G., Zarowitz, H., and Akgun, S.: *N. Engl. J. Med.,* **262**:403, 1960.
128. Taylor, R. M., Milton, R. M., Powers, M. J., and Winbury, M. M.: *Pharmacologist,* **2**:58, 1961.
129. Black, J.: *Ann. N. Y. Acad. Sci.,* **150**:194, 1968.
130. Tabachnick, I. I. A., Gulbenkian, A., and Seidman, F.: *Diabetes,* **13**:408, 1964.
131. Anysley-Green, A., and Alberti, K. G.: *Diabetologia,* **9**:34, 1973.
132. Weller, J. M., and Borondy, M.: *Metabolism,* **16**:532, 1967.
133. Dollery, C. T., Pentecost, B. L., and Samaan, N. A.: *Lancet,* **2**:735, 1962.

134. Graber, A. L., Porte, D., and Williams, R. H.: *Diabetes,* **15**:143, 1966.
135. Seltzer, H. S., and Allen, E. W.: *Diabetes,* **14**:439, 1965.
136. Fajans, S. S., Floyd, J. C., Thiffault, C. A., Knopf, R. F., Harrison, T. S., and Conn, J. W.: *Ann. N. Y. Acad. Sci.,* **150**:261, 1968.
137. Fajans, S. S., Floyd, J. C., Knopf, R. F., Rull, J., Gunstsche, E. M., and Conn, J. W.: *J. Clin. Invest.,* **45**:481, 1966.
138. Senft, G.: *Ann. N. Y. Acad. Sci.,* **150**:242, 1968.
139. Rubin, A. D., Roth, F. E., Taylor, R. M., and Rosenkilde, H.: *J. Pharmacol. Exp. Ther.,* **136**:344, 1962.
140. Preziosi, P., Bianchi, A., Loscalzo, B., and DeSchaepdryber, A. F.: *Arch. Int. Pharmacodyn.,* **118**:467, 1959.
141. Seltzer, H. S., and Crout, J. R.: *Ann. N. Y. Acad. Sci.,* **150**:309, 1968.
142. Runyan, J. W.: *N. Engl. J. Med.,* **267**:541, 1962.
143. Drash, A., Kenny, F., Field, J., Blizzard, R., Langs, H., and Wolff, F.: *Ann. N. Y. Acad. Sci.,* **150**:337, 1968.
144. Drash, A., and Wolff, F.: *Metabolism,* **13**:487, 1964.
145. Marks, V., Rose, F. C., and Samols, E.: *Proc. Roy. Soc. Med.,* **58**:577, 1965.
146. Frericks, H., Gerber, R., and Creutzfeldt, W.: *Diabetologia,* **2**:269, 1966.
147. Seltzer, H. S., and Crout, J. R.: *Diabetes,* **15**:523, 1966.
148. Wolff, F. W.: *Clin. Med.,* **72**:309, 1965.
149. Tabachnick, I. I. A., Gulbenkian, A., Zeman, W., and Black, J.: *Diabetes,* **12**:354, 1963.
150. Staquet, M., Nabwangu, J., and Wolff, F.: *Metabolism,* **14**:1307, 1965.
151. Tabachnick, I. I. A., and Gulbenkian, A.: *Ann. N. Y. Acad. Sci.,* **150**:204, 1968.
152. Kvam, D. C., and Stanton, A. C.: *Diabetes,* **13**:639, 1966.
153. Zarday, Z., Viktora, J., and Wolff, F.: *Metabolism,* **15**:257, 1966.
154. Graber, A. L.: *Diabetes,* **15**:143, 1966.
155. Wolff, F. W., Hirsch, E., Wales, J., and Viktora, J.: *Ann. N. Y. Acad. Sci.,* **150**:429, 1968.
156. Lukens, F. D. W., and Kennedy, W. B.: *Proc. Soc. Exp. Biol. Med.* **70**:113, 1949.
157. Okamoto, K.: *Tr. Soc. Pathol. Jap.,* **32**:99, 1942.
158. Okamoto, K.: *Tr. Soc. Pathol. Jap.,* **33**:247, 1943.
159. Kadota, I.: *J. Lab. Clin. Med.,* **35**:568, 1950.
160. Kadota, I., and Abe, T.: *J. Lab. Clin. Med.,* **43**:375, 1954.
161. Kadota, I., and Kawachi, Y.: *Proc. Soc. Exp. Biol. Med.,* **101**:365, 1959.
162. Root, M. A., and Chen, K. K.: *J. Pharmacol. Exp. Ther.,* **104**:404, 1952.
163. Creutzfeldt, W., Creutzfeldt, C., Frericks, H., Perings, E., and Sickinger, K.: *Horm. Metab. Res.,* **1**:53, 1969.
164. Lazaris, Y. A., Bavelsky, Z. E., and Boguslavskaya, D. M.: *Probl. Endokrinol.,* **21**:91, 1975.
165. Stone, C. A., Wenger, H. C., Ludden, C. T., Stavorski, J. M., and Ross, C. A.: *J. Pharmacol. Exp. Ther.,* **131**:73, 1961.
166. Lavenstein, A. F., Dacaney, E. P., Lasagna, L., and VanMetre, T. E.: *JAMA,* **180**:912, 1962.
167. Drash, A., Elliott, J., Langs, H., Lavenstein, A. F., and Cooke, R. E.: *Clin. Pharmacol. Ther.,* **7**:340, 1966.
168. Stiel, J. N., Liddle, G. W., and Lacy, W. W.: *Metabolism,* **19**:192, 1970.
169. Bergen, S. S.: *Amer. J. Dis. Child.,* **108**:270, 1964.
170. Wold, J. S., Longnecker, D. S., and Fischer, L. J.: *Toxicol. Appl. Pharmacol.,* **19**:188, 1971.
171. Longnecker, D. S., Wold, J. S., and Fischer, L. J.: *Diabetes,* **21**:71, 1972.
172. Richardson, B. P., McDaniel, M. L., and Lacy, P. E.: *Diabetes,* **24**:836, 1975.
173. Capizzi, R. L., Bertino, J. R., Skeel, R. T., Creasey, W. A., Zanes, R., Olayon, C., Peterson, R. G., and Handschumacher, R. E.: *Ann. Int. Med.,* **74**:893, 1971.
174. Gailani, S., Nussbaum, A., Ohnuma, T., and Freeman, A.: *Clin. Pharmacol. Ther.,* **12**:487, 1971.
175. Ohnuma, T., Holland, J. F., Freeman, A., and Sinks, L. F.: *Cancer Res.,* **30**:2297, 1970.
176. Whitecar, J. P., Bodey, G. P., Harris, J. E., and Freireich, E. J.: *N. Engl. J. Med.,* **282**:732, 1970.
177. Whitecar, J. P., Bodey, G. P., Hill, C. S., and Samaan, N. A.: *Metabolism,* **19**:581, 1970.
178. Prager, M. D., and Bachynsky, N.: *Arch. Biochem. Biophys.,* **127**:645, 1968.

179. McCoy, T. A., and Maxwell, M.: *J. Nat. Cancer Inst.*, **23**:385, 1959.
180. Haley, E. E., Fischer, G. A., and Welch, A. D.: *Cancer Res.*, **21**:532, 1961.
181. Khan, A., Adachi, M., and Hill, J. M.: *J. Clin. Endocrinol. Metab.*, **29**:1373, 1969.
182. Sokal, J. E.: In: *Diabetes Mellitus: Therapy and Practice.* Edited by M. Ellenberg and H. Rifkin. McGraw Hill, New York, 1970, p. 112.
183. Assan, R., Attali, R., Ballerio, G., Geraid, J. R., Hautecourverture, M., Kervran, A., Plouin, P. F., Slama, G., Soufflet, E., Tcholeroutsky, G., and Trengo, A.: In: *Diabetes, 8th Congress of International Diabetes Federation.* Excerpta Medica, Amsterdam, 1973, p. 144.
184. Unger, R. H.: *Diabetes*, **25**:136, 1976.
185. Eaton, R. P.: *Diabetes*, **24**:523, 1975.
186. Collip, J. B.: *Amer. J. Physiol.*, **63**:391, 1923.
187. Kimball, C. P., and Murlin, J. R.: *J. Biol. Chem.*, **58**:337, 1923.
188. Behrens, O. K., and Bromer, W. W.: *Vit. Horm.*, **16**:263, 1958.
189. Eisentraut, A., Ohneda, A., Parada, E., and Unger, R. H.: *Diabetes*, **17**:321, 1968.
190. Unger, R. H., Eisentraut, A. M., McCall, M. S., Keller, S., Lanz, H. C., and Madison, L. L.: *Proc. Soc. Exp. Biol. Med.*, **102**:631, 1959.
191. Unger, R. H., Eisentraut, A. M., McCall, M. S., and Madison, L. L.: *J. Clin. Invest.*, **41**:682, 1962.
192. Yoshinaga, T., Okuno, G., Shinji, Y., Tsujii, T., and Nishikawa, M.: *Diabetes*, **15**:709, 1966.
193. Mallinson, C. N., Bloom, S. R., Warin, A. P., Salmon, P. R., and Cox, B.: *Lancet*, **1**:1, 1974.
194. Ketterer, H., Eisentraut, A. M., and Unger, R. H.: *Diabetes*, **16**:283, 1967.
195. Logothetopoulos, J., Sharma, B. B., Salter, J. M., and Best, C. H.: *Diabetes*, **9**:278, 1960.
196. Butterfield, W. J. H.: *Guys Hosp. Rep.*, **109**:95, 1960.
197. Shipp, J. C., Delcher, H. K., and Munroe, J. F.: *Diabetes*, **13**:645, 1964.
198. Salter, J. M., Davidson, I. W. F., and Best, C. H.: *Diabetes*, **6**:248, 1957.
199. Cavallero, C., and Malandra, B.: *Acta Endocrinol.*, **13**:79, 1953.
200. Lazarus, S. S., and Volk, B. W.: *Endocrinol.*, **63**:359, 1958.
201. Samols, E., Marri, G., and Marks, V.: *Lancet*, **2**:415, 1965.
202. Grodsky, G. M., and Bennett, L. L.: *Prog. 26th Ann. Meet. Amer. Diabetes Assoc.*, **18,** 1966.
203. Aguilar-Parada, E., Eisentraut, A. M., and Unger, R. H.: *Amer. J. Med. Sci.*, **257**:415, 1969.
204. Muller, W. A., Faloona, G. R., Aguilar-Parada, E., and Unger, R. H.: *N. Engl. J. Med.*, **283**:109, 1970.
205. Unger, R. H., Aguilar-Parada, E., Muller, W. A., *et al.: J. Clin. Invest.*, **49**:837, 1970.
206. Koerker, D., Ruck, W., Chidickel, E., Palmer, J., Goodner, C. J., Ensinck, J., and Gale, C.: *Clin. Res.*, **22**:129, 1974.
207. Gerich, J. E., Lorenzi, M., Schneider, V., Karam, J. H., Rivier, J., Guillemin, R., and Forsham, P. H.: *N. Engl. J. Med.*, **291**:544, 1974.
208. Gerich, J. E., Lorenzi, M., Bier, D. M., Schneider, V., Tsalikian, E., Karam, J. H., and Forsham, P. H.: *N. Engl. J. Med.*, **292**:985, 1975.
209. Sokal, J. E., and Ezdinli, E. Z.: *J. Clin. Invest.*, **46**:778, 1967.
210. Miller, L. L.: *Rec. Progr. Horm. Res.*, **17**:539, 1961.
211. Miller, L. L.: *Nature (London)*, **185**:248, 1960.
212. Kalant, N.: *Proc. Soc. Exp. Biol. Med.*, **86**:617, 1954.
213. Chiassom, J. L., Liljenquist, J. E., Sinclair-Smith, B. C., and Lacy, W. W.: *Diabetes*, **24**:574, 1975.
214. Exton, J. H., and Park, C. R.: *Pharmacol. Rev.*, **18**:181, 1966.
215. Steinberg, D. M., Shafrir, E., and Vaughan, M.: *Clin. Res.*, **7**:250, 1959.
216. Schade, D. S., and Eaton, R. P.: *Diabetes*, **24**:502, 1975.
217. Schade, D. S., and Eaton, R. P.: *J. Clin. Invest.*, **56**:1340, 1971.
218. Heimberg, M., Weinstein, I., and Kohout, M.: *J. Biol. Chem.*, **244**:5131, 1969.
219. Parrilla, R., Goodman, M. N., and Toews, C. J.: *Diabetes*, **23**:725, 1974.
220. Logothetopoulos, J., Sharma, B. B., Salter, J. M., and Best, C. H.: *Diabetes*, **9**:278, 1960.
221. Logothetopoulos, J., Sharma, B. B., Salter, J. M., and Best, C. H.: *N. Engl. J. Med.*, **261**:423, 1959.

222. DeBodo, R. C., and Altszuler, N.: *Physiol. Rev.,* **38**:389, 1958.

223. Randle, P. J., and Morgan, H. E.: *Vit. Horm.,* **20**:199, 1962.

224. Randle, P. J.: *Ann. Rev. Physiol.,* **25**:291, 1963.

225. Young, F. G.: *Rec. Prog. Horm. Res.,* **8**:471, 1953.

226. Altszuler, N.: In: *Handbook of Physiology,* Sect. 7, Vol. 4, part 2. Edited by R. O. Greep, E. B. Astwood, E. Knobil, W. H. Sawyer, and S. R. Geiger. *Amer. Physiol. Soc.,* Washington, 1974, p. 233.

227. Engle, F. L., and Kostyo, J. L.: In: *The Hormones: Physiology, Chemistry and Applications.* Edited by G. Pincus, K. V. Thimann, and E. B. Astwood, Academic Press, New York/London, Vol. 5, 1964, p. 69.

228. Houssay, B. A., and Biasotti, A.: *C. R. Soc. Biol.,* **104**:407, 1930.

229. Young, F. G.: *Lancet,* **2**:372, 1937.

230. Ham, A. W., and Haist, R. E.: *Amer. J. Pathol.,* **17**:787, 1941.

231. Young, F. G.: *Biochem. J.,* **32**:513, 1938.

232. Best, C. H., Campbell, J., Haist, R. E., and Ham, A. W.: *J. Physiol.,* **101**:17, 1942.

233. Evans, H. M., Meyer, K., Simpson, M. E., and Reichert, F. L.: *Proc. Soc. Exp. Biol. Med.,* **29**:857, 1931.

234. Lukens, F. D. W., and Dohan, F. C.: *Endocrinology,* **30**:175, 1942.

235. Cotes, P. M., Reid, E., and Young, F. G.: *Nature (London),* **164**:209, 1949.

236. Houssay, B. A., and Anderson, E.: *Endocrinology,* **45**:627, 1949.

237. Mirsky, A., Gitelson, S., and Perisutti, G.: *Ann. N. Y. Acad. Sci.,* **74**:499, 1959.

238. Zierler, K. L., and Rabinowitz, D.: *Medicine,* **42**:385, 1963.

239. Ikkos, D., and Luft, R.: *Lancet,* **2**:897, 1960.

240. Ikkos, D., and Luft, R.: In: *Human Pituitary Hormones, CIBA Foundation on Endocrinology.* Edited by G. E. W. Wolstenholme, and C. M. O'Connor. Vol. 13:106, 1960.

241. Ikkos, D., Luft, R., Gemzell, C. A., and Almquist, S.: *Acta Endocrinol.,* **39**:547, 1962.

242. Daughaday, W. H.: In: *Textbook of Endocrinology.* Edited by R. H. Williams. Saunders, Philadelphia, 162, p. 11.

243. Luft, R., Cerasi, E., and Hamberger, C. A.: *Acta Endocrinol.,* **56**:593, 1967.

244. Luft, R., and Cerasi, E.: *Diabetologia,* **4**:1, 1968.

245. Bates, R. W.: In: *Diabetes, Proceedings of the 7th Congress of the International Diabetes Federation.* Edited by R. R. Rodriguez, and J. Vallance-Owen. Excerpta Medica, New York, 1971, p. 757.

246. Bates, R. W., and Garrison, M. M.: *Endocrinology,* **81**:527, 1967.

247. Bishop, J. S., Steele, R., Altszuler, N., Rathgeb, I., Bjerknes, C., and DeBodo, R. C.: *Amer. J. Physiol.,* **212**:272, 1967.

248. Altszuler, N., Steele, R., Dunn, A., Wall, J. S., and DeBodo, R. C.: *Amer. J. Physiol.,* **196**:231, 1959.

249. Kipnis, D. M.: *Ann. N. Y. Acad. Sci.,* **82**:354, 1959.

250. Morgan, H. E., Regen, D. M., Henderson, M. J., Sawyer, T. K., and Park, C. R.: *J. Biol. Chem.,* **236**:2162, 1961.

251. Altszuler, N., Steele, R., Wall, J. S., Dunn, A., and DeBodo, R. C.: *Amer. J. Physiol.,* **196**:121, 1959.

252. Altszuler, N., Rathgeb, I., Winkler, B., and DeBodo, R. C.: *Ann. N. Y. Acad. Sci.,* **148**:441, 1968.

253. Skosey, J. L.: In: *Protein and Polypeptide Hormones.* Edited by J. Margoulies. Excerpta Medica, Amsterdam, 1969, p. 116.

254. Conn, J. W., and Fajans, S. S.: *Metabolism,* **5**:114, 1956.

255. Thorn, G. W., Renold, A. E., and Cahill, G. F.: *Diabetes,* **8**:337, 1959.

256. Beck, J. C., and McGarry, E. E.: *Brit. Med. Bull.,* **18**:134, 1962.

257. Hartman, F. A., and Brownell, K. A.: *Proc. Soc. Exp. Biol. Med.,* **31**:834, 1934.

258. Long, C. N. H., and Lukens, F. D. W.: *J. Exp. Med.,* **63**:465, 1936.

259. Long, C. N. H., Lukens, F. D. W., and Dohan, F. C.: *Proc. Soc. Exp. Biol. Med.,* **36**:553, 1937.

260. Bierry, H., and Mallorizel, L.: *C. R. Soc. Biol.,* **65**:232, 1908.

261. Porges, O.: *Z. Kin. Med.,* **69**:341, 1909.

262. Long, C. N. H., Katzin, B., and Fry, E. G.: *Endocrinology*, **26**:309, 1940.
263. Sprague, R. G., Hayles, A. B., Power, M. H., Mason, H. L., and Bennett, W. A.: *J. Clin. Endocrinol.*, **10**:289, 1950.
264. Plotz, C. M., Knowlton, A. I., and Ragan, C.: *Amer. J. Med.*, **13**:597, 1952.
265. Volk, B. W., and Lazarus, S. S.: *Diabetes*, **12**:162, 1963.
266. Kobernick, S. D., and More, R. H.: *Proc. Soc. Exp. Biol. Med.*, **74**:602, 1950.
267. Ingle, D. J., and Thorn, G. W.: *Amer. J. Physiol.*, **132**:670, 1941.
268. Abelove, W. A., and Paschkis, K. E.: *Endocrinology*, **55**:637, 1954.
269. Pincus, J. B., Natelson, S., and Logovoy, J. K.: *Proc. Soc. Exp. Biol. Med.*, **78**:24, 1951.
270. Hausberger, F. X., and Ramsay, A. J.: *Endocrinology*, **53**:423, 1953.
271. Campbell, J., Rastogi, K. S., and Hausler, H. R.: *Endocrinol.*, **79**:749, 1966.
272. Lazarus, S. S., and Bencosme, S. A.: *Proc. Soc. Exp. Biol. Med.*, **89**:114, 1955.
273. Azuma, T., and Eisenstein, A. B.: *Endocrinol.*, **75**:521, 1964.
274. Sirek, O. V., and Best, C. H.: *Proc. Soc. Exp. Biol. Med.*, **80**:594, 1952.
275. Spellacy, W. N., and Carlson, K. L.: *Amer. J. Obstet. Gynecol.*, **95**:474, 1966.
276. Conn, J. W., Louis, L. H., and Johnston, M. W.: *J. Lab. Clin Med.*, **34**:255, 1947.
277. Bunim, J. J., Kaltman, A. J., and McEwen, C.: *Amer. J. Med.*, **12**:125, 1952.
278. Welt, I. D., Stetten, D., Ingle, D. J., and Morley, E. H.: *J. Biol. Chem.*, **197**:57, 1952.
279. Uete, T., and Ashmore, J.: *J. Biol. Chem.*, **238**:2906, 1963.
280. Haynes, R. C.: *Endocrinology*, **71**:399, 1962.
281. Glenn, E. M., Bowman, B. J., Bayer, R. B., and Meyer, C. E.: *Endocrinology*, **68**:386, 1961.
282. Munck, A.: *Biochim, Biophys. Acta*, **57**:318, 1962.
283. Kupperman, H. S., Persky, M., Linsk, J., Isaacs, M., and Rosenbluth, M.: *Ann. N. Y. Acad. Sci.*, **61**:494, 1955.
284. Persky, M., Linsk, J., Isaacs, M., Jenkins, J. P., Rosenbluth, M., and Kupperman, H. S.: *J. Clin. Endocrinol. Med.*, **15**:1247, 1955.
285. Burns, T. W., Engel, F. L., Viau, A., Scott, J. L., Hollingsworth, D. R., and Werk, E.: *J. Clin. Invest.*, **32**:781, 1953.
286. Lazarus, S. S., and Bencosme, S. A.: *Amer. J. Clin. Pathol.*, **26**:1146, 1956.
287. Volk, B. W., and Lazarus, S. S.: *Amer. J. Pathol.*, **34**:121, 1958.
288. Hausberger, F. X., and Ramsay, A. J.: *Endocrinology*, **56**:533, 1955.
289. Houssay, B. A., Hartman, L. F., and Cardeza, A. F.: *Proc. Soc. Exp. Biol. Med.*, **30**:33, 1954.
290. Abrams, G. D., Baker, B. L., Ingle, D. J., and Li, C. H.: *Endocrinol.*, **53**:252, 1953.
291. Thorn, G. W., Renold, A. E., and Cahill, C. F.: *Diabetes*, **8**:337, 1959.
292. Himms-Hagen, J.: *Pharmacol. Rev.*, **19**:367, 1967.
293. DeBodo, R. C., and Altszuler, N.: *Physiol. Rev.*, **38**:389, 1958.
294. Ellis, S.: *Pharmacol. Rev.*, **8**:485, 1956.
295. Hillestad, L., and Brodwall, E.: *Acta Med. Scand.*, **187**:313, 1970.
296. Spergel, G., Bleicher, S. J., and Ertel, N. H.: *N. Engl. J. Med.*, **278**:803, 1968.
297. Duncan, L. E., Semans, J. H., and Howard, J. E.: *Ann. Int. Med.*, **20**:815, 1944.
298. Goldner, M. G.: *J. Clin. Endo. Med.*, **7**:716, 1947.
299. Bloom, W. L., and Russell, J. A.: *Amer. J. Physiol.*, **183**:356, 1955.
300. Cori, C. F., and Cori, G. T.: *J. Biol. Chem.*, **84**:699, 1929.
301. Altschule, M. D., Siegel, E., and Mora-Castaneda, F.: *Arch. Neurol. Psychiat.*, **65**:589, 1951.
302. Anderson, J., and Chen, K. K.: *J. Amer. Pharmacol. Assoc. Sci. Ed.*, **23**:290, 1934.
303. Cori, C. F., Cori, G. T., and Buchwald, K. W.: *Amer. J. Physiol.*, **93**:273, 1930.
304. Coore, H. G., and Randle, P. J.: *Biochem. J.*, **93**:66, 1964.
305. Robertson, R. P., and Porte, D.: *Diabetes*, **22**:1, 1973.
306. Porte, D., and Robertson, R. P.: *Fed. Proc.*, **32**:1792, 1973.
307. Altszuler, N., Steele, R., Rathgeb, I., and DeBodo, R. C.: *Amer. J. Physiol.*, **212**:677, 1967.
308. Loubatieres, A., Mariani, M. M., Chapal, J., Taylor, J., Houareau, M. H., and Rondot, A. M.: *Diabetologia*, **1**:13, 1965.
309. Chatonnet, J., Minaire, Y., Pernod, A., and Vincent-Falquet, J. C.: *J. Appl. Physiol.*, **32**:170, 1972.
310. Kipnis, D. M., Helmreich, E., and Cori, C. F.: *J. Biol. Chem.*, **234**:165, 1959.

311. Kipnis, D. M., and Cori, C. F.: *J. Biol. Chem.,* **234**:171, 1959.
312. Crane, R. K., and Sols, A.: *J. Biol. Chem.,* **210**:597, 1954.
313. Fritz, I. B., Shatton, J., Morton, J. V., and Levine, R.: *Amer. J. Physiol.,* **189**:57, 1959.
314. Haist, R. E.: *Meth. Horm. Res.,* **4**:193, 1965.
315. Gerich, J. E., Lorenzi, M., Tsalikian, E., and Karam, J. H.: *Diabetes,* **25**:65, 1976.
316. Kalkhoff, R. K.: *Ann. Rev. Med.,* **23**:429, 1972.
317. Spellacy, W. N.: *Amer. J. Obstet. Gynecol.,* **104**:448, 1969.
318. Beck, P.: *Metabolism,* **22**:841, 1973.
319. Mauvais-Jarvis, P., and Plouin, P. F.: *Nouv. Presse Med.,* **4**:341, 1975.
320. Goldman, J. A., and Ovadia, J. L.: *Amer. J. Obstet. Gynecol.,* **103**:172, 1969.
321. Gershberg, H., Javier, Z., and Hulse, M.: *Diabetes,* **13**:378, 1964.
322. Javier, Z., Gershberg, H., and Hulse, M.: *Metabolism,* **17**:443, 1968.
323. Posner, N. A., Silverstone, F. A., Tobin, E. H., and Breuer, J.: *Amer. J. Obstet. Gynecol.,* **123**:119, 1975.
324. Buchler, D., and Warren, J. C.: *Amer. J. Obstet. Gynecol.,* **95**:479, 1966.
325. Starup, J., Date, J., and Deckert, T.: *Acta Endocrinol.,* **58**:537, 1968.
326. Puchulu, Jr., F., DiPaola, G., Marti, M. L., Robin, M., Nicholson, R., and Groppa, S.: *Exc. Med.,* **140**:122, 1967.
327. Pyörälä, K., Pyörälä, T., Lampinen, V.: *Lancet,* **2**:776, 1967.
328. Benjamin, F., and Casper, D. J.: *Amer. J. Obstet. Gynecol.,* **94**:991, 1966.
329. Yen, S. S. C., and Vela, P.: *J. Clin. Endocrinol. Metab.,* **28**:1564, 1968.
330. Danowski, T. S., Sabeh, G., Alley, R. A., Robbins, T. J., Tsai, C. T., and Sekaran, K.: *Clin. Pharmacol. Ther.,* **9**:223, 1968.
331. Burt, R. L.: *Diabetes,* **11**:227, 1962.
332. Hurwitz, D., and Jensen, D.: *N. Engl. J. Med.,* **234**:327, 1946.
333. Carrington, E. E., and Messick, R. R.: *Amer. J. Obstet. Gynecol.,* **85**:669, 1963.
334. Baker, D. P., Hutchison, J. R., and Vaughn, D. L.: *Obstet. Gynecol.,* **31**:475, 1968.
335. Houssay, B. A.: *Brit. Med. J.,* **2**:505, 1951.
336. Lewis, J. T., Foglia, V. G., and Rodriguez, R. R.: *Endocrinology,* **46**:111, 1950.
337. Ingle, D. J.: *Endocrinology,* **29**:838, 1941.
338. Sloan, J. M., and Oliver, I. M.: *Diabetes,* **24**:337, 1975.
339. Costrini, N. V., and Kalkhoff, R. K.: *J. Clin. Invest.,* **50**:992, 1971.
340. Beck, P.; *Diabetes,* **18**:146, 1969.

Chapter 19

Viral Diabetes

John E. Craighead

A viral etiology for diabetes mellitus was first proposed some 50 years ago by Gunderson,[1] who documented an association between community outbreaks of mumps and the occurrence of the juvenile form of the disease (JODY).[2] Since that time, epidemiologic observations and annotations in the literature have repeatedly emphasized the role of mumps virus in the causation of diabetes.[3-8] More recently, other common human viruses have been implicated in its pathogenesis.[9-13]

Many features of JODY are consistent with a viral etiology. The disease often is abrupt in onset, and clinicians often note a preceding episode of viral-like illness.[14] Numerous studies have documented seasonal differences in the prevalence of new cases, observations suggesting a relationship to viral out-breaks in the community.[15-18] Geographic temporal clustering of cases also has been recorded.[19,20] Based on their studies of identical twins in which one member of the pair had JODY, Tattersall and Pyke[21] implicated environmental factors in the causation of the disease in a substantial number of cases.

Although heritable factors appear to influence the occurrence of at least some cases of JODY, a genetic predisposition is not as clearly defined as in the maturity-onset form of the disease.[21,22] Recent studies have documented an association between certain histocompatibility antigens and JODY.[23-26] These antigens might affect B cell susceptibility, or they could be linked to genes that control immunologic mechanisms triggered by infection. The demonstration of specific humoral antibodies[27,28] and cell-mediated immunity directed against B cells in patients with JODY is not inconsistent with a viral pathogenesis.[29,30] Indeed, the immune response to B cell antigens might be only a secondary phenomenon, having little pathologic importance, or it could serve to further damage insular tissue during convalescence from infection. The insulitis so frequently observed in the pancreases of children with the abrupt onset form of diabetes mellitus[31-35] may be an expression of a viral infection or an immunopathologic event, or both.

In recent years the experimental observation that certain viruses appear to attack preferentially cells of the islets of Langerhans has provided support for

John E. Craighead • University of Vermont, Burlington, Vermont.

the hypothetical considerations cited above. This chapter will review these experimental findings with particular emphasis directed to their relevance to diabetes in man. We will consider here models of the disease produced with specific viruses.

Encephalomyocarditis (EMC) Virus

Studies with EMC have provided concrete evidence that viruses possess the capacity to attack specifically B cells in the islets of Langerhans. The tropism of this virus is affected by heritable influences as well as by a number of complex constitutional factors. Experimental studies in several different laboratories now have provided critical information on the biologic mechanisms involved and the metabolic alterations that develop in this unique model system.

EMC is a small RNA-containing virus biologically similar to the picornaviruses that commonly infect man.[36] Its pathogenetic properties strikingly resemble the human group B coxsackie viruses and the foot-and-mouth disease viruses of ungulates. EMC infections appear to occur commonly in the wild inasmuch as the virus has been recovered from a diversity of animals, and members of a number of species possess naturally acquired serum antibodies.[37-39] Interestingly enough, an occasional human also has specific antibodies to this or to an antigenically related agent.[40,41]

EMC has long been the subject of laboratory investigation. In animals, most strains exhibit tropism for the myocardium or the central nervous system, or both. Although they infect the pancreas and other zymogen organs, the lesions produced by laboratory strains usually are confined to the acinar tissue.[42] Similar lesions also develop in animals infected with the group B coxsackie and foot-and-mouth disease viruses.[43-46] The neural tropism of most strains of EMC appears to be, at least in part, an artifact of laboratory study, probably resulting from the repeated transmission of brain tissue from animal to animal, using the intracerebral route of inoculation.

In the late 1950's, Murnane *et al.*[47] recovered a wild strain of EMC virus from swine dying with myocarditis in the Republic of Panama. This agent was infectious for mice but caused a relatively subtle disease when passaged at low concentrations by peripheral routes. Intracerebral inoculation of the virus produced lesions of the central nervous system, whereas subcutaneous introduction led primarily to myocardial inflammation and necrosis. In an effort to elucidate the factors involved in these differing pathologic lesions, Craighead isolated encephalotropic and myocardiotropic variants from the Panama strain.[48] This work yielded two viruses—E (encephalotropic) and M (myocardiotropic)—annotations referring to the organs primarily affected by the virus. Further study showed that the E variant caused severe coagulation necrosis of the acinar cells of zymogen organs prior to the development of lesions in the central nervous system. In contrast, myocarditis and changes in the islets of Langerhans of the pancreas were observed in animals infected with the M variant. More detailed studies showed that viral antigens were confined to the acinar pancreas of E variant-infected mice, whereas antigen was present only in the B cells of the islets of Langerhans in animals receiving the M variant. To this date, the basis for this unique viral tropism remains obscure.

As will be discussed in detail below, the effect of M variant on the islets of Langerhans is strongly influenced by heritable factors in the mouse. Thus, this review initially will be concerned with observations on CD-1, SJL, and DBA/2 mice, strains that develop prominent insular lesions consequent to infection with the virus. Subsequently, the influence of host factors on viral pathogenicity will be considered.

Insular Changes during Acute Stages of Infection

After subcutaneous inoculation, EMC multiplies in connective tissue at the site of inoculation. It then circulates in the blood. After 48 hr, it is found in the pancreas. Titers of virus in the pancreatic tissue increase during the following 24 to 72 hr, and by the 5th day the virus content of the organ is approximately 10^5 to 10^6 infectious units (Fig. 1). At this time, lesions of the islets and localization of antigen within B cells are clearly demonstratable (Fig. 2).[49] Subsequently, resolution of the infection occurs. By 18 days, EMC can no longer be recovered from pancreatic tissue, and high titers of serum antibody are present in the blood. On the basis of existing information, it appears that the pathological changes in the islets of Langerhans are consequent to direct viral damage to the islets, occurring during the time of replication in the tissue.[50,51]

A spectrum of alterations is found in B cells of the islets during the acute stages of infection.[51-54] The extent and severity of the lesion varies from one islet to another and between different animals in the same experiment. Many B cells exhibit rarefaction of the cytoplasmic matrix and focal areas of cytoplasmic degeneration (Figs. 3–5). Necrosis of scattered, individual B cells is observed by 4 days after virus inoculation, at which time infiltrating mononuclear cells frequently are found phagocytizing cellular debris (Figs. 5–7). Often plasma membranes adjacent to capillaries are indistinct and somewhat fragmented.

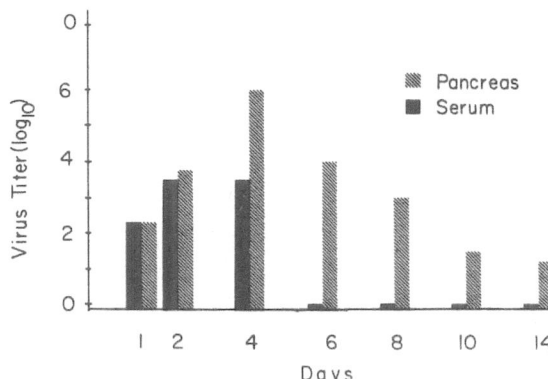

Figure 1. EMC virus in pancreas and blood serum of CD-1 mice at intervals after subcutaneous inoculation.

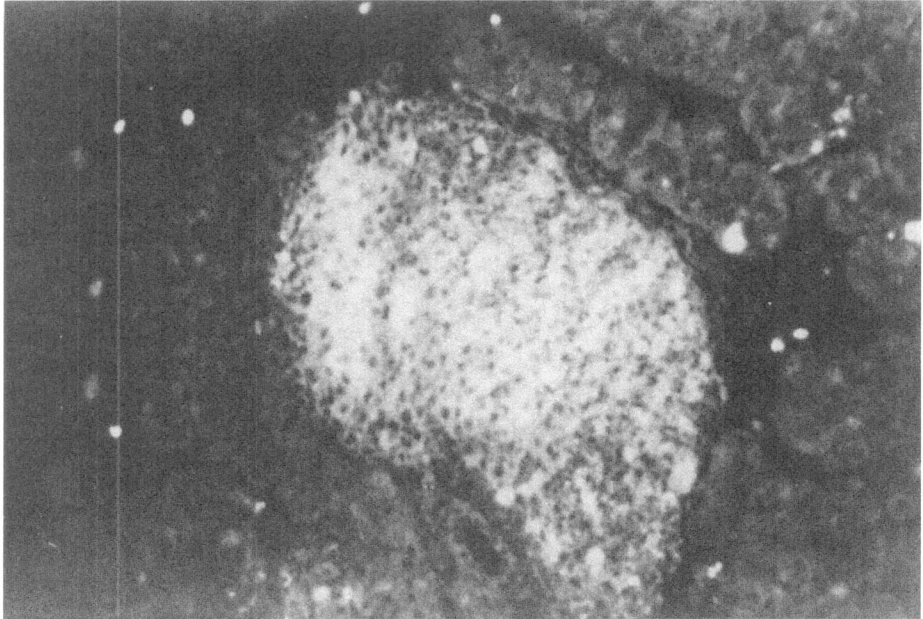

Figure 2. EMC virus antigen in cells of the islets of Langerhans of a DBA/2 mouse 3 days after inoculation, as demonstrated by immunofluorescence. Note the absence of antigen in pancreatic acinar tissue and the relative paucity of fluorescence in the cells at the periphery of the islets. The latter observation suggests that α cells that cluster at the margin of the islet are not infected. (Courtesy of Dr. Abner Notkins).

(Unless otherwise noted, ultrastructural illustrations were prepared from gluteraldehyde-osmium tetroxide fixed, uranylacetate–lead citrate stained tissue. Light micrographs of animal tissue were prepared from specimens fixed in Bouin's solution and stained with hematoxylin and eosin.)

   After 4 to 6 days, the majority of the B cells in the islets are degranulated (Fig. 8). Usually they appear contracted and assume a polygonal configuration when examined ultrastructurally. Interestingly enough, the cytoplasmic organelles of these degranulated cells appear largely intact. By light microscopy, the islets often are shrunken, and aldehyde fuchsin stains confirm the complete degranulation demonstrated by electron microscopy (Fig. 9). At this time immunofluorescence studies demonstrate the presence of viral antigens in the cytoplasm of most B cells (Fig. 2).[51] Although a critical evaluation of A cells has not been carried out as yet, ultrastructurally these elements appear unaltered and granulated (Fig. 10).
   Prominent changes are observed in insular capillaries as early as 2 days after inoculation. The endothelial cells are enlarged and swollen and exhibit an apparent increase in cytoplasmic matrix. Projections often are evident on the surfaces of these cells, and the fenestrae appear obliterated (Fig. 11). Although

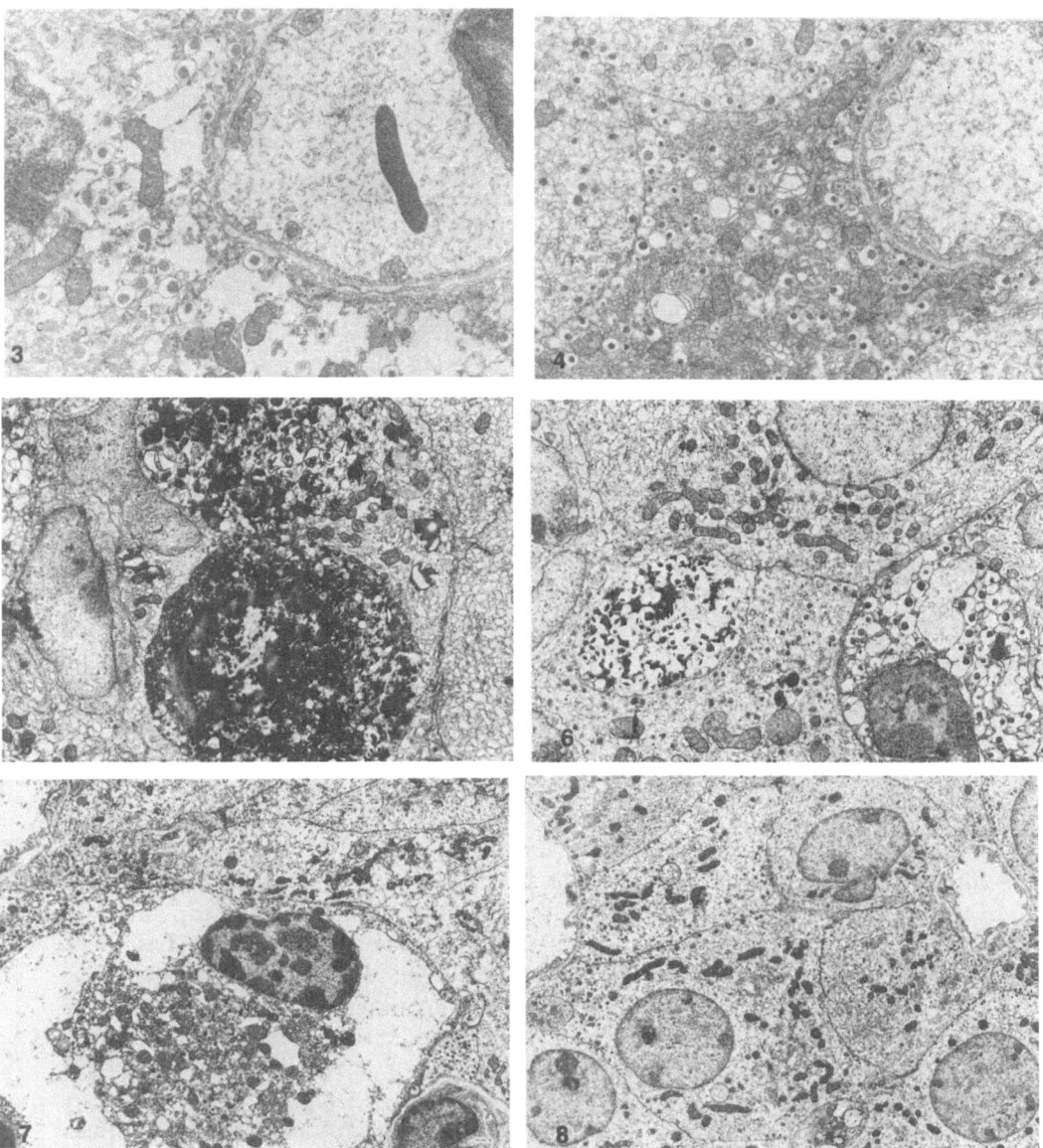

Figures 3 and 4. Selected B cells in the islets of Langerhans of EMC-virus-infected CD-1 mice killed during the first week of the infection. Note the cytoplasmic rarefication in Fig. 3 and the condensation of cytoplasmic matrix in Fig. 4. Figures 5, 6, and 7. Necrosis of scattered B cells is noted in the islets of Langerhans of EMC-infected CD-1 mice 6 days after inoculation. Note the focal areas of cytoplasmic degeneration in Fig. 5. Also in Fig. 5, the necrotic B cells are adjacent to, or encompassed by, infiltrating mononuclear phagocytes. Note the degranulation of intact adjacent B cells. Figure 8. Degranulation of B cells in pancreas of CD-1 mouse 7 days after EMC inoculation. The majority of B cells in most islets are degranulated and contracted and exhibit a polygonal configuration.

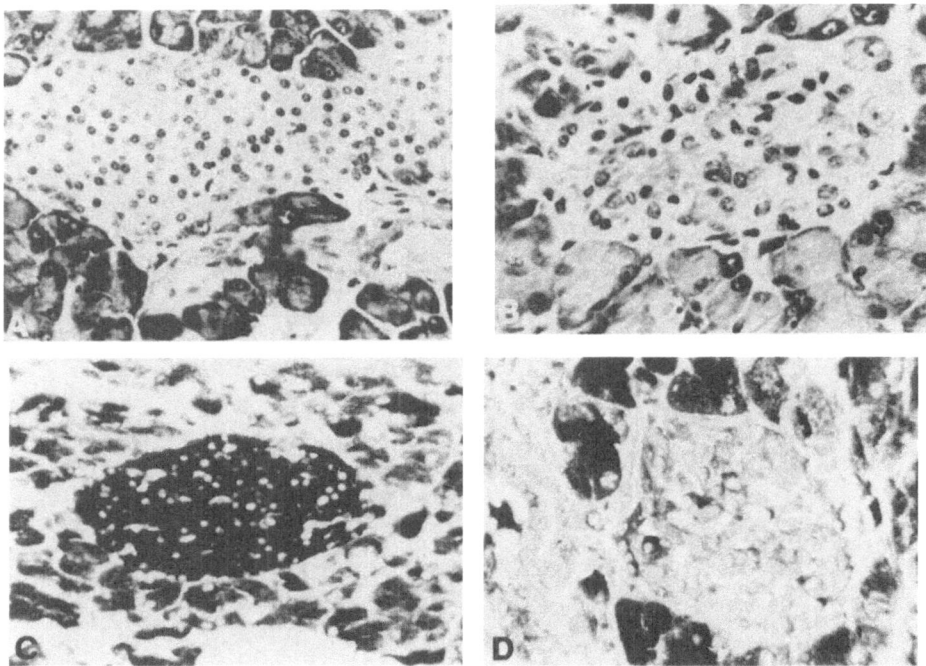

Figure 9. Hematoxylin and eosin (A, B) and aldehyde fuchsin (C, D) stained islets of Langerhans from an uninfected CD-1 mouse (A, C) and an animal killed 5 days after EMC virus inoculation (B, D). Note the disorganized architecture and focal infiltrate of mononuclear cells in the islet in Fig. 9B. Degranulation of the B cell is evident in Fig. 9D. (Published with permission of *Science*.)

interendothelial cell junctions are intact, the basement membranes of occasional capillaries are indistinct and slightly fragmented. Changes in the capillaries of the islets become prominent with the passage of time. By the 6th day, basement membranes vary in electron density and thickness; focally, they are folded into bizarre irregular whorls and exhibit elaborate, complex patterns (Fig. 12). It is unclear whether or not these changes are consequent to a direct effect of the virus and the associated insular inflammation, or a result of the seemingly abrupt degranulation of adjacent B cells.

During the 2nd week of the infection, interstitial and periinsular infiltrates of lymphocytes are found in and around some, but not all, degranulated islets (Figs. 10–13).[55,56] These cells often approximate individual B cells in an intimate fashion. The infiltrates usually persist until no longer than the end of the 2nd week, at which time fibroblast-like cells are often found in the tissue immediately surrounding the islets (Fig. 14).

A variety of cytologic alterations is evident in the islets 12 to 24 days after the inoculation of virus. Often degranulated B cells exhibit proliferation of the endoplasmic reticulum and clumping of ribosomes. Although the capillary lesions described above are evident, perivascular and periinsular fibroblastic

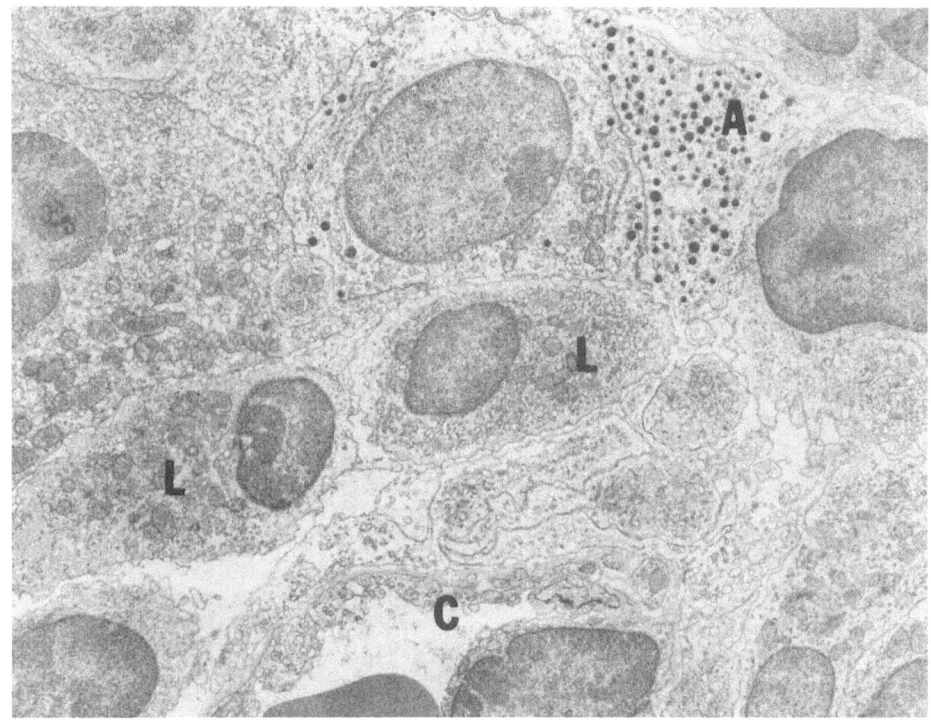

Figure 10. Lymphocyte (L) infiltrate in islet of Langerhans of EMC-infected CD-1 mouse killed 6 days after inoculation. Note the changes in B cells adjacent to a lymphocyte and the granulated A cell (A). Capillary (C).

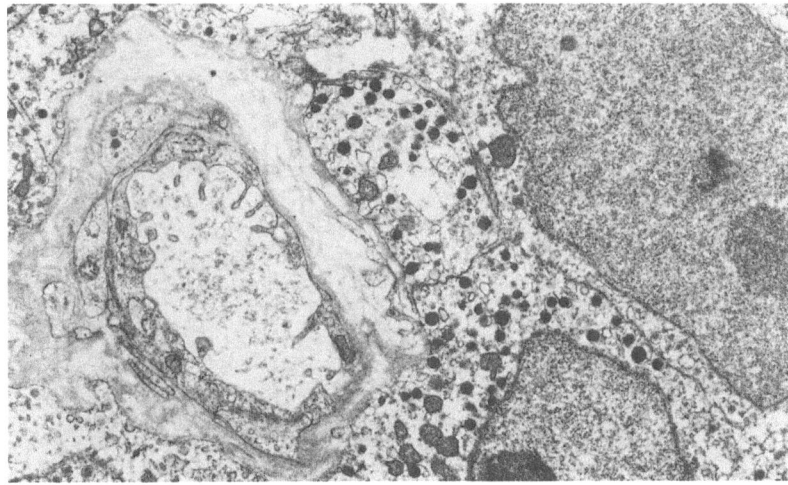

Figure 11. Capillary and an adjacent A cell in the islet of an EMC-infected CD-1 mouse 6 days after inoculation. Note the finger-like excrescences on the luminal surface of the endothelial cells and the marked pericapillary edema.

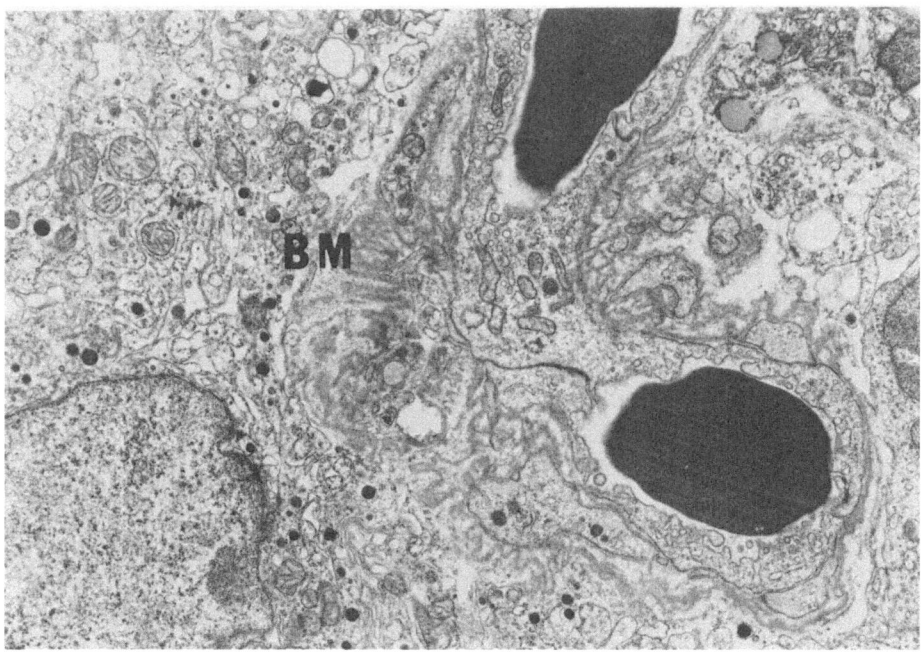

Figure 12. Alterations of capillary basement membranes (BM) are noted in this islet from an EMC-infected CD-1 mouse 6 days after inoculation. Prominent changes are present in the adjacent parenchymal cells.

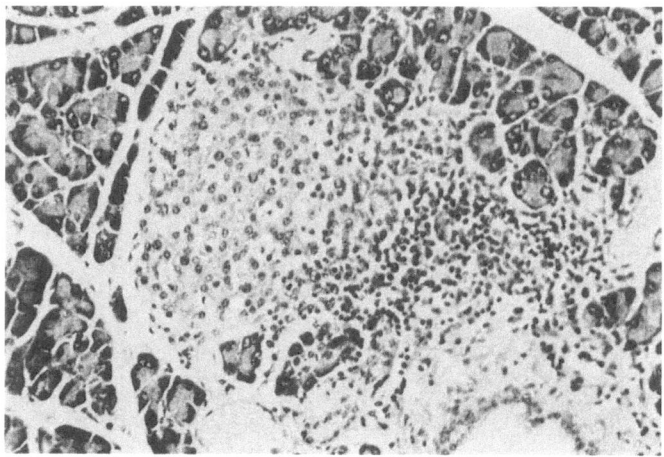

Figure 13. Infiltrates of mononuclear cells, largely lymphocytes, within and adjacent to an islet of Langerhans from CD-1 mouse sacrificed 8 days after inoculation of EMC virus. Note the subtle alterations in insular structure. Acinar tissue appears edematous, but otherwise intact.

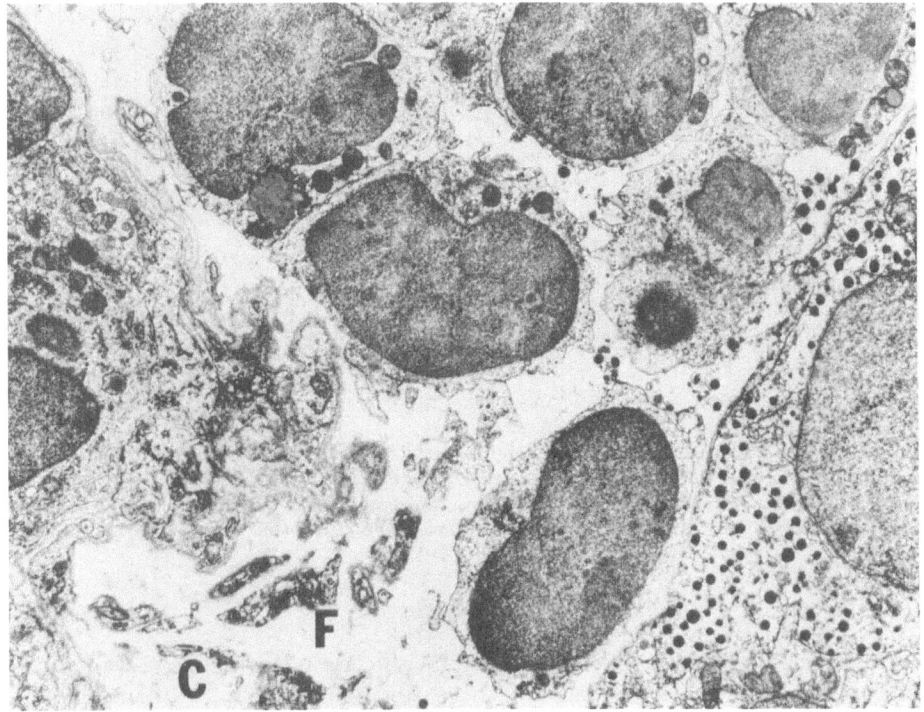

Figure 14. Lymphocyte infiltrate adjacent to the insular parenchyma of animal sacrificed 13 days after inoculation of EMC virus. Cytoplasmic processes of fibroblasts (F) are associated with collagen (C), and reticulin fibers often are found adjacent to the islets at this time. Note the endocrine granules free in the interstitial tissue.

activity and collagen deposition is seen. During the early convalescent period, dense accumulations of endoplasmic reticulum and increased numbers of mitochondria are found in the cytoplasm of many B cells. Aldehyde fuchsin stains at this time also show granulation of B cells in scattered islets.

Metabolic Abnormalities during Acute Stages of Infection

Prominent aberrations in carbohydrate metabolism develop in association with the appearance of the structural alterations of the islets described above.[50,53,57] Initially, necrosis and degranulation of B cells during the early stages of infection are accompanied by a relative hypoglycemia, at least in some animals. As might be expected, pancreatic depletion of insulin results in a hypoinsulinemia and hyperglycemia that persists for varying periods of time (Fig. 15). Since infected animals are often inappetent, and their liver glycogen is often depleted, the severity of the metabolic changes occasionally is obscured. However, during the first week after virus inoculation, tests of glucose tolerance consistently demonstrated abnormalities. Glucagon metabolism during EMC virus infection has not been studied as yet.

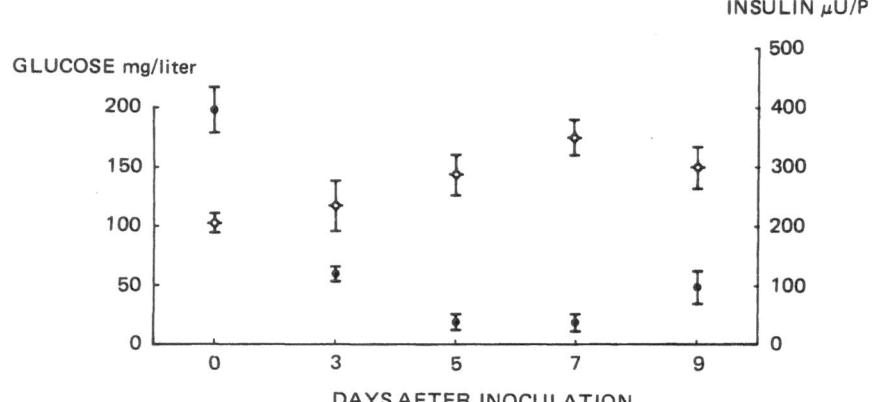

Figure 15. Blood glucose and pancreatic immunologically reactive insulin concentrations in CD-1 mice at intervals after EMC inoculation. The pancreatic insulin concentration decreases concomitant with virus replication in the B cells. Blood glucose concentrations are elevated in many, but not all, animals during this period. (± Standard error of mean.) (Published with permission of S. Karger.)

Changes during Convalescence from Infection

A variable number of infected animals succumb during the 2-week period after virus inoculation. Death of these mice appears to be consequent to myocarditis and not a direct result of the metabolic alterations described above. Thus, studies during convalescence may be conducted on animals that sustained a relatively mild infection from which they survived. Four forms of structural and metabolic abnormalities are observed in the convalescent period.[50] Some animals fail to develop pancreatic insular lesions, and tests for carbohydrate tolerance yield normal results. In others, the islets appear unremarkable when examined by light and electron microscopy, yet abnormalities are observed when glucose tolerance is tested.[57] A third group has varying degrees of nonfasting hyperglycemia and demonstrates a spectrum of structural alterations of the insular tissue. Finally, about 10% of convalescent mice manifest profound hypoinsulinemia and hyperglycemia accompanied by striking changes in the structure of the islets. In the laboratory of this author, the relative proportion of animals with these different forms of pathophysiologic abnormality varies from one experiment to another. As will be discussed below, genetic, constitutional, and environmental factors influence the long-term outcome of the infection.

Figure 16 summarizes data on several selected hyperglycemic mice sacrificed 3 weeks after inoculation.[50] The results of studies on additional mice with marked hyperglycemia and weight loss are recorded in Table 1.[50] Members of this latter group of animals were killed when moribund 2 to 3 months later. Examination of the pancreatic tissue from these mice reveals a paucity of islets which, when present, are shrunken and distorted (Fig.17). It is apparent that the B cell reserves of these chronically hyperglycemic mice are depleted. The picture resembles strikingly the pancreas of some children with JODY.

Animals with persistent, but less severe degrees of hyperglycemia or abnormal glucose tolerance usually survive for indefinite periods. Often they are hyperphagic but maintain a stable weight. Morphologic examination of the pancreatic tissue reveals a diversity of alterations. In many animals the islets appear normal, whereas in others they are shrunken or distorted in configuration. Mitosis and an apparent metaplasia of the surrounding acinar cells are occasionally observed (Fig.18). Scattered B cells are enlarged and exhibit an abundant endoplasmic reticulum but a paucity of granules, whereas adjacent cells are contracted and appear to lack functional integrity (Fig. 19). The structural features of the islets during convalescence suggest a compensatory response of the endocrine elements to metabolic demands.

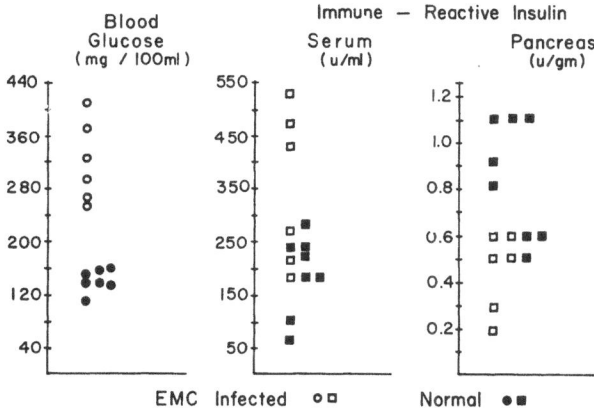

Figure 16. Concentrations of immunologically reactive insulin in blood serum and pancreas with associated alterations in blood glucose concentration in selected CD-1 mice 3 weeks after inoculation of EMC virus. In animals with severe hyperglycemia the pancreatic insulin concentrations are relatively reduced. Although circulating insulin levels in some animals are elevated, the amounts of insulin would appear to be insufficient to reduce the blood glucose concentrations to a normal range.

Table 1.   Results of Metabolic Studies on CD-1 Mice with Diabetes-Mellitus-Like Disease 3 Months after Infection

Mice	Age (months)	Nonfasting blood glucose (mg/100 ml)	IRI	
			Plasma (μU/ml)	Pancreas (μU/mg)
Infected	8	$\geqslant$500	10	0.13
	9	$\geqslant$500	22	0.08
	11	$\geqslant$500	5	0.33
Control	10	141	40	1.71
	10	149	10	1.16
	12.5	158	55	1.44
	12.5	183	30	1.28
	13.5	130	38	1.11
	13.5	144	23	2.34

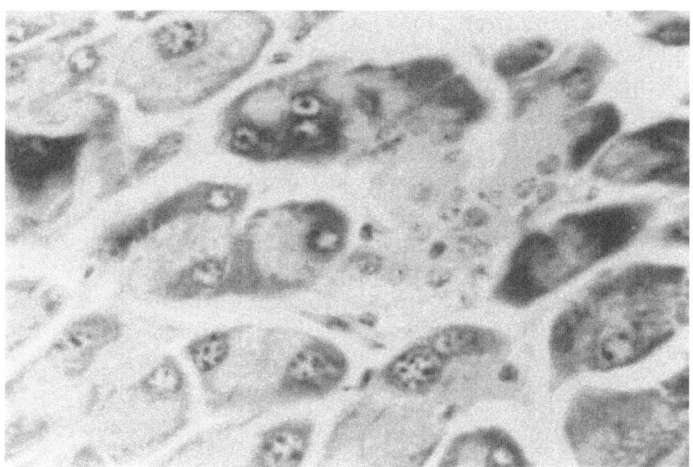

Figure 17. Shrunken and distorted islet of Langerhans in the pancreas of a chronically hypergly-cemic CD-1 mouse killed 3 months after inoculation of EMC virus. The β cells vary in size and configuration and are degranular as demonstrated by aldehyde fuchsin staining.

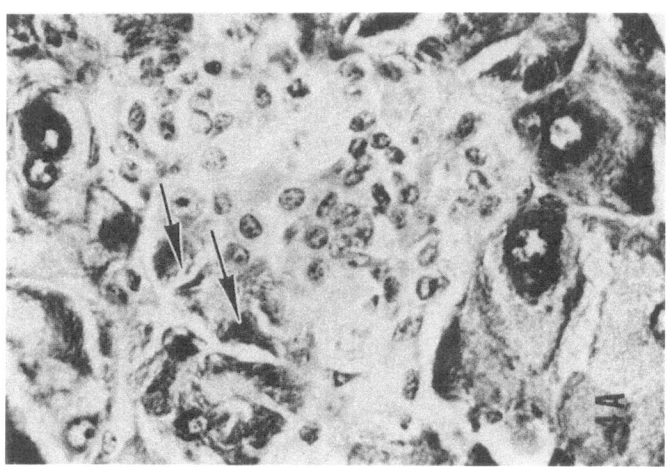

Figure 18. Islet of Langerhans from chronically hyperglycemic DBA/2 mouse sacrificed about 9 months after inoculation of EMC virus. Note the distortion in the configuration of the islet and the altered arrangement of β cells. Acinar-like elements at the periphery of the islet often exhibit evidence of hyperplasia and metaplasia to a structure resembling B cells.

Influences on Insular Structure and Function during Infection

The pathophysiologic changes described above reflect studies conducted on CD-1, SJL, and DBA/2 adult male mice. Female animals of two of these strains are relatively resistant to the diabetogenic effects of the virus, even though they develop a systemic infection.[59] When male DBA/2 animals are

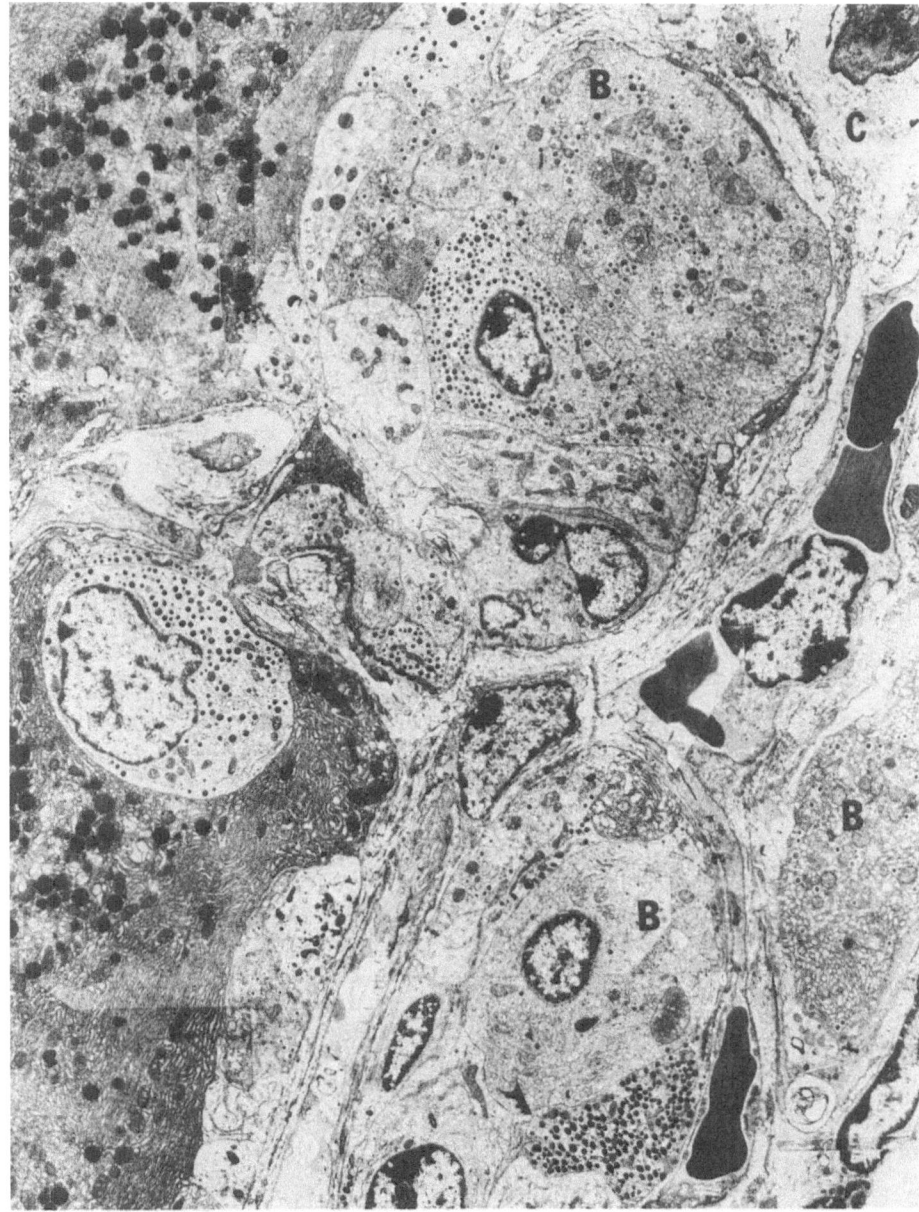

Figure 19. Ultrastructure of a portion of a selected islet from a chronically hyperglycemic DBA/2 mouse sacrificed about 9 months after inoculation of EMC virus. Note the distorted configuration and arrangement of B cells. Adjacent acinar elements are also altered. A portion of the cytoplasm of a fully granulated, presumptive A cell is observed. Collagen bundles (C) in and around the islet are present.

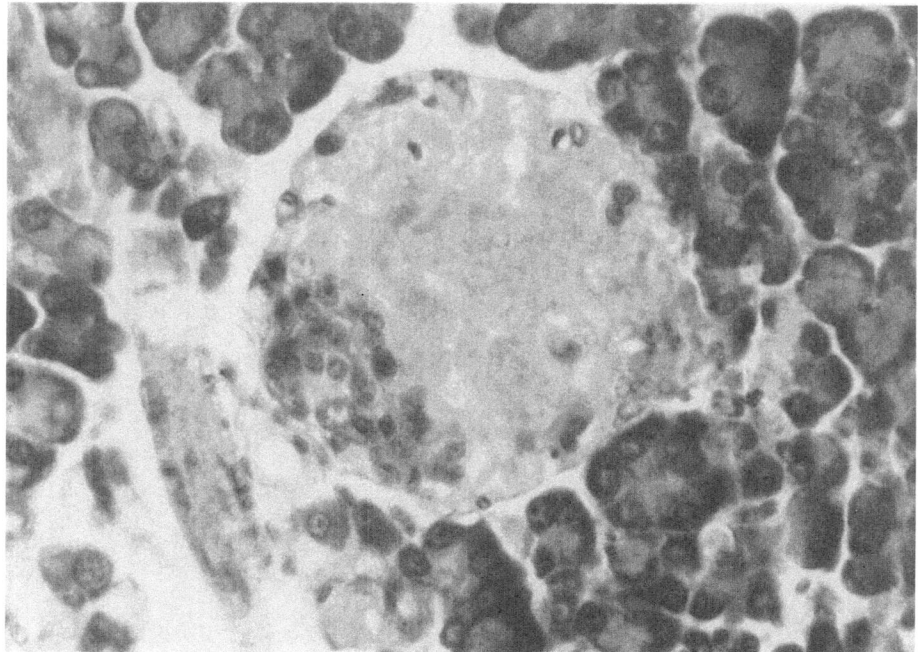

Figure 20. Islet of Langerhans in EMC infected mouse 7 days after inoculation. The animal was treated with 1 mg/day of cortisone. Note the extensive necrosis of B cells and the intact acinar tissue.

castrated and inoculated with EMC, a systemic infection also occurs, but metabolic abnormalities fail to develop. On the other hand, administration of testosterone to both castrate male and female mice results in an infection that is accompanied by insular degranulation and hyperglycemia. The basis for this effect of the male sex hormone is at present unclear.[60]

Administration of adrenal corticosteroids in high, nonphysiologic dosages before and after virus inoculation results in a fatal infection in which frank coagulative necrosis of the islets consistently occurs (Fig. 20). As might be expected, the animals are frankly hyperglycemic. Detailed studies of this phenomenon have not yet been carried out. Because of the diversity of complex metabolic effects of the steroid, one can only speculate as to the functional basis for this striking lesion.[61]

Obesity and the resulting hyperplasia of the pancreatic islets in CD-1 mice also enhances the severity of the B cell alterations and the associated hyperglycemia. This question was evaluated in the laboratory of this author by studying animals that had been infected after the administration of gold-thioglucose, a chemical that damages the satiety center of the hypothalamus and, in this way, causes hyperphagia and obesity.[62] Mice inoculated with virus 30 weeks after the administration of gold-thioglucose develop prominent lesions of the insular tissue and marked hyperglycemia. The work carried out thus far, although limited in scope, suggests that hyperfunction or hyperplasia of the B cell mass, or both, increases susceptibility to the virus.[55]

Detailed studies by Ross *et al.*[63] have shown that environmental factors peculiar to the housing of experimental animals influence the severity of the metabolic abnormalities after infection. They noted significant cage-to-cage differences when the degree of hyperglycemia was evaluated. Since variability among cage mates was relatively small, the observations suggest that social interactions between mice influence the diabetogenic effect of the virus. Although the basis for this finding is obscure, one might speculate that subtle physiologic alterations play a role.

Studies by Craighead and Higgins,[64] Ross *et al.*[63] and Kromman *et al.*[65] indicate that heritable influences have a dramatic effect on the susceptibility of mice to the diabetogenic effect of the virus. Inbred strains differ strikingly, as was shown in a survey conducted by Boucher *et al.*[59] (Table 2). Moreover, hyperglycemia develops in female animals of some strains, whereas they are consistently resistant in others. Classical genetic studies using selected strains of

Table 2.   Metabolic Abnormalities in Selected Inbred Strains of Mice Inoculated with EMC Virus

Strain	Sex	Hyperglycemic animals (%)	Animals with abnormal glucose tolerance test (%)
DBA/2	Male	65	90
SWR	"	53	100
SJL	"	52	80
DBA/1	"	50	—
C57L	"	23	46
A/He	"	4	66
C58	"	0	90
RF	"	0	90
AKR	"	0	0
BALB/c	"	5	0
CBA	"	0	0
CE	"	0	0
C3H/He	"	0	0
CeHeB/Fe	"	0	0
LP	"	0	0
C57BL/6	"	0	—
C57BL/Ks	"	7	—
C57BL/10SN	"	0	—
B10-D2/0SN	"	0	—
DBA/2	Female	14	64
SWR	"	54	100
SJL	"	100	60
CBA	"	0	10
C3H/He	"	4	0

inbred mice demonstrate a recessive pattern of inheritance, most probably a reflection of the influence of two or more genes.[63,64] It is evident from this work that the genetic influences are independent of the H-2 locus, the murine histocompatibility marker.

The basis for this heritable effect was explored by Yoon and Notkins,[66] using B cells isolated from the pancreatic tissue of selected strains of mice. It was possible to show that cells from mice susceptible to the diabetogenic effects of the virus support the growth of EMC and undergo necrosis and degranulation, whereas B cells from insusceptible strains are relatively resistant to infection. Inasmuch as cultures prepared from tissues other than pancreas sustain an infection of equal severity when challenged with EMC virus, the genetic influence appears to reflect a unique property of individual B cell virus. Either receptors are lacking from the membranes of the resistant cells, or these cells fail to support the production of infectious virus. A considerable body of virologic evidence supports the receptor hypothesis.

Group B Coxsackie Viruses

Lesions of the pancreas have been observed in infants dying with disseminated group B coxsackie virus infections (Fig. 21).[67–69] Seroepidemiologic

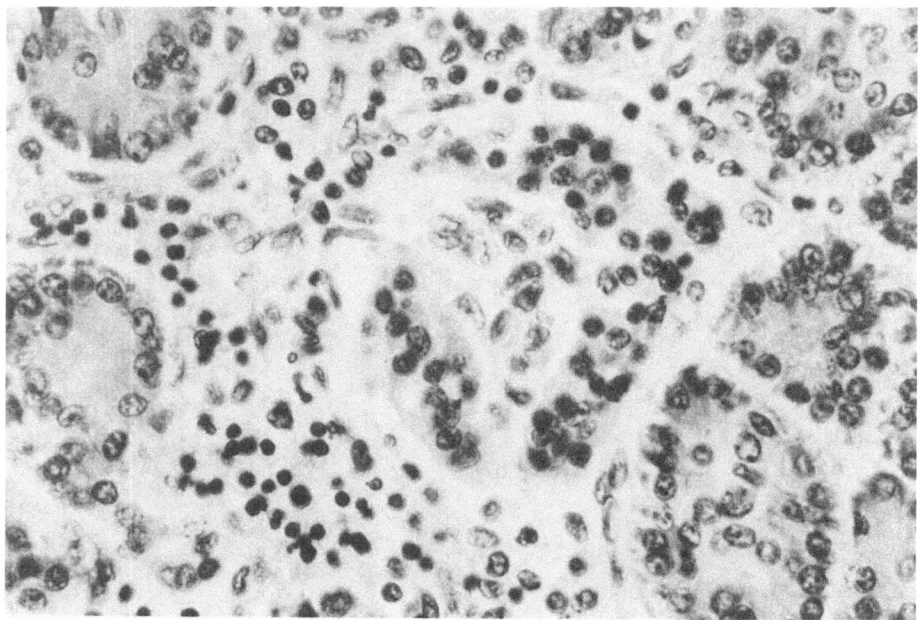

Figure 21. Islet of Langerhans from the pancreas of a 14-day-old infant with a disseminated coxsackie virus, group B, type 4 infection. In addition to the pancreas, lesions were found in the central nervous system, heart, and adrenal gland. The illustration demonstrates an interstitial and periinsular infiltrate of mononuclear cells, many of which are lymphocytes. (Courtesy of William A. Newton, M.D.)

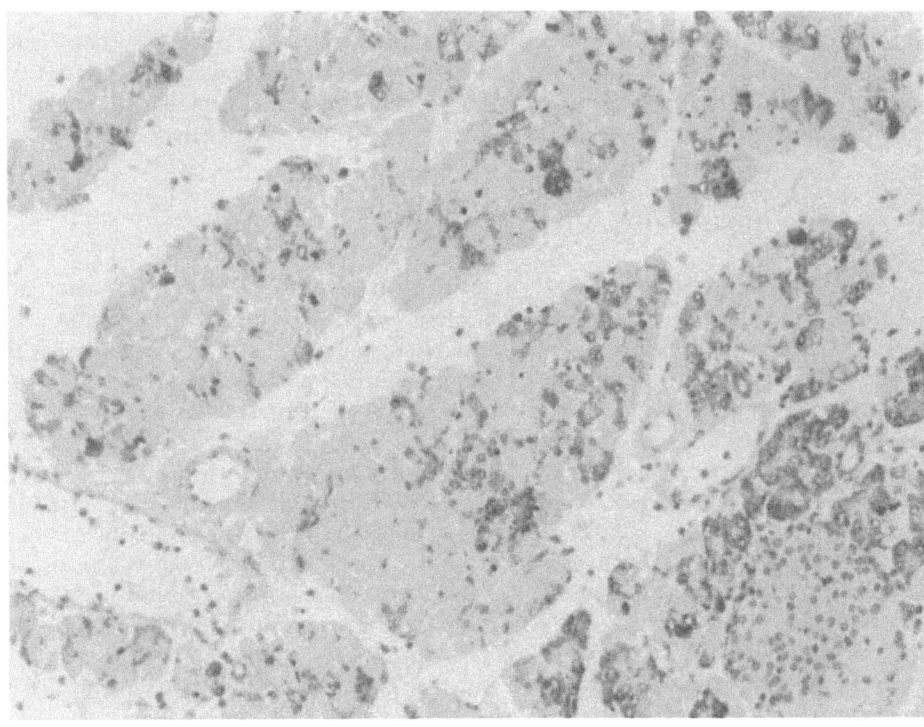

Figure 22. Pancreatic tissue of adult mouse infected with a group B coxsackie virus. Note the frank coagulation necrosis of the acinar pancreas and the preservation of the islet. The pancreas is edematous and infiltrated focally with mononuclear cells.

studies by Gamble *et al.*[13] suggest that viruses of this group may play a role in the etiology of at least some cases of insulin-dependent diabetes mellitus. Although evidence relating group B coxsackie viruses to diabetes in man is equivocal, considerable experimental work has been centered on this question.

In mice and hamsters, group B coxsackie viruses replicate in the pancreas and cause coagulation necrosis of the exocrine tissue (Fig. 22)[43,44,70] Although focal cytolytic and degenerative changes in the islets of Langerhans have been reported, they are neither prominent nor consistently present.[71,72] The passage history of the virus in animals influences its pathogenic properties and the occurrence of acinar lesions. Genetic factors in the mouse also appear to play a role, as was recently shown by Webb and his associates.[73]

Coleman *el al.*[74] reported the induction of a diabetes-like syndrome in CD-1 mice infected with an "unadapted" coxsackie virus, group B, type 4. Islets in the pancreases of these animals showed B cell degeneration accompanied by a mononuclear cell infiltrate. By 15 to 20 days, the animals were hyperglycemic and glucose tolerance tests abnormal. Ross and Notkins,[75] Loria and his associates,[76] and this author have all attempted unsuccessfully to confirm the observations of Coleman and associates. Although subsequent attempts by Coleman *et al.*[76] to reproduce their initial findings were also unsuccessful, Webb *et al.*[76]

demonstrated glucose intolerance in several CD-1 strain mice 20 weeks after inoculation of a "pancreatotropic" strain of coxsackie virus, group B, type 4. As this is written, the role of group B coxsackie viruses in the pathogenesis of insular lesions and diabetes in experimental animals is unsettled.

Venezuelan Encephalitis Virus (VEV)

VEV, a member of the arbor virus group, multiplies in the pancreatic tissue of laboratory rodents during the course of a systemic infection. Acinar lesions have been demonstrated in experimentally infected animals of several types.[77-80] Although this virus and related members of the arbor virus group have not been implicated in the pathogenesis of human diabetes, VEV is a potentially useful agent for experimental studies.

Rayfield *et al.*[81,82] studied Syrian hamsters infected with a highly virulent and an attenuated vaccine strain of VEV. With the virulent "Trinidad" strain, pancreatic replication of the virus is associated with the development of focal cytolytic alterations in both the acinar and insular components of the tissue. Localization of virus in these cells can be documented by both immunofluorescence and electron microscopy. Inasmuch as the virulent strain develops lethal infections in hamsters, Rayfield and his associates focused attention on the attenuated infection caused by the TC-83 vaccine strain. This virus multiplies in pancreatic tissue during the acute stages of infection but causes only focal pathologic changes. Because titers are relatively low, localization of virus by immunofluorescence and electron microscopy is not possible. Although these animals fail to develop changes in glucose metabolism during the acute stages, carbohydrate intolerance can be demonstrated during the convalescent period. These changes are associated with a severely diminished insulin response to a glucose challenge.

The work of Rayfield and his associates provides an additional model of pancreatic viral disease in which alterations in carbohydrate metabolism develop. However, there is doubt as to its applicability to the study of human diabetes, inasmuch as the alterations in B cell function are accompanied by lesions of the exocrine pancreas. Moreover, based on epidemiological considerations, it seems unlikely that arbor viruses play a significant role in the pathogenesis of the disease in man.

Cytomegalovirus (CMV)

Autopsy studies on infants and adults dying with generalized cytomegalic inclusion disease sporadically reveal the typical inclusions of CMV in cells of the islets of Langerhans (Fig. 23).[83-87] Although exocrine tissue of the pancreas also is affected, the extent of involvement of the insular cells is noteworthy. Both Hultquist[88] and Gepts[89] found viral particles by electron microscopy in presumptive α cells of the islets in infants with fatal, generalized CMV infections.

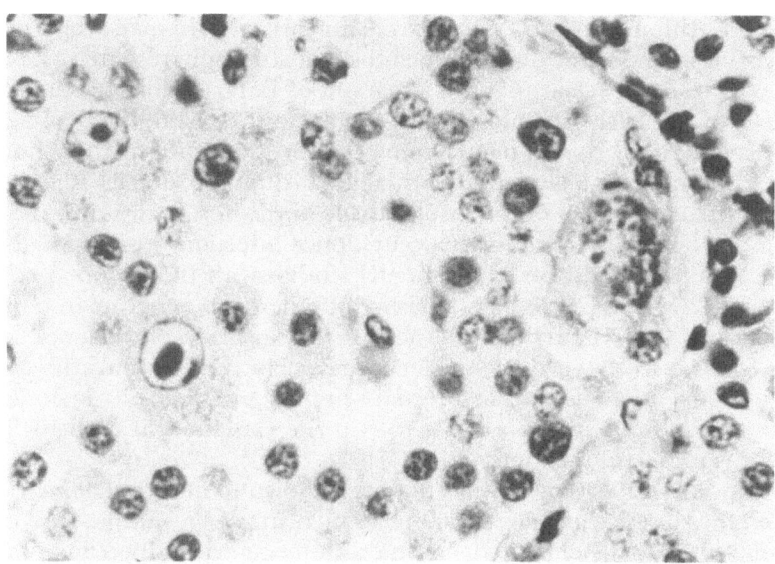

Figure 23. Islet of Langerhans from pancreas of a 34-year-old man with generalized cytomegalic inclusion disease. The β cells exhibit the enlargement and intranuclear inclusions typical of this viral infection. (Courtesy of R. E. Kanich, M.D.)

Insular lesions have been demonstrated in immunosuppressed mice infected with a murine strain of CMV in the laboratory of the writer. Animals treated with antilymphocyte serum develop a generalized infection and frequently succumb with pneumonia 3 to 4 weeks after virus innoculation.[90] The typical intranuclear inclusions of CMV are regularly found in scattered B cells of the pancreas in moribund animals, and ultrastructural studies demonstrate viral particles in various stages of the replicative cycle. Although infected B cells are degranulated, evidence of widespread cell injury in the islets is not observed. Thus far, we have failed to demonstrate hyperglycemia in these animals.[87]

Human and murine strains of CMV appear to have a specific tropism for cells of the islets of Langerhans. Because of the common occurrence of clinically apparent and generalized subclinical CMV infections in man, the possible occurrence of associated endocrine abnormalities deserves careful investigation. As yet, definitive studies remain to be carried out.

Concluding Remarks

The notion that viruses play an etiologic role in human diabetes is an intriguing, but unproven concept. It is supported by clinical and epidemiological observations in man and the experimental work summarized here.

In this chapter, studies in mice using the M variants of EMC virus were emphasized. Although a pathogenetic role for this agent in man seems unlikely, EMC provides a model of diabetes mellitus that strikingly resembles its human counterpart. It is now clear that the M variant of EMC exhibits specific tropism for B cells of the islets of Langerhans. Regardless, constitutional and genetic factors play a critical role in determining the severity of the pathologic lesions and the consequent metabolic abnormalities. Although details remain to be clarified, the susceptibility of the insular tissue of the host to the virus ultimately determines whether or not disease occurs, once infection is established.

The significance of the experimental studies with the group B coxsackie viruses and VEV remains to be established. Both agents replicate in pancreatic tissue, causing lesions of both the acinar and insular components. Specific tropism for B cells thus would appear to be lacking. Because of the common occurrence of systemic coxsackie infections in man and the biologic similarity of these viruses to EMC, their possible role in the causation of diabetes in man must be given careful scrutiny.

Although cytomegalovirus has not been shown to induce diabetes, experimental studies in mice and observations in man suggest a specific viral tropism for insular tissue. Disseminated chronic cytomegalovirus infections are now known to occur in most humans. Thus, one might speculate that pancreatic involvement occurs more commonly than has heretofore been recognized. Interestingly enough, there is postmortem evidence suggesting involvement of α cells in humans.

Experimental work of the type considered in this chapter is in its infancy. Many viruses other than those few considered here are known to infect the pancreas.[67] Future studies focusing on metabolic alterations and their associated structural lesions should yield rewarding insights.

References

1. Gunderson, E.: *J. Infect. Dis.*, **41**:197, 1927.
2. Tattersall, R. B., and Fajans, S.S.: *Diabetes*, **24**:44, 1974.
3. Harris, H. F.: *Boston Med. Surg. J.*, **140**:465, 1899.
4. Patrick, A.: *Brit. Med. J.*, **2**:802, 1924.
5. Kremer, H. U.: *Amer. J. Med.*, **3**:257, 1947.
6. Hinden, E.: *Lancet*, **1**:1381, 1962.
7. Kahana, D., and Berant, M.: *Clin. Pediat.*, **6**:124, 1967.
8. Sultz, H. A., Hart, B. A., Zielezny, M., and Schlesinger, E. R.: *J. Ped.*, **86**:654, 1975.
9. Plotkin, S. A., and Kaye, R.: *Pediatrics*, **46**:650, 1970.
10. Johnson, G. M., and Tudor, R. B.: *Amer. J. Dis. Child.*, **120**:453, 1970.
11. Forrest, J. M., Menser, M. A., and Burgess, J. A.: *Lancet*, **2**:332, 1971.
12. Adi, F. C.: *Brit. Med. J.*, **1**:183, 1974.
13. Gamble, D. R., Kinsley, M. L., Fitzgerald, M. G., Bolton, R., and Taylor, K. W.: *Brit. Med. J.*, **3**:627, 1969.
14. John, H. S.: *J. Pediat.*, **35**:723, 1949.
15. Adams, S. F.: *Arch. Int. Med.*, **37**:861, 1926.
16. Danowski, T. S.: *Diabetes Mellitus With Emphasis on Children and Young Adults*. Williams & Wilkins, Baltimore, 1957, p. 129.
17. Gamble, D. R.: *Postgrad. Med. J., (Suppl. 3)* **50**:538, 1974.

18. Gleason, R., Funk, I., and Craighead, J. E.: Unpublished data.
19. Bloom, A., Hayes, T. M., and Gamble, D. R.: *Brit. Med. J.,* **2**:580, 1975.
20. Huff, J. C., Hierholzer, J. C., and Farris, W. A.: *Amer. J. Epidemiol.,* **100**:277, 1974.
21. Tattersall, R. B., and Pyke, D. A.: *Lancet,* **2**:1120, 1972.
22. Gottlieb, M. S., and Root, H. F.: *Diabetes,* **17**:693, 1968.
23. Singal, D. P., and Blajchman, M. A.: *Diabetes,* **22**:429, 1973.
24. Nerup, J., Platz, P., Andersen, O. O., Christy, M., Lyngsoe, J., Poulsen, J. E., Ryder, L. P., Thomsen, M., Neilson, L. S., and Svejgaard, A.: *Lancet,* **2**:864, 1974.
25. Nelson, P. G., Pyke, D. A., Cudworth, A. G., Woodrow, J. C., and Batchelor, J. R.: *Lancet,* **2**:193, 1975.
26. Garovoy, M. R., Carpenter, C. B., Myrberg, S. M., Gleason, R. E., Funk, I. B., and Craighead, J. E.: *Transplant. Proc.,* **9**(1):177, 1977.
27. Lendrum R., Walker, G., and Gamble, D. R.: *Lancet,* **1**:880, 1975.
28. Maclaren, N. K., Huang, S. E., and Fogh, J.: *Lancet,* **1**:997, 1975.
29. MacCuish, A. C., Jordan, J., Campbell, C. J., Cuncan, L. J. P., and Irvine, W. J.: *Diabetes,* **24**:36, 1975.
30. Maclaren, N. K., and Huang, S. W.: *Science,* **192**:64, 1976.
31. Stansfield, O. H., and Warren, S.: *N. Engl. J. Med.,* **198**:686, 1928.
32. von Meyenburg, H.: *Schweiz. Med. Wochenschr.,* **70**:554, 1940.
33. LeCompte, P. M.: *Arch. Pathol.* **66**:450, 1958.
34. Steiner, H.: *Klin. Wochenschr.,* **46**:417, 1968.
35. Gepts, W.: *Diabetes,* **14**:619, 1965.
36. Andrews, C., and Pereira, H. G.: *Viruses of Vertebrates.* Barlliere, Tindall, & Cassell, London, 1967.
37. Kissling, R. E., Vanella, J. M., and Schaeffer, M.: *Proc. Soc. Exp. Biol. Med.,* **91**:148, 1956.
38. Warren, J., Russ, S. B., and Jeffries, H.: *Proc. Soc. Exp. Biol. Med.,* **71**:376, 1949.
39. Gainer, J. H., and Murchison, T. E.: *Vet. Med.,* **56**:173, 1961.
40. Craighead, J. E., Peralta, P. H., and Shelokov, A.: *Proc. Soc. Exp. Biol. Med.,* **114**:500, 1963.
41. Zonkers, A. H.: *Amer. J. Trop. Med. Hyg.,* **10**:593, 1961.
42. Craighead, J. E.: *Nature (London)* **207**:1268, 1965.
43. Pappenheimer, A. M., Kunz, L. J., and Richardson, S.: *J. Exp. Med.,* **94**:45, 1951.
44. Godman, G. C., Bunting, H., and Melnick, J. L.: *Amer. J. Pathol.,* **28**:223, 1952.
45. Platt, H.: *Virology,* **9**:484, 1959.
46. Platt, H.: *J. Pathol. Bacteriol.,* **75**:119, 1958.
47. Murnane, T. G., Craighead, J. E., Mondragon, H., and Shelokov, A.: *Science,* **131**:498, 1960.
48. Craighead, J. E.: *Amer. J. Pathol.* **48**:333, 1966.
49. Craighead, J. E., Kanich, R. E., and Kessler, J. B.: *Amer. J. Pathol.,* **74**:287, 1974.
50. Craighead, J. E., and Steinke, J.: *Amer. J. Pathol.,* **63**:119, 1971.
51. Hayashi, K., Boucher, D. W., and Notkins, A. L.: *Amer. J. Pathol.,* **75**:91, 1974.
52. Boucher, D. W. and Notkins, A. L.: *J. Exp. Med.,* **137**:1226, 1973.
53. Wellmann, K. F., Amsterdam, D., Brancato, P., and Volk, B. W.: *Diabetologia,* **8**:349, 1972.
54. Müntefering, H., Schmidt, W. A. K., and Körber, W.: *Dtsch. Med. Wochenschr.,* **96**:693, 1971.
55. Craighead, J. E.: In: *Immunity and Autoimmunity in Diabetes Mellitus. Proceedings of the Francqui Foundation Colloquia.* Edited by P. A. Bastenie Elsevier, Excerpta Medica, Amsterdam, 1974, p. 227.
56. Müntefering, H.: *Virchow's Arch. Pathol. Anat.,* **356**:207, 1972.
57. Hayashi, K., Boucher, D. W., and Notkins, A. L.: *Amer. J. Pathol.* **75**:91, 1974.
58. Wellmann, K. F., Amsterdam, D., Brooks, S. E., and Volk, B. W.: *Proc. Soc. Exp. Biol. Med.,* **148**:261, 1975.
59. Boucher, D. W., Hayashi, K., Rosenthal, J., and Notkins, A. L.: *J. Infect. Dis.,* **131**:462, 1975.
60. Morrow, P., Freedman, A., and Craighead, J. E.: *Testosterone affect on diabetes in mice induced with EMC virus.* In preparation.
61. Craighead, J. E.: *Amer. J. Pathol.,* **48**:375, 1966.
62. Debons, A. F., Krimsky, I., Likuski, H. J., From, A., and Cloutier, R. J.: *Amer. J. Physiol.,* **214**:652, 1968.

63. Ross, M. E., Ondera, T., Brown, K. S., and Notkins, A. L.: *Diabetes,* **25**:190, 1976.
64. Craighead, J. E., and Higgins, D.: *J. Exp. Med.,* **139**:414, 1974.
65. Kromann, I., Vestergaard, B. F., and Nerup, J.: *Acta Endocrinol.,* **76**:670, 1974.
66. Yoon, Y. W., and Notkins, A. L.: *J. Exp. Med.,* **143**:1170, 1976.
67. Kibrick, S., and Benirschke, K.: *N. Engl. J. Med.,* **255**:883, 1956.
68. Sussman, M. L., Strauss, L., and Hodes, H. L.: *Amer. J. Dis. Child.,* **97**:183, 1959.
69. Craighead, J. E.: In: *Handbook of Physiology.* Sect. 7, *Endocrinology.* Vol. 1, *Endocrine Pancreas.* Edited by R. O. Greep, E. B. Astwood, D. F., Steiner, N. Freinkel, and S. R. Geiger. Amer. Physiol. Soc., Washington, Chapt. 19, 1972, p. 315.
70. Harrison, A. K., Bauer, S. P., and Murphy, F. A.: *Exp. Mol. Pathol.,* **17**:206, 1972.
71. Burch, G. E., Tsui, C. Y., Harb, J. M., and Colcolough, H. L.: *Arch. Int. Med.,* **128**:40, 1971.
72. Burch, G. E., Tsui, C. Y., and Harb, J. M.: *Experientia,* **28**:310, 1972.
73. Webb, S. R., Loria, R. M., Madge, G. E., and Kibrick, S.: *J. Exp. Med.,* **143**:1239, 1976.
74. Coleman, T. J., Taylor, K. W., and Gamble, D. R.: *Diabetologia,* **10**:755, 1974.
75. Ross, M. E., and Notkins, A. L.: *Brit. Med. J.,* **2**:226, 1974.
76. Personal communications from R. Louria.
77. Kundin, W. D., Liu, C., and Rodina, P.: *J. Immunol.,* **96**:39, 1966.
78. Jahrling, P. B., and Scherer, W. F.: *Amer. J. Pathol.* **72**:25, 1973.
79. Gorelkin, L. and Jahrling, P. B.: *Amer. J. Pathol.,* **75**:349, 1974.
80. Rodriguez, G.: *Patologia,* **13**:297, 1975.
81. Rayfield, E. J., Jahrling, P. B., Gorelkin, L., and Curnow, R. T.: *Diabetes,* **23**:345, 1974.
82. Rayfield, E. J., Gorelkin, L., Curnow, R. T., and Jahrling, P. B.: *Diabetes,* 1977 (in press).
83. Smith, M. G., and Vellios, F.: *Arch. Pathol.,* **50**:862, 1950.
84. Worth, W. A., and Howard, H. L.: *Amer. J. Pathol.* **26**:17, 1950.
85. Wyatt, J. P., Saxton, J., Lee, R. S., and Pinkerton, H.: *J. Pediat.,* **36**:271, 1950.
86. Kissane, J. M., and Smith, M. G.: *Pathology of Infancy and Childhood.* C. V. Mosby, St. Louis, 1967, p. 92.
87. Craighead, J. E.: *Prog. Med. Virol.,* **19**:161, 1975.
88. Hultquist, G., Nordvall, S., and Sundstrom, C.: *Upsal. J. Med. Sci.,* **78**:139, 1973.
89. Gepts, W.: Personal communication.
90. Brody, A. R., and Craighead, J. E.: *J. Infect. Dis.,* **129**:677, 1974.

Chapter 20

Effects of Sulfonylureas on the Pancreas

Auguste Loubatières

In 1942 Janbon and his collaborators[1,2] reported that during clinical tests with *p*-aminobenzenesulfamidoisopropylthiodiazole (2254 RP), its administration in high doses (up to 12 g/day orally) produced, in some patients with typhoid fever, hypoglycemic manifestations and sometimes fatalities.

At the same time Loubatières *et al.*[3] undertook the study of the physiological and pharmacological effects of this substance and of some of its congeners. In a series of papers[4–6] and in his Thesis for the Doctorate in Sciences (Fig. 1) the following facts were established: (a) 2254 RP produces in the normal dog, whatever the route of administration, a progressive lowering of the blood glucose level; (b) the time course of the hypoglycemia produced by the sulfonamides resembles that produced by the administration of insulin; (c) in totally pancreatectomized animals 2254 RP fails to act on the blood glucose concentration (Fig. 2); (d) it suffices to leave in place only a fraction of the pancreas (a tenth and sometimes much less) for the hypoglycemic action of 2254 RP to manifest itself; (e) injection of 2254 RP stimulates the β cells to liberate increased quantities of endogenous insulin into the venous blood of the pancreas; and (f) this liberation of endogenous insulin can be proved by cross-circulation experiments between a donor dog that has been given sulfonamide and a receiver dog that reacts with intense hypoglycemia when it receives the donor's blood.[6]

The stimulating action of the sulfonamides on the β cells and on the secretion of insulin has been designated the pancreatotropic and betacytotropic action of this substance.[7–9] The major therapeutic usefulness of the hypoglycemic sulfonamides has been based on this action.

As stated in 1946[5:77*]:

> It was logical to think that such hypoglycemic substances could, to a certain extent at least, be utilized in the treatment of certain forms of diabetes mellitus. Indeed one can admit a priori that besides the diabetes that results from the more or less severe anatomical alteration of the islets of Langer-

---

*Reference and page number therein.

Auguste Loubatières • Late of the Faculté de Médecine de Montpellier, Montpellier, France.

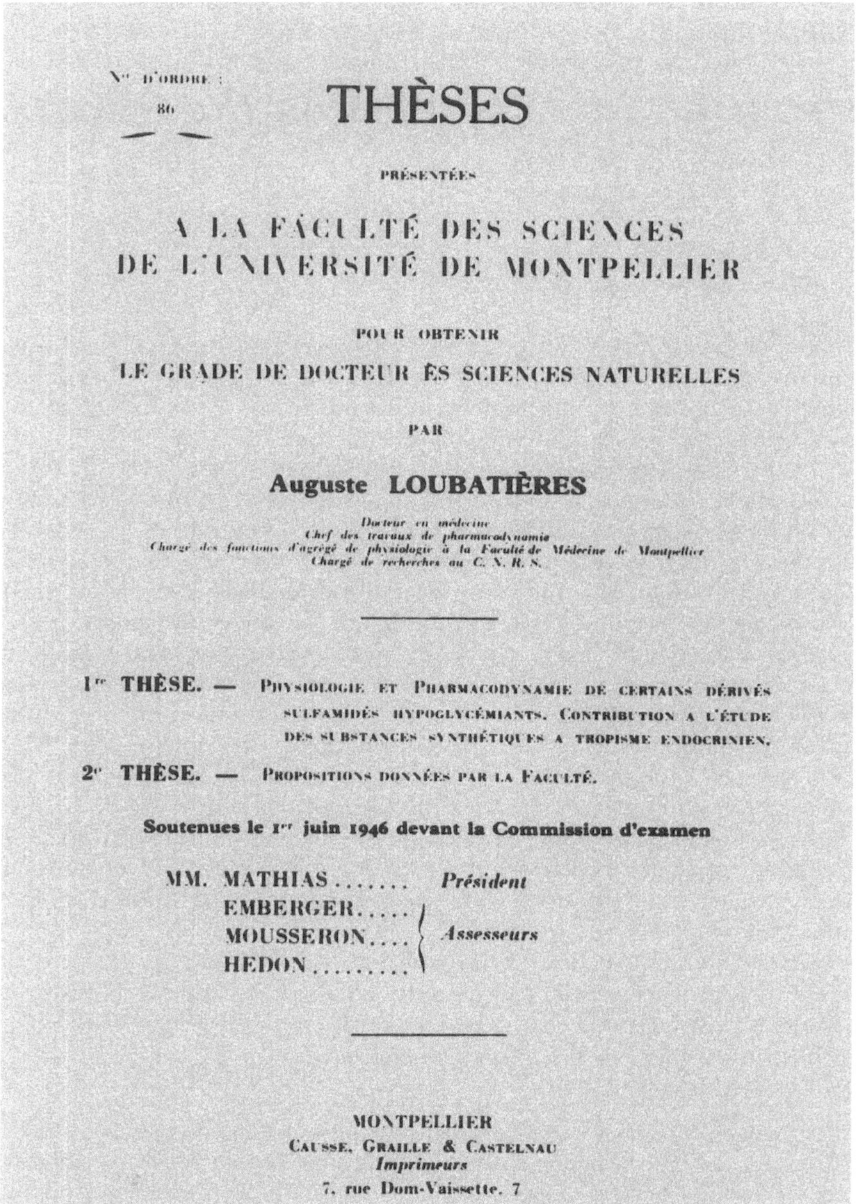

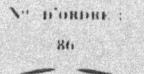

THÈSES

PRÉSENTÉES

À LA FACULTÉ DES SCIENCES
DE L'UNIVERSITÉ DE MONTPELLIER

POUR OBTENIR

LE GRADE DE DOCTEUR ÈS SCIENCES NATURELLES

PAR

Auguste LOUBATIÈRES

Docteur en médecine
Chef des travaux de pharmacodynamie
Chargé des fonctions d'agrégé de physiologie à la Faculté de Médecine de Montpellier
Chargé de recherches au C. N. R. S.

1ʳᵉ THÈSE. — PHYSIOLOGIE ET PHARMACODYNAMIE DE CERTAINS DÉRIVÉS
SULFAMIDÉS HYPOGLYCÉMIANTS. CONTRIBUTION A L'ÉTUDE
DES SUBSTANCES SYNTHÉTIQUES A TROPISME ENDOCRINIEN.

2ᵉ THÈSE. — PROPOSITIONS DONNÉES PAR LA FACULTÉ.

Soutenues le 1ᵉʳ juin 1946 devant la Commission d'examen

MM. MATHIAS.......   *Président*
    EMBERGER.....
    MOUSSERON....   *Assesseurs*
    HEDON........

MONTPELLIER
CAUSSE, GRAILLE & CASTELNAU
Imprimeurs
7, rue Dom-Vaissette, 7

Figure 1. Photograph of the first page of the Thesis for the Doctorate of Sciences presented on the 1st of June, 1946.

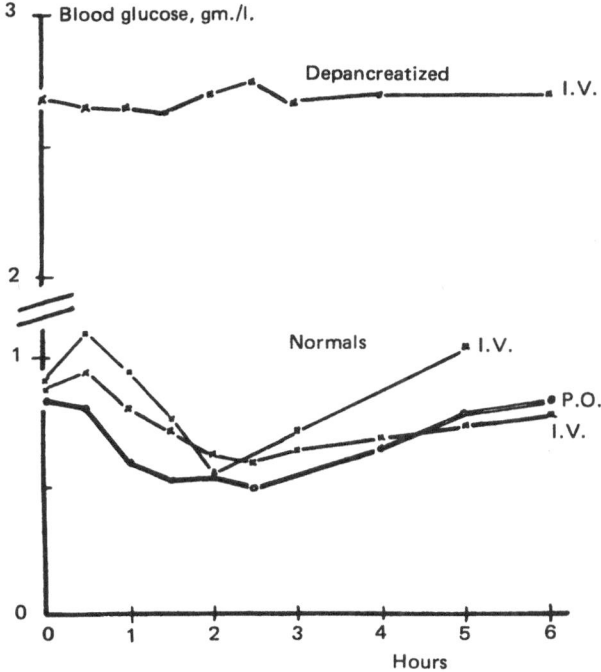

Figure 2. Hypoglycemic action of 2254 RP in the normal dog. Dose: 0.4 g/kg by mouth (p.o.) or by vein (i.v.). Note the lack of effect in the depancreatized animal (upper curve). Reproduced with permission of *N.Y. Acad. Sci.*[24]

hans, there are other kinds of diabetes that can be qualified as functional and which are the consequence of a sluggishness of the insulin-secretory mechanisms. In this case, the cells of the islets of Langerhans appear histologically normal although they possess a supranormal excitation threshold and consequently liberate less insulin than is necessary to assure the maintenance of the blood glucose equilibrium. It is in this type of diabetes that it would be logical to use the sulfonamide compounds which are the object of our work.

Furthermore, the idea was expressed[5:86] that

> ... insulin secreting hypoglycemic sulfonamides could be used for the diagnosis of certain diabetic conditions and also to assess the state of the insulin reserves and the functional capacity of the pancreas to secrete insulin.

This test is presently called the tolbutamide test.

Although this author initially anticipated that the hypoglycemic sulfonamides could, due to their stimulating action on the β cells, eventually provoke exhaustion, degeneration, and severe damage of these cells, chronic administration of 2254 RP instead produced hyperplasia of the islets of Langerhans.[5:80]

He later demonstrated that the hypoglycemic sulfonamides facilitate the formation of new β cells.[8-10] This action was called by the author the betacytotrophic action. These new β cells arise from cells located at the terminal branches of the excretory canaliculi or even from the centroacinar cells, that is, those intermediary cells that are not yet completely differentiated into either exocrine or endocrime types.

The betacytotrophic action of the hypoglycemic sulfonamides was used to retard the appearance or to prevent the onset of diabetes mellitus in animals sensitized or predisposed to diabetes by having been deprived of nine-tenths of their pancreas.[11]

As early as 1958 it was suggested by Loubatières[9] that the hypoglycemic sulfonamides might be used to prevent diabetes in human subjects predisposed to this disease.

In 1956 Loubatières and his collaborators discovered that the sulfonamides potentiate the hypoglycemic effects of exogenous insulin[12] (Fig. 3). This action, confirmed by others,[13] was shown in the totally pancreatectomized dog, thus excluding action of the sulfonamides on the β cells. A detailed report of these facts may be found in several publications.[14-17]

Even though a few therapeutic trials of the hypoglycemic sulfonamides had been conducted for human diabetes as early as 1943, it was in 1955 that Franke and Fuchs[18] as well as Bertram *et al.*[19] made use of these drugs, notably carbutamide, a derivative of sulfonylurea, in a large number of diabetic patients. In 1955, Loubatières also treated a large number of diabetic subjects with a hypoglycemic sulfonamide (*p*-aminobenzenesulfamidoisopro-

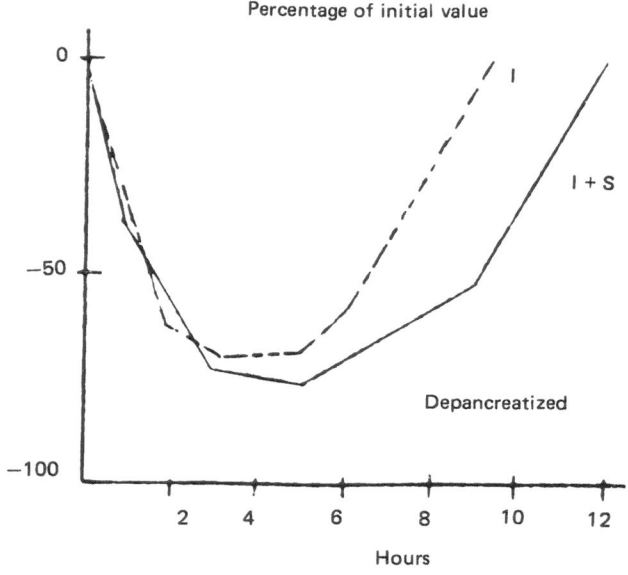

Figure 3. Hypoglycemic action of insulin (I) and of insulin plus 2254 RP (I + S) in a depancreatized dog. Dose: insulin, 0.5 U/kg, s.c.; 2254 RP, 0.25 g/kg, i.v. immediately before insulin. Reproduced with permission of *N.Y. Acad. Sci.*[24]

pylthiodiazole, 2254 RP) the mechanism of action of which he had reported.[14,20-22]

Tolbutamide, which is a hypoglycemic sulfonamide that does not possess the NH_2 radical on the benzene ring, was made the object of research by Bänder and his colleagues in 1956.[23] This product, which is a sulfonylurea, has no bacteriostatic action.

The hypoglycemic sulfonamides, no matter whether they are the derivatives of sulfathiazole or sulfonylurea, possess practically the same fundamental structure (Fig. 4). Experimentally, however, they did not have the same degree of hypoglycemic activity; glibenclamide is presently the most active of them all (Figs. 5 and 6).

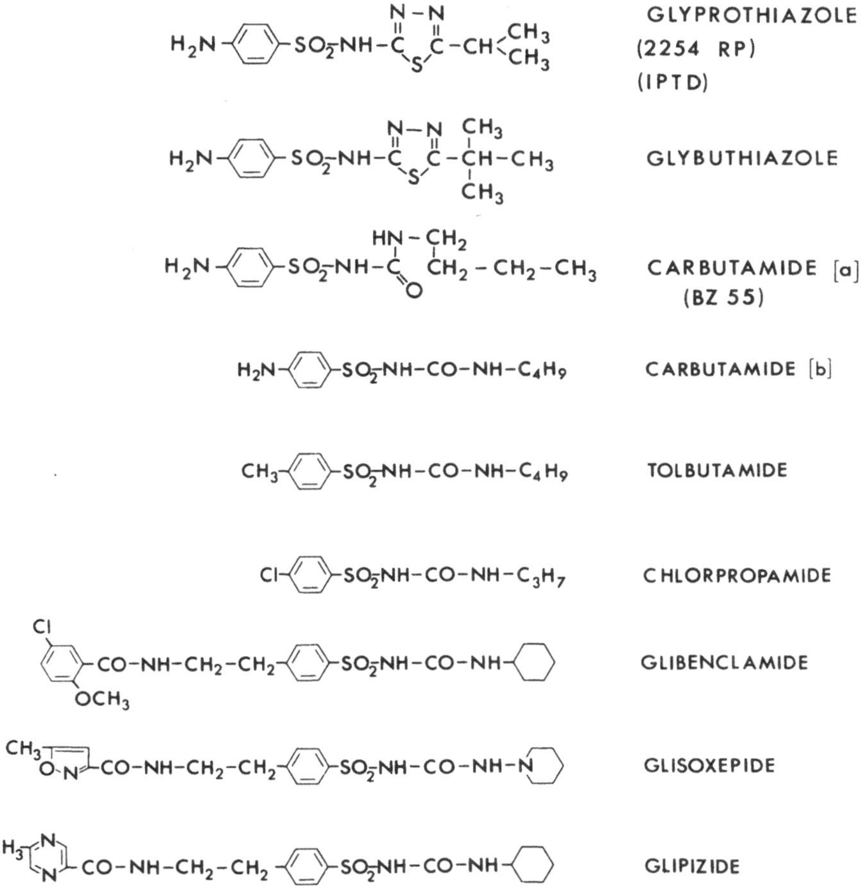

Figure 4. Sulfathiazoles and sulfonylureas. The sulfathiazoles and the sulfonylureas show similarity of chemical structure. This similarity is evident when one examines the two presentations of the formula of carbutamide.

Glyprothiazole, glybuthiazole, carbutamide, and tolbutamide are first generation sulfonamides. Chlorpropamide is a transition compound. Glibenclamide, glisoxepide, and glipizide are second generation sulfonamides. Reproduced with permission of *Med. Hyg.*[43]

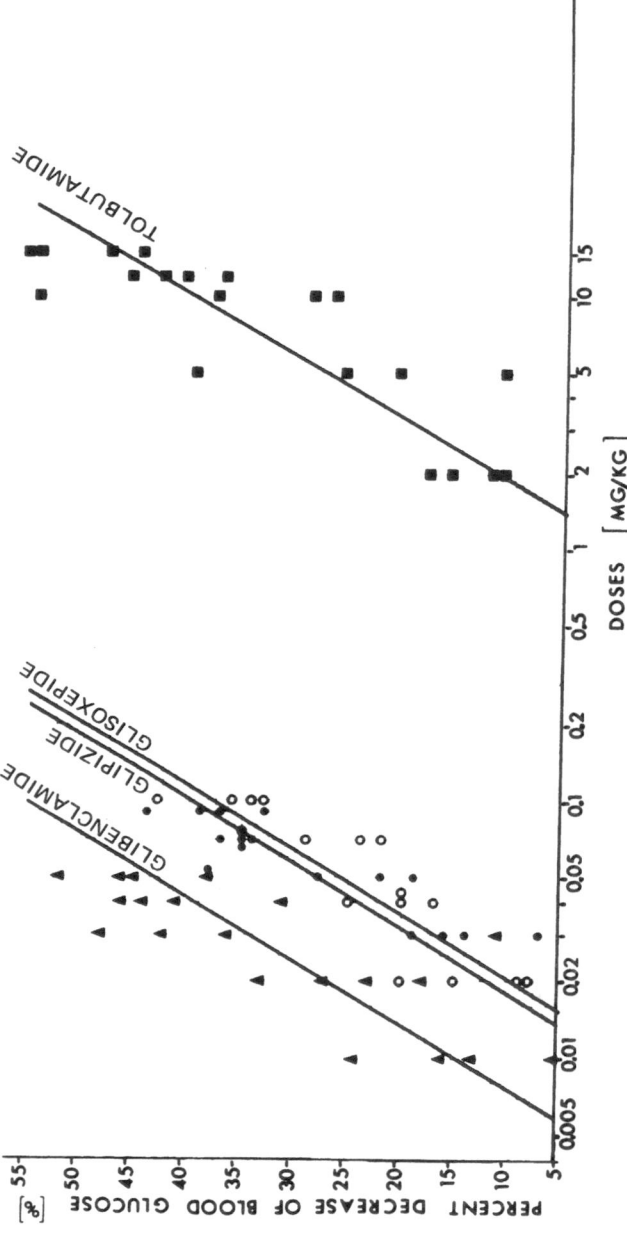

Figure 5. Comparative study of glibenclamide, glipizide, glisoxepide, and tolbutamide with regard to their relative hypoglycemic potency in the normal, conscious dog after intravenous administration. Doses (mg/kg) are expressed on a logarithmic scale on the abscissa. Ordinates represent the percent blood glucose reduction. Each point indicates the maximal blood glucose drop obtained in each animal after administration of one dose. Reproduced with permission of *Med. Hyg.*[43]

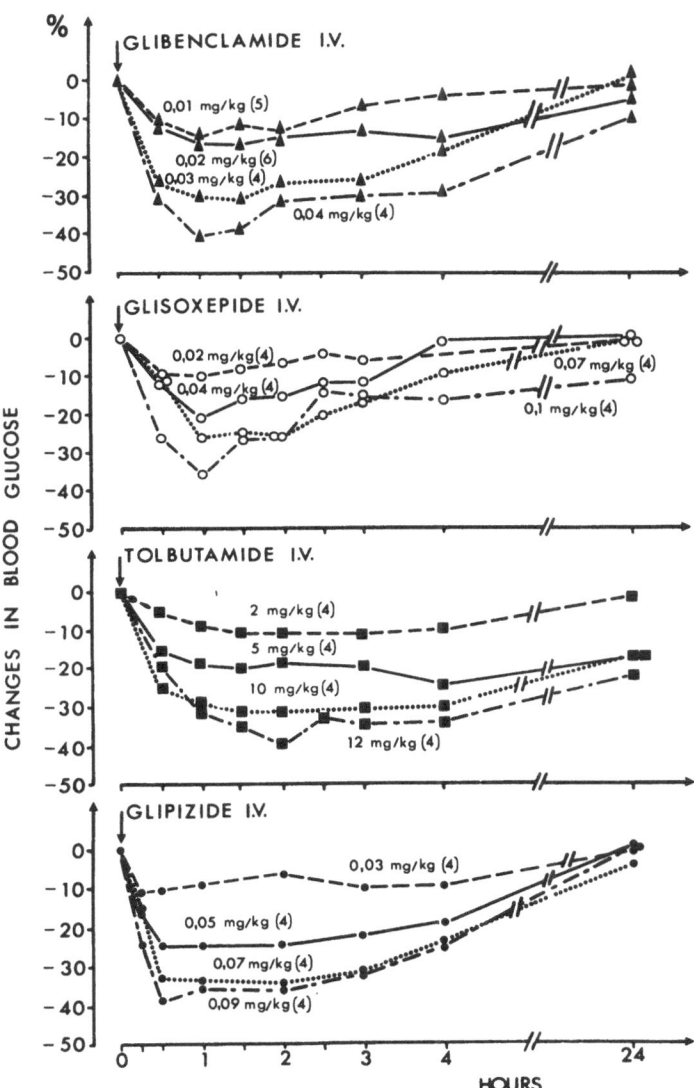

Figure 6. Effects of increasing doses of intravenously administered glibenclamide, glisoxepide, tolbutamide, and glipizide on the glycemia of the normal conscious dog. The changes are expressed as percentages of the value at time zero. The doses used in each series of experiments are indicated on the corresponding curve. The number of animals used in each case is indicated in parentheses. Reproduced with permission of *Med. Hyg.* [43]

The Necessity of the Endocrine Pancreas for the Manifestation of Hypoglycemic Action

Loubatières first reported, and it has since been confirmed, that the pancreas plays an essential role in the mechanism of the hypoglycemic action of these substances. Thus, he has demonstrated that the hypoglycemic sulfonamides are active in dogs possessing an intact pancreas.[4-6] This fact was later confirmed in other species of animals (cat, monkey, guinea pig, toad, snake, and hamster) as well as in man. On the other hand, he has shown that these sulfonamides fail to effect the glycemic levels of totally pancreatectomized animals.[4-6] However, if a fragment of pancreatic tissue is kept in the abdomen (for example, one-tenth of the initial weight of the pancreas in contact with the duodenum), the hypoglycemic action of the sulfonamides can still be observed. Loubatières has found that these substances are capable of lowering glycemia as long as a small quantity of pancreatic tissue enclosing cells capable of secreting insulin remains in the organism.

It can therefore be stated that, for the hypoglycemic effect of sulfonamide to manifest itself, the organism must contain a minimal amount of pancreatic endocrine tissue. In dogs and cats with simultaneous removal of the pancreas and the pituitary gland, the sulfonamides do not have a hypoglycemic effect. These facts favor the conclusion, advanced as early as 1944, that the presence of the endocrine pancreas is essential for the production of the hypoglycemic action manifested by the sulfonamides. Loubatières has also shown that endocrine glands, other than the pancreas, such as the adrenals, thyroid, parathyroids, gonads, and pituitary, are not necessary for the production of hypoglycemia by the sulfonamides[4-6,24,25] (Fig. 7).

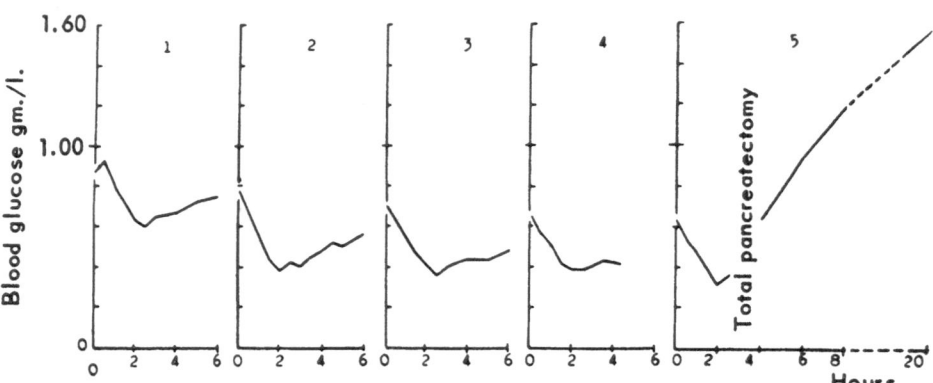

Figure 7. Effects of 2254 RP, 0.2 g/kg, i.v., on the blood sugar of a dog subjected successively to various procedures: (1) normal control; (2) after bilateral adrenalectomy; (3) after subsequent thyroparathyroidectomy and gonadectomy; (4) after total hypophysectomy; and (5) after total pancreatectomy. Note the immediate interruption of the hypoglycemic effect of the drug by total pancreatectomy. Reproduced with permission of *N.Y. Acad. Sci.*[24]

In 1944, convincing proof permitted the confirmation that the insulin secretory stimulus provoked by the sulfonamide is not mediated by the pneumogastrics, nerves which are considered to stimulate insulin secretion; in effect, atropinization of the animal or transsection of the two pneumogastric nerves do not abolish the hypoglycemic effect of sulfonamides.[4,5] These facts have been confirmed *in vitro* (unpublished experiments). On the other hand, the blockage of β-adrenergic receptors by propranolol does not diminish *in vitro* and *in vivo* its hypoglycemic action.[26,27]

The Role of the Liver

The presence of the liver does not appear to be indispensible for the production of hypoglycemia of the sulfonamides. In fact, in the totally hepatectomized dog where glycemia is maintained at normal levels by continuous perfusion with a glucose solution, the sulfonamides completely preserve their hypoglycemic action, provided that the pancreas remains intact.[28] On the other hand, the hypoglycemic sulfonamides are inactive in the eviscerated animal, in whom the pancreas is absent. It must be concluded that the presence of the liver is not immediately essential for the manifestation of the hypoglycemic action of the sulfonamides. However, the presence of the pancreas is absolutely necessary. This does not signify that the liver does not play a role in the sulfonamide-induced hypoglycemia of the intact animal. One part of this hypoglycemia is explained by the fact that insulin secreted in excess into the portal vein affects directly the hepatic cells.

The Primary Role of the β Insulin Secretory Cells of the Islets of Langerhans

For a certain period of time it was thought that the hypoglycemic action of the sulfonamides is due to a destructive action on the α cells of the islets of Langerhans, which would prevent glucagon from exercising its normal role in the control of glycemia.

Meanwhile, as the result of various experimental, histological, physiological, pharmacological, and clinical observations by a number of researchers, and even by the authors of this theory,[19] this hypothesis had to be discarded.

The hypothesis that tolbutamide not only stimulates the secretion of insulin but also inhibits the secretion of glucagon has not been confirmed. Loubatières *et al.*[29-32] have shown *in vitro* in the isolated and perfused rat pancreas, and *in vivo* in the dog, that the two hypoglycemic sulfonamides, tolbutamide and glibenclamide, do not inhibit the secretion of glucagon. This conclusion has since largely been confirmed.

Numerous experiments have demonstrated that the hypoglycemic sulfonamides act directly on the β cells of the islets of Langerhans by stimulating and liberating an excess of endogenous insulin into the efferent blood of the pancreas. In fact, the hypoglycemic sulfonamides are slightly active in the animal with moderate-intensity *m*-alloxanic diabetes. In this case a few β cells have survived the toxic action of alloxan. However, if the *m*-alloxanic diabetes is intense (which indicates that practically all the β cells have been destroyed), the sulfonamides are inactive.[14]

Other arguments based on histologic and histopathologic observations also favor the theory of action of the hypoglycemic sulfonamides on the β cells and their stimulating action on the secretion of insulin.

Administration of a hypoglycemic sulfonamide to a normal animal (dog, cat, rabbit, and calf) produces a significant degranulation of the β cells of the islets of Langerhans.[33] It has been demonstrated with the aid of the electron microscope that administration of a hypoglycemic sulfonamide is followed by a certain depletion of β cell granules, which are secreted by way of pinocytosis.

This degranulation is functional, not toxic, and reversible. In a few hours, the insulin-containing granules are reformed and are again present in normal numbers. This migratory phenomenon of the insulin granules which are ejected from the β cells and the resulting final degranulation are most striking in the cells which are closest to blood vessels.

The ultrastructural modifications produced by tolbutamide in the β cells of the rat have been studied by Williamson *et al.*,[34] Lacy,[35,36] and Orci *et al.*[37]

Lacy has put forward the hypothesis that the microtubular system permits the transport of β granules to the cellular membrane where they are liberated by emiocytosis. The stimulus which acts on the microtubular system could depend on glucose metabolism with the formation of ATP and resulting contraction of the microtubules. It also takes into account ionic exchanges and, in particular, the movements of ionized Ca^{2+} and of Na. The role of the microfilamentous system does not seem to have been definitely established.

The process of emiocytosis is probably not the only mechanism by which the hypoglycemic sulfonamides provoke the extrusion of insulin from the β cells. It is also possible that a certain quantity of soluble insulin present in the cytoplasm crosses the membrane of the β cell and flows into the intercellular space.

Demonstration of Excess Endogenous Insulin Secretion in the Blood

Experiments in Vivo

By experiments *in vivo* utilizing pancreaticojugular anastomosis and cross circulations between a donor dog treated with sulfonamide and a dog receiving the pancreatic blood of the donor, Loubatières,[6] in 1946, demonstrated the passage of excess endogenous insulin secreted into the blood of the recipient dog from the donor animal treated with sulfonamide.

Proof also exists for the increase of "plasma insulin activity" in the efferent venous blood of the pancreas in the animal treated with hypoglycemic sulfonamides. Experiments have proved that in dog, rat, and man, "insulin activity of the serum" increases considerably after intravenous administration of hypogly-cemic sulfonamides.[38,39]

This fact was established by utilization of an immunological method which was both sensitive to and specific for measuring the quantity of human plasma insulin.[40] It has thus been shown that the concentration of endogenous insulin in peripheral blood increases in man and in the normal animal after oral or intravenous administration of tolbutamide. Similar results can also be observed in middle-aged diabetics (around 45 to 50 years) who are sensitive to the hypoglycemic sulfonamides.

The problem was to determine whether the action of hypoglycemic sulfon-amides was of short or long duration. In experiments performed on the dog,[41,42] the animal was prepared the day before the experiment. Aseptically and under general anesthesia with nembutal, a polyethylene catheter was introduced into the pancreaticoduodenal vein. With this preparation, it was possible to take blood samples for measurement and to compare the duration of action of the different hypoglycemic sulfonamides. It was thus shown that 0.05 mg/kg of glibenclamide administered intravenously acted as a powerful insulin secretory agent, the effect of which persisted during numerous hours under experimental conditions of prolonged starvation[42] (Fig. 8).

Oral administration of glibenclamide in the dog, at a dose of 2 mg/kg, is

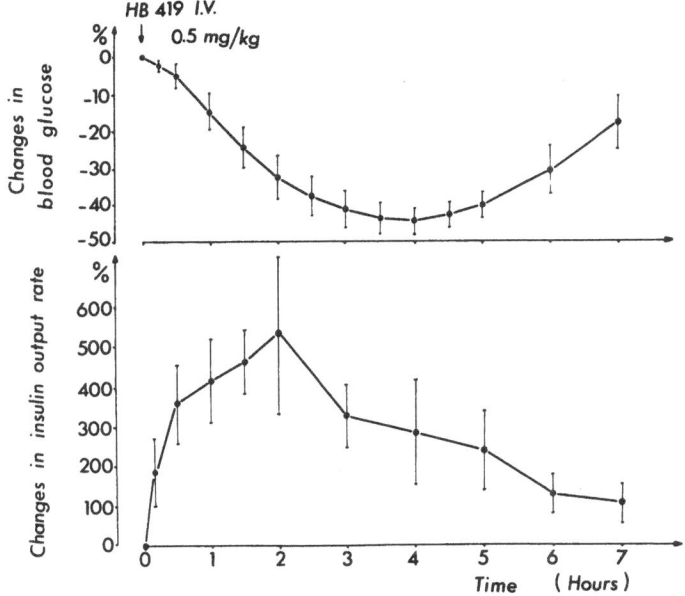

Figure 8. Changes of the glycemia in a peripheral vein and changes of insulin output rate in the blood of the pancreaticoduodenal vein of five anesthetized dogs, each having received 0.5 mg/kg of HB 419 intravenously. The changes are expressed as percentage of the value of time zero. Each point represents the mean of the values, with the standard error of the mean. Reproduced with permission from Springer-Verlag.[42]

followed by an increase in insulin secretion which attains in 4 hr a maximum of
five times that of the level of the initial secretion. After this release of insulin,
the intensity of secretion diminishes. Nevertheless, from 6 to 24 hr after
administration, the plasma insulin concentration still represents two to three
times the initial level.[41-44] Figure 9 represents the experiments comparing the
effects of the different hypoglycemic sulfonamides on glycemia and insulin-
emia. (Refer to Figs. 5 and 6 concerning the action of sulfonylureas on blood
glucose levels when administered intravenously.) After oral administration of

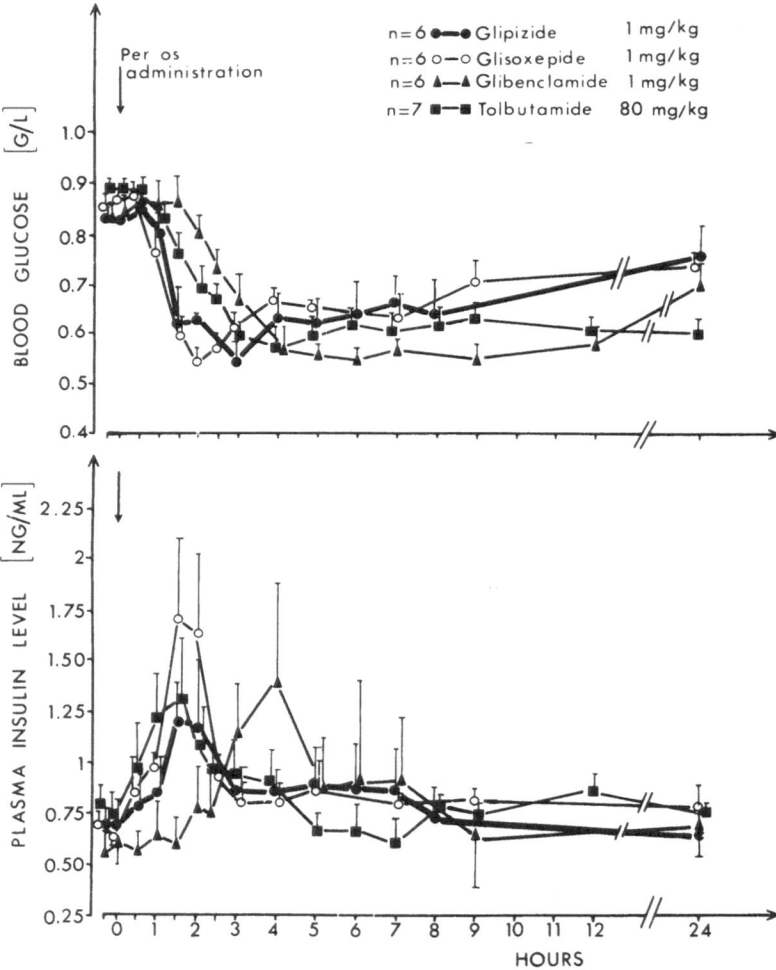

Figure 9. Changes in blood glucose and plasma insulin levels in the peripheral venous blood of
normal conscious dogs after oral administration of glipizide, glisoxepide, glibenclamide, and
tolbutamide. Each point represents the mean of the values, with the standard error of the mean. n,
number of animals. Reproduced with permission of *Med. Hyg.*[43]

the product, the glibenclamide concentration in the blood increases to attain its maximum 1 to 2 hr after ingestion. Following this the concentration drops. The same phenomenon has been produced in man.

It has thus been confirmed that the hypoglycemic sulfonamides possess *in vivo* a tropism for the β cells of the islets of Langerhans (betacytotropic activity) and that they stimulate the β cells and insulin secretion in a powerful manner (insulin secretory action).

Experiments in Vitro

The *in vitro* action of the sulfonylureas on the insulin secretion of the perfused rat pancreas has been studied by different authors.

During experiments performed on isolated and perfused rat pancreas preparations (after excluding all gastrointestinal tissue, omental and splenic, in contrast to the preparation used by Grodsky,[45] in which not only the pancreas was conserved but also parts of the stomach, duodenum and spleen, which experimentally does not correspond to a really isolated pancreas) the following results were obtained[46,47]:

Tolbutamide, in the absence of glucose in the perfusate, increases the basal secretion of insulin by the pancreas. After having rapidly attained a peak of elevated secretion (first phase) which lasts 3 to 5 min, the rhythm of secretion diminishes progressively and then maintains itself (second phase) (Fig. 10A); at the end of the experiment the insulin output remains higher than that observed before tolbutamide was added to the perfusate. When the concentration of glucose is maintained at 1.50 g/liter, the second phase of insulin secretion lasts as long as tolbutamide and glucose are present (Fig. 10B).[48]

In the presence of increasing concentrations of glucose, and in the presence of tolbutamide, the quantity of insulin secreted per unit of time is very high. Figure 11 shows that insulin secretion, while the concentration of glucose alone is augmented, increases very rapidly and takes on a sigmoid curve for values between 0 and 5 g glucose/liter. For 3 g glucose/liter, the insulin output is equal to or greater than 100 times the basal secretion obtained in the absence of glucose. At a concentration of 5 g glucose/liter, the secretion is only slightly superior to that obtained with 3 g/liter. Therefore, a maximum of secretion seems to have been obtained with 3 g glucose/liter (Fig. 11). In the presence of the same concentrations of glucose as those used in the preceding experiment, the addition of 100 mg tolbutamide provokes a still greater increase in insulin secretion.[47]

If, as has been shown in Fig. 11, one plots on the abscissa, on one hand, the effects of glucose alone, and on the other, the simultaneous action of both glucose and tolbutamide on the same pancreas, it can be seen that the two curves representing insulin secretion with glucose alone and with glucose and tolbutamide are sigmoid. The difference between them represents the supplementary insulin secretion per minute due to the presence of tolbutamide.[46-49] This supplementary output of insulin increases, at the same time, with the concentration of glucose, until a maximum is attained at 2 g glucose/liter. It

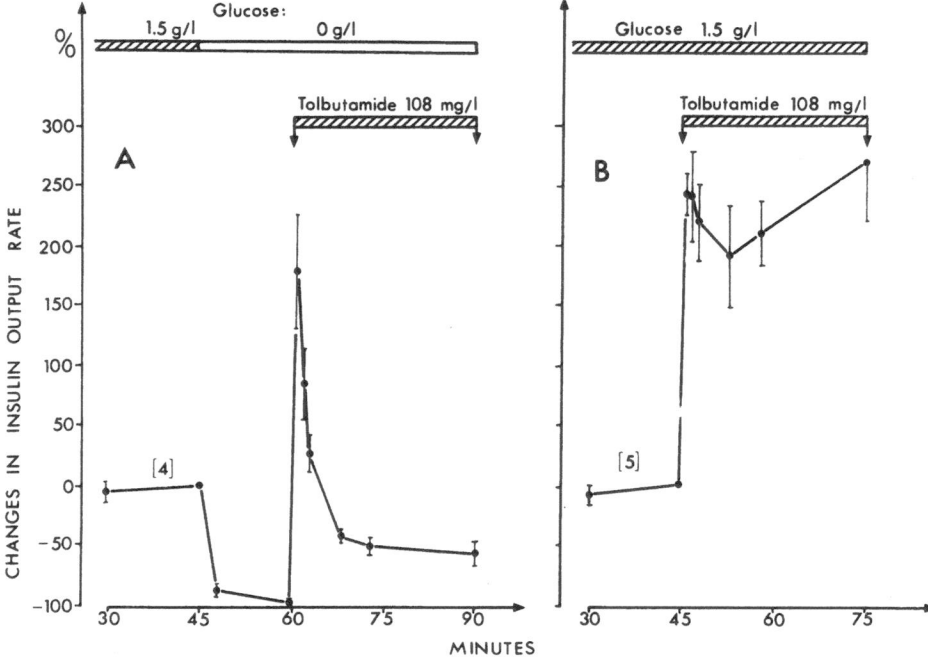

Figure 10. Effect of 0.4 mM tolbutamide (108 mg/liter) on the secretion of insulin by the isolated perfused rat pancreas, in the absence of glucose in the perfusion medium (Graph A), and in the presence of glucose (1.5 g/liter) (Graph B). Each point represents the mean of the values obtained, with the standard error of the mean. The number of experiments is indicated in parentheses. Reproduced with permission of Springer-Verlag.[48]

decreases subsequently at a concentration of 3 g glucose/liter and practically disappears at 5 g/liter (Fig. 11). The quantity of insulin secreted by the combined effects of glucose and tolbutamide depends, therefore, on the concentration of glucose present in the perfusing fluid.

There obviously exists a synergistic effect between glucose and tolbutamide. As has been shown,[46,47] this synergistic effect is not additive (that is to say, it is not the result of the simple addition of the respective effects of these two substances), but it is a potentializing synergy (in the sense that the combined effects of the two substances are greater than the addition of their individual effects). This suggests that the synergistic actions of glucose and tolbutamide increase the capacity of the normal β cell to secrete insulin. Under their conjugated influence, insulin is secreted more rapidly and, by unit of time, in greater quantity.[49] It is by this mechanism that the hypoglycemic sulfonamides act in the presence of hyperglycemia in certain diabetics possessing low-functioning β cells. The β cells of these diabetics secrete insulin less rapidly and in quantities less than normal. They are capable, however, of responding to a sulfonamide stimulation, as is the case in 60 to 70% of maturity-onset diabetics or in prediabetics.

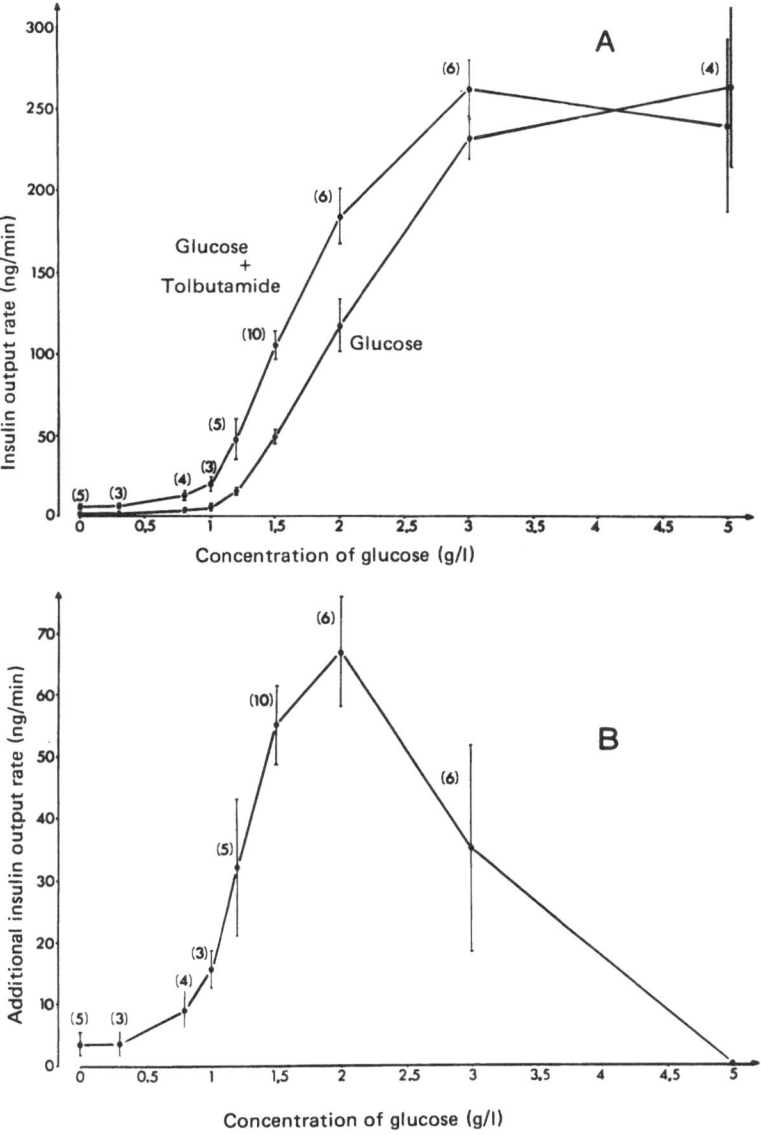

Figure 11. (Graph A) The insulin output of the isolated pancreas as a function of the concentration of glucose, in the presence of glucose alone, and in the presence of glucose and tolbutamide. (Graph B) The difference in insulin output rates, as a function of the concentration of glucose, obtained on the same pancreases, in the presence and in the absence of tolbutamide (100 mg/liter). Each point represents the mean value, with the standard error of the mean. Number of pancreases is indicated in parentheses. Reproduced with permission from Springer-Verlag.[47,49]

Even though it has been intensely investigated, the precise cause of this secretory difficulty which touches the β cells of certain diabetic patients is not known. It is perhaps due to the inability of the β cells to fully recognize glucose as its physiological stimulant because of an allosteric structural modification. It is possibly due to a diminution in the sensitivity of glucoreceptors, probably in the membrane, because of a deficiency of one or more of the enzymes implicated in the formation of glucose metabolites in the cell. It is also possible that there exists a deficiency of cellular 3'5' cyclic AMP synthesis (a component seemingly playing an important role in insulin secretion) or else excessive activation of the phosphodiesterase enzyme which hydrolyzes it. There may also exist a secretory deficiency of multiple hormones, some of gastrointestinal origin, which seem implicated in insulin secretion. One can really think of, as a factor of insulin inhibition, the activation of catecholamine secretion at the terminals of orthosympathetic fibers which innervate the islets of Langerhans, since it is known that these catecholamines (adrenalin, noradrenalin) are, at very low concentrations (1 μg/liter), inhibitors of insulin secretion[50] when they activate α adrenergic receptors in the β insulin secretory cells. Insulin secretory deficiency could also be due to structural modifications of the cellular membranes, which occur frequently in diabetes, and which could involve the β cells as well. These modifications could result in disturbances of β cell membrane permeability β to glucose in one sense (that is to say, as a stimulating agent) or to insulin in another (that is to say, the hormone resulting from the stimulation). Whatever the cause may be, it is certain that in diabetes, the organism suffers from a relative or an absolute deficiency of insulin.

The sensitivity of β cells to the sulfonylureas is, for some of these substances, e.g., glibenclamide, glisoxepide, and glipizide, considerable.[44,51] The β cells respond by an increased insulin secretion to a concentration of these substances as low as 0.5 μg/liter. In the isolated and perfused rat pancreas, in the presence of glucose (1.5 g/liter), glibenclamide, when perfused for 15 min at a concentration of 50 μg/liter, provokes a very abundant insulin secretion which lasts for 60 min after the termination of the perfusion (Fig. 12). This differentiates the action of glibenclamide from that of tolbutamide on insulin secretion.[41,42,46,49,52,53]

It thus appears that the action of the hypoglycemic sulfonamides is not only acute, but is also persistent for some of them. Under the influence of several of these drugs (especially glibenclamide) and in the presence of glucose, the β cells are maintained in a state of prolonged stimulation for a certain time (Fig. 12). This state persists even when the sulfonamide stimulation is terminated.[52,53] This was observed first by this author in 1968[52] and then reconfirmed by him in 1969,[42,53] by Grodsky in 1969,[45] by Pfeiffer in 1969,[54] and by others.

Other methods more or less physiological than the isolated perfused rat pancreas have been utilized to explore insulin secretion resulting from the action of the hypoglycemic sulfonamides, for example: pancreatic fragments of rats and rabbits, microdissected isolated islets, islets isolated by methods using collagenase, or cultures of embryonic pancreas of the rat. In all of these experiments the hypoglycemic sulfonamides have been shown to be powerful agents which stimulate insulin secretion.

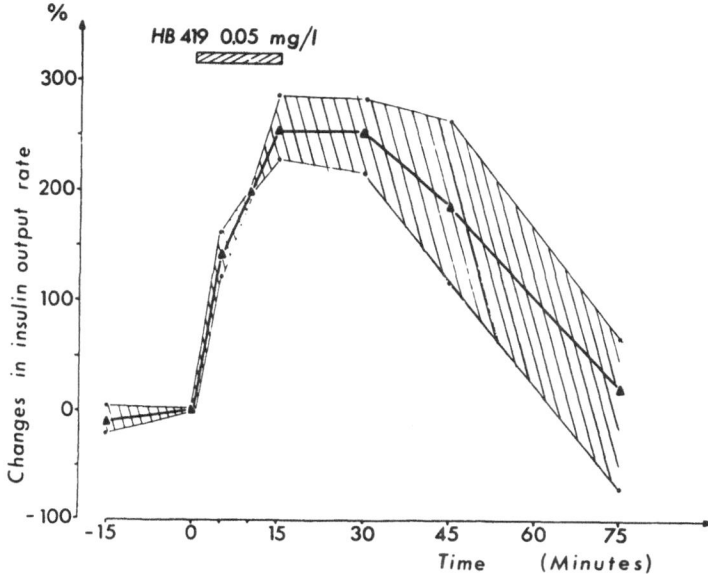

Figure 12. Variations in insulin output rate due to glibenclamide (HB 419) on the isolated rat pancreas, perfused with a physiological solution containing glucose (1.5 g/liter). The variations are expressed in percentages of the value registered immediately before the addition of the substance. ▲——▲ shows the mean value obtained in four experiments, and the shaded area is the range. Note that the secretion of insulin persists long after the suppression of glibenclamide from the perfusion liquid. Reproduced with permission of Casa Editrice "IL PONTE."[52]

It is not known definitely whether the initial stimulating action of tolbutamide is mediated through the pathway of the adenylcyclase–3'5'-cyclic AMP–phosphodiesterase system. It is known that in the presence of glucose, theophylline, an inhibitor of phosphodiesterase, considerably reinforces the insulin secretory effects of tolbutamide.[55] (Fig. 13).

In an early study of Levey *et al.*[56] on tolbutamide in a particular preparation of an islet cell adenoma, concentrations of 5×10^{-5} M and 10^{-4} M tolbutamide stimulated adenylate cyclase activity. A similar effect was reported by Kuo *et al.*[57] using 5×10^{-4} M tolbutamide. An alternative explanation for the stimulating effect of tolbutamide on insulin release is suggested by the tolbutamide inhibition of cyclic nucleotide phosphodiesterase from an islet cell tumor of Syrian hamsters.[58] Consideration of the dose–response characteristics of these two enzyme systems will be necessary in order to determine the primary action of tolbutamide. Studies using intact tissue in another system, the toad bladder, suggest that the major effect of sulfonylureas may be exerted on adenylate cyclase.[59] The recent results obtained by Bowen and Lazarus[60] are in agreement with the conclusions that the sulfonylureas (tolbutamide, glibenclamide) exert their pharmacological action by interacting with the plasma membrane. Their action would be transmitted by the pathway of the enzyme, adenylate cyclase.

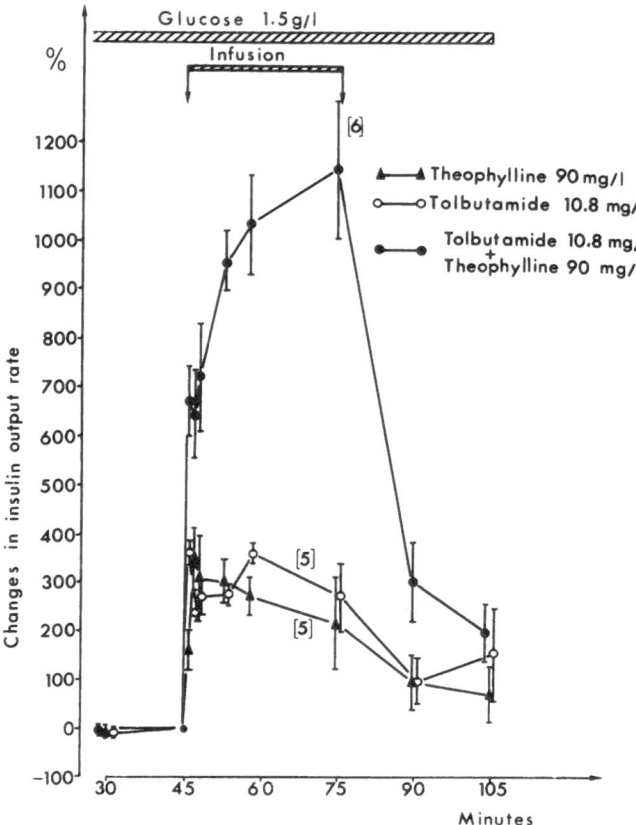

Figure 13. Effects on the insulin output of the isolated perfused rat pancreas: of tolbutamide alone, of theophylline alone, and of tolbutamide and theophylline. Each point represents the mean of the values, with the standard error of the mean. The number of experiments is indicated in parentheses. Reproduced with permission from *C. R. Soc. Biol.*[55]

A convincing argument in favor of the tropism of the hypoglycemic sulfonamides for β cells has been furnished by Matthews and Dean,[61] who demonstrated the direct stimulating action of the hypoglycemic sulfonamides on the β cells. These authors, working on the rat, exposed the islets by microdissection. They observed that tolbutamide is capable of provoking the appearance of action potentials in the β cells. The production of action potentials in the β cells by tolbutamide (as well as by adequate concentrations of glucose) strongly suggests a selective effect on cellular membrane permeability by ionic exchange.

More recently, the effect of a "square wave" stimulation with glucose or glibenclamide on the electrical activity of β cells has been studied by Meissner and Atwater[62] with microelectrode techniques in isolated perifused mouse β cells. The results obtained by them are represented in Fig. 14.

Since glibenclamide evokes a permanent depolarization of the membrane with a continuous spike activity, it could be speculated that glibenclamide has an inhibitory effect on the sodium pump. This speculation is supported by the observation that glibenclamide reduces the ATP content of β cells.[63] On the other hand, it is possible that glibenclamide increases the passive permeability of the cell membrane to sodium and/or calcium. This would depolarize the membrane and counteract the hyperpolarizing effect of the sodium pump. The prolonged electrical activity following removal of glibenclamide is consistent with the idea that there is a relatively strong binding of the drug to the plasma membrane.[64] The results suggest that sulfonylureas are bound reversibly to islet tissue, but are normally restricted to the outside of the β cells. The electrophysiology of β cells, therefore, confirms the extremely prolonged stimulating action of glibenclamide described for the first time by Loubatières.[41,52]

On sections of rabbit pancreas, the reduction of potassium concentration to 1 mM provokes an inhibition of the insulin secretory response to glucose and to tolbutamide. Conversely, an augmentation of potassium of 5 to 10 mM increases the speed of insulin liberation in response to these two stimuli.

It was shown in the isolated perfused rat pancreas that calcium is necessary for the secretion of insulin, induced by glucose and tolbutamide, to manifest itself. In fragments of rabbit pancreas incubated *in vitro,* extracellular sodium

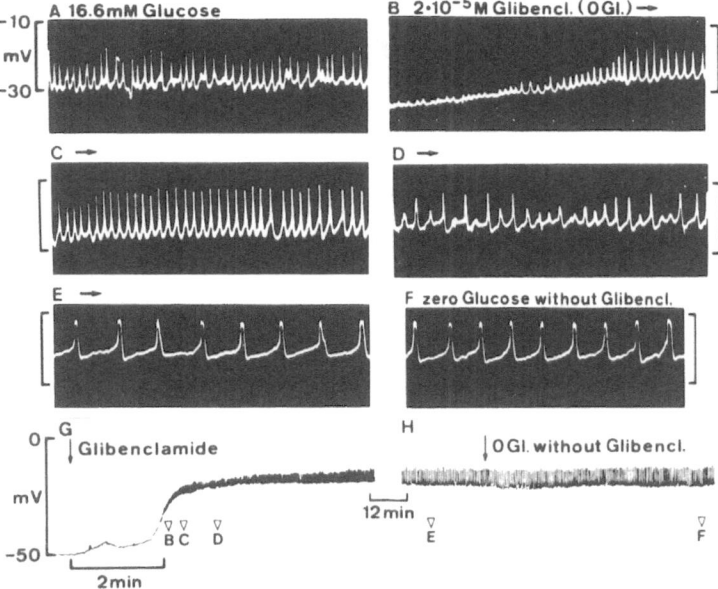

Figure 14. Effect of glibenclamide on the membrane potential of a single β cell perifused with a glucose-free medium. (A) Control of spike activity during plateau phase elicited by 16.6 mM glucose (prior to treatment with glibenclamide). (B–F) Oscilloscope records of electrical activity taken with triangles in G and H. (G, H) Chart recordings of time course of membrane potential: glibenclamide ($2.10^{-5}M$) added at arrow in G, removed at arrow in H. Reproduced with permission from the author and Georg Thieme Verlag.[62]

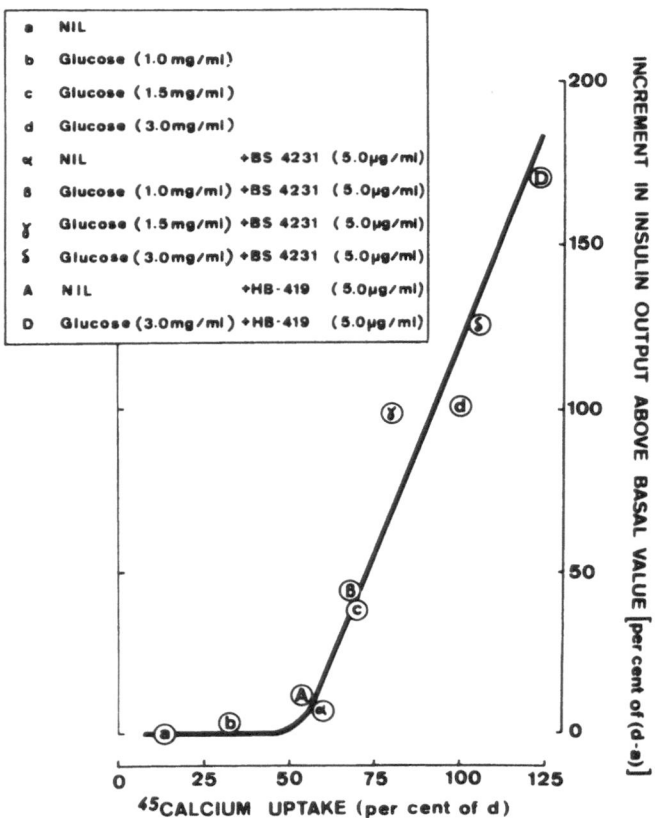

Figure 15. Relationship between the increment in insulin output above basal value induced by glucose and sulfonylureas in pieces of pancreatic tissue, and the corresponding values for calcium uptake by isolated islets of Langerhans. Both parameters are expressed in percent of the control value found at high glucose concentration [3.0 mg/ml (d)]. All incubations were carried out at 37°C for 60 min. Each point represents the mean of 13 or more individual observations. Reproduced with permission from the author and *Arch. Int. Pharmacodyn.*[65]

and calcium are necessary for the stimulation of insulin secretion by glucose and tolbutamide.

The necessity of ions for insulin secretion suggests that the uptake of calcium by the β cell is a fundamental component in the process by which numerous stimuli act to increase insulin liberation. In fact, the sulfonylurea, glibenclamide, stimulates the uptake of calcium by the isolated islets of Langerhans[65] (Fig. 15).

In two recent publications, Alric and co-workers[66,67] described a kind of nonsaturable cooperative binding of labeled tolbutamide to rat islets of Langerhans isolated with collagenase. The inflexion of the binding isotherm is situated in the range of tolbutamide concentrations which exert a graded stimulating effect on the secretion of insulin. This cooperation shows organ specificity, being much less apparent in the binding of tolbutamide to the exocrine pancreas. Unlabeled tolbutamide at an almost maximally effective concentration as well as equally active concentrations of chlorpropamide or carbutamide and an exactly antagonistic concentration of diazoxide cancel the synergism when added to the labeled drug. Such a cooperative pattern, which reflects a variation in the affinity and, therefore, in the physical properties of the binding structures, as a consequence of the binding itself, could be a direct evidence of the cell perturbation involved in the stimulating action of this drug on hormone secretion (Fig. 16).

From the results which have been obtained, as well as from *in vitro* studies with tolbutamide on the isolated perfused rat pancreas (as was shown also *in vivo* with glibenclamide in the normal anesthetized dog), it became apparent that propranolol does not modify, by its β adrenergic blocking action, the insulin secretory action of these hypoglycemic sulfonamides. Based on the available pharmacological evidence, the β adrenergic receptors do not seem to be directly implicated in the stimulating action of these sulfonylureas on the β cells of the islets of Langerhans.[26,27]

Also, the hypoglycemic sulfonamides do not exert their stimulating action on insulin secretion by activating the cholinergic receptors of the β cell. In fact, atropine does not modify it, as has been demonstrated both *in vivo*[4,5] and *in*

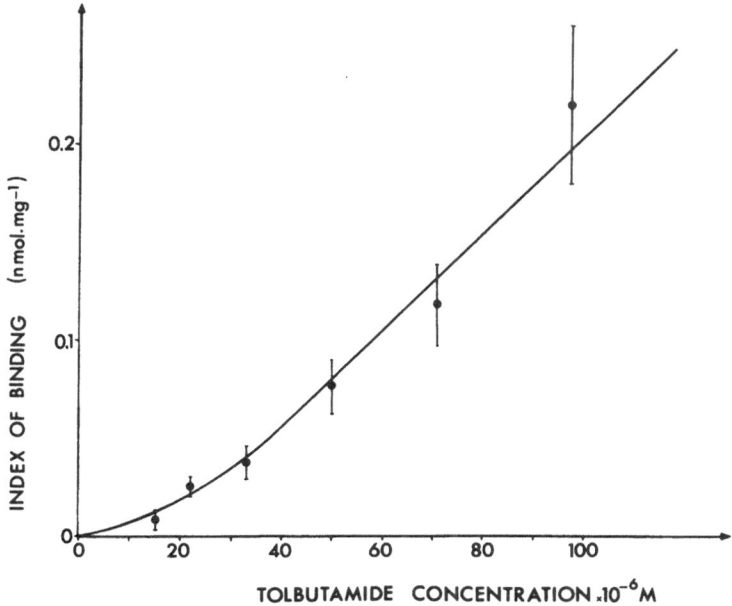

Figure 16. Isotherm (37°C) of tolbutamide binding to rat isolated islets of Langerhans. Each point represents the mean of six experiments, with the standard error of the mean, after subtraction of the variation between experiments. From Alric *et al.*[66]

vitro (Loubatières *et al.,* unpublished data). It can be thought that, considering its action on the β cells of the islets and in particular on the pancreas, gliben-clamide should be concentrated in this organ in great quantities. However, it appears that this drug is concentrated above all in the liver, clearly less so in the kidney, the heart, and the brain, and to a very limited degree in the pancreas.[68] This demonstrates again the extreme sensitivity of the β cell to the hypogly-cemic sulfonamides.

Reinforcement of the Action of Insulin by the Hypoglycemic Sulfonamides

Over and above their stimulating action on the β cell, the hypoglycemic sulfonamides reinforce the effects of exogenous and endogenous insulin on glycemia, even in the completely pancreatectomized animal[12,13] (Fig. 3).

β Cytotrophic and Antidiabetic Action of the Hypoglycemic Sulfonamides

If hypoglycemic sulfonamides are administered for a few consecutive days to the normal rat, rabbit, or dog, hyperplasia of the islets of Langerhans is provoked as well as formation of new β cells secreting insulin.[5,9] This phenome-non has been labeled the betacytotrophic action of the hypoglycemic sulfon-amides[7-9] because the action of these substances can be compared to those of certain hormones, e.g., the pituitary trophins, acting on certain endocrine glands. The result of this action is the production of an intense neogenesis of β cells from the cells of the excretory ductules, from the centroacinar cells, and from incompletely differentiated cells. Mitoses of the β cells are also observed.[10]

Qualitative histological analysis of this betacytotrophic action has been supplemented by quantitative studies in the rat and mouse. These studies have led to the conclusion that various hypoglycemic sulfonamides (*p*-aminoben-zenesulfamidoisopropylthiodiazole, 2254 RP), glybuthiazol (2259 RP), carbu-tamide, tolbutamide, chlorpropamide, azepinamide, glibenclamide (HB 419), glisoxepide, and glipizide, administered orally for 35 to 45 days to the rat or mouse, produce a considerable increase in the total volume of the islets of Langerhans, an increase in the total weight of the islets, and at the same time an increase in the proportion of islet volume to total pancreatic volume[44,51,69,70] (Fig. 17).

In the work of Chick,[71] rat pancreatic cell cultures were utilized to study the effects of glucose, tolbutamide, and other drugs (dexamethazone phosphate, bovine growth hormone, and porcine glucagon) on β cell replication. Replica-tion was estimated by determining the frequency of labeling of aldehyde-thionine-positive cells in stained radioautographs. Both glucose (3 mg/ml medium) and tolbutamide (100 μg/ml) caused a three- to fourfold increase in labeling compared to controls. Both glucose and tolbutamide increased insulin release; dexamethazone decreased insulin release, while growth hormone and glucagon produced no significant effects.

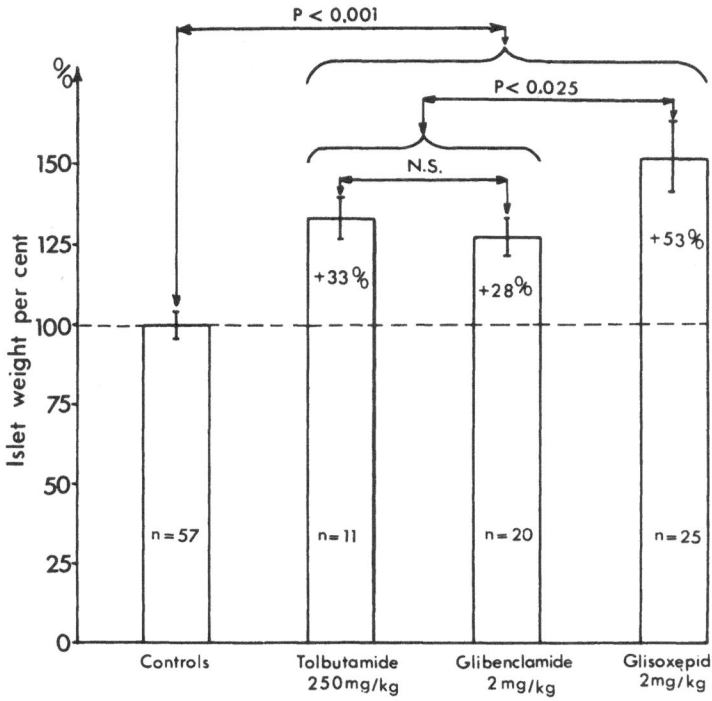

Figure 17. Changes in weight of pancreatic islets in mice treated orally with tolbutamide, gliben-clamide, or glisoxepide for 35 days. The results are evaluated in percentages in reference to the control animals. Each column represents the mean islet weight ± the standard error of the mean. The number, *n*, of animals is indicated for each group. Reproduced with permission from *Israel J. Med. Sci.*[69]

These data suggest that agents which stimulate insulin release can trigger β cell replication *in vitro*. In addition, since growth hormone, glucocorticoid, and glucagon stimulate β cell replication *in vivo* but not *in vitro*, this action *in vivo* may be mediated by effects on other tissues rather than by direct action on the β cell.

The results of these studies indicate that the replicating action of glucose or of tolbutamide are due to a direct action on the β cell.

The DNA synthesis of isolated pancreatic islets has been determined after culture *in vitro* of the islets for 5 days in a medium containing either various glucose concentrations or tolbutamide. The results showed that glucose stimulated the replication of DNA, whereas tolbutamide was without effect. In fact, tolbutamide failed to enhance the DNA synthesis of the islet cells, despite being used at a concentration high enough for stimulation of insulin release both *in vivo* and *in vitro*. The author concludes that this would agree with the hypothesis of Loubatières,[17] suggesting that if the sulfonylureas have a cytotrophic effect, it manifests itself as β cell neogenesis from nonendocrine pancreatic cells rather than by proliferation of already existing β cells.[72] It is possible, however, that the increase of the number of β cells provoked by tolbutamide is due to two mechanisms, the new formation of certain β cells and the neogenesis of β cells from potentially endocrine pancreatic cells.

It is important to note that in the intact animal the excess endogenous insulin secreted and the hypoglycemia produced by sulfonamide β cell stimulation does not inhibit the normal growth of the islets of Langerhans, as can be produced after repeated injections of exogenous insulin.

The betacytotrophic action of hypoglycemic sulfonamides probably explains their "antidiabetic" action. This statement implies that the hypoglycemic sulfonamides could, under certain conditions, reduce in part the underlying cause of the diabetic condition, that is, the functional and possibly the numeric deficiency of the β cells, and thus perhaps aid in the prevention of the diabetic state.

The Antagonism between the Hypoglycemic Sulfonamides and Diazoxide

Loubatières, in 1944[73] and 1946,[5] described three groups of sulfonamides: some were hypoglycemic, others had no influence on blood glucose level, and the last group were hyperglycemic. The principal hyperglycemic agent is diazoxide (3-methyl-7-chloro-1,2,4 benzothiadiazine-1, 1-dioxide).

The hyperglycemic action of diazoxide is due to a number of mechanisms described by Loubatières *et al.*[74,75] as well as by Seltzer and Crout.[76] It seems that the inhibitory action of the substance on insulin secretion plays an essential role in the production of hyperglycemia. In the normal anesthetized dog Loubatières *et al.*[74,75] demonstrated that the administration of diazoxide produces in the pancreaticoduodenal venous blood a prolonged and spectacular reduction of the secretion of insulin by 80 to 100%, compared with a control. This decrease of insulin release persists in the animal deprived of its adrenal glands.[75]

To determine whether this inhibitory effect is the consequence of a direct action of diazoxide on the β cells of the islets, Loubatières *et al.*[74,75] used the isolated whole rat pancreas and found that perfusion with diazoxide considerably reduces the secretion of insulin provoked by glucose at a concentration of 1.5 g/liter. These findings furnished proof that diazoxide exerts a direct inhibitory action on the secretion of endogenous insulin. This interpretation was confirmed by the work of Frerichs *et al.*,[77] who showed that the β cells of rats treated for 3 days with 500 mg diazoxide/kg orally twice daily, contained numerous multigranular sacs filled with β granules and granular material, suggesting cellular digestion of granules. In rats fed for 2 weeks with diazoxide, the total number of β cell granules was decreased, while multigranular sacs and electron-dense bodies, probably the residues of digested granules, were still present. It therefore appeared to be important to study, in the isolated perfused rat pancreas, the eventual antagonistic effects on the secretion of insulin between a hypoglycemic sulfonamide (an insulin-secretory stimulator: tolbutamide or glibenclamide) and a hyperglycemic sulfonamide (diazoxide, an

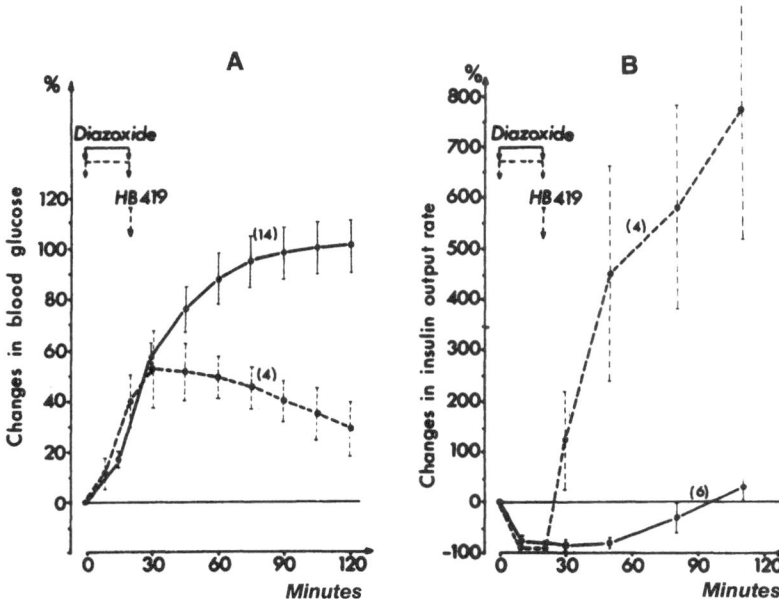

Figure 18. Indication of the antagonism of glibenclamide (HB 419) with respect to diazoxide on the blood sugar level (A) and on the insulin output rate in the pancreatocoduodenal vein (B) in the anesthetized dog. Variations are estimated in percentages in reference to values at time 0. Each point represents the mean of the values obtained, with the standard error of the mean; number of dogs used to establish each curve is indicated in parentheses. Animals of first group (·——·) received only diazoxide intravenously, 1 mg/kg/min for 20 min; the other group (·······) received, at the end of the diazoxide perfusion, an intravenous injection of 0.5 mg/kg of glibenclamide (HB 419). Reproduced with permission from Springer-Verlag.[42]

inhibitor of this secretion). Such an antagonism has previously been demonstrated.[74,75] These results were confirmed by the authors in *in vivo* studies, in which the administration of glibenclamide to anesthetized dogs provoked cessation of the hyperglycemia produced by diazoxide[42] (Fig. 18).

References

1. Janbon, M., Chaptal, J., Vedel, A., and Schaap, J.: *Montpellier Méd.*, **21–22**:441, 1942.
2. Janbon, M., Lazergues, P., and Metropolitanski, J. H.: *Montpellier Méd.*, **21–22**:489, 1942.
3. Loubatières, A., Goldstein, L., Metropolitanski, J., and Schaap, J.: In: *43ème Congrè Médecins Aliénistes et Neurologistes de France et des Pays de Langue Francaise.* Edited by Masson. Montpellier, Paris. 1942, p. 415.
4. Loubatières, A.: *C. R. Soc. Biol.*, **138**:766, 1944.
5. Loubatières, A.: Thèse Doctorat ès-Sciences naturelles. Montpellier, Causse, Graille et Castelnau, 1946.
6. Loubatières, A.: *Arch. Int. Physiol.*, **54**:174, 1946.
7. Loubatières, A.: *Arch. Int. Pharmacodyn.*, **140**:127, 1962.

8. Loubatières, A.: In: *Perspectives in Biology.* Edited by C. F. Cori, V. G. Foglia, L. F. Leloir, and S. Ochoa. Elsevier, Amsterdam, 1963, p. 117.
9. Loubatières, A.: In: *Diabetes Mellitus.* Edited by K. Oberdisse and K. Jahnke. Georg Thieme Verlag, Stuttgart, 1958, p. 279.
10. Fruteau de Laclos, C., and Loubatières, A.: *Bull. Assoc. Anat.,* **106**:261, 1960.
11. Loubatières, A.: In: *The Structure and Metabolism of the Pancreatic Islet.* Edited by S. E. Brolin, B. Hellman, and H. Knutson. Pergamon Press, Oxford, 1964, p. 437.
12. Loubatières, A., Bouyard, P., Fruteau de Laclos, C., Sassine, A., and Alric, R.: *C. R. Soc. Biol.,* **150**:1601, 1956.
13. Houssay, B. A., Penhos, J. C., Urgoiti, E., Teodosio, N., Apelbaum, J., and Bowket, J.: *Ann. N.Y. Acad. Sci.,* **71**:25, 1957.
14. Loubatières, A.: *Presse Méd.,* **63**:1701, 1955.
15. Loubatières, A.: *Ann. N.Y. Acad. Sci.,* **71**:4, 1957.
16. Loubatières, A.: In: *Pharmacokinetics and Mode of Action of Oral Hypoglycemic Agents.* Edited by A. Loubatières and A. E. Renold. Acta Diabetologica Latina, Milan, Suppl. 1, 1969, p. 20.
17. Loubatières, A.: In: *Pharmacokinetics and Mode of Action of Oral Hypoglycemic Agents.* Edited by A. Loubatières and A. E. Renold. Acta Diabetologica Latina, Milan, Suppl. 1, 1969, p. 216.
18. Franke, J., and Fuchs, J.: *Dtsch. Med. Wachenschr.,* **80**:1449, 1955.
19. Bertram, F., Bendfeldt, E., and Otto, H.: *Dtsch. Med. Wochenschr.,* **80**:1455, 1955.
20. Loubatières, A.: *C. R. Acad. Sci.,* **241**:1422, 1955.
21. Loubatières, A.: *Méd. Hyg.,* **13**:495, 1955.
22. Loubatières, A., Bouyard, P., and Fruteau de Laclos, C.: *Sem. Hôp. Paris,* **32**:RM 47, 1956.
23. Bänder, A., Creutzfeldt, W., Dorfmüller, T., Ehrhart, H., Marx, R., Maske, H., Meier, W., Mohnike, G., Pfeiffer, E. F., Schlaginweit, S., Schöffling, K., Scholz, J., Seidler, I., Steigerwald, H., Stich, W., Stötter, G., and Ulrich, H.: *Dtsch. Med. Wochenschr.,* **81**:823, 1956.
24. Loubatières, A.: *Ann. N.Y. Acad. Sci.,* **71**:192, 1957.
25. Loubatières, A.: *Diabetes,* **6**:408, 1957.
26. Loubatières, A., Mariani, M. M., Ribes, G., and Chapal, J.: *C.R. Soc. Biol.,* **169**:1392, 1971.
27. Loubatières, A., Loubatières-Mariani, M. M., Ribes, G., and Chapal, J.: *Diabetologia,* **9**:79, 1973.
28. Levine, R., and Fritz, I. B.: *Diabetes,* **5**:209, 1956.
29. Loubatières, A., Alric, R., Loubatières-Mariani, M. M., and Puech, R.: *C.R. Soc. Biol.,* **166**:1761, 1972.
30. Loubatières, A., Loubatières-Mariani, M. M., Ribes, G., and Alric, R.: *C.R. Soc. Biol.,* **166**:1757, 1972.
31. Loubatières, A., Loubatières-Mariani, M. M., Alric, R., and Ribes, G.: *Diabetologia,* **10**:271, 1974.
32. Loubatières, A., Loubatières-Mariani, M. M., Chapal, J., and Blayac, J. P.: *C.R. Soc. Biol.,* **169**:1568, 1975.
33. Volk, B. W., Goldner, M. G., Weisenfeld, S., and Lazarus, S. S.: *Ann. N. Y. Acad. Sci.,* **71**:141, 1957.
34. Williamson, J. R., Lacy, P. E., and Grisham, J. W.: *Diabetes,* **10**:460, 1961.
35. Lacy, P. E.: *Diabetes,* **11**:509, 1962.
36. Lacy, P. E.: In: *Mechanism and Regulation of Insulin Secretion.* Edited by R. Levine and E. F. Pfeiffer. Acta Diabetologica Latina, Milan, Suppl. 1, 1968, p. 436.
37. Orci, L., Stauffacher, W., Don Beaven, Lambert, A. E., Renold, A. E., and Rouiller, C.: In: *Pharmacokinetics and Mode of Action of Oral Hypoglycemic Agents.* Edited by A. Loubatières and A. E. Renold. Acta Diabetologica Latina, Milan, Suppl. 1, 1969, p. 271.
38. Pfeiffer, E. F., Renold, A. E., Martin, D. B., Dagenais, Y., Meakin, J. W., Nelson, D. H., Shoemaker, G., and Thorn, G. W.: In: *Diabetes Mellitus.* Edited by K. Oberdisse and K. Jahnke. Georg Thieme Verlag, Stuttgart, 1958, p. 298.
39. Pfeiffer, E. F., Schöffling, K., and Ditschuneit, H.: In: *Handbuch des Diabetes Mellitus.* Edited by E. F. Pfeiffer. J. F. Lehmanns Verlag, Munich, 1969, p. 636.
40. Yalow, R. W., Black, H., Villazon, M., and Berson, S. A.: *Diabetes,* **9**:356, 1960.
41. Loubatières, A., and Mariani, M. M.: *C.R. Acad. Sci.,* **265**:643, 1967.

42. Loubatières, A., Mariani, M. M., Ribes, G., De Malbosc, H., and Chapal, J. *Diabetologia*, 5:1, 1969.
43. Loubatières, A.: In: *Medecine et Hygiène*. Edited by B. Glasson and A. Benakis. Geneva, 1974, p. 179.
44. Loubatières, A., Loubatières-Mariani, M. M., Alric, R., Ribes, G., Sorel, G., and Tarasco, A.: *Diab. Mét.*, 1:13, 1975.
45. Grodsky, G. M., Curry, D., Landahl, A., and Bennett, L.: In: *Pharmacokinetics and Mode of Action of Oral Hypoglycemic Agents*. Edited by A. Loubatières and A. E. Renold. Acta Diabetologica Latina, Milan, Suppl. 1, 1969, p. 554.
46. Loubatières, A., Mariani, M.M., and Chapal, J.: *C.R. Acad. Sci.*, 267:123, 1968.
47. Loubatières, A., Mariani, M. M., and Chapal, J.: *Diabetologia*, 6:457, 1970.
48. Loubatières-Mariani, M. M., Loubatières, A., and Chapal, J.: *Diabetologia*, 9:152, 1973.
49. Loubatières, A., Mariani, M. M., and Chapal, J.: *C.R. Acad. Sci.*, 269:1460, 1969.
50. Loubatières, A., Mariani, M. M., and Chapal, J.: *Diabetologia*, 6:533, 1970.
51. Loubatières, A., Mariani, M. M., Ribes, G., and Alric, R.: *Acta Diabetologia Latina*, 10:261, 1973.
52. Loubatières, A.: In: *Mechanism and Regulation of Insulin Secretion*. Edited by R. Levine and E. F. Pfeiffer. Acta Diabetologia Latina, Milan, Suppl. 1, 1968, p. 220.
53. Mariani, M. M.: In: *Pharmacokinetics and Mode of Action of Oral Hypoglycemic Agents*. Edited by A. Loubatières and A. E. Renold. Acta Diabetologia Latina, Milan, Suppl. 1, 1969, p. 256.
54. Pfeiffer, E. F.: In: *Pharmacokinetics and Mode of Action of Oral Hypoglycemic Agents*. Edited by A. Loubatières and A. E. Renold. Acta Diabetologia Latina, Milan, Suppl. 1, 1969, p. 477.
55. Loubatières, A., Loubatières-Mariani, M. M., and Chapal, J.: *C.R. Sec. Biol.*, 167:1892, 1973.
56. Levey, G. E., Schmidt, W. M. I., and Mintz, D. H.: *Metabolism*, 21:93, 1972.
57. Kuo, W. N., Hodgins, D. S., and Kuo, J. F.: *J. Biol. Chem.*, 248:2705, 1973.
58. Rosen, O. M., Hirsch, A. M., and Goren, E. N.: *Arch. Biochem. Biophys.*, 146:660, 1971.
59. Ozer, A., and Sharp, G. W. G.: *Europ. J. Pharmacol.* 22:227, 1973.
60. Bowen, V. and Lazarus, N. R.: *Biochem. J.*, 142:385, 1974.
61. Matthews, E. K., and Dean, P. M.: In: *The Structure and Metabolism of the Pancreatic Islets*. Edited by S. Falkmer, B. Hellman, I. B. Taljedal. Pergamon Press, Oxford, 1970, p. 305.
62. Meissner, H. P., and Atwater, I. J.: *Horm. Metab. Res.*, 8:11, 1976.
63. Hellman, B., Idahl, L. A., and Danielsson, A.: *Diabetes*, 18:509, 1969.
64. Hellman, B., Sehlin, J., and Taljedal, I. B.: *Diabetologia*, 9:210, 1973.
65. Malaisse, W. J., Mahy, M., and Malaisse-Lagae, F.: *Arch. Int. Pharmacodyn.*, 192:205, 1971.
66. Alric, R., Manteghetti, M., Puech, R., Lignon, F., and Loubatières, A.: *C. R. Acad. Sci.*, 281:2029, 1975.
67. Alric, R., Manteghetti, M., Puech, R., Lignon, F., and Loubatières, A.: *C. R. Acad. Sci.*, 283:283, 1976.
68. Somogyi, J., Vincze, I., Willig, F., and Schmidt, F. H.: *Horm. Metab. Res.*, 6:181, 1974.
69. Loubatières, A.: *Israel J. Med. Sci.*, 8:682, 1972.
70. Loubatières, A., Mariani, M. M., Alric, R., Ribes, G., De Malbosc, H., and Houareau, M. H.: *Diabetologia*, 5:219, 1969.
71. Chick, W. L.: *Diabetes*, 22:687, 1973.
72. Andersson, A.: *Endocrinology*, 96:1051, 1975.
73. Loubatières, A.: *C. R. Soc. Biol.*, 138:830, 1944.
74. Loubatières, A., Mariani, M. M., and Alric, R.: *Ann. N.Y. Acad. Sci.*, 150:226, 1968.
75. Loubatières, A., Mariani, M. M., Alric, R., and Chapal, J.: In: *Tolbutamide after Ten Years*. Edited by W. J. H. Butterfield and W. Van Westering. Excerpta Medica, New York, 1967, p. 100.
76. Seltzer, H. S., and Crout, J. R.: *Diabetes*, 15:523, 1966.
77. Frerichs, H., Creutzfeldt, C., and Creutzfeldt, W.: In: *Mechanism and Regulation of Insulin Secretion*. Edited by R. Levine and E. F. Pfeiffer. Acta Diabetologica Latina, Milan, Suppl. 1, 1968, p. 105.

Chapter 21

Islet Transplantation

Orion D. Hegre and Arnold Lazarow

Early investigations of the effects of pancreatic transplantation[1,2] combined with results obtained from pancreatectomy studies[3] provided definitive evidence for the involvement of the pancreas in diabetes mellitus. The hypothesis of the endocrine nature of the islets of Langerhans[4] was confirmed by subsequent duct-ligation experiments demonstrating the role of the islet tissue component in diabetes mellitus.[5,6] The discovery and extraction of insulin and its clinical application in the successful control of diabetes[7] for a time lessened interest in pancreatic transplantation. However, the subsequent realization that insulin therapy alone was apparently insufficient to completely reverse the consequences of diabetes—the associated vascular lesions—generated renewed interest. As with other organs, immunological barriers complicated studies on the feasibility of pancreatic transplantation. This problem could be partially or even completely circumvented in the laboratory by immunosuppression, irradiation, autotransplantation, or the use of immunologically privileged sites or highly inbred strains of experimental animals. However, pancreatic transplantation has been, in addition, further complicated by the morphological nature of the mammalian pancreas itself. With the islet tissue distributed throughout the exocrine organ as small islands[8] comprising only 1–2% of the gland,[9–14] the question of how best to provide the diabetic recipient with a new complement of functioning islet tissue has been approached from two aspects.

In the more direct approach, investigators have attempted to replace islet function by transplanting the whole organ with vascular anastomosis between donor and recipient, in much the same manner that has been successfully utilized with other organs. Surgical techniques, first developed in the research laboratory, have provided ample evidence of successful endocrine function in such transplants; these techniques have been successfully applied clinically to man. A number of reviews have summarized the current status of progress in the field.[15–20] It is clear that one of the major problems limiting the long-term functional success of whole organ pancreatic transplants has been the presence of the acinar component of the graft and its enzymatic secretions.

Concurrent with the development of whole organ transplantation, an

---

Orion D. Hegre and Arnold Lazarow • University of Minnesota, Minneapolis, Minnesota. A.L. is deceased.

alternative approach has been pursued—that of islet cell transplantation. The duct-ligation studies of Ssobolew demonstrated that it was only the islet component of the pancreas that was necessary to prevent diabetes and he suggested in 1902 the possibility of islet cell transplantation as an alternative to the whole organ approach.[6] Although the idea of replacing only the desired endocrine component, and thereby circumventing the problems associated with the acinar gland, was theoretically very appealing, here again the morphological nature of the dispersed islet within the mammalian pancreas provided a practical hurdle. The problem of obtaining relatively pure preparations of mammalian islets was resolved by drawing on the information gained and the techniques developed in a number of islet research areas. Within the past few years a definitive and reproducible reversal of experimentally induced diabetes has been attained, with such islet cell preparations resulting in greatly expanded interest in the islet cell transplantation approach.

Sources of Donor Islet Tissue

Fetal and Neonatal Islet Tissue

Studies of the fetal and neonatal rat pancreas demonstrate separate patterns for the differentiation and growth of the acinar and endocrine compo-

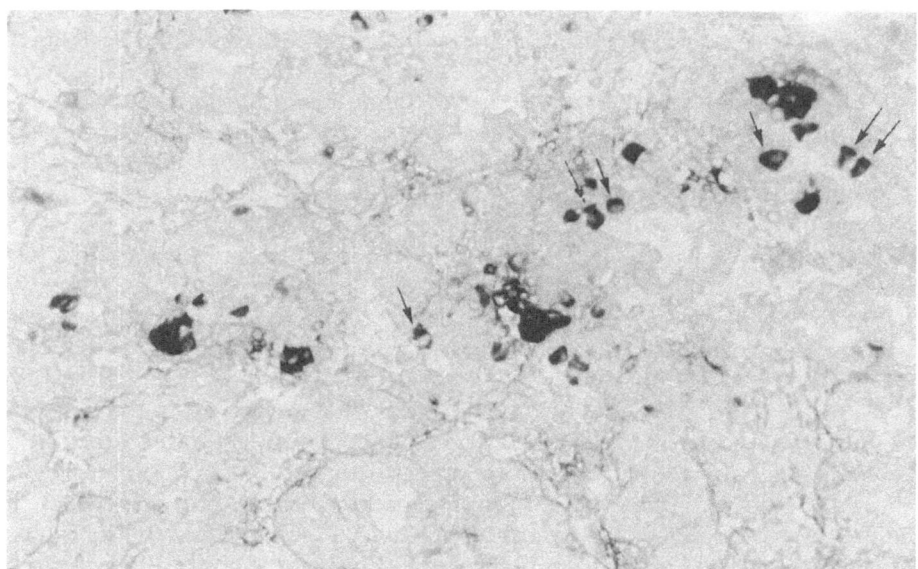

Figure 1. Immunocytochemical localization of insulin in the fetal rat pancreas (18 days postcoitum) reveals developing β cells in small groups associated with the ductal elements or as single cells which frequently lie within the duct walls (arrows). The acinar cells are relatively undifferentiated at this stage of pancreatic development. Unlabeled antibody enzyme method. Aniline blue. ×175.

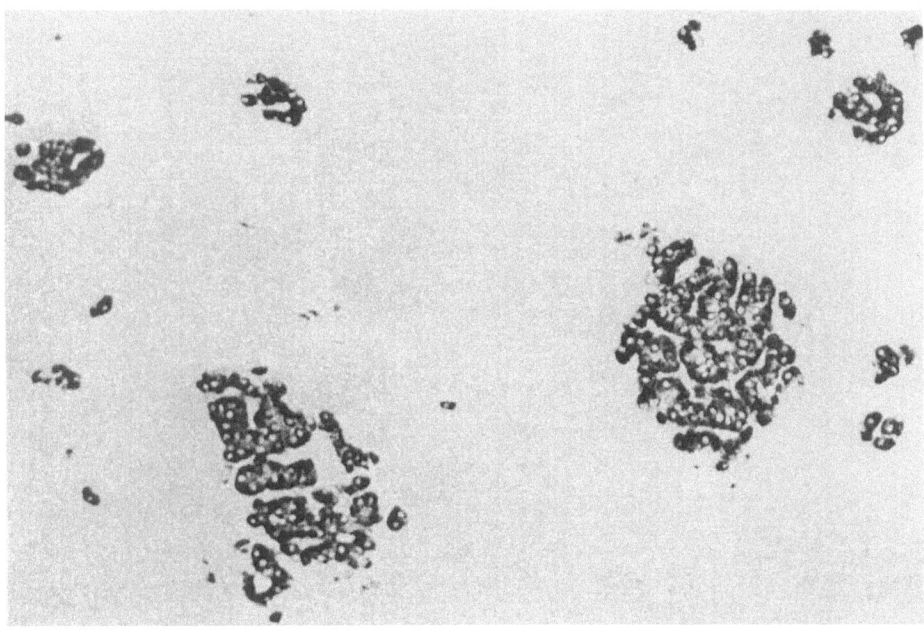

Figure 2. Immunocytochemical localization of insulin in the neonatal rat pancreas (5 days postpartum) demonstrates the relatively large concentration of islets present, representing nearly 5% of the total gland. Differentiated acinar cells are present, comprising the majority of the pancreas; however, their content of exocrine enzymes is low compared to levels in the adult gland. Unlabeled antibody enzyme method. ×175.

nents.[21-25] Endocrine cells appear early in ontogenesis (Fig. 1), and the ability of islets to synthesize glucagon and insulin can be shown at a time when acinar cells are still relatively undifferentiated.[21-29] The high growth potential of these endocrine cells has been demonstrated *in vitro*.[24,26,28] During the early neonatal period, the pancreatic islet volume and insulin content of the pancreas are high (Fig. 2),[30-36] while the acinar cell component and enzyme content are reduced in comparison with adult levels.[36-38] Thus, by choosing the appropriate aged neonatal or fetal pancreas, tissue can be obtained which is relatively rich in functioning islets or which possesses a high islet tissue growth potential.

Cellular dispersion techniques used in tissue culture studies have been successfully applied to the pancreas. With enzymatic and mechanical disruption of the pancreas, preparations of dispersed cells derived from the entire pancreatic gland can be obtained (Fig. 3).[39-43] Subsequent growth of the dispersate in monolayer culture has established the viability of the endocrine cells as well as cells derived from the ductal and connective tissue components of the gland. Although the acinar cells in the dispersed pancreas are not physically separated from the endocrine component, these cells dedifferentiate or fail to survive *in vitro*.[40,41,43] The physiological responsiveness of the endocrine cells in such

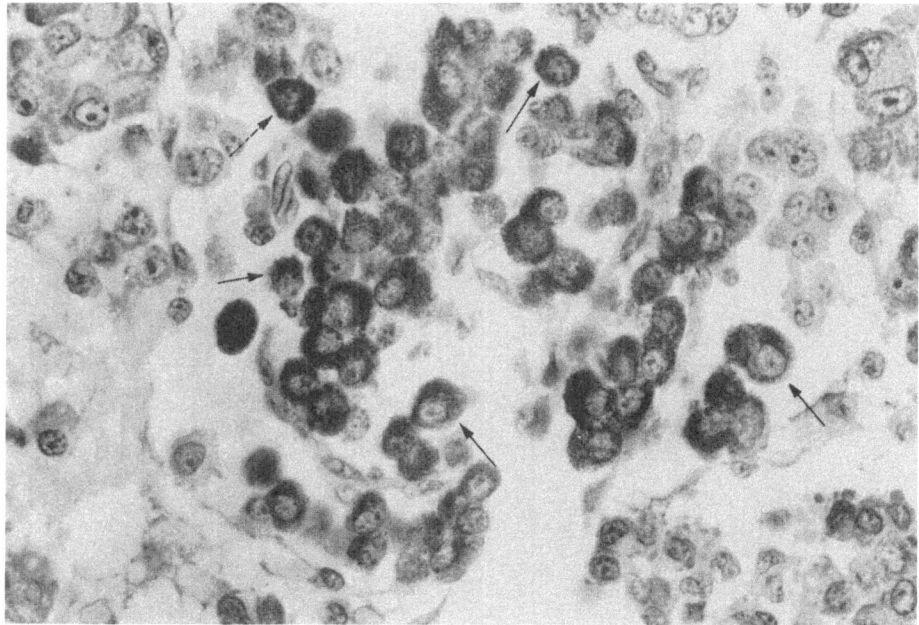

Figure 3. Enzymatic treatment with mechanical agitation of the pancreas results in a disaggregation of the cells. Histologic examination (following centrifugation and sectioning of the pellet) of dispersed 9-day neonatal pancreas reveals intact islet β cells either in clumps or as single cells (arrows) as well as cells derived from the other tissues of the pancreas. Aldehyde fuchsin–Ponceau de xylidine. ×700.

preparations to appropriate stimuli is evidenced by secretion of insulin and glucagon.[40,42] Although estimates of overall cell viability can be made following the initial dispersion procedure, the yield of viable endocrine cells is yet to be determined. With this technique, a mixed cell preparation can be obtained containing viable endocrine cells and apparently nonviable acinar cells.

Adult Islet Tissue

Enzymatic treatment of the adult pancreas can be employed as a means of separating the endocrine and acinar components.[44–46] With limited enzymatic digestion and subsequent hand-picking or density gradient centrifugation,[47] whole islets can be isolated from the remainder of the gland (Fig. 4). Approximately 200–400 islets can be isolated from an adult rat pancreas routinely by this method. Based on estimates of total islet number,[31,32] this represents about a 5–10% yield. The morphological and physiological integrity of the islets can be demonstrated *in vitro*.[47–52] Despite the more fibrous nature of the primate pancreas, the technique has been successfully applied to monkey[53] and human[54-57] glands with similar results. The physical separation of pancreatic components with this technique results in a pure preparation of viable mammalian islets.

Duct ligation of the pancreas *in vivo* results in a selective loss of the acinar component of the pancreas over a period of weeks.[58-61] The endocrine component remains morphologically intact, enmeshed in a connective tissue stroma and associated ductal elements (Fig. 5). Continued function of the islets is confirmed by the fact that the duct-ligated animals are not diabetic. In addition, portions of such pancreases can be successfully grown *in vitro* with continued survival and function of the islets.[62] With this preparation, although the islet tissue is not separated from the gland, a selective destruction of the acinar cells results in an adult islet preparation which is somewhat analogous to fetal and neonatal pancreas.

Each of these techniques for the acquisition of purified preparations of mammalian islet tissue has been successfully utilized in recent transplantation studies to affect a reversal of experimentally induced diabetes in animal models.

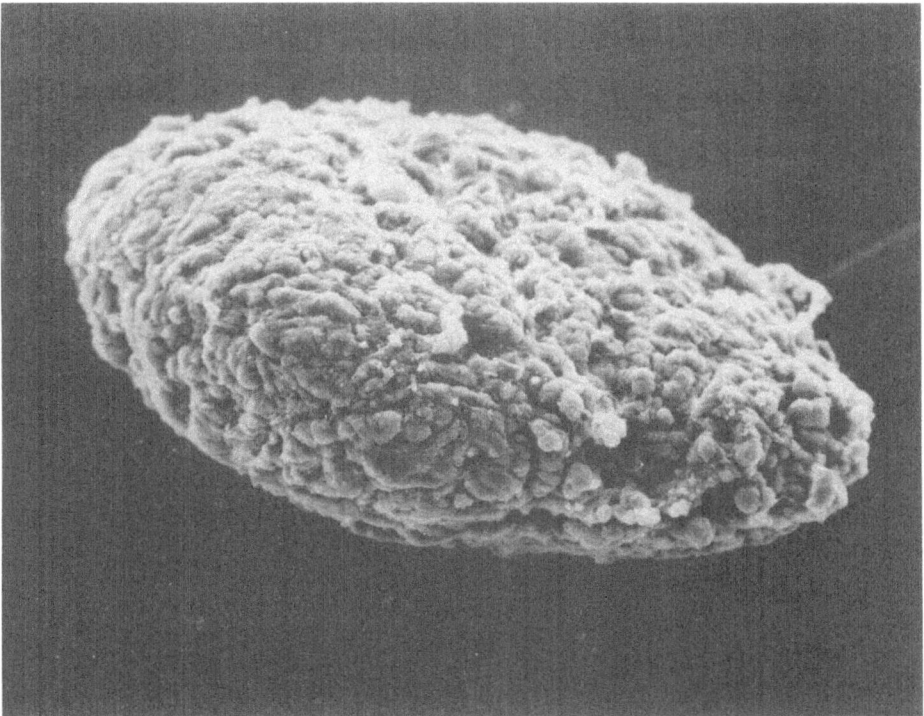

Figure 4. Scanning electron micrograph of a rat islet isolated by the collagenase technique. (Courtesy of Paul E. Lacy.)

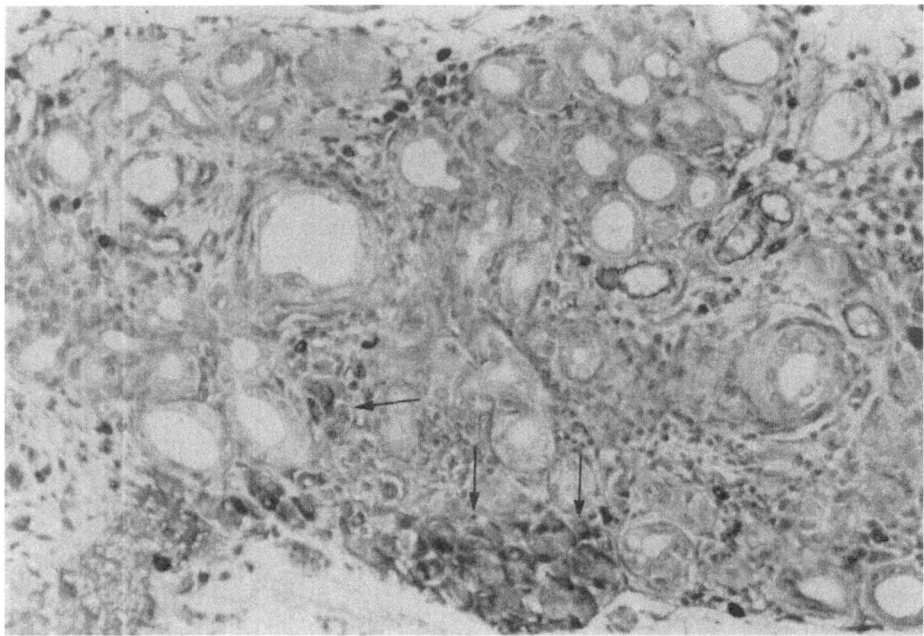

Figure 5. Histologic examination of adult rat pancreas, 6 weeks following pancreatic duct ligation, reveals an absence of acinar cells but the persistence of both ductal and islet (arrows) components distributed within the connective tissue stroma. Aldehyde fuchsin–Ponceau de xylidine. ×240.

Isogenic Transplantation Studies

The utilization of inbred strains of experimental animals, thus circumventing the immunological effects of the host on graft survival and function, has permitted the investigation of islet cell transplantation with a number of different preparations at a variety of transplantation sites. These studies have established the efficacy of the islet cell transplantation approach (Fig. 6).

Adult Isolated Islets

The amelioration of streptozotocin-induced diabetes in the rat by intraperitoneal isotransplantation of enzymatically separated isolated islets was first reported by Ballinger and Lacy in 1972.[63] The majority of recipients, receiving 400–600 isolated islets, exhibited a reduction in polyuria, glycosuria, and hyperglycemia accompanied by stabilization of weight and prolonged survival. In some recipients, with mild diabetes, a complete and persistent reversal of the diabetic state was attained. The ability of intraperitoneally transplanted islets to ameliorate the diabetic state was confirmed in subsequent studies on moderate[64-71] and severely diabetic (ketotic) rats[72] and mice.[73] A relationship between the amount of islet tissue transplanted and the degree of amelioration attainable was demonstrated in studies involving the transplantation of large numbers of rat islets (800–1800) to the intraperitoneal site. The majority of these recipients demonstrated an apparent permanent normalization of metabolic parameters.[68,71] A normal response to standard glucose tolerance tests (0.5 g/kg i.v.) was observed in these recipients.[71] However, higher doses of glucose (1.0 g/ kg oral) produced an abnormal response,[68] suggesting a reduced insulin reserve (islet mass) in the reversed recipients. Over a period of months a significant number of recovered or ameliorated recipients returned to their pretransplant diabetic state.[66-68,73] The incidence of recurring diabetes was related to the initial number of islets transplanted and suggested that minimal numbers of transplanted adult islets may eventually fail at the intraperitoneal site, perhaps due to exhaustion by overstimulation.[68] The nature of the intraperitoneal site makes complete removal of the transplanted islet impossible.

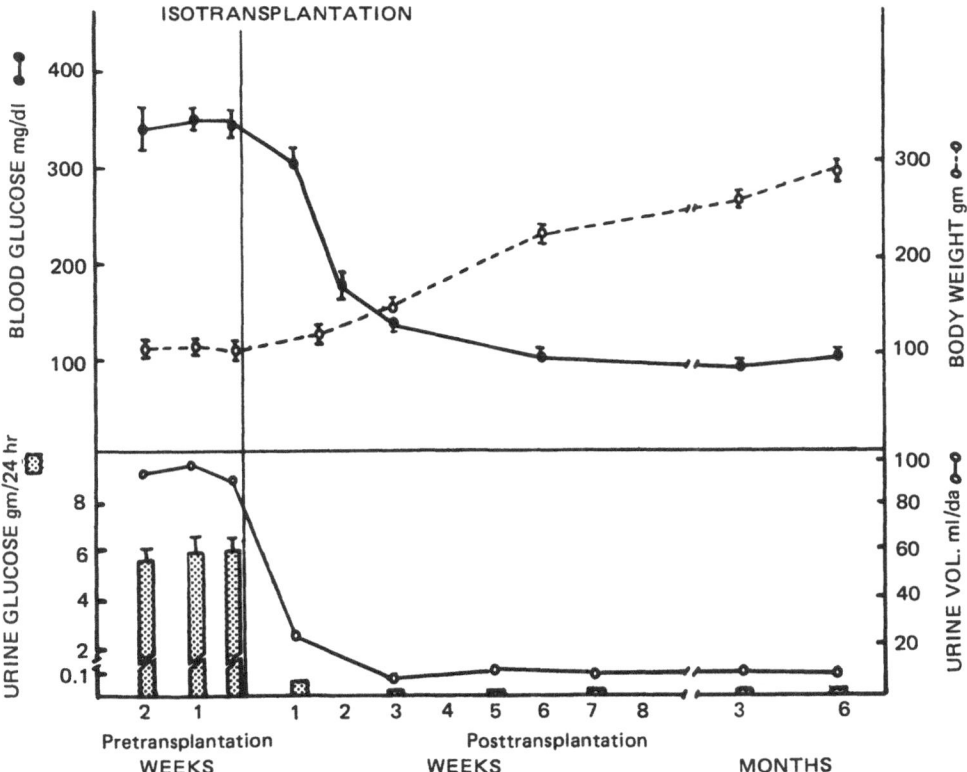

Figure 6. Reversal of the diabetic state in isologous rat recipients following intraperitoneal transplantation of dispersed neonatal pancreas. Similar results can be demonstrated in diabetic recipients receiving donor islet tissue derived from isolated adult islets, duct-ligated pancreas, and whole fetal pancreases transplanted at various sites.

However, morphological evidence of surviving transplanted islets has been obtained.[71] Immunofluorescent localization of insulin and glucagon in the recovered islets confirmed the presence of both β and α cells. Histological examination of the recipient's own pancreases at times following successful reversal of the diabetic state revealed pancreatic islets characteristic of streptozotocin diabetes and gave no evidence of spontaneous recovery on the part of the recipient.[63,65] Thus, it is clear that the transplanted islets were responsible for the improvement in the diabetic state.

Although transplantation to the peritoneal cavity approximates an orthotopic site, assurance of islet implantation on the visceral peritoneum and, therefore, portal venous drainage of secreted insulin and other islet hormones cannot be guaranteed. The small mass of the isolated islet preparation, however, has permitted its injection into the portal vein with subsequent embolism to the liver.[66] This alternative site assures that hormones released from the transplanted islets will reach the liver in high concentrations and in this manner will more closely stimulate the *in vivo* condition. The intraportal injections of isolated islets, introduced by Kemp *et al.*,[66,67] has been successfully utilized by a number of other investigators to attain long-term reversal of experimentally induced diabetes.[68,71,74−79] In the majority of rats receiving from 400–600 to 1000–2500 isolated islets, prompt reversal of the diabetic state occurred, as evidenced by a return to normoglycemia and aglycosuria, initiation of weight gain, and normal circulating insulin levels. "Reversed" animals have been followed for from 2 to 6 months[66,71,75,76] to over 1 year,[74,78] and return to the diabetic state has not been reported. Glucose tolerance tests in these animals, although dramatically improved over untreated diabetics, were still abnormal.[74] When greater numbers of isolated islets were transplanted to the liver site (1000–2500), representing the replacement of 10–30% of the normal islet number in an adult rat,[31,32] reversed recipients had a normal glucose response curve following intravenous glucose tolerance test.[71,79] Their blood insulin curves were elevated, however, indicating a nonphysiological response to glucose challenge.[79] Histological examination of the liver from recipients revealed islets in the terminal hepatic portal venules and in the connective tissue of the portal ducts (Fig. 7).[66,74,77,80−82] The islets appeared fully vascularized by day 8 posttransplantation[81] and were comprised primarily of heavily granulated β cells.[66,82] Both insulin and glucagon could be demonstrated in such islets by immunofluorescent techniques,[71] and by immunoassay of homogenates of isletbearing livers.[77] Ultrastructural examination confirmed the presence of α cells within the hepatic islets as well as δ cells.[81] The presence of the islets within the liver appeared to have little if any adverse effect on hepatic morphology[81,82] or function[80] and did not initiate portal vein hypertension.[80] Increased glycogen and lipid in hepatocytes were noted in the early phases following transplantation, but they disappeared with time.[81]

Isolated rat islets have been placed at a number of other sites in diabetic recipients with varying degrees of success. Injection of isologous islets into the systemic venous system has been without effect[68] or produced only transitory amelioration of the diabetic state.[67] Isotransplantation of 200[64] or 400–600[63]

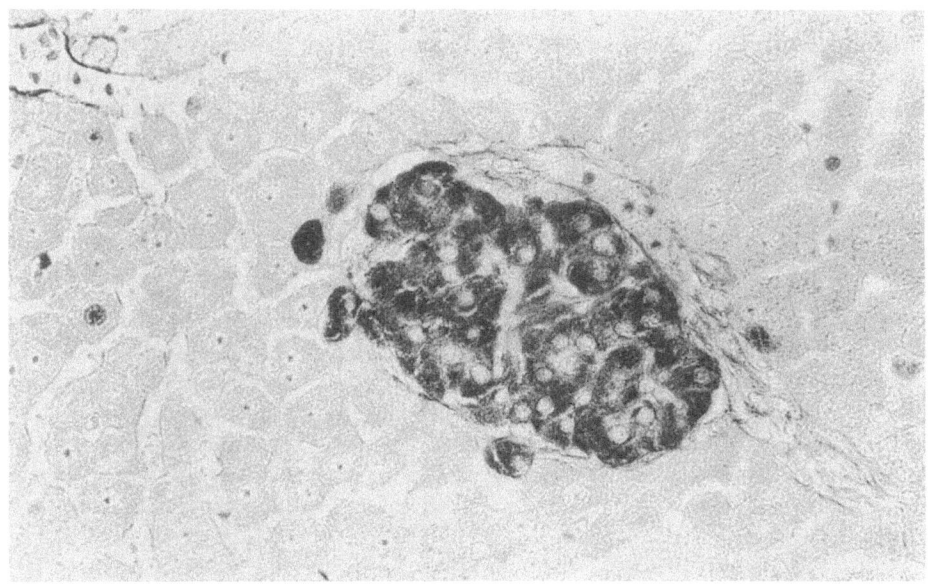

Figure 7. Following injection of adult isolated rat islets into the portal vein, histologically intact islets can be found in the terminal portal venules of the recipient's liver. The hepatic islets in reversed recipients are comprised primarily of heavily granulated β cells. Aldehyde fuchsin. × 420. (Courtesy of Paul E. Lacy.)

islets intramuscularly was without measurable effect on recipient hypergly-cemia, glycosuria, or body weight. A decreased mortality in animals receiving 400–600 islets, however, suggested some beneficial effect of the transplant.[63] Intramuscular transplantation of large numbers of isolated islets (850) to ketotic recipients resulted in the disappearance of ketonemia, amelioration of hyperglycemia, and prolonged survival.[72] In one animal, transitory reversal of the diabetes was obtained. The localized nature of the islets permitted their subsequent recovery and histological examination. Degranulated β cells were observed within surviving islets, a morphological response consistent with the hyperglycemic state of these recipients and suggestive of insulin release.[63,72] Transplantation of isolated islets to subcutaneous sites has so far proved ineffective in altering the diabetic state in the rat, even though large numbers of islets (890) were transplanted in some cases.[66,67] Small numbers of isolated islets (200) also proved ineffective when placed within the testicle or beneath the kidney or splenic capsule.[64] However, more recent evidence suggests that the spleen may be a suitable site for implantation if large enough numbers of islets are transplanted.[83] When 800 isolated islets were injected into the substance of the spleen, amelioration of diabetes was obtained. Following splenectomy, a return to pretransplant blood glucose levels occurred. Histological evidence of surviving islets, consisting of degranulated β cells, was obtained, and mitotic figures were observed within the transplanted islet tissue.

In summary, adult isolated islets have proven effective as an islet cell transplant source. The severity of the diabetic state determines the number of islets required for reversal.[72] The transplanted islets survive and function at a number of different sites, and at present the hepatic site appears advantageous in that fewer islets are required, a greater percentage of recipients are reversed, and the effectiveness of the transplanted islet is more permanent.[75]

Adult Duct-Ligated Pancreas

To date the duct-ligated preparation has had limited trial as a source of donor islet tissue for isotransplantation studies.[84,85] Four minced adult mouse pancreases, removed 6–8 weeks following duct ligation, successfully reversed experimental diabetes in isogenic recipients when transplanted subcutaneously.[84] Histologically identifiable islets with aldehyde-fuchsin-positive β cells were observed in the transplants recovered from the subcutaneous site. Intraperitoneal transplantation of duct-ligated pancreas resulted in a significant amelioration of the diabetic state; however, complete reversal was not obtained.[85]

The time required to reach normoglycemia following subcutaneous transplantation was related to the severity of the pretransplant diabetes. In less severely diabetic animals (streptozotocin induced) normoglycemia was attained in the majority of recipients by 5 weeks posttransplantation. With more severely alloxan-diabetic animals, fewer recipients recovered and longer periods were required for decreases in blood glucose to become apparent.[84] A similar delay of 4–8 weeks before recovery was reported in pancreatectomized dogs receiving an autotransplant of duct-ligated pancreas.[86]

The role of the transplanted β cells in reversal of diabetes was demonstrated by the failure to reverse the diabetic state when duct-ligated fragments from streptozotocin- or alloxan-diabetic donors were used.[85] Interestingly, over 7 to 8 months following such transplantation, amelioration of the diabetic state did occur in 80% of the recipients. Although spontaneous recovery on the part of these animals cannot be excluded in these preliminary experiments, the slow amelioration in the recipients suggests the possibility of proliferation of surviving β cells or the regeneration of new β cells from surviving precursors within the grafts. Support for the hypothesis may be found in reports of islet regeneration from ductal precursors in duct-ligated pancreas *in vivo*,[58,61] in organ culture,[62] and in transplants of duct-ligated pancreas to the anterior eye chamber,[87–89] and it may in fact offer an explanation for the delay periods routinely observed with this type of islet cell preparation.

Thus, minced fragments of duct-ligated pancreas have proven to be effective in reversing diabetes in the mouse. To date, the subcutaneous site, which has the advantage of easy accessibility, has proved most suitable for vascularization and subsequent function of this preparation. The peritoneal site appears less favorable, although not incompatible. Testing of other sites in isogenic recipients has not been reported.

Dispersed Islet Cells

Successful reversal of experimental diabetes utilizing an islet cell preparation derived from enzymatically dispersed neonatal rat pancreas was initially reported by Leonard *et al.* in 1973.[90,91] Subsequent studies have confirmed the suitability of both fetal and neonatal dispersed pancreatic cells for transplantation.[92–100] Since the nonendocrine components within the dispersate are included, the transplantation of relatively large quantities of tissue has been required (approximately 20–40 neonatal donor pancreases). The peritoneal cavity has been used in the majority of studies, offering the advantage of a large surface area for implantation and subsequent vascularization.[90–99] Following intraperitoneal injection of the dispersed cell population, the majority of diabetic recipients demonstrated a return to normoglycemia and aglycosuria, and the disappearance of polyuria.[94,95,97] Near-normal weight gain has been documented in these recipients, as well as normal levels of circulating insulin.[98] In some cases, hyperinsulinemia has been reported.[94,96] Blood glucose responses following intravenous glucose tolerance testing (0.5–3.0 g/kg) were normal in reversed recipients, as were insulin responses in most groups studied (Fig. 8).[90,91,94,95,98] Again, in some groups of animals receiving large quantities of dispersed islet tissue, a hyperinsulinemic response during glucose tolerance

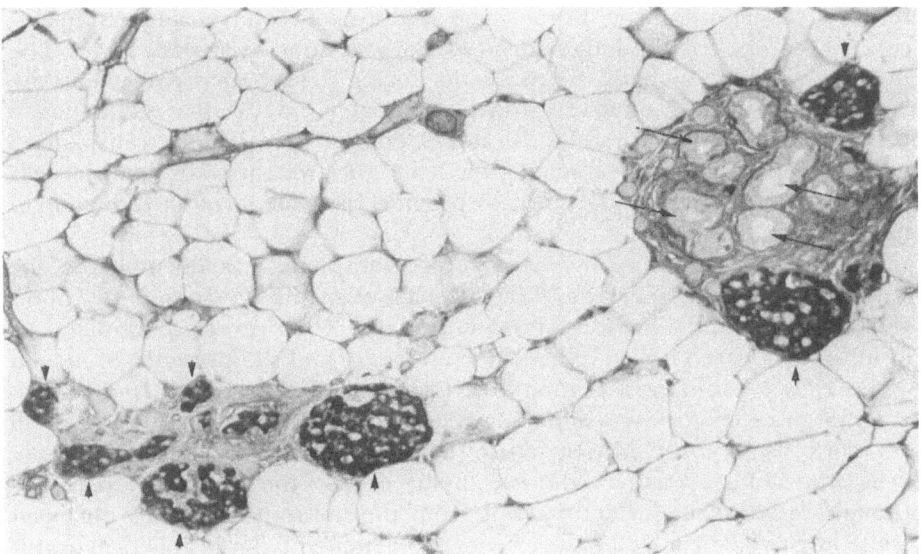

Figure 8. In recipients reversed of alloxan diabetes by intraperitoneal injection of dispersed neonatal pancreas, histologically identifiable transplanted islets can be recovered from the parietal and visceral peritoneum. Such islets (arrow heads) appear to consist primarily of heavily granulated β cells. Large accumulations of adipose tissue are routinely found in the areas of surviving islet tissue. While ductal elements (arrows) are also frequently observed in such grafts, acinar cells appear not to survive. Aldehyde fuchsin–Ponceau de xylidine. ×490.

testing was observed.[94] Successfully reversed animals have been followed from 6 months[90,91,94,95] to over a year,[98] and a return to the diabetic state has not been reported.

As observed with the isolated islet preparation, a relationship exists between the severity of the diabetes and the amount of dispersed islet tissue required to reverse the diabetic state.[90,91] In addition, the age of the donor tissue with this type of islet cell transplant appears to be critical. Use of adult tissue has been unsuccessful.[63,92] A nearly 100% success rate was obtained with early neonatal (1 day postpartum) or fetal dispersed pancreatic tissue, while reduced success was observed with older neonatal donor sources.[92] Fetal tissue appears to be the most effective source of donor cells in that less tissue is required to attain the same degree of success.[92,98]

As observed with the duct-ligated preparation, delays between the time of transplantation and reversal of the diabetic state were frequently seen with the dispersed islet cell preparation.[90,98,99] The length of time appeared to be related to both the amount of islet transplanted and to the age of the donor pancreas. When small amounts of neonatal donor pancreas were used, periods of more than 10 weeks were required before normoglycemia was attained.[98] In contrast, transplantation of small amounts of differentiated fetal pancreas was accompanied by a relatively short delay before normoglycemia was reached.[98] Although the time required for vascularization of the newly transplanted islet tissue may offer an explanation for the shorter delay periods between transplantation and recovery, reasons for the longer delay periods are not completely clear. The progressive improvement of the recipients during the recovery period and the relationship of its duration to the growth potential of the transplanted tissue are consistent with the hypothesis that while not enough islet tissue is transplanted initially to reverse the diabetic state, growth and differentiation of new islet cells during the transplant period eventually provide adequate insulin production to control the diabetes.[90,98]

Histological examination of recovered transplants has documented the failure of acinar tissue survival.[90,91,95,98] Ductal elements are frequently found associated with the surviving islet tissue. (Fig. 9).[90,97] In reversed recipients, β cells in the recovered islets are heavily granulated, and the presence of insulin in these cells is confirmed by immunocytochemical localization.[98] In addition, glucagon- and somatostatin-containing cells are present, demonstrating that all these islet cells survive.[98] Mitotic figures have been observed in recovered islet β cells, indicating growth of the islet tissue during the transplant period.[90] Although removal of the entire graft from the peritoneal site has not been possible due to its dispersed nature, evidence obtained from histological examination of recipients' own pancreases confirms the assertion that the transplanted dispersed islet cells were responsible for the normalization of the host (Fig. 10).[90,98]

Recent evidence suggests that the intraportal site can also be successfully combined with transplantation of small quantities of enzymatically dispersed neonatal pancreas.[101] Reversal of streptozotocin-induced diabetes was obtained in a high percentage of recipients and persisted for as long as 1 year. Data

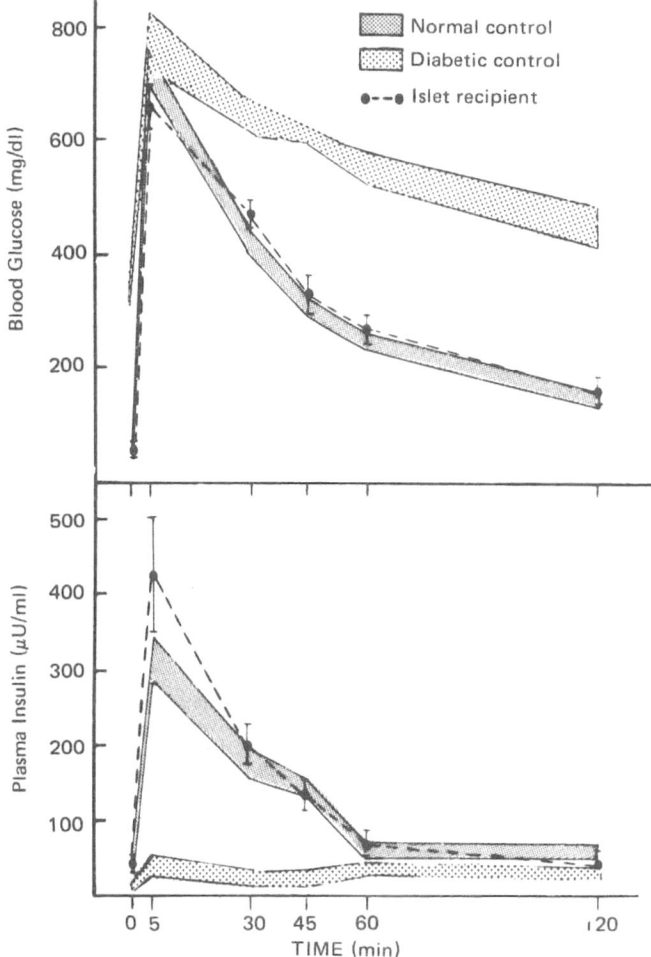

Figure 9. Intravenous glucose tolerance testing (3.0 g/kg) of reversed rat recipients 6 months following intraperitoneal isotransplantation of dispersed neonatal pancreas reveals both a normal blood glucose as well as plasma insulin response. The existence of an insulin reserve in reversed recipients following isotransplantation of isolated islets or fetal pancreas can also be demonstrated and suggests the survival of relatively large amounts of transplanted islet tissue.

suggest that as little as one neonatal pancreas can be effective in reversing the diabetic state if minimal damage is done during the dispersion procedure.

Successful reversal of the diabetic state has also been accomplished following subcutaneous transplantation of mechanically (nonenzymatically) disaggregated fetal pancreatic anlage.[100] Endocrine tissue composed almost exclusively of histochemically identifiable β cells, associated with ductal elements as well as acinar-like cells, was identified in recovered tissue 4 weeks after transplantation.[102,103] Severely diabetic rats (ketotic) maintained on insulin therapy in the

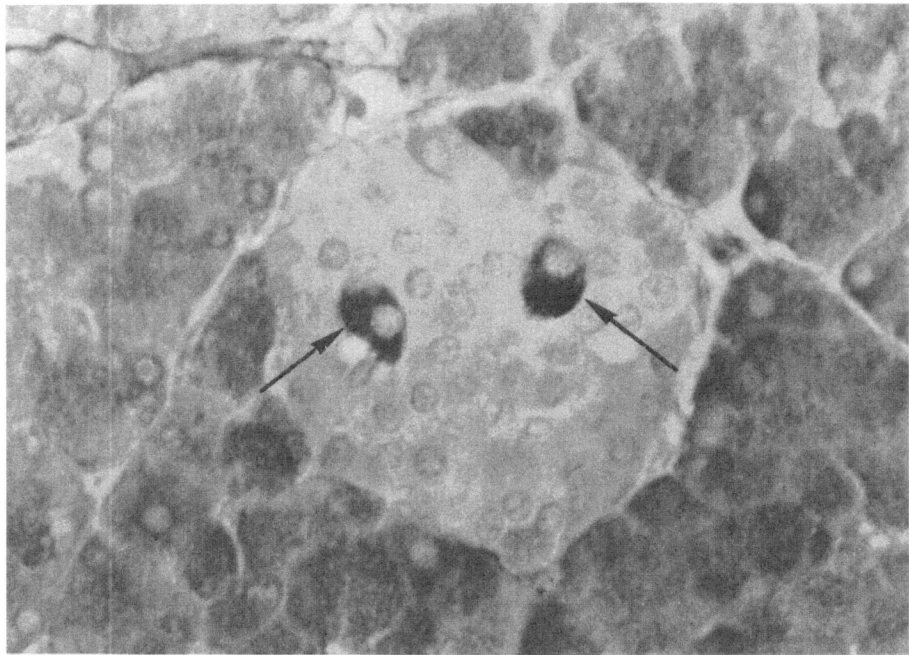

Figure 10. Following reversal of the alloxan-diabetic state, examination of the recipient's own pancreas reveals little evidence of β cell regeneration. The β cells which still survive (arrows) in these islets appear fully granulated, reflecting the normoglycemic condition of the recipient. However, the islets remain small and the total β cell mass of the recipient's pancreas is less than 3% of that in a normal adult pancreas. Aldehyde fuchsin–Ponceau de xylidine. ×710.

posttransplantation period exhibited a progressive improvement in their diabetic state, reaching normoglycemia around 3 to 4 months posttransplantation, and remained reversed following cessation of insulin therapy for over 1 year. Removal of the transplant resulted in a return to the diabetic state.[100]

In summary, the dispersed pancreatic islet cell preparation has proven to be an effective source of islet cells for transplantation studies in a number of sites, including the peritoneal cavity, subcutaneous tissue, and the liver. This preparation has the advantage of not requiring prior separation of nonislet component and thus permits the use of fetal tissue. The disadvantages include the inability to use adult pancreatic sources and, in addition, the necessity of exposing the cells to proteolytic enzyme treatment (as is also the case with whole islet transplantation), which undoubtedly damages some of the islet cells.

Pancreatic Slices

Early studies demonstrated that whole neonatal murine pancreases, when placed at a subcutaneous site in isogenic alloxan diabetic recipients, would significantly reduce glycosuria.[104] Transplantation of fetal pancreas was less effective but did prolong survival time in the majority of recipients. Definitive evidence of successful reversal of streptozotocin-induced diabetes was reported by Brown *et al.* in 1974 following the transplantation of relatively undifferentiated isologous fetal pancreas at the renal subcapsular site.[105] Recipients exhibited a normalization of parameters measuring glucose homeostasis, including a normal glucose and insulin response following standard intravenous glucose tolerance test.[105,106] Histologically, islets and ducts associated with a large accumulation of adipose tissue were observed in the recovered grafts (Fig. 11). Acinar cells were absent. Morphologically intact β and α cells were observed by ultrastructural techniques.[106] Removal of the grafts resulted in a return to the diabetic state in the majority of recipients, confirming the role of the transplant in reversal of the diabetic state.[105,106] The effectiveness of the transplanted fetal tissue in reversal of the diabetic state was related to the age of the pancreas at the time of transplantation, and to the number of pancreases (mass of islet tissue) transplanted, thus offering a probable explanation for previously reported unsuccessful attempts with fetal tissue.[65,104] Four to six fetal pancreases transplanted at a stage prior to complete acinar cell differentiation were most effective. The diabetic state in the recipients was ameliorated with exogenous insulin administration during the 1st week posttransplantation, with the suggestion that such treatment had a beneficial effect on subsequent trans-

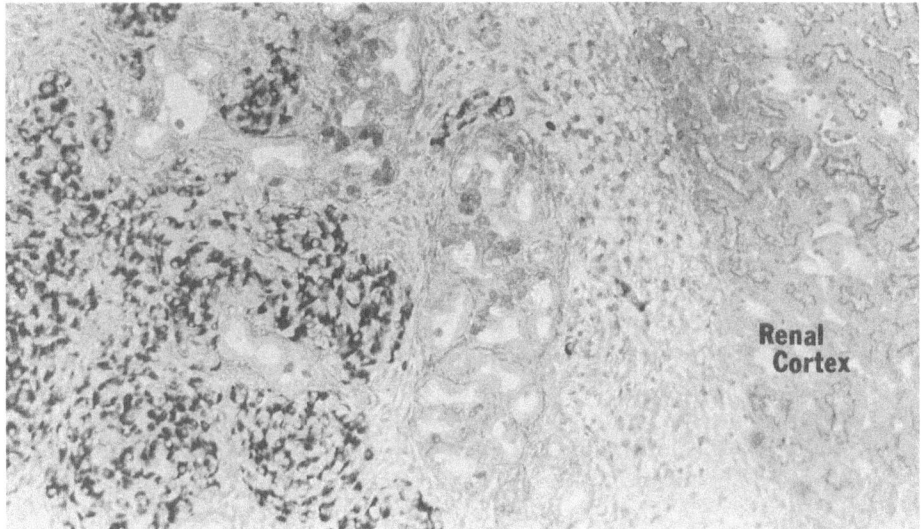

Figure 11. Histological examination of transplanted fetal rat pancreases recovered from the renal subcapsular site in reversed isologous recipients reveals the survival of both the islet and ductal components of the pancreas. Only occasional acinar cells can be identified in such grafts after 3 weeks at the transplant site. The presence of large numbers of β cells in such transplants (left) when compared with the number of cells present at the time of transplantation (cf. Fig. 1) indicates the continued growth and differentiation of these islet cells during the transplantation period. Aldehyde fuchsin–Ponceau de xylidine. ×155.

planted islet tissue function.[106] The beneficial effect of hypoglycemic agents on transplanted islet survival during the immediate posttransplantation phase has been previously suggested.[107,108] Increased growth and prolonged survival of the islet tissue in neonatal transplants was previously reported, when diabetic recipients were treated with insulin during the transplant period. Increased islet cell mitoses were observed in transplanted islet tissue recovered from tolbutamide-treated recipients.[108] Quantitative morphological studies have demonstrated that the fetal endocrine component (primarily the β cells) will continue to differentiate and grow when implanted into normal recipients.[91,98,109] Whether this promotion of islet tissue survival and growth is related to the insulin levels or to the glucose levels in the milieu of the transplanted islet is unclear at present. Recent data demonstrating that only one fetal pancreas is required to reverse the diabetic state, but only if it is first grown at the renal site in a normal adult for 3 weeks prior to transplantation to the diabetic recipient,[110] provides further evidence of the beneficial effects of a normal environment on subsequent islet transplant function.

Thus, untreated slices of whole fetal pancreas provide an effective source of donor tissue for isotransplantation studies. The small size of the pancreas and the inherent growth potential of the endocrine component permits the use of extremely small amounts of tissue. Advantage can be taken of the fact that the acinar component of the fetal pancreas fails to survive following transplantation, thus making prior treatment (enzymatic or duct ligation) unnecessary. The transplantation of the fetal pancreas itself acts as the means for obtaining the purified islet preparation, as was suggested by the studies of a number of earlier investigators.[111,112] It is interesting to note that this type of islet cell preparation was the one initially suggested by Ssobolew in 1902.[6]

Allogenic Transplantation Studies

The effectiveness of islet cell preparations, similar to those just described, has also been investigated in allogenic diabetic recipients. Although studies of whole organ pancreatic transplantation via vascular anastomosis suggested that islet tissue may be less immunogenic than some other organs,[18] allotransplantation experience with islet cells has consistently demonstrated that islet tissue provokes the expected immune response. Although short-term successful reversal of diabetes has been attained, allografts of islet tissue are rejected and a return to the diabetic state in the recipients occurs (Fig. 12).

Isolated Islets

In noninbred pancreatectomized rats receiving 600–1000 islets[113] and in partially inbred streptozotocin-diabetic animals receiving 100–600 islets[114] at a subcutaneous, epididymal fat pad site or muscle pocket, aglycosuria and an improved tolerance to glucose were observed during the first few weeks follow-

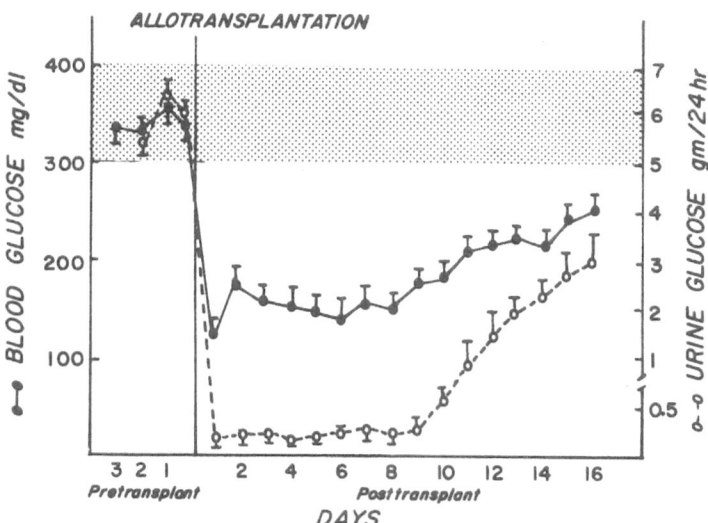

Figure 12. Temporary amelioration of experimentally induced diabetes can be accomplished following intraperitoneal allotransplantation of dispersed neonatal pancreas. However, within 2 weeks posttransplantation a progressive return to the diabetic state is observed. Similar short-term reversal of hyperglycemia and glycosuria has been observed with the isolated islet preparation.

ing transplantation. Although these allogenic recipients eventually returned to the prediabetic state, as a group they exhibited prolonged survival when compared with untreated diabetic controls.

Intraperitoneal allotransplantation of large numbers of isolated adult islets has also resulted in a transitory amelioration of the diabetic state.[64,65,68,113–115] The extent of amelioration was found to be related to the genetic compatibility of host and donor.[64,65,68] When donor and recipient differed at the major rat histocompatibility locus (*AgB*), transitory amelioration of the diabetes was seen to last less than 3 days. In contrast, normoglycemia could be maintained with allografts for an average of 8 days when donor and recipient were compatible at the *AgB* locus but incompatible at other, weaker histocompatibility loci. Rejection of the islets was confirmed, since sensitization of such recipients could be demonstrated by accelerated rejection of a subsequent skin graft from the same donor strain.[65,68] Similar results were obtained with a highly purified islet preparation, thus eliminating immunogenic effects of acinar cell contamination.[68] Further investigation of the factors related to islet failure in allogenic recipients indicates that islet tissue is vulnerable to both humoral as well as cellular immune response—more vulnerable than skin.[78]

Injection of islets into the systemic venous sytem of allogenic diabetic recipients resulted in a transitory amelioration of the diabetes. The effectiveness of isolated islets transplanted in this manner appeared to be more prolonged than at perivascular sites.[114]

Intraportal vein injection of allogenic isolated islets has also resulted in transitory amelioration of the diabetic state.[68,74,75,116] Crossing weak histocompatibility loci, 50% of recipients receiving isolated islets intraportally remained normoglycemic for approximately 30 days before rejection occurred, compared to only a 12-day period of reversal when the intraperitoneal site was used, suggesting an advantage to the liver site.[116] When differences at the *AgB* locus existed between donor and recipient, no advantage in the liver site was observed. Allotransplants of islets at the liver, as at other sites, sensitized the recipients as evidenced by accelerated second set skin graft rejection[75] and morphological studies of such intrahepatic islets, allotransplanted to normal and diabetic recipients across major histocompatibility barriers, show early signs of rejection.[82] The advantages of the liver site from an immunological standpoint require further elucidation.

Dispersed Cells

Transient reversal of experimental diabetes has also been attained with allotransplantation of dispersed pancreatic cells. Prior to the immunological response on the part of the recipient, clinical parameters of glucose homeostasis indicated effective function of the allotransplanted neonatal rat islet tissue.[90,91,97,98] Following reversal of the diabetes, a slow return to the prediabetic state was observed, beginning around 8–10 days[90] or even more rapidly, beginning at 4–5 days posttransplantation.[97] Histologic examination of grafts recovered from the peritoneal lining within the 1st week following transplantation indicated islet cell survival,[90,97] including evidence of islet cell division,[90] while grafts recovered at later times provided evidence of round cell infiltration and β cell destruction in the islets.[90,97] Xenotransplantation of dispersed rat pancreatic cells to diabetic mice has also been reported with results similar to those described above.[97]

Duct-Ligated Adult Pancreas

No improvement in streptozotocin-induced diabetes was observed when minced tissue obtained from three duct-ligated pancreases were allotransplanted subcutaneously to mouse recipients differing at the major histocompatibility locus.[85] Recipients remained hyperglycemic during the 18-week period of observation.

Pancreatic Slices

Early studies indicated that fragments of adult, neonatal, or fetal pancreas were ineffective as transplants to allogenic recipients.[104,117] Transplantation antigens appear early in ontogenesis[118]; however, some evidence suggests that fetal tissue may be less immunogenic than adult.[119–121] Fetal pancreas does appear to be immunogenic, since sensitization of recipients was observed following transplantation across weak histocompatibility barriers.[68] Nevertheless, a brief report indicating the histological survival of fetal pancreas in the majority of incompatible (differing at *AgB* locus) allogenic recipients 1 and 2 months posttransplantation[122] suggests further investigation of this islet cell preparation be pursued.

Improved Transplantability of Islet Tissue Allografts

Abrogation of Recipients' Immune Response

Efforts have been directed toward improving the survival and function of allo- or xenotransplanted islet tissue by recipient modification utilizing immunologically privileged sites, immunosuppressive therapy, induced tolerance, or irradiation.

Immunologically Privileged Sites. Circumvention of or at least a weakening of the recipient's immune response to allotransplanted islet tissue can be accomplished by utilization of immunologically privileged sites.[123] The anterior chamber of the eye,[104,112,124] the testis,[111,125] and the hamster cheek pouch[107,108,126,127] were utilized to provide the first definitive evidence of the survival and function of transplanted islet cell preparations. Morphological study of allotransplanted pancreatic fragments in a number of species demonstrated selective survival of the islet and ductal components accompanied by the loss of acinar tissue.[104,107,108,111,125-127] Additional studies demonstrated that better islet survival and growth at the transplant site was attained with immature donor pancreases (fetal and neonatal),[104,127] thus confirming observations with other organs.[128,129] Islet tissue at these sites survived for extended periods, in some cases (anterior chamber) for over 1 year.[112] In general, morphological examination revealed islet tissue consisting almost exclusively of β cells.[104,107,108,111,125] Degranulation of the β cells occurred in transplants to diabetic recipients, suggesting physiological responsiveness of the cells.[107,127] The demonstration of insulin-like activity (ILA) in the recovered grafts[111,125,126] and in medium following *in vitro* incubation of recovered grafts[126] confirmed the survival of the β cells. Increases in allograft ILA following transplantation of fetal pancreas correlated with observation of continued differentiation and growth of the islet tissue during the transplant period.[111,125] Though relatively small amounts of islet tissue were transplanted in these studies, transitory amelioration or normalization of hyperglycemia was obtained in some groups of diabetic allogenic recipients.[125,130]

Although slices of adult pancreas are unsuccessful,[104] other adult islet cell preparations have been shown to survive and function at immunologically privileged sites in allogenic recipients. Six months following allotransplantation to the anterior chamber site nearly 25 % of duct-ligated pancreatic fragments had morphologically identifiable islet tissue.[88,89] Evidence of islet growth was noted, including the suggestion of neogenesis of islet from duct elements.[87] α and δ (A_1) cells, along with β cells, were identified by light and electron microscopy.[87,88] Although amelioration of the diabetic state has not been reported, evidence of β cell degranulation in duct-ligated grafts recovered from these recipients suggests functional responsiveness of the islet tissue. Adult isolated islets also survive for extended periods when allotransplanted to an immunologically privileged site (testis).[131-133] Guinea pig islets, recovered 1 to 2 weeks following allotransplantation to normal recipients consisted of both α and partially degranulated β cells.[131,132] Mitoses were observed in both these cell populations. Lymphocytic infiltration was not observed. When transplanted for longer periods, varying degrees of lymphocytic infiltration were observed within the testicular islets.[133] Allotransplantation of adult isolated islets to immunologically privileged sites in diabetic recipients has not yet been reported.

Immunosuppression. The studies on the effects of immunosuppression in islet cell recipients have, to date, shown no adverse effects on implantation and function of isogenically transplanted islets,[43] while immunosuppression in allogenic recipients has been shown to have a beneficial effect on transplanted islet tissue function and survival.

Early studies demonstrated a beneficial effect of cortisone on allografts of neonatal hamster pancreas transplanted to the cheek pouch.[107,108] Better growth and survival of the islet cells within the transplants and reduced lymphocytic infiltration were reported in normal or insulin-treated diabetic recipients.[107]

Azathioprine effectively prolonged allograft survival and function in recipients of rat isolated islets.[63] Animals demonstrated an amelioration of hyperglycemia, polyuria, and glycosuria, accompanied by stabilization of weight for 5 weeks following intraperitoneal transplantation. Intramuscular or intraperitoneal allotransplantation of isolated porcine islets to immunosuppressed pancreatectomized recipients resulted in a prolongation of survival time, amelioration of hyperglycemia in some recipients, and increases in circulating insulin.[55]

Antilymphocytic serum (ALS) has also been successfully employed in prolonging survival and function of allotransplanted islet tissue. ALS treatment of allogenic rat recipients ensured longer function of isolated islets transplanted via the portal vein[74,134] or to the peritoneal site,[65] with normoglycemia maintained for up to 220 days.[134] At the peritoneal site ALS was effective only in transplants compatible at the major AgB locus.[65] In such recipients, ALS given for 5 days prior to transplantation prolonged normoglycemia threefold with some animals remaining reversed of their diabetes for over 3 months. When comparing these results to skin grafts, ALS was less effective in prolonging islet survival, confirming marked immunogenicity of isolated islet preparations.[65]

Induced Tolerance. House *et al.* reported that allotransplantation of neonatal hamster pancreas to the cheek pouch of nondiabetic adult thymectomized recipients resulted in greatly increased growth of the implants and increased numbers of surviving, heavily granulated β cells.[135] These results, however, have not been confirmed or extended. More recently, pretreatment of recipients with ALS prior to allogenic islet transplantation (across weak histocompatibility barriers) has resulted in the ability of the recipients to accept skin grafts of the same donor strain 4–9 months later, suggesting induction of tolerance.[68]

ALS treatment in combination with the injection of bone marrow cells prior to transplantation of the streptozotocin diabetic recipients with incompatible islet tissue led to prolongation of normoglycemia for up to 16 weeks, providing preliminary evidence that abrogation of the immune response in adult animals by the induction of tolerance (or enhancement) may be useful in studies of islet cell allotransplantation.[136]

Irradiation. Sublethal irradiation of rats prior to intraperitoneal xeno-transplantation of teleost islet tissue resulted in a temporary (24 hr) amelioration of hyperglycemia in the majority of recipients.[137] Experiments in mice have demonstrated the ability of duct-ligated pancreatic tissue to reverse experimental diabetes when subcutaneously transplanted to diabetic allogenic radiation chimeras.[85] In these experiments the immunocompetent cells of lethally irradiated mice were replaced by injection of allogenic bone marrow. Following induction of diabetes by streptozotocin, these chimeras receiving either allogenic or isogenic duct-ligated pancreas demonstrated a progressive fall in blood glucose, approaching normal levels over a period of weeks.

Modification of Donor Tissue

Attempts have been made to improve the survival and function of allo- or xenotransplants by modification of the donor islet preparation, prior to transplantation, by the use of artificial chambers or by *in vitro* incubation. Success has been limited.

Artificial Chambers. Based on experiences with other endocrine tissues,[138–140] a number of investigators have pursued the feasibility of sequestering transplanted islets in artificial chambers as a means of prolonging their function and survival in allogenic recipients. Amelioration of hyperglycemia was not observed in diabetic mice receiving 300 isogenic isolated islets enclosed in a Millipore chamber at a subcutaneous site,[141] nor in rats receiving a similar transplant of 500–1000 isologous islets intraperitoneally.[67] Although diabetic rats receiving an intraperitoneal allotransplant of 600–1000 islets enclosed with a Millipore chamber did exhibit a temporary amelioration of glycosuria, the overall response of these animals to allotransplantation was no better nor more prolonged than that in animals receiving islet tissue directly to other sites.[113] As observed by earlier investigators, an adverse host response to the chamber, in this case the elaboration of a thick fibrous layer around the implanted Millipore capsule, may have interfered with vascularization and/or secretory capacity of islet grafts. Xenotransplantation of teleost islets encased in Millipore chambers or dialysis envelopes resulted in a transitory reduction in hyperglycemia in diabetic rat recipients, usually lasting only a matter of hours, but under certain conditions persisting up to 5 days.[137]

Despite this limited success with experimentally diabetic animals, the ability of chamber-enclosed isolated islets to survive and function has been demonstrated in transplantation studies to nondiabetic animals. Murine islets enclosed in a Millipore chamber continued to demonstrate insulin responsiveness to glucose stimulation *in vitro* following a 1-week transplantation period at a subcutaneous site in normal isogenic recipients.[141] When chambers containing about 200 normal murine islets were transplanted intraperitoneally to mice with genetic obese hyperglycemic syndrome (NZO or *ob/ob*), amelioration of the syndrome was observed.[142-144] These animals, although hyperglycemic, also exhibit hyperinsulinemia. The normalization of blood glucose, reduction in hyperinsulinism, and reduction in body weight which occurred during the transplantation period were reversed when the chamber was removed from the animal, confirming that the isolated islets could maintain function for as long as 45 to 70 days. A well-vascularized tissue encapsulation was observed around chambers removed from successfully ameliorated animals after 45 days. Islets in chambers removed 10 weeks following intraperitoneal transplantation were still viable, as indicated by their ability to release insulin in response to glucose stimulation *in vitro*.[143,144]

The survival and function of chamber-enclosed islets in nondiabetic recipients[141-144] suggests that the diabetic state itself may be deleterious to the implantation and vascularization of the chamber. Studies involving the amelioration of the diabetic state during the initial posttransplantation period may permit further investigation concerning the feasibility of utilizing chamber-enclosed islet tissue as a means of inducing prolonged reversal of experimental diabetes in allogenic recipients.

Organ Culture. Based on reported experience with a number of endocrine organs[145-147] and tumor cells,[148-153] the effects of a period *in vitro* have been tested on the immunogenicity of subsequently transplanted islet tissue. To date, unequivocal demonstration of prolonged islet allograft survival following incubation *in vitro* has not been attained. Fetal pancreatic slices cultured for 10 days prior to transplantation at the kidney capsule of normal allogenic recipients did not survive beyond 10–14 days.[98] Allogenic adult isolated islets maintained in tissue culture for 8 days prior to injection into the portal vein did not significantly increase survival time of diabetic recipients, and the tissue was rejected.[74] Human islet cells grown in monolayer for 8 weeks demonstrated identical HL-A type with lymphocytes from the original cadaver donor, indicating no change in their cellular antigens during culture.[154] One brief report has appeared in which prolonged reversal of the diabetic state was reported following organ culture of isolated islets prior to intraperitoneal allotransplantation.[155] However, these results have not been confirmed, and the possibility of fortuitous matching of histocompatibility loci cannot be ruled out, since animals used in the study were from an outbred strain.

Transplantation of in Vitro Preserved Islet Tissue

In light of the small mass of islet tissue present in mammalian pancreas and the difficulties in obtaining high yields of such islets, numerous studies have been directed toward developing means of preserving quantities of viable islet tissue which might eventually be utilized for transplantation.

Cryopreservation techniques have been applied to islet tissue. The limited data to date suggest that while enzymatically isolated rat[156] and canine islets[157] can be maintained at 4°C for 48 hr with only minor effects on insulin release in response to secretogogues, longer periods of storage are deleterious. More recent evidence demonstrates that β cell-rich *ob/ob* mouse islets can be successfully stored at 8°C for up to 1 week and still maintain normal insulin responsiveness to glucose stimulation.[158] Transplantation of cryopreserved islets has not been reported.

Tissue and organ culture (37°C) of islet prior to transplantation as a means of islet tissue storage has been successfully utilized in conjunction with transplantation studies (Fig. 13). Despite an early report of the unsuccessful survival

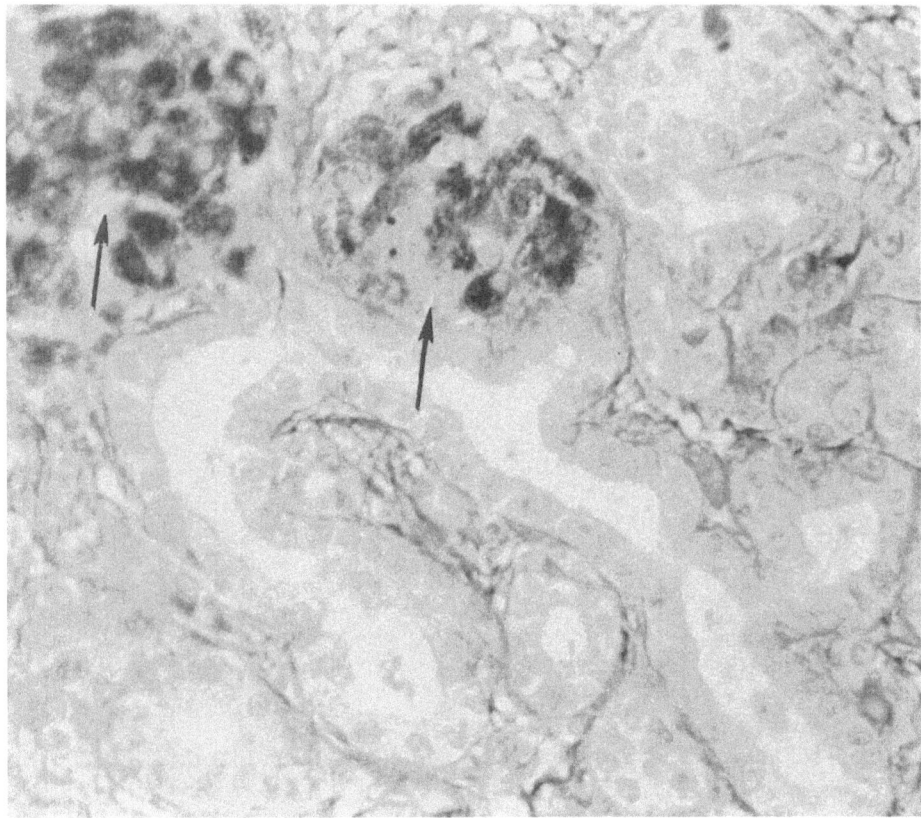

Figure 13. Histologic examination of neonatal pancreas grown in organ culture for 9 days reveals the continued survival of islet tissue (arrows). The presence of increased levels of insulin in the incubation medium following glucose stimulation of such explants suggests the continued physiological integrity of the islet β cells. Aldehyde fuchsin–Ponceau de xylidine. × 565.

and function of allotransplanted-organ-cultured fragments of either fetal or
duct-ligated canine pancreas,[159] more recent evidence demonstrates that the
explants of organ-cultured fetal rat pancreas can be successfully allotransplanted for up to 10 days.[91,109,160,161] Taking advantage of the selective survival
of islet tissue and accompanying degeneration of the acinar component *in
vitro*,[24,162] β cells in such cultured islet tissue appear to be responsive to glucose
stimulation in the diabetic recipients, as evidenced by degranulation of the β
cells and transitory amelioration of the recipient hyperglycemia.[91,160,161] In
addition, growth and differentiation of the β cells in cultured transplants
continued following transplantation.[109] Adult guinea pig isolated islets maintained in organ culture for 1 to 2 weeks remained viable for periods of up to 14
days when allotransplanted to a number of sites in normal recipients.[131,132]
Cultured adult rat isologous islets, maintained *in vitro* for up to 3 weeks,
reversed streptozotocin-induced diabetes when transplanted to liver via the
portal vein route.[163] Animals maintained normal glucose homeostasis for the 3-
month period of observation. Dispersed neonatal pancreatic cells, prepared

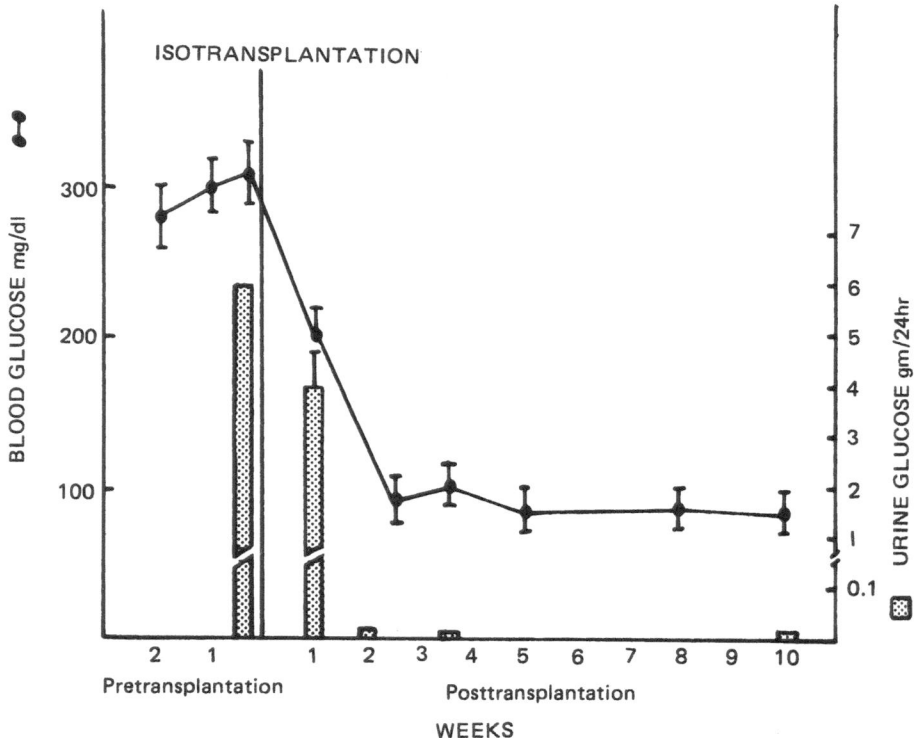

Figure 14. Organ-cultured neonatal pancreas maintained *in vitro* for 9 days prior to intraperitoneal
transplantation proved to be an effective source of donor islet tissue. The pattern of reversal of
experimental diabetes in isologous recipients of the dispersed preparation was similar to animals
receiving uncultured material (cf. Fig. 6).

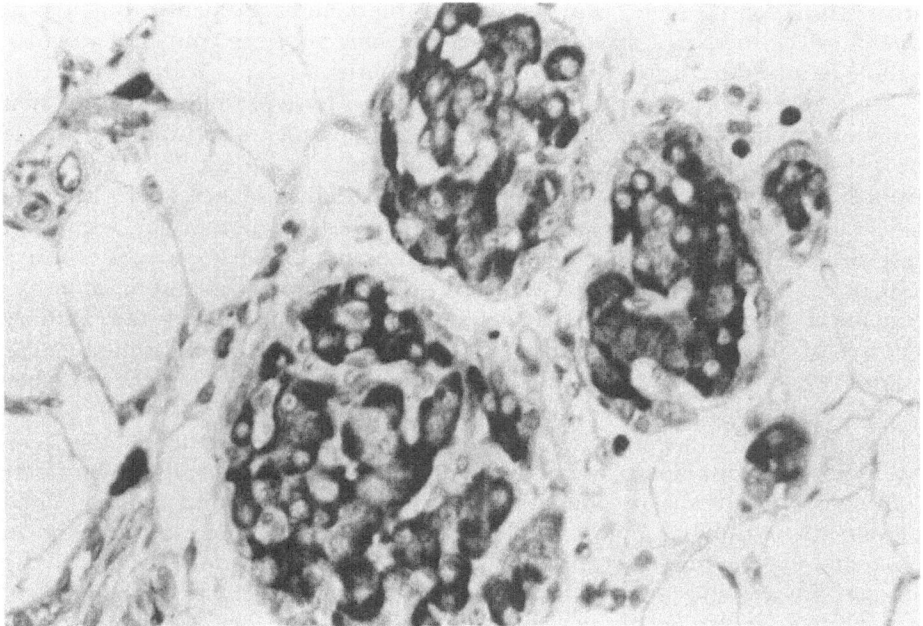

Figure 15. Transplants of organ-cultured dispersed neonatal pancreas could be recovered from the peritoneum of reversed recipients. Histologic examination revealed well-defined islets consisting primarily of heavily granulated β cells, associated with regions of adipose tissue. Aldehyde fuchsin–Ponceau de xylidine. ×440.

from explants incubated for 24 hr[95] or grown in organ culture for 2 to 9 days[98,164] have resulted in complete reversal of experimental diabetes in isologous recipients (Fig. 14). The time required for normalization of blood glucose following transplantation appeared to be related to the amount of islet mass transplanted, as was the case with uncultured tissue.[98,164] Morphological evidence of islet tissue survival was obtained following recovery of transplanted islets from the peritoneal cavity (Fig. 15). Normalization of recipients was observed for over 6 months, with no evidence of islet cell regeneration in the recipients' own pancreas.

Thus, the storage of islet tissue *in vitro* either by cryopreservation for short periods or in organ/tissue culture for more extended time periods prior to transplantation seems feasible from the standpoint of islet tissue survival and continued function.

Effects of Islet Cell Transplantation on Renal Glomerular Lesions in the Rat

From a clinical standpoint, pancreatic transplantation is visualized as an alternative to exogenous insulin therapy, with the hope that the replacement of normal functioning islets, providing a fine moment-to-moment physiological control of the metabolic state of the diabetic, may alter the course of vascular pathology associated with human diabetes mellitus.

Successful islet cell transplantation techniques have permitted investigation of the effects of reversal of the diabetic state by endogenous insulin release on the glomerular lesions of experimental diabetes in the rat.[165,166] Following reversal of diabetes by intraperitoneal transplantation of neonatal dispersed pancreatic endocrine cells, a regression or arrest of glomerular lesions in streptozotocin-induced diabetic rats was observed.[165] While diabetic control animals continued to demonstrate progressive morphological and immunohistochemical evidence of glomerular pathology, about half of the animals reversed of diabetes for 3 months had no further progression of the glomerular lesions, while the remainder actually demonstrated improvement. Further studies on the rate of regression of the glomerular lesion indicated that significant improvement in the kidney mesangium of long-term diabetic rats receiving islet cell transplants was apparent 2 weeks following transplantation.[166] Complement (C_3) was no longer detectable at 3 weeks, and only minimal staining for immunoglobulins was noted at 9 weeks. Although a reduction in mesangial thickening was apparent by 6–9 weeks posttransplantation, the abnormality was still present. Interestingly, one-third of the transplant recipients exhibited improved glomerular morphology during early phases posttransplantation when hyperglycemia was still present. These animals, however, did have normal insulin levels, suggesting that insulin or its effects, other than reduction of hyperglycemia, may play an important role in improvement of the glomerular lesions.[166] Further improvement was not observed in light-microscopical glomerular lesions examined at later times following reversal of the diabetes. Although these are the only reports to date concerning the effectiveness of islet cell transplantation on development and regression of vascular lesions in experimentally induced diabetes, similar observations have subsequently been reported using alternative experimental designs.[167,168] Evidence for the reversal of diabetic glomerular lesions has been reported when kidneys from diabetic rats were transplanted to normal recipients of the same strain,[167] and a similar decrease in the incidence and severity of morphological and immunohistochemical glomerular pathology has been observed following whole organ transplantation of the pancreas to diabetic rats.[168]

Islet Cell Transplantation Studies in Humans and Other Primates

The development of improved methods for the procurement of isolated islets from the fibrous primate pancreas has resulted in islet yields that have permitted initial studies of the effects of islet cell transplantation on diabetic primates.

Subhuman Primates

Rhesus monkeys made diabetic by a combination of partial pancreatectomy and streptozotocin received an intraportal allotransplant of isolated islets derived from a single donor and were maintained on immunosuppressive agents.[53] Although complete reversal of the diabetic state was not attained, improvement in the diabetes of five recipients was indicated by decreases in hyperglycemia, polyphagia, polyuria, and polydipsia. Recipients demonstrated an improved glucose tolerance test accompanied by an obtunded yet significant insulin response. One animal was reported still normoglycemic at 6 weeks posttransplantation.

Humans

The availability of viable human cadaver pancreases has been a limiting factor in these studies. In addition, the size as well as the histological structure of human pancreas have made separation of islet component from surrounding fibrous stroma and exocrine tissue difficult. However, technical advances have made such human isolated islet preparations available.[54-57] Although yields are inconsistent and generally low, morphological and biochemical evidence has indicated that relatively purified preparations of human islets can be obtained. The recent report of the successful isolation and maintenance of viable adult human islets in culture provides definitive evidence of the viability of such preparations.[57] β and α cells were preserved by ultrastructural criteria, and such islets were responsive to glucose and theophylline stimulation after 1 week in tissue culture. Monolayer cultures developed from isolated adult human islets have also been maintained up to 5 weeks *in vitro* and continued to release insulin into the medium.[154] Fetal human pancreases offered another possible source of islet tissue for transplantation. Studies have indicated that such pancreases can be successfully maintained *in vitro* for extended periods with continued survival and function of the islet β cells (Fig. 16).[91,169] Continued investigation of human pancreas *in vitro* may permit the future establishment of "islet banks" for use in conjunction with islet cell transplantation.[91]

While the effectiveness of whole organ pancreatic transplantation with vascular anastomosis in humans has been extensively investigated (see reviews cited earlier) only limited experience in humans has been reported with the transplantation of islet cell preparations. In 1938, Stone *et al.* reported an unsuccessful attempt at amelioration of human diabetes by islet cell transplantation.[146] On two occasions, grafts of cultured human embryonic pancreas were made; however, no beneficial effect was reported. In 1959, Brooks and Gifford reported experience with intramuscular transplantation of minced pancreatic fragments obtained from stillborn infants.[117] In six clinical trials the tissue was transplanted back to the diabetic mother; however, in only one case was a transitory reduction in recipient insulin requirement observed. Human islet cell adenomas have been tested for their effectiveness in ameliorating juvenile diabetes. In the earliest report, a benign islet adenoma was maintained in hanging drop culture for 3 weeks in medium derived from prospective recipient serum prior to subcutaneous implantation.[170] No effect upon the patient in terms of blood or urine glucose levels or insulin requirement was observed during the 3-month period of observation. In the second report, in which a pancreatic insulinoma was transplanted directly to an intramuscular site in an

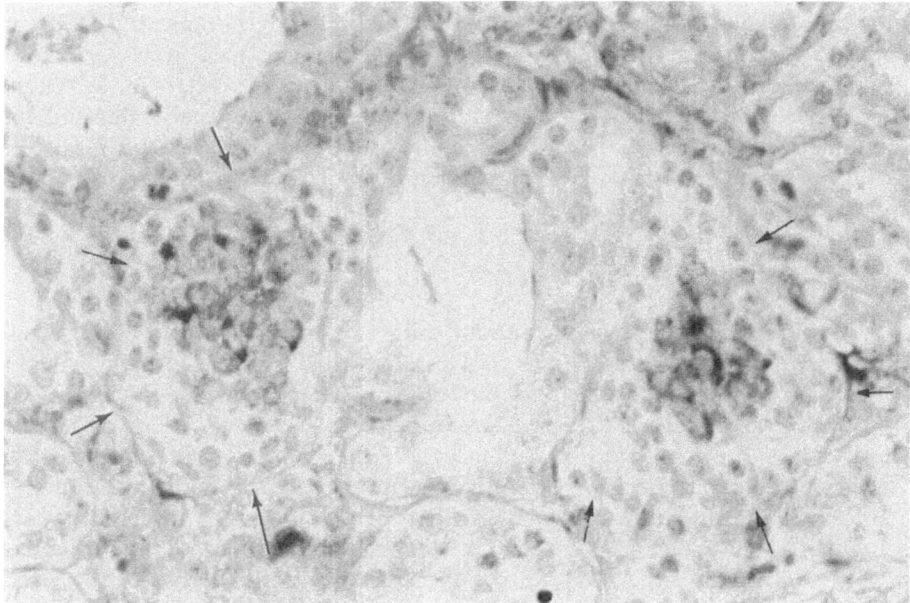

Figure 16. Histologic examination of 13-week gestation human fetal pancreas maintained in organ culture for 3 weeks revealed the presence of ductal elements and associated islets (arrows). Acinar cells were not present. Centrally located β cells as well as peripherally distributed non-β islet cells were identifiable, demonstrating the ability of the human fetal islet tissue to survive for extended periods *in vitro*. Aldehyde fuchsin–Ponceau de xylidine. × 440.

insulin resistant juvenile diabetic, temporary function of the grafted islet tissue was suggested.[171]

In light of the successful experience in reversing the metabolic parameters of diabetes in experimental animals, limited preliminary studies have been carried out to test the efficacy and safety of isolated islet transplantation to man.[172] The recipients were already on immunosuppressive therapy following renal allotransplantation for end-stage nephropathy. Isolated human cadaver islets, representing an estimated 1–14% of normal adult islet mass, were placed at various sites, including peritoneal cavity, liver via portal vein, and subcutaneously. Transitory decreases in exogenous insulin requirement to about 50% of pretransplant level were observed in 60% of the patients receiving transplants. In one recipient receiving infant islet tissue to the liver site, a more prolonged reduction in daily insulin requirement from 72 to 32 U was reported over a 14-month period.

Conclusions

Transplantation of islet tissue apart from its normal relationships within the acinar pancreas is feasible. Such islet cell transplants can reverse experimental diabetes, as measured by parameters of glucose metabolism, under a variety of experimental conditions. Adult isolated islets, dispersed neonatal and fetal pancreatic cells, fragments of adult duct-ligated pancreas, as well as slices of fetal pancreas and explants of cultured neonatal pancreas have all proven effective. In addition, a multiplicity of transplantation sites appear suitable, including subcutaneous and intramuscular sites, peritoneum, liver, spleen, and kidney capsule. The list can be expanded if one includes sites which have proven suitable for islet cell survival even though not yet successfully utilized in the reversal of the diabetic state. Indeed, it would seem that if one can prepare a viable preparation of islet tissue and transplant adequate quantities of the cells to a recipient site where vascularization is assured, normal glucose homeostasis can be attained. The goal of islet cell transplantation is to correct the hormonal deficiencies and imbalances in the experimentally diabetic recipient. While the parameters of glucose metabolism reflect an aspect of the hormonal status, direct evidence regarding insulin and glucagon as well as the other islet hormone levels in the various groups of successfully reversed recipients will be required to assess how "normal" the animals are. Evidence of persistent hyper-glucagonemia,[96] hyperinsulinemia,[94,96] and an abnormal pattern of insulin response to glucose tolerance testing[79,94] in some groups of islet cell recipients indicates that while animals may be successfully reversed of their diabetes, they may still be abnormal with respect to circulating levels of islet hormones. How important is the maintenance of the normal morphological relationships of the cells within the islet organ in terms of its hormonal function following trans-plantation? What are the effects of heterotopic transplantation of the hormone-secreting cells of the islet—thus altering the normal circulating levels of the various islet hormones—on the rest of the organism? Answers to these and other questions will be required before one can assess the best site or the most effective islet tissue preparation for transplantation.

The immunological aspects of islet cell transplantation are twofold. First, allogenic transplantation studies have provided evidence that islet tissue is immunogenic. Continued study utilizing experimental techniques seeking to alter the allograft rejection response may improve upon what up to now has been limited success. In addition, the mounting evidence favoring an immuno-logical etiology in insulin-dependent human diabetics—perhaps of an autoim-mune nature—raises some questions as to the eventual applicability of islet cell transplantation in these patients. These problems seem solvable only with major advances in transplantation biology and immunology in general.

On the more positive side, the evidence of a beneficial effect of islet cell transplantation on the regression of the kidney pathology seen in experimen-tally diabetic rats does provide the encouragement that islet cell transplantation may fulfill the goal of altering the progression of vascular complications associ-ated with human diabetes. In addition, the ability to maintain human islet tissue *in vitro* and the demonstration that such storage conditions do not alter the subsequent effectiveness of rat islet tissue as a transplantation donor source suggest that solutions to the problem of obtaining adequate amounts of islet tissue for human transplantation may be found.

References

1. Minkowski, O.: *Berlin Klin. Wochenschr.*, **29**:90, 1892.
2. Hedon, E.: *C. R. Soc. Biol.*, **44**:678, 1892.
3. Von Mering, J., and Minkowski, O.: *Arch. Exp. Pathol. Pharmakol.*, **26**:371, 1889.
4. Laguesse, E.: *C. R. Soc. Biol.*, **45**:819, 1893.
5. Schulze, W.: *Arch. F. Mikros. Anat. Entwick.*, **56**:491, 1900.
6. Ssobolew, L. W.: *Virchows Arch. Pathol. Anat.*, **168**:91, 1902.
7. Banting, F. G., Best, C. H., Collip, J. B., Campbell, W. R., and Fletcher, A. A.: *Canad. Med. Assoc. J.*, **12**:141, 1922.
8. Langerhans, P.: Thesis, Berlin, G. Lange, 1869.
9. Clark, E.: *Anat. Anz.*, **43**:81, 1913.
10. Hellman, B., and Ogilvie, R. F.: *Quart. J. Med.*, **6**:287, 1937.
11. Gepts, W.: *Ann. Soc. Roy. Sci. Med. Nat. Brux.*, **10**:5, 1957.
12. Lazarow, A., Carpenter, A.-M., Morgan, C., and Wright, D.: *Diabetes*, **11**:103, 1962.
13. Richardson, A. C., and Young, F. G.: *J. Physiol.*, **91**:352, 1937.
14. Haist, R. E., and Pugh, E. J.: *Amer. J. Physiol.*, **152**:36, 1948.
15. Garick, E. I.: *Johns Hopkins Med. J.*, **127**:294, 1970.
16. Lillehei, R. C., Simmons, R. L., Najarian, J. S., Weil, R., Uchida, H., Ruiz, J. O., Kjellstrand, C. M., and Goetz, F. C.: *Acta Diab. Lat.*, **7**:909, 1970.
17. Podelsky, S.: In: *Joslin's Diabetes Mellitus*. Edited by A. Marble, P. White, R. Bradley, and L. Krall. Lea & Febiger, Philadelphia, 1971, p. 750.
18. Lillehei, R. C., Simmons, R. L., Najarian, J. S., Kjellstrand, C. M., and Goetz, F. D.: *Trans. Proc.*, **3**:318, 1971.
19. Goetz, F. C.: *Metabolism*, **23**:875, 1974.
20. Barker, C. F.: *Diabetes*, **24**:766, 1975.
21. Rutter, W. J., Kemp, J. D., Bradshaw, W. S., Clark, W. R., Ronzio, R. A., and Sanders, T. G.: *J. Cell Physiol.*, *(Suppl. 1)* **72**:1, 1968.
22. Pictet, R. L., Clark, W. R., Williams, R. H., and Rutter, W. J.: *Dev. Biol.*, **29**:436, 1972.
23. Clark, W. R., and Rutter, W. J.: *Dev. Biol.*, **29**:468, 1972.
24. Hegre, O. D., McEvoy, R. C., Bachelder, V., and Lazarow, A.: *Diabetes*, **22**:577, 1973.
25. McEvoy, R. C., Hegre, O. D., Leonard, R. J., and Lazarow, A.: *Diabetes*, **22**:584, 1973.
26. Murrell, L. R.: *Exp. Cell Res.*, **41**:350, 1966.
27. Murrell, L. R., Morgan, C. R., and Lazarow, A.: *Exp. Cell Res.*, **41**:365, 1966.
28. Lambert, A., Vecchio, D., Gonet, A., Jeanrenaud, B., and Renold, A. E.: In: *Tolbutamide after Ten Years*. Edited by W. J. H. Butterfield and W. Van Westering. Excerpta Medica, Amsterdam, 1967, p. 61.
29. Girard, J. R., Kervran, A., Soufflet, E., and Assan, R.: *Diabetes*, **23**:310, 1973.
30. Bensley, R. R.: *Amer. J. Anat.*, **12**:297, 1911.
31. Overholser, M. D.: *Endocrinology*, **9**:493, 1925.
32. Hess, W. N., and Root, C. W.: *Amer. J. Anat.*, **63**:489, 1938.
33. Hellman, B.: *Acta Endocrinol.*, **32**:63, 1959.
34. Hellman, B.: *Acta Pathol. Microbiol. Scand.*, **47**:35, 1959.
35. Hellman, B., Hellerström, C., and Petersson, B.: *Diabetes*, **10**:470, 1961.
36. Leonard, R. J., Lazarow, A., McEvoy, R. C., and Hegre, O. D.: *Kidney Inter. (Suppl. 1)* **6**:S169, 1974.
37. Robberecht, P., Deschodt-Lanckman, M., Camus, J. Bruylands, J., and Christophe, J.: *Amer. J. Physiol.*, **221**:376, 1971.
38. Snook, J. T.: *Amer. J. Physiol.*, **221**:1388, 1971.
39. Hilwig, I., Schuster, S., Heptner, W., and Wasielewski, E.: *Z. Zellforsch.*, **90**:333, 1968.
40. Lambert, A. E., Blondel, B., Kanazawa, Y., Orci, L., and Renold, A. E.: *Endocrinology*, **90**:239, 1972.
41. Chick, W. L., Lauris, V., Flewelling, J. H., Andrews, K. A., and Woodruff, J. M.: *Endocrinology*, **92**:212, 1973.

42. Marliss, E. B., Wollheim, C. B., Blondel, B., Orci, L., Lambert, A. E., Stauffacher, V., Like, A. A., and Renold, A. E.: *Eur. J. Clin. Invest.,* **3**:16, 1973.
43. Orci, L., Like, A. A., Amherdt, M., Blondel, B., Kanazawa, Y., Marliss, E. B., Lambert, A. E., Wollheim, C. B., and Reynold, A. E.: *J. Ultrastruct. Res.,* **43**:270, 1973.
44. Moskalewski, S.: *Gen. Comp. Endocrinol.* **5**:342, 1965.
45. Lacy, P. E., and Kostianovsky, M.: *Diabetes,* **16**:846, 1967.
46. Howell, S. L., and Taylor, A. W.: *Biochem. J.,* **108**:17, 1968.
47. Scharp, D. W., Kemp, C. B., Knight, M. J., Ballinger, W. F., and Lacy, P. E.: *Transplant. Proc.,* **16**:686, 1973.
48. Lacy, P. E., Young, D. A., and Fink, C. J.: *Endocrinology,* **83**:1155, 1968.
49. Andersson, A., and Hellerström, C.: *Diabetes (Suppl. 2),* **21**:546, 1972.
50. Thomas, D. R., Fox, M., and Grieve, A.: *Transplant. Proc.,* **5**:765, 1973.
51. Andersson, A., Westman, J., and Hellerström, C.: *Diabetologia,* **10**;743, 1974.
52. Kostianovsky, M. L., McDaniel, M. F., Codilla, R. C., and Lacy, P. E.: *Diabetologia,* **10**:337, 1975.
53. Scharp, D. W., Murphy, J. J., Newton, W. T., Ballinger, W. F., and Lacy, P. E.: *Surgery,* **77**:100, 1975.
54. Aschcroft, S. J. H., Bassett, J. M., and Randle, P. J.: *Lancet,* **1**:888, 1971.
55. Sutherland, D. E., Steffes, M. W., Bauer, G. E., McManus, D., Noe, B. D., and Najarian, J. S.: *J. Surg. Res.,* **16**:102, 1974.
56. Najarian, J. S., Sutherland, D. E., and Steffes, M. W.: *Transplant. Proc. (Suppl. 1),* **7**:611, 1975.
57. Andersson, A., Borg, H., Groth, C.-G., Gunnarsson, R., Hellerström, C., Lundgren, G., Westman, J., and Ostman, J.: *J. Clin. Invest.,* **57**:1295, 1976.
58. Edstrom, C.: *Umea Univ. Med. Diss.,* **10**, 1972.
59. Edstrom, C., and Falkmer, S.: *Acta. Soc. Med. Upsal.* **72**:376, 1967.
60. Jonsson, L. E.: *Acta Soc. Med. Upsal.,* **73**:61, 1968
61. Boquist, L., and Edstrom, C.: *Virchows Arch. Pathol. Anat.,* **349**:69, 1970.
62. Hultquist, G., and Ponten, J.: *Upsal. J. Med. Sci.,* **79**:21, 1974.
63. Ballinger, W. F., and Lacy, P. E.: *Surgery,* **72**:175, 1972.
64. Reckard, C. R., and Barker, C. F.: *Transplant. Proc.,* **5**:761, 1973.
65. Reckard, C. R., Ziegler, M. M., and Barker, C. F.: *Surgery,* **74**:91, 1973.
66. Kemp, C. B., Knight, M. J., Scharp, D. W., Ballinger, W. F., and Lacy, P. E.: *Diabetologia,* **9**:468, 1973.
67. Kemp, C. B., Scharp, D. W., Knight, M. J., Ballinger, W. F., and Lacy, P. E.: *Surg. For.,* **24**:297, 1973.
68. Ziegler, M. M., Reckard, C. R., and Barker, C. F.: *J. Surg. Res.,* **16**:575, 1973.
69. Lorenz, V. D., Petermann, J., Becker, R., Rosenbaum, K.-D., and Dorn, A.: *Z. Exp. Chir.,* **8**:135, 1975.
70. Lorenz, V. D., Petermann, J., Rosenbaum, K.-D., Beckert, R., Ziegler, M., and Dorn, A.: *Acta Histochem.,* **52**:324, 1975.
71. Lorenz, V. D., Petermann, J., Beckert, R., Rosebaum, K.-D., Ziegler, M., and Dorn, A.: *Acta Diabet. Lat.,* **12**:30, 1975.
72. Koncz, L., Davidoff, F., DeLellis, R. A., Selby, M., and Zimmerman, C. E.: *Metabolism,* **25**:147, 1976.
73. Panijayanoud, P., Soroff, H. S., and Monaco, A. P: *Surg. For.,* **24**:329, 1973.
74. Scharp, D. W., Kemp, C. B., Knight, M. J., Murphy, J. J., Newton, W. T., Ballinger, W. F., and Lacy, P. E.: *Diabetes (Suppl. 1),* **23**:359, 1974.
75. Barker, C. F., Reckard, C. R., Ziegler, M. M., Galbut, D. L., and Naji, A.: *Diabetes (Suppl. 1),* **23**:359, 1974.
76. Amamoo, D. G., Woods, J. E., and Donovan, J. L.: *Mayo Clin. Proc.,* **49**:289, 1974.
77. Pipeleers, D., Pipeleers-Marichal, M., and Kipnis, D.: *Diabetes (Suppl. 2),* **24**:420, 1975.
78. Naji, A., Reckard, C. R., Ziegler, M. M., and Barker, C. F.: *Surg. For.,* **26**:459, 1975.
79. Lacy, P. E.: Personal communication.
80. Amamoo, D. G., Woods, J. E., and Holley, K. E.: *Mayo Clin. Proc.,* **50**:416, 1975.

81. Griffith, R. C., Scharp, D. W., Ballinger, W. F., and Lacy, P. E.: *Diabetes (Suppl. 2)*, **24**:419, 1975.

82. Slater, D., Manganall, Y., Smythe, A., and Fox, M.: In: *Immunological Aspects of Diabetes Mellitus.* Edited by O. O. Anderson, T. Deckert, and J. Nerup. *Acta Endocrinol. (Kbh) (Suppl. 205)*, Gentofte, 1975, p. 295.

83. Koncz, L., Zimmerman, C. E., DeLellis, R. A., and Davidoff, F.: *Transplant. Proc.*, **21**:427, 1976.

84. Kramp, R. C., Congdon, C. C., and Smith, L. H.: *Diabetes*, **23**:183, 1974.

85. Kramp, R. C., Congdon, C. C., and Smith, L. H.: *Eur. J. Clin. Invest.*, **5**:249, 1975.

86. Swan, H., and Rundles, W. R.: *Trans. Bull.*, **4**:53, 1957.

87. Hultquist, G.: *Upsal. J. Med. Sci.*, **77**:8, 1972.

88. Grimelius, L., Hultquist, G., Thorell, J., and Winbladh, L.: In: *Structure and Metabolism of the Pancreatic Islets.* Edited by S. E. Brolin, B. Hellman, and H. Knutson. Pergamon Press, Oxford, 1964, p. 173.

89. Hultquist, G., and Thorell, J.: *Acta Soc. Med. Upsal.*, **69**:291, 1964.

90. Leonard, R. J., Lazarow, A., and Hegre, O. D.: *Diabetes*, **22**:413, 1973.

91. Lazarow, A., Wells, L. J., Carpenter, A.-M., Hegre, O. D., Leonard, R. J., and McEvoy, R. C.: *Diabetes*, **22**:877, 1973.

92. Leonard, R. J., Hegre, O. D., and Lazarow, A.: *Diabetes (Suppl. 2)*, **24**:419, 1975.

93. Steffes, M. W., Sutherland, D. E. R., Mauer, S. M., Najarian, J. S., and Brown, D. M.: *Transplant. Proc.*, **19**:449, 1975.

94. Steffes, M. W., Sutherland, D. E. R., Mauer, S. M., Leonard, R. J., Najarian, J. S., and Brown, D. M.: *J. Lab. Clin. Med.*, **85**:75, 1975.

95. Weber, C., Weil, R., McIntosh, R., and Reemtsma, K.: *Transplant. Proc.*, **19**:442, 1975.

96. Weber, C., Lerner, R. L., Felig, P., Hardy, M. A., and Reemtsma, K.: *Surg. For.*, **26**:192, 1975.

97. Weber, C., Zatriqi, A., Weil, R., McIntosh, R., Hardy, M. A., and Reemtsma, K.: *Surgery*, **79**:144, 1976.

98. Hegre, O. D., Leonard, R. J., Erlandsen, S. L., McEvoy, R. C., Parsons, J. A., and Elde, R. P.: In: *Immunological Aspects of Diabetes Mellitus.* Edited by O. O. Anderson, T. Deckert, and J. Nerup. *Acta Endocrinol. (Kbh) (Suppl. 205)*, Gentofte, 1975, p. 257.

99. Matas, A. J., Sutherland, D. E. R., Steffes, M. W., and Najarian, J. S.: *J. Surg. Res.*, **20**:143, 1976.

100. Usadel, K. H., Schwedes, U., Bastert, G. P., and Schöffling, K.: *Diabetologia.*, 1977 (in press).

101. Matas, A. J., Sutherland, D. E. R., Steffes, M. W., and Najarian, J. S.: *Transplant. Proc.*, **22**:71, 1976.

102. Usadel, K. H., Rockert, H., Obert, I., and Schöffling, K.: *Klin. Wochenschro*, **48**:1417, 1970.

103. Usadel, K. H., Schwedes, U., Leuschner, U., and Schöffling, K.: *Acta Endocrinol. (Suppl. 184):* 97, 1974.

104. Browning, H., and Resnik, P.: *Yale J. Biol. Med.*, **24**:141, 1951–52.

105. Brown, J., Molnar, I. G., Clark, W., and Mullen, Y.: *Science*, **184**:1378, 1974.

106. Brown, J., Clark, W., Molnar, I. G., and Mullen, Y.: *Diabetes*, **25**:56, 1976.

107. Pansky, B., House, E. L., and Jacobs, M. S.: *Amer. J. Physiol.*, **203**:487, 1962.

108. Sak, M. F., Macchi, I. A., and Beaser, S. B.: *Diabetes*, **15**:51, 1966.

109. Hegre, O. D., Leonard, R. J., Rusin, J. D., and Lazarow, A.: *Anat. Rec.*, **185**:209, 1976.

110. Molnar, I. G., Mullen, Y., Clark, W., and Brown, J.: *Diabetes (Suppl. 1)*, **25**:338, 1976.

111. Gonet, A. E.: In: *Structure and Metabolism of the Pancreatic Islets.* Edited by S. E. Brolin, B. Hellman, and H. Knutson. Pergamon Press, Oxford, 1964, p. 179.

112. Coupland, R. D.: *J. Endocrinol.*, **20**:69, 1960.

113. Helmke, K., Slijepcevic, M., and Federlin, K.: *Horm. Metab. Res.*, **7**:210, 1975.

114. Slijepcevic, M., Helmke, K., and Federlin, K.: *Horm. Metab. Res.*, **7**:456, 1975.

115. Younoszai, R., Sorenson, R. L., and Lindall, A. W.: *Diabetes (Suppl. 1)*, **19**:406, 1970.

116. Barker, C. F., Reckard, C. R., Ziegler, M. M., and Naji, A.: *Diabetes (Suppl. 2)*, **24**:418, 1975.

117. Brooks, J. R., and Gifford, G. H.: *Transplant. Bull.*, **6**:91, 1959.

118. Billingham, R., and Silvers, W.: *The Immunobiology of Transplantation*. Prentice-Hall, New Jersey, 1971, p. 56.
119. Wachtel, S. S., and Silvers, W. F.: *J. Exp. Med.*, **133**:921, 1971.
120. Heslop, B. F.: *Transplant. Proc.*, **1**:560, 1969.
121. Heslop, B. F., Carter, J. M., and Hornibrook, J.: *Transplant. Proc.*, **5**:149, 1973.
122. Obando, M., Peale, A., Noval, J., Rao, N., Chang, K., Reichle, R., and Reichle, F.: *Diabetes, (Suppl. 2)* **24**:420, 1975.
123. Billingham, R., and Silvers, W.: *The Immunobiology of Transplantation*. Prentice-Hall, New Jersey, 1971, p. 64.
124. Coupland, R.: *Nature (London)*, **179**:51, 1957.
125. Gonet, A. E., and Renold, A. E.: *Diabetologia*, **1**:91, 1965.
126. Sak, M. F., and Macchi, I. A.: *Amer. Zool.*, **2**:443, 1962.
127. House, E. L., Jacobs, M. S., and Pansky, B.: *Transplant. Bull.*, **28**:435, 1961.
128. Browning, H. C.: *Cancer*, **2**:646, 1949.
129. May, R. M.: *Ann. N.Y. Acad. Sci.*, **64**:937, 1957.
130. House, E. L., Pansky, B., and Jacobs, M. S.: *Anat. Rec.*, **140**:341, 1961.
131. Moskalewski, S.: *Proc. Kon. Med. Akad. Wet.*, **72**:157, 1969.
132. Moskalewski, S.: In: *The Structure and Metabolism of the Pancreatic Islets*. Edited by S. Falkmer, B. Hellman, and I.-A. Taljedal. Pergamon Press, Oxford, 1970, p. 69.
133. Ferguson, J., and Scothorne, R. J.: *Brit. J. Surg.*, **59**:316, 1972.
134. Gray, B. N., and Watkins, E.: *Surg. For.*, **25**:382, 1974.
135. House, E. L., Pansky, B., Jacobs, M. S., Palmer, J., Ostrower, V., Strebel, R., and Payan, H.: *Ann. N.Y. Acad. Sci.*, **120**:652, 1964.
136. Panijayanoud, P., and Monaco, A. P.: *Surg. For.* **25**:379, 1974.
137. Weber, C., Weil, R., McIntosh, R., Hogle, H., Warden, G., and Reemtsma, K.: *Surgery*, **77**:208, 1975.
138. Hallin, R. W., and Swan, H.: *Surg. For.*, **9**:628, 1958.
139. Potter, J. F., and Haverbock, C. Z.: *Ann. Surg.*, **151**:460, 1960.
140. Gough, M. H., Pugh, D. E., and Brook, J. R.: *Surgery*, **52**:144, 1962.
141. Buschard, K.: *Horm. Metab. Res.*, **7**:441, 1975.
142. Strautz, R. L.: *Diabetologia*, **6**:306, 1970.
143. Gates, R. J., Hunt, M. I., Smith, R., and Lazarus, N. R.: *Lancet*, **1**:561, 1972.
144. Gates, R. J., Hunt, M. I., and Lazarus, N. R.: *Diabetologia*, **10**:401, 1974.
145. Stone, H. B., Owings, J. C., and Gey, G. O.: *Calif. West. Med.*, **38**:409, 1933.
146. Stone, H. B., Owings, J. C., and Gey, G. O.: *Miss. Doc. J.*, **15**:6, 1937–38.
147. Lafferty, K. J., Cooley, M. A., Woolnough, J., and Walker, K. Z.: *Science*, **188**:259, 1975.
148. Foley, G. E., Handler, A. H., McCarthy, R., and Adams, R. A.: *Quart. Rev. Pediat.*, **16**:14, 1961.
149. Rabotti, G. F., Geldner, J., and Hoffner, W.: *Cancer Res.*, **23**:165, 1963.
150. Miller, E. E.: *Transplant. Proc.*, **5**:1528, 1967.
151. Jacobs, B. B., and Huseby, R. A.: *Transplant. Proc.*, **5**:410, 1967.
152. Jacobs, B. B., and Huseby, R. A.: *Proc. Soc. Exp. Biol. Med.*, **127**:957, 1968.
153. Jacobs, B. B.: *J. Nat. Cancer Inst.*, **42**:537, 1969.
154. Lawson, R. K., and Poutala, S. D.: *Surg. For.*, **25**:377, 1974.
155. Boyles, R. R., and Seltzer, H. S.: *Diabetes (Suppl. 2)*, **24**:420, 1975.
156. Knight, M. J., Scharp, D. W., Kemp, C. B., Ballinger, W. F., and Lacy, P. E.: *Cryobiology*, **10**:89, 1973.
157. Payne, J. E., Kumar, D., Garobedian, J. V., and Berne, T. V.: *Diabetes (Suppl. 1)*, **22**:326, 1973.
158. Frankel, B. J., Gylfe, E., Hellman, B., and Taljedal, I.-A.: *J. Clin. Invest.*, **57**:47, 1976.
159. Selle, W. A.: *Amer. J. Physiol.*, **113**:118, 1935.
160. Hegre, O. D., Wells, L. J., and Lazarow, A.: *Diabetes*, **19**:906, 1970.
161. Hegre, O. D., Wells, L. J., and Lazarow, A.: *Diabetes*, **21**:193, 1972.
162. Hegre, O. D., McEvoy, R. D., Bachelder, V., and Lazarow, A.: *In Vitro*, **7**:366, 1972.
163. Scharp, D. W., White, D. J., Ballinger, W. F., and Lacy, P. E.: *In Vitro*, **9**:364, 1974.

164. Hegre, O. D., Leonard, R. J., Schmitt, R. V., and Lazarow, A.: *Diabetes,* **25**:180, 1976.
165. Mauer, S. M., Sutherland, D. E. R., Steffes, M. W., Leonard, R. J., Najarian, J. S., Michael, A. F., and Brown, D. M.: *Diabetes,* **23**:748, 1974.
166. Mauer, S. M., Steffes, M. W., Sutherland, D. E. R., Najarian, J. S., Michael, A. F., and Brown, D. M.: *Diabetes,* **24**:280, 1975.
167. Lee, C. S., Mauer, S. M., Brown, D. M., Sutherland, D. E. R., Michael, A. F., and Najarian, J. S.: *J. Exp. Med.,* **139**:793, 1974.
168. Weil, R., Nozawa, M., Koss, M., Weber, C., and Reemtsma, K.: *Surgery,* **78**:142, 1975.
169. Leach, F. N., Ashworth, M. A., Barson, A. J., and Milner, R. D. G.: *J. Endocrinol.,* **59**:65, 1973.
170. Murray, M. R., and Bradley, C. F.: *Amer. J. Cancer,* **25**:98, 1935.
171. Urca, I., Kott, I., and Lev-Ran, A.: *Diabetes,* **19**:182, 1970.
172. Najarian, J. S., Sutherland, D. E. R., Matas, A. J., Steffes, M. W., Simmons, P. L., and Goetz, F. C.: *Trans. Proc.,* **9**:233, 1977.

Chapter 22

Endocrine Tumors of the Pancreas

Werner Creutzfeldt

Prevalence and Categorization

The endocrine tumors of the pancreas are usually called islet cell tumors (adenomas or carcinomas of islets of Langerhans). This name implies their origin from the pancreatic islets. However, this assumption is not justified. The histologic structure of the endocrine pancreatic tumors is not markedly different from other endocrine tumors, and not all hormones produced by these tumors are normal products of the islets of Langerhans. The still controversial question of the origin of the pancreatic tumors will be discussed later. Any nomenclature anticipating this undecided problem should be avoided. This applies also to the term "nesidioblastoma," introduced in 1938 by Laidlaw.[1] Laidlaw named the cells that differentiate from the duct epithelium to form islets "nesidioblasts," their proliferation "nesidioblastosis," and their tumors "nesidioblastomas."

When in 1902 the first "adenoma of the pancreas arising from an island of Langerhans" was described by Nicholls,[2] no clinical symptoms were related to this tumor. Accordingly, Heiberg[3] stated in his handbook on "The Diseases of the Pancreas" in 1914 that "the adenomata of the pancreatic islets are without clinical significance and therefore not further discussed."

The first recognition of hypoglycemia caused by an endocrine tumor of the pancreas dates back to 1927, when Wilder *et al.*[4] demonstrated the blood glucose lowering potency of tumor extracts. Since this description the attribute "functional" or "nonfunctional" has been added to endocrine pancreatic tumors. Only when the clinician had observed hypoglycemia was the tumor regarded as functional. It soon became apparent that "functioning" endocrine tumors of the pancreas were extremely rare, while many more tumors of the same histologic structure were found incidently, if the pancreas was investigated carefully at autopsy. The prevalence of islet tumors in an unselected autopsy material according to such investigations is between 0.5 and 1.5%.[5-8] However, the justification for calling the majority of these tumors nonfunction-

Werner Creutzfeldt • Medizinische Klinik und Poliklinik der Universität Göttingen, West Germany.

ing is highly debatable. Nonfunctioning endocrine ("islet") tumor meant, until 20 years ago, that clinically no hypoglycemia had been observed. Zollinger and Ellison,[9] in 1955, postulated that a humoral factor was responsible for the existence of recurrent ulcer disease, gastric hypersection, and pancreatic tumor, and that therefore these conditions had to be excluded before the pathologist was justified to speak of a nonfunctioning pancreatic tumor. In 1958, Verner and Morrison [10] broadened the clinical spectrum of functioning "islet" tumors by the description of the syndrome of watery diarrhea, hypokalemia, and hypochlorhydria (WDHH syndrome). The clinical symptoms accompanying a glucagon-producing pancreatic tumor (diabetes and a characteristic skin disease named "necrolytic migratory erythema") were correctly described by McGavran in 1966[11]; however, they were not recognized as a clinical entity until Mallinson *et al.*[12] published a series of nine such cases in 1974.

The clinical symptoms mentioned are frequent and, therefore, nonspecific for pancreatic endocrine tumors. Retrospectively, they can rarely be used as an argument for hormone secretion of a pancreatic tumor found incidently during autopsy. In addition, the rate of hormone secretion of endocrine tumors varies greatly and is not related to their size. Possibly, also the threshold for the appearance of clinical symptoms varies individually. Elevated hormone levels may be compensated for some time by regulatory hypersecretion of other hormones. This subclinical state may last for years or even decades because the growth of the tumors is usually extremely slow if they are of the nonmetastasizing benign variety.

As the historical development demonstrates, further clinical syndromes can be expected to be related to hormone production of pancreatic tumors. Recently, it has been realized that the pancreas of man and animals produces two further hormones, somatostatin [13-16] and pancreatic polypeptide.[17] Both hormones have been demonstrated already by immunochemical methods in endocrine pancreatic tumors.[18,19] However, no clinical symptoms have, as yet, been related to the overproduction of these hormones.

A last complicating factor lies in the observation that pancreatic tumors are a preferential site of ectopic hormone production, i.e., they can produce peptides which are normally not found in the pancreas. Examples for this are ACTH,[20,21] MSH,[20] parathormone, and calcitonin.[22]

Our knowledge about endocrine pancreatic tumors has greatly increased in the last decade. Methods have been developed for the estimation of peptide hormones in blood and tissue extracts by Berson and Yalow, and immunohistological techniques allow an exact and specific localization of hormone production. The ultrastructural analysis of the tumor cells made the recognition of specific secretory products possible. Thus, the diagnosis of "nonfunctioning islet cell tumor" should become less frequent, if the skills of the investigator and the methodological spectrum applied by him undergo improvement. In summary, then, one has to conclude that endocrine tumors of the pancreas are not as uncommon as is usually thought. Rare are tumors leading to major clinical symptoms because the classical tumor-induced clinical syndromes indeed occur infrequently. If, however, any hormone production of these tumors is accepted as endocrine activity, then the actual number of functioning pancreatic tumors will increase considerably. One has only to accept that a tumor can function below the threshold level of clinical symptomatology.

A correct categorization of these tumors can only be made if: (1) the tumor tissue is immediately fixed or frozen; (2) very careful morphological and biochemical investigations are performed; and (3) the clinical data are supported by a battery of endocrinological investigations. This may not be possible in most cases, either because the techniques are not available or the material is not properly preserved (autopsy material is seldom suitable). In such situations the reason should be stated why hormone production could not be demonstrated, rather than the tumor being called "nonfunctioning."

If hormone production has been demonstrated biochemically and/or by specific staining techniques, the tumor is named after the identified hormone. If more than one hormone is produced by a tumor, then the latter is named after the hormone which is responsible for the clinical symptoms. Otherwise, the tumor is called "multiple hormone producing." If multiple tumors are found which produce different hormones, the entity is named the multiple endocrine neoplasia (MEN) or adenomatosis (MEA) syndrome, which may occur sporadically or as a familial disease.[23]

Table 1 demonstrates systematically the endocrine tumors of the pancreas, their relationship to recognized clinical syndromes, and some of their morphological and endocrine characteristics.

Common Features of Pancreatic Endocrine Tumors

The localization of the endocrine tumors of the pancreas is almost evenly distributed over the gland. This statement is based on substantial statistics of insulinomas,[24,25] gastrinomas,[26] and diarrheogenic tumors.[27] Multiple tumors are found rarely in hyperinsulinism and frequently in the Zollinger-Ellison syndrome. Gross clinical symptomatology does not usually occur in tumors below 0.5 g; otherwise, the size of the tumor is not related to the severity of the clinical syndrome. In cases of malignancy, metastases are usually found in the regional lymph nodes around the pancreas, the duodenum, and the portal tract, and in the liver.

Warren[28] has set up light-microscopic criteria for the recognition of an endocrine adenoma of the pancreas, such as resemblance in morphology and arrangement of the cells to those of normal islets, encapsulation with compression of adjacent pancreatic tissue, and a diameter of at least 1 mm. The close resemblance to normal islets is only fulfilled for the ribbon-like type of endocrine pancreatic tumors. It is now agreed that structurally endocrine pancreatic tumors exhibit no distinct differences from other endocrine tumors. Three growth patterns are usually distinguished.[1,29,30] They are: (1) a trabecular, ribbon-like, or gyriform pattern closely resembling arrangements of the normal

Table 1. Categorization and Features of Endocrine Tumors of the Pancreas

Name	Insulin-producing tumor, Insulinoma	Glucagon-producing tumor, Glucagonoma	Ulcerogenic tumor, Gastrin-producing tumor, Gastrinoma	Diarrheogenic tumor
Clinical symptoms	Fasting hypoglycemia	Necrolytic, migratory erythema, Diabetes, Anemia (Glucagonoma syndrome)	Gastric hypersecretion, Recurrent ulcer disease, Steatorrhea (Zollinger–Ellison syndrome)	Watery diarrhea, Hypokalemia, Gastric hyposecretion (Verner–Morrison syndrome)
Hormone responsible	Insulin	Glucagon	Gastrin	VIP GIP? Secretin?
Predominant cell types	B Type IV (D_1) EC	A Type IV (D_1)	G Type IV (D_1) EC	Type IV (D_1)
Rate of malignancy	<10%	>80%	>90%	>50%
Other hormones frequently found	Pancreatic polypeptide	Pancreatic polypeptide, Somatostatin, Gastrin	Insulin, Pancreatic polypeptide, ACTH	Pancreatic polypeptide
Extrapancreatic localization	Rare	Rare	Frequent	Rare

islets of Langerhans with their rich capillary network bordered by rows of columnar and cuboidal cells (Fig. 1); (2) a rosette-like arrangement of cells around capillaries. This growth pattern has also been called glandular, alveolar or pseudoacinose (Fig. 2); and (3) a medullary, solid, or diffuse growth pattern (Fig. 3).

It has been claimed that the growth pattern has some diagnostic significance regarding the hormone production. Tumors characterized by a trabecular (gyriform) pattern of growth were found to be insulinomas or glucagonomas, and tumors containing glandular formations were either gastrinomas or diarrheogenic tumors.[30] In the author's series of 50 insulinomas, 20 gastrinomas, 4 glucagonomas, and 4 diarrheogenic tumors this could not be confirmed. Tumors of each variety frequently revealed more than one growth pattern if investigated at different sites. Immunohistological investigations showed that this was not due to different hormone production in different areas of the tumor. A certain prevalence of the trabecular growth pattern in insulinomas and a prevalence of the glandular and also medullary growth pattern in gastrinomas present also in the author's material was of no diagnostic significance.

Independent of the growth pattern and the hormone production of the tumor, the amount of vascular stroma and connective tissue varies considerably,

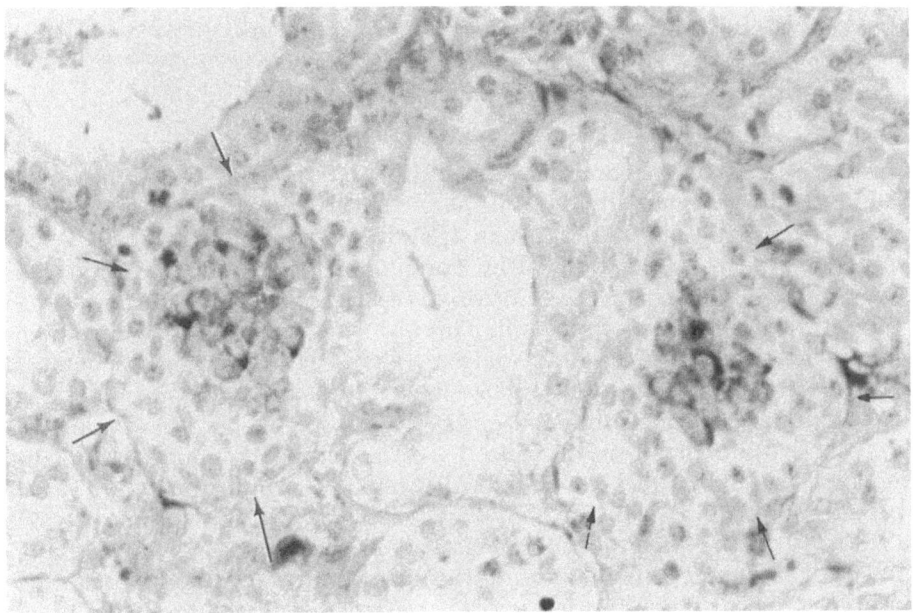

Figure 1. Trabecular or ribbon-like pattern of tumor growth. The hormone concentration (peroxidase-positive dark material) of the single cell varies considerably. Insulinoma (pat. Lang.). Bouin fixation. Paraffin embedding. Incubation with 1/20 diluted antiinsulin serum, after washing incubation with 1/20 diluted peroxidase-labeled antiguinea-pig γ-globulin from rabbit. ×400.

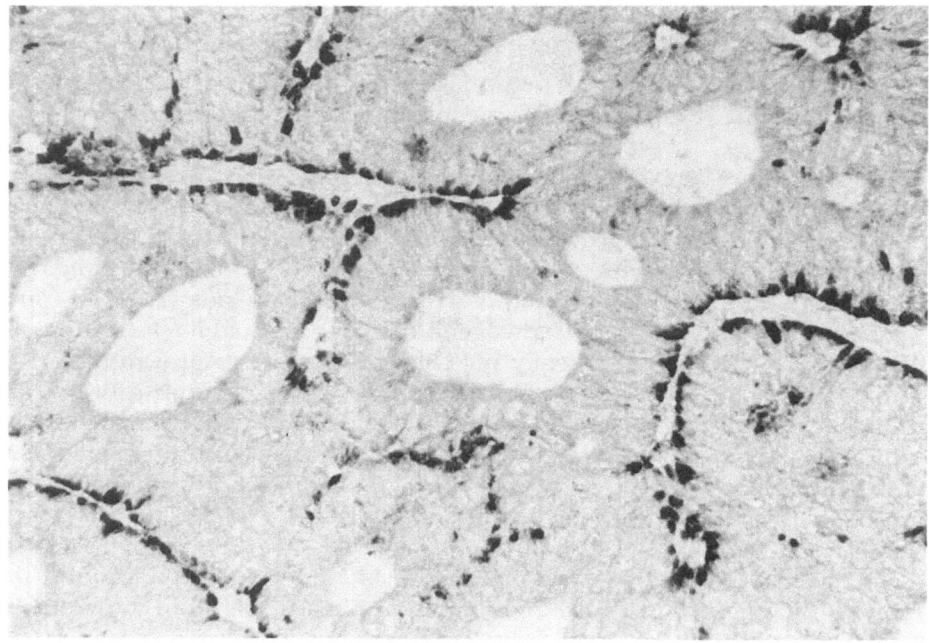

Figure 2. Rosette or glandular pattern of tumor growth. The hormone is stored exclusively at the basal poles of the cells (black peroxidase reaction). Gastrinoma (pat. Duc.). Bouin fixation. Paraffin embedding. Incubation with 1/20 diluted antigastrin serum, after washing incubation with 1/50 diluted peroxidase labeled antirabbit γ-globulin from sheep. ×400. Reproduced at 105%.

sometimes constituting more than half of the total tumor mass. Hyaline degeneration is found frequently in the tumors[29]; sometimes throughout the whole tumor, and sometimes only in certain areas (Fig. 4).

It has first been pointed out by Porta *et al.*[31] that the hyaline substance found in insulinomas has the tinctorial reactions and ultrastructurally the typical fibrillar structure of amyloid. This has been confirmed for insulinomas and gastrinomas.[32–34] According to Pearse *et al.*[34] this amyloid is chemically different from immunamyloid and is, therefore, called apudamyloid. In the author's material the investigation of Congo-red-stained sections in polarized light revealed in most of the hyalinized areas of different endocrine tumors of the pancreas the presence of amyloid. Also, ultrastructurally the typical fibrillar structure of amyloid located around capillaries and intracytoplasmically could be demonstrated in many insulinomas and gastrinomas (Fig. 5). Nothing is known yet about the genesis and the nature of the amyloid in endocrine tumors not only of the pancreas, but also of other endocrine neoplasms.

In some tumors round intracytoplasmic inclusions have been observed.[33,35–38] They are usually homogeneous and eosinophilic and are often larger than the nucleus. The ultrastructure of these globular inclusions is fibrillar,[37,41] (Fig. 6) suggesting intracellular amyloid.[33,37] However, these inclusions are found regardless of whether pericapillary hyaline and amyloid are

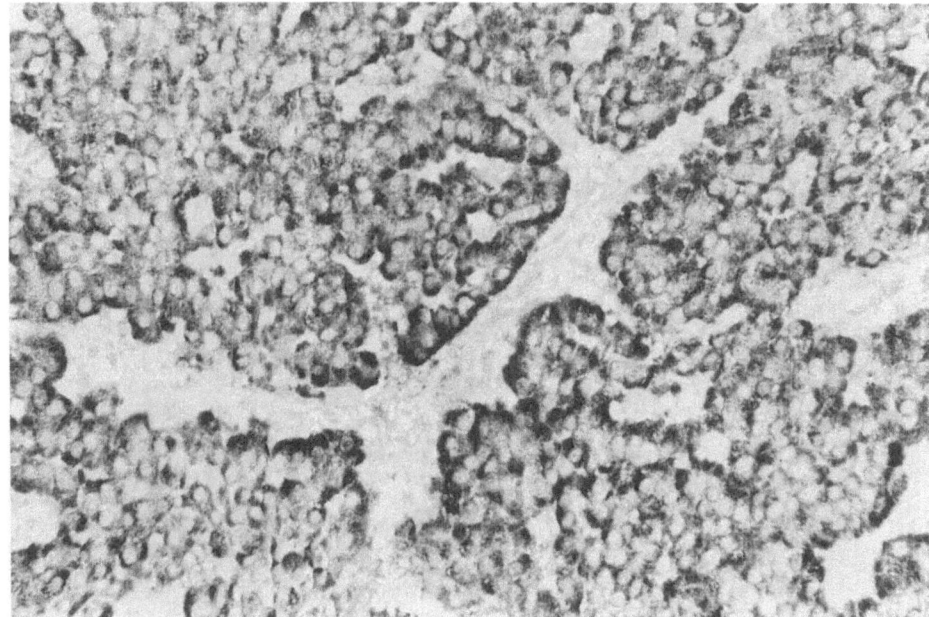

Figure 3. Medullary or solid pattern of tumor growth. Hormone-containing cells are evenly distributed (black peroxidase reaction). Gastrinoma (pat. Bru.). Technique as in Fig. 2. ×240. Reproduced at 105%.

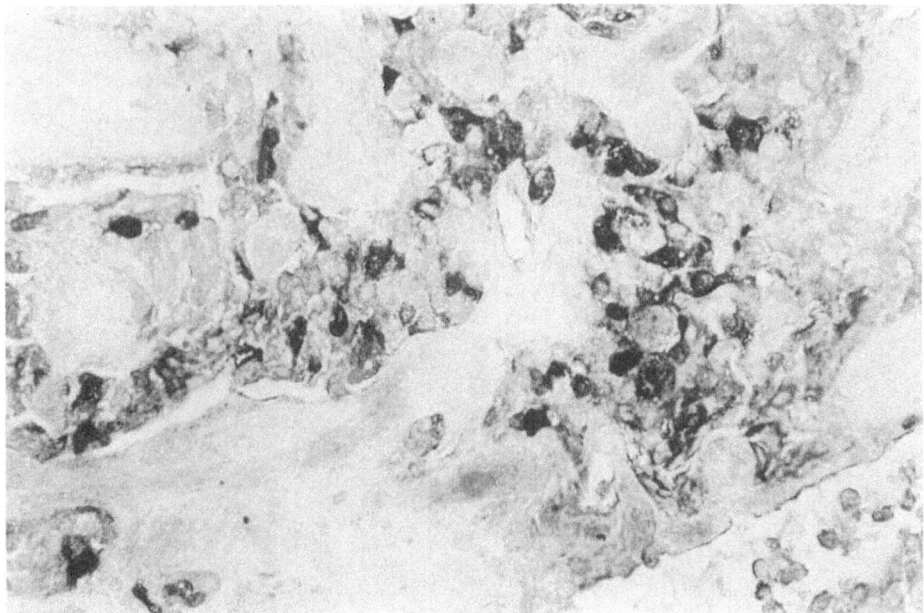

Figure 4. Extensive hyaline deposits around the tumor cells which contain a variable amount of hormone (black peroxidase reaction). Insulinoma (pat. Frau.). Technique as in Fig. 1. ×400. Reproduced at 105%.

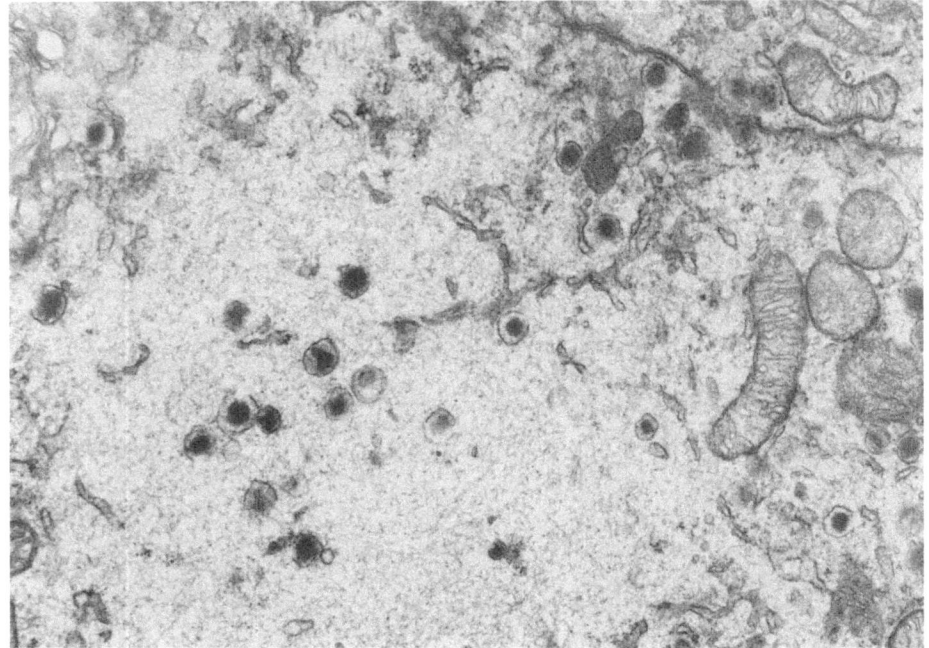

Figure 5. Parts of tumor cells containing typical β granules. The cells are surrounded by a medium electron-dense material with the fibrillar structure of amyloid. Insulinoma (pat. Kö.). Karnovsky fixation. Postfixation with osmium. Vestopal embedding. × 24,000. Reproduced at 75%.

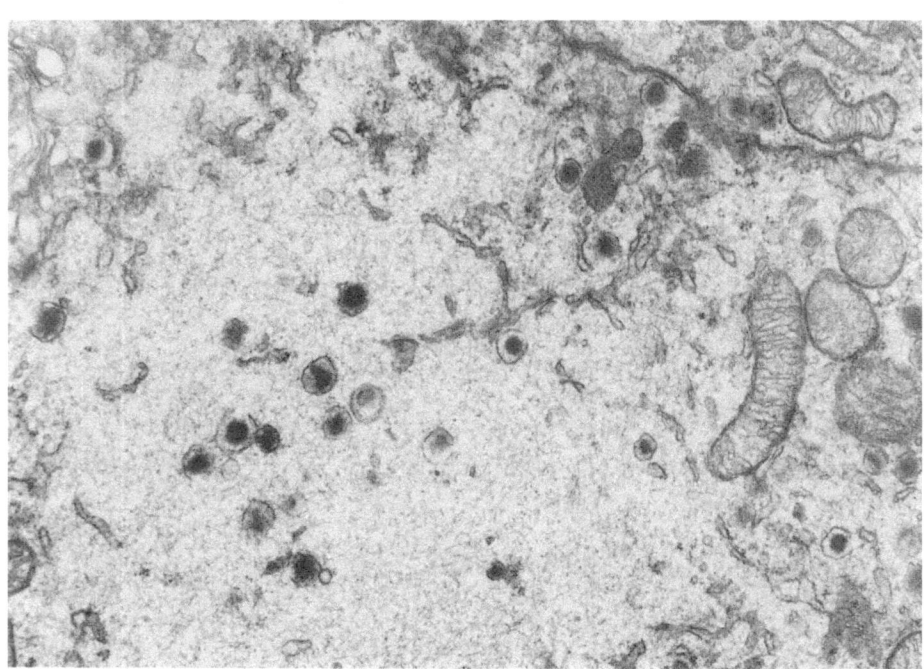

Figure 6. Inclusion of fibrillar material suggesting intracellular amyloid. Insulinoma cell (pat. Miel.). Technique as in Fig. 5. × 30,000. Reproduced at 75%.

present. The occurrence of ductular structures in endocrine tumors of the pancreas, or their close connection to hyperplastic ducts (Fig. 7), has been observed by many authors,[1,28,38–41] and is of interest for the discussion of the origin of these tumors.

Encapsulation of the tumors by connective tissue is a frequent finding. However, the capsule is nearly always incomplete and lacking in most of the smaller tumors. This may be misinterpreted as an infiltrating growth which is usually regarded as a sign of malignancy. The trapping or engulfing of cells by the tumor is a feature of benign tumors almost as frequently as of malignant ones. Also, nuclear pleomorphism and nucleolar prominence are found in benign and malignant tumors. Therefore, most authors agree that the diagnosis of carcinoma can rarely be made on histologic grounds[29,30,42] and has to be based on the observation of gross invasion and/or metastases into lymph nodes or the liver. Persistence of elevated serum hormone levels after tumor extirpation are indicative of metastases overlooked during operation. The possibility of measuring gastrin radioimmunologically has changed our view on the frequency of malignant gastrinomas considerably.[43]

A battery of staining methods, silver impregnation techniques, and histochemical methods has been applied for the differentiation of the endocrine tumors of the pancreas.[27,30,39,44–46] These methods allow the recognition of endocrine tumors, since they give positive reactions in cells of the so-called apud cell system of Pearse.[47,48] However, they are not true and specific histo-

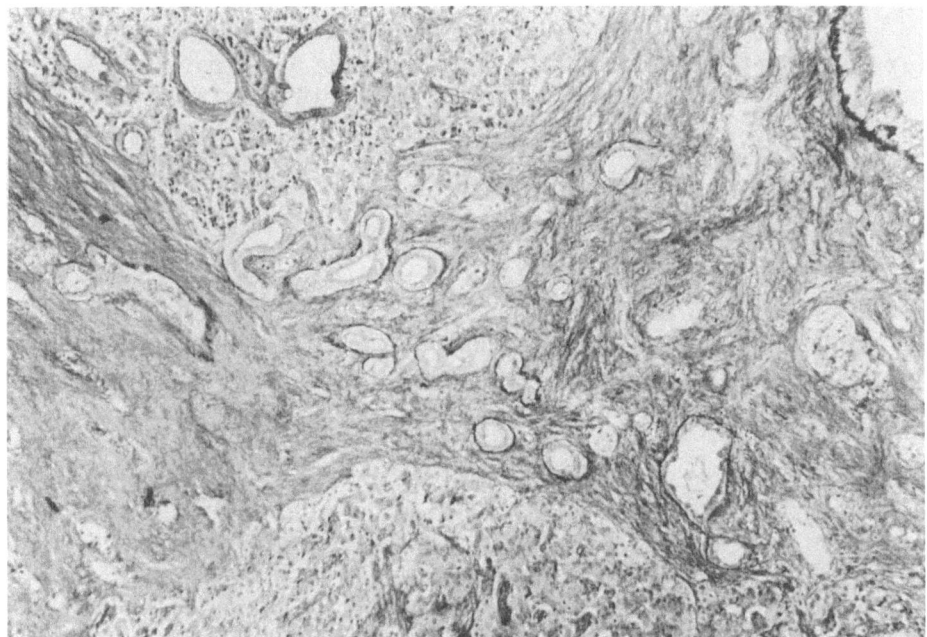

Figure 7. Ductular structure and proliferation of ducts in and around an insulinoma (pat. Jan.). The tumor tissue is visible at the top and the bottom of the figure. Bouin fixation. Paraffin embedding. Aldehyde-thionin stain. ×100. Reproduced at 105%.

chemical methods, and do not usually provide the diagnosis of a specific hormone production. Controversies about the staining properties of the so-called non-B-cell tumors of the pancreas only reflect the low specificity and the unreliability of these methods and do not clarify the nature of the tumors. The following reactions are semispecific for the characterization of some pancreatic endocrine cells: aldehyde-thionin[49] for the insulin-producing B cell, silver impregnation after Hellerström and Hellman[50] for the somatostatin-producing D cell, Fontana–Masson for the enterochromaffin (EC) cell, and silver impregnation after Grimelius[51] for islet A cells, G cells, and D_1 (type IV) cells. For practical purposes the following reactions, preferably after Bouin fixation, can be recommended for the characterization of endocrine tumors of the pancreas[46]: aldehyde-thionin staining for demonstration of β granules, Grimelius'[51] silver impregnation for A, G, and type IV cells, and Hellerström–Hellman's silver impregnation for D cells.

The final decision about the type of endocrine cell has to be made by immunohistological and immunochemical investigations. Only these highly specific methods allow the diagnosis and categorization of an endocrine tumor of the pancreas. Today, immunohistological and radioimmunological methods are available for the demonstration of insulin, glucagon, somatostatin, pancreatic polypeptide, VIP (vasoactive intestinal polypeptide), GIP (gastric inhibitory polypeptide), secretin, and CCK (cholecystokinin). The following sections about well-defined endocrine tumors of the pancreas are based on such immunohistological methods and on the radioimmunological identification of hormones in tumor tissue extracts.

The ultrastructural analysis of the type of secretory granules can also help in establishing the diagnosis of an endocrine tumor of the pancreas. A certain percentage of insulinomas, glucagonomas, and gastrinomas contain tumor cells revealing the characteristic structure of their secretory granules as found in the normal B, A, and G cells. However, each of these tumors may contain, in addition to or exclusively, atypical secretory granules.[38,43] Thus, in the ultrastructural analysis of tumor tissue, only a positive finding is of diagnostic help.

Caution is necessary if multiple tumors are found because each tumor may produce a different hormone. It is only if the immunochemical, immunohistological and ultrastructural analyses have been performed on the same piece of tissue that these parameters can be related to one another. The same holds true for solitary large tumors because hormone production may vary from area to area.

Insulinomas

Morphological Findings

The size of insulinomas at the time of diagnosis varies considerably and is not related to the severity of the clinical symptoms.[24] The smallest insulinoma producing clinical symptoms in our material weighed 0.5 g. Of our 50 patients, 6 had tumors weighing less than 1.0 g. The largest tumor weighed 25.0 g (two carcinomas with liver metastasis excepted). Also, in our patients the severity of the hypoglycemia was independent of the tumor size.

Insulinomas are rarely malignant. In the collective statistical analysis of Howard et al.,[24] 9.3% of 398 cases had metastases, which are the only reliable parameters for malignancy in endocrine tumors of the pancreas. If one excludes 14 nonfunctioning carcinomas, the rate of malignancy would be even lower. In the more recent report of Stefanini et al.[25] on 951 completely documented cases of insulinoma with clinical hypoglycemia, metastases were found in only 5%. This figure is in agreement with the author's experience, since of 50 patients with insulinomas only 2 had a metastasizing carcinoma.

If staining procedures specific for the normal islet B cell (e.g., aldehyde-fuchsin, aldehyde-thionin) are applied to insulinomas, a positive reaction can be found in only about three-fourths of the tumors. The number of tumor cells containing stainable secretory granules varies considerably, and so does the number of granules per cell. Sometimes only very few tumor cells reveal a scarce specific granulation. The granule density of normal islet B cells is hardly found in tumor cells. This suggests that the tumor cells store less insulin than normal B cells and that the insulin concentration of insulinoma tissue is lower than in normal islet tissue.

Immunohistology using fluorescein or peroxidase-labeled insulin antibodies and tissue fixed in Bouin's solution gives the most reliable results.[52] Some tumors which did not react with the aldehyde-thionin stain did react positively with the peroxidase-labeled antibody, indicating the superiority of immunohistology in identifying insulin-producing tumor cells (Table 2). Tumors with insulin concentrations below 1.0 U/g had a negative immunohistological reaction. As with the aldehyde-thionin staining, a variable number of tumor cells reacted positively with the peroxidase-labeled antibody, indicating a different insulin content of the cells (Figs. 1 and 4). A similar reaction was achieved with porcine C-peptide antisera, despite the fact that human and porcine C-peptide differ in eight positions in their amino acid sequences.[52] None of the insulinomas reacted positively with glucagon or gastrin antiserum.

Table 2.   Insulin Concentration and Stainability of Insulinomas Categorized According to the Ultrastructural Type of Secretory Granules[58]

		Number of cases	Mean IRI concentration (U/g) (range)	Stainable with aldehyde-thionin	Immunohistological reaction for insulin
I.	Tumors with typical β granules	18	28.2 (3.6–88.9)	+	+
II.	Tumors with typical β granules and atypical granules	11	27.9 (2.8–111.2)	+	+
III.	Tumors with atypical granules only	5	8.6 (1.7–16.3)	−	+
IV.	Virtually agranular tumors	4	0.5 (0.01–1.1)	−	−

Ultrastructurally, both typical β granules[39–41,53,54] and atypical secretory granules[37,40,41,55] have been described in insulinoma cells. These reports are confined to a single case or to a few cases. In the author's laboratory, 50 insulinomas were investigated ultrastructurally. The ultrastructural appearance of the tumors was not uniform. Even in individual cases the cells differed sometimes considerably in different areas of the tumor. According to their ultrastructure, insulinomas can be categorized into the following four types[38] (Fig. 8): tumors with cells containing secretory granules typical for human islet B cells (type I); tumors with cells containing typical β granules and atypical secretory granules (type II); tumors with cells containing only atypical secretory granules (type III); and tumors which contain only virtually agranular cells (type IV).

In types III and IV, the diagnosis of an insulinoma is not possible on ultrastructural grounds or with granule stains. Table 2 shows the frequency with which the different ultrastructural types were found. In addition, the IRI concentration is listed. From this it is concluded that in type I and II tumors, which are the most frequent, the IRI concentration is the highest. Type IV tumors have the lowest insulin concentration, and that of type III lies between these extremes. A correlation between ultrastructural findings and IRI concentration is more evident if the number of agranular cells is also accounted for; the more virtually agranular cells in a tumor, the lower the IRI concentration.

The frequent finding of atypical secretory granules in insulinoma cells is difficult to explain. Atypical granules are small spherical granules of high electron density and different diameter, usually much smaller than the secretory granules of the well-defined islet cells (A, B, and D cells). They occur with or without an encompassing membrane, which is either tightly fitting or is associated with a small electron-lucent space. Figure 9 demonstrates tumor cells with atypical secretory granules from a type III insulinoma. Only recently has a similar cell been described in normal human pancreatic islets; it has been called the type IV cell[56] or D_1 cell.[45] Nothing is known about the function of this rare cell type. It has also not yet been decided if the atypical secretory granules contain biologically active peptide hormones. The low insulin content of type III insulinomas (Table 2) suggests that no insulin is stored in these atypical granules. This and the frequent occurrence of cells with similar granules in tumors producing different hormones suggests that we are dealing with an immature cell type.

In several instances tumor cells with very unusual pleomorphic secretory granules (rod-like or comma-shaped) were observed (Fig. 10). Such granules were never found in normal human pancreatic islets.

Other islet cells (A and D cells) were not identified in insulinomas. However, in many tumors single cells were observed which resembled the enterochromaffin cells (EC cells) found in the gastrointestinal mucosa and in carcinoid tumors. These EC cells were most frequent in two carcinomas with extensive metastases.

The silver method of Hellerström and Hellman[50] impregnates the islet D (or A_1) cells, and the Grimelius silver technique[51] stains the glucagon-producing

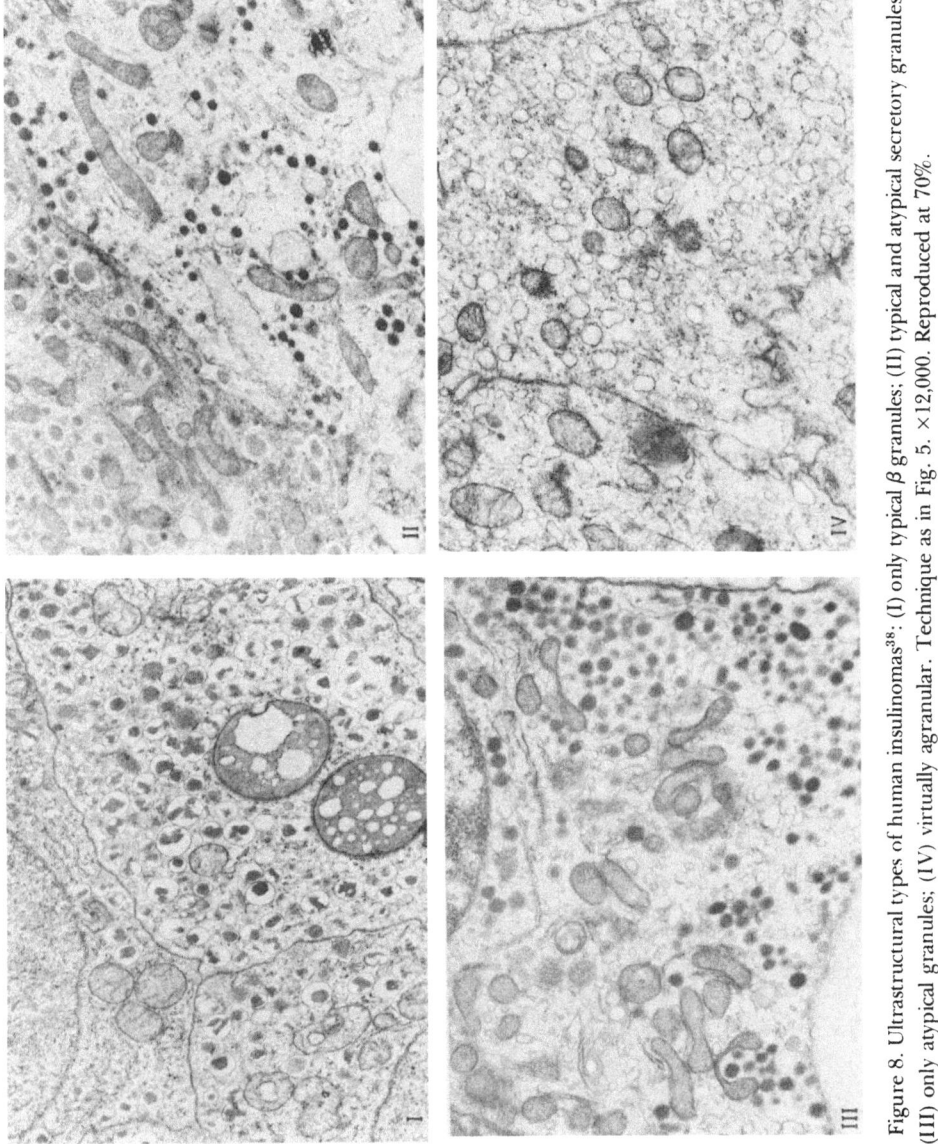

Figure 8. Ultrastructural types of human insulinomas[38]: (I) only typical β granules; (II) typical and atypical secretory granules; (III) only atypical granules; (IV) virtually agranular. Technique as in Fig. 5. ×12,000. Reproduced at 70%.

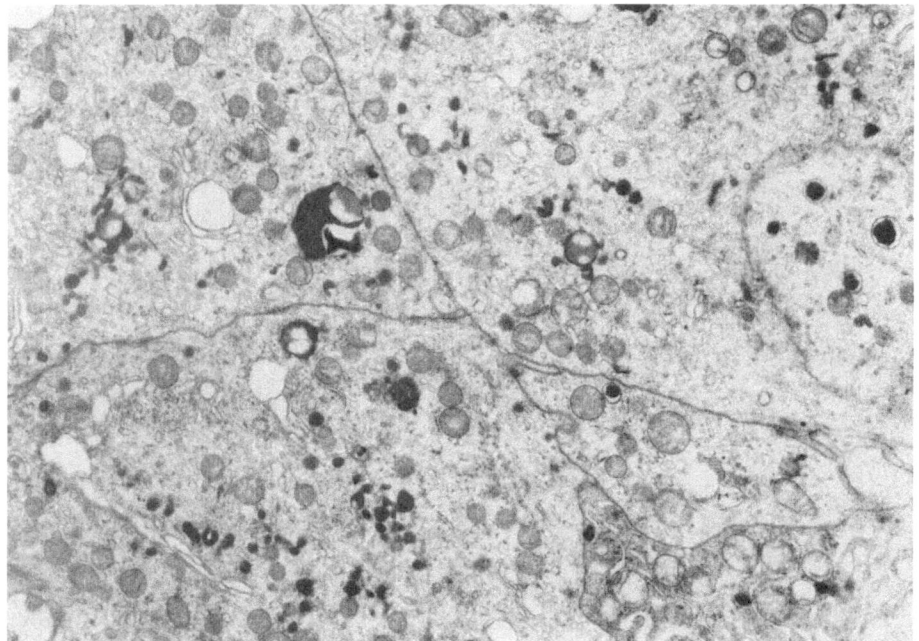

Figure 9. Part of tumor cells containing only small electron-dense ("atypical") secretory granules. Type III insulinoma (pat Dra.). Technique as in Fig. 5. ×24,000. Reproduced at 75%.

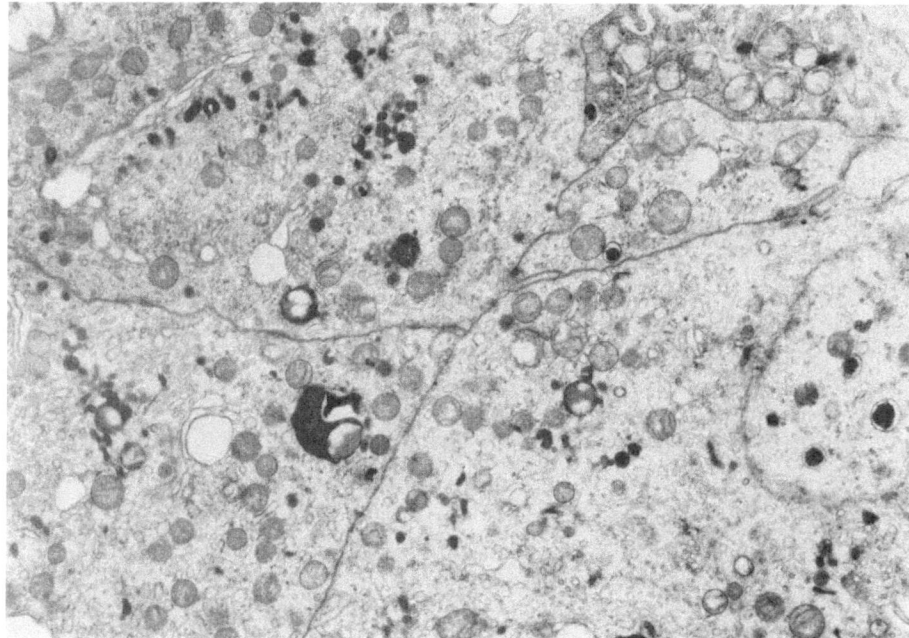

Figure 10. Part of tumor cells containing pleomorphic secretory granules of high electron density. Type II insulinoma (pat. Ruh.). Technique as in Fig. 5. ×18,000. Reproduced at 75%.

A (or A_2) cells and less distinctly the antral gastrin-producing G cells.[57] The insulin-producing B cells are silver-negative with both methods. Surprisingly, in 40% of our 50 insulinomas, at least some tumor cells were Grimelius silver positive. In another series, 4 of 11 insulinomas also gave a positive reaction with the Grimelius silver stain.[75] Since the normal islet B cell is Grimelius silver-negative, this finding is difficult to understand. A clarification of this question may help to explain the presence and the function of atypical secretory granules in tumor cells.

Insulinomas of ultrastructural type I were usually Grimelius negative, or only occasional cells were impregnated, while all type III and type IV tumors displayed a positive reaction. The findings in type II tumors varied greatly. Generally, the intensity of the silver reaction and the number of impregnated cells were negatively correlated with the IRI concentration of the respective insulinoma. This suggests that the tumor cells with atypical granules and/or virtually agranular tumor cells were reacting with silver salts. Figure 11 demonstrates strongly Grimelius-positive cells in a type III insulinoma with a very low IRI content (2.2 U/g). In serial sections stained with antiinsulin serum and impregnated with Grimelius silver it was not possible to decide with certainty if the same cells react with antiinsulin serum and silver salts.[58] However, more cells were silver positive than reacted with antiinsulin serum.

Silver grains can be localized ultrastructurally in the secretory granules.[59] In normal human pancreatic islets, only the granules of the A cells (especially

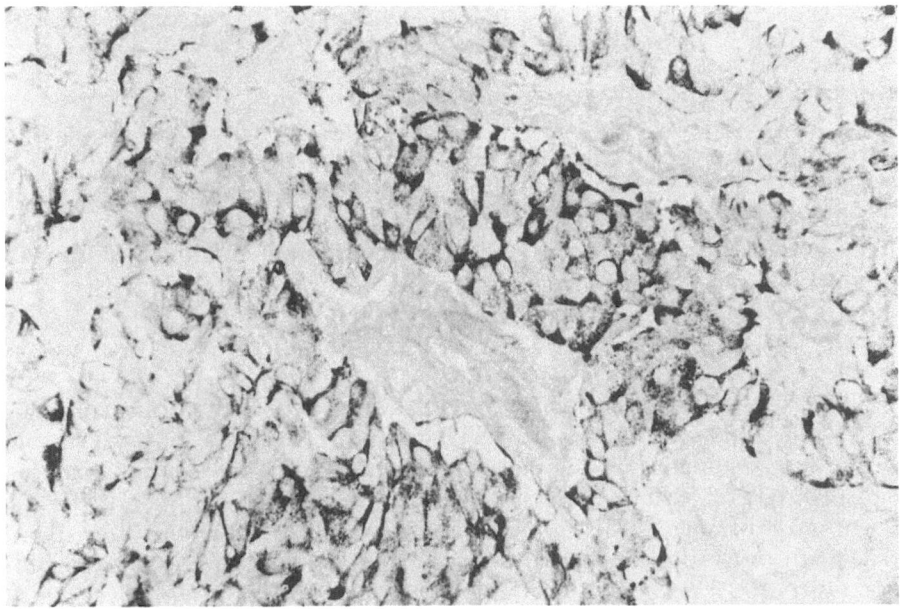

Figure 11. Silver-reactive cells in a type III insulinoma (pat. Dra.). Bouin fixation. Silver impregnation after Grimelius.[51] ×400.

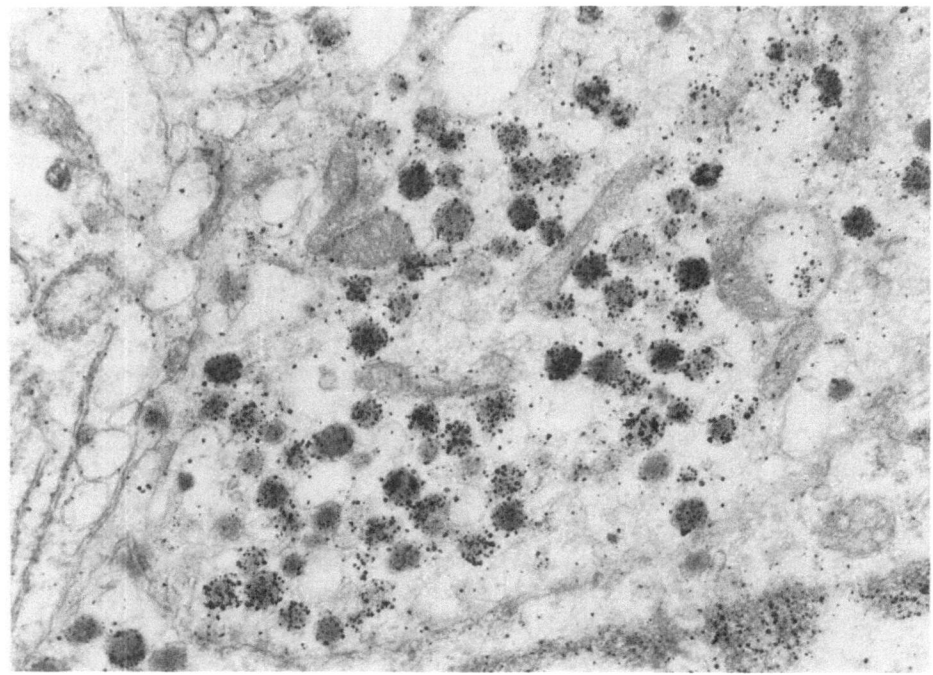

Figure 12. Grimelius silver stain of a type III insulinoma (pat. Dra.). The atypical secretory granules are covered with silver grains. Technique according to Vassallo *et al.*[59] ×24,000.

their electron-opaque halo) are covered with silver grains, whereas the granules of the B and D cells are free of silver grains. The ultrastructural investigation of Grimelius-positive type II insulinomas revealed that tumor cells with typical crystalline secretory granules did not react with silver, while atypical granules were silver positive.[58] Figure 12 shows that all secretory granules of a type III insulinoma are covered with silver grains if impregnated with the Grimelius technique.

Insulin Concentration

The fact that insulinoma cells contain less insulin than normal human B cells[60-63] was confirmed in the author's laboratory.[38,58] Table 3 shows the insulin concentration estimated in our material. Assuming that the average pancreas weighs 100 g and that the islet tissue comprises 1% of the gland, the IRI concentration in normal islet tissue could be considered to lie between 49 and 485 U/g. In only 10 out of 40 insulinomas the IRI concentration was in this range (40.1–199 U/g). In 30 insulinomas the concentration was lower (0.01–37.8 U/g), and in 24 of these it was below 20.0 U/g. The mean total insulin content of the insulinomas (78.6 U) was lower than the mean insulin content of

Table 3. Total Extractable Immunoreactive Insulin (IRI) Concentration (U/g) and
IRI Content (U) of Insulinoma Tissue and Noninvolved Pancreas[117]

		Mean	Range	No. investigated
Insulinoma	U/g	21.9	(0.8–92.5)[a]	42
	U	78.6	(2.1–267.0)[b]	40
Insulinoma[c]	U/g	0.2	0.01	2
	U	100	5	
Pancreas	U/g	1.93	(0.5–4.9)	28

[a]In one 0.9 g tumor 199 U/g were found.
[b]One 12 g tumor contained 454 U of IRI.
[c]Metastasizing carcinomas.

the pancreases of these patients (200 ± 20 U). No tumor contained more insulin than the pancreas with the highest insulin content. These data are incompatible with the idea that hyperinsulinism in insulinoma patients is simply the consequence of insulin overproduction.

Proinsulin Concentration

Since the discovery of proinsulin, different studies have demonstrated that patients with insulinomas have a higher percentage of proinsulin in their serum than do normal persons.[38,64–68] Thus far, however, the insulinoma proinsulin content has been reported in only three cases.[66,68,69] The percentage of proinsulin was estimated by column chromatography of the pancreas or tumor extracts upon Sephadex G-50.[38] The average proinsulin percentage in the pancreatic tissue of 12 cases was 2.5% (range: 1.7–4.8) and in 22 insulinomas, 15.1% (range: 5.3–40.8). A near normal proinsulin concentration (5.3%) was estimated in the tumor with the highest insulin concentration.

Generally, the highest proinsulin percentages were found in the tumors with the lowest IRI concentration. The levels of proinsulin were much higher in the sera than in the tumors of the same patients, which can be explained by the longer half-life of proinsulin compared to insulin in plasma.[70]

Correlation of Morphological and Biochemical Findings

As stated above, histologically (aldehyde-thionin stain), immunohistologically, and ultrastructurally, a variable number of tumor cells contained only few and often no β granules. The number of granulated tumor cells was positively correlated with the insulin concentration and negatively correlated with the proinsulin concentration in the extracts.[38] The virtually agranular (type IV) tumors had the lowest insulin concentrations and the highest proinsulin percentages.

These findings suggest that the major defect in insulinomas is a decreased storage capacity, resulting in uncontrolled insulin release in a proportion of the tumor cells. Since the conversion of proinsulin to insulin takes place only in the Golgi apparatus and in the secretory granules,[71] a defective storage capacity (i.e., reduced granule population) should lead to increased proinsulin levels.

The hypothesis of a decreased storage capacity of insulinoma cells is supported by subcellular fractionation and *in vitro* incorporation studies with [³H]leucine in 10 insulinomas, demonstrating that tumor cells have the capacity for a higher turnover of proinsulin and insulin when compared to pancreatic islets.[72,73]

The concept of the major defect of insulinoma cells having a decreased storage capacity explains all clinical, morphological, and biochemical facts known so far. The tumor cell has the ability to synthesize the hormone and also frequently the ability to react to known stimuli with hormone discharge. However, it has lost partially or completely, varying from case to case, the ability to retain its product when it is not needed by the organism. In the normal B cell a low blood glucose level turns off insulin release; in the tumor cell this mechanism does not operate properly. The hormone "leaks out" permanently and, thus, produces the clinical disease.

Gastrinoma

Morphological Findings

Solitary pancreatic tumors are found in less than 30% of patients with the Zollinger–Ellison syndrome (ZES).[26] Frequently, multiple tumors are present. Of 249 tumors, 61% were malignant.[26] However, in reality this percentage is probably much higher.[43,76] Metastases and/or the primary lesion may often be overlooked during surgery and even at autopsy. Only if elevated serum gastrin levels decrease to normal after extirpation of a gastrinoma can metastases be excluded. Older statistics do not fulfill this condition because radioimmunoassay has been available for only a few years and only in a limited number of institutions. Only 1 of the 30 patients investigated in the author's laboratory showed normal serum gastrin levels after tumor extirpation and total gastrectomy. And even in this patient a lymph node metastasis had been extirpated together with the (duodenal) gastrinoma. Therefore, the rate of malignancy for gastrinomas has been indicated as 90% in Table 1.

Hyperplasia of the pancreatic islets, which has been regarded as a cause of ZES in 10% of all cases,[26] is a doubtful explanation for hypergastrinemia. Gastrin has not been demonstrated in pancreatic extracts or immunohistologically in the islets of these cases.

Islet hyperplasia has been described in the presence of a pancreatic and also an extrapancreatic gastrinoma,[43,77,78] and if found alone may be due to an overlooked gastrinoma. It has been suggested that hypergastrinemia stimulates islet growth.[43] Since the description of Zollinger and Ellison,[9] an increasing number of reports have appeared of gastrinomas localized outside the pancreas. Tumors have been found in the stomach and the duodenum (cf. Creutzfeldt *et al.*[43] and Isenberg *et al.*[76]). These tumors may be small and, therefore, are easily overlooked. Recent data from the Zollinger–Ellison tumor registry disclosed 103 patients with duodenal wall tumors.[76] Of the 20 gastrinomas investigated by the author, 6 originated in the duodenum. Cytological signs of malignancy were rare, despite proven metastases in all. Infiltration into the surrounding tissue was more frequent.

As pointed out above, controversies about the staining properties of the so-called non-B-cell tumors reflect only the low specificity and the unreliability of the applied methods. Therefore, these controversies[30,43–46] will not be discussed here. All 20 tumors of the author were negative with the Davenport silver impregnation (modification of Hellerström and Hellman) which stains the islet D (or A_1) cells. Since the islet D cells are Hellerström–Hellman silver positive,[50] it appears that gastrinomas are not D cell tumors. This fits in with the modern view that the islet D cells produce somatostatin (see above) and not gastrin. The Grimelius[51] silver technique which impregnates the islet A (or A_2) cells and the antral G cells[45,57] gave positive results in most of the cells of 19 of the 20 tumors investigated by the author (Fig. 13). The only Grimelius-negative tumor was immunohistologically an insulinoma with low gastrin content.

Since one-third of the insulinomas, the Verner–Morrison tumors, the glucagonomas, and the parathyroid tumors studied in this laboratory are also Grimelius positive, this method cannot be regarded as specific for gastrinomas.

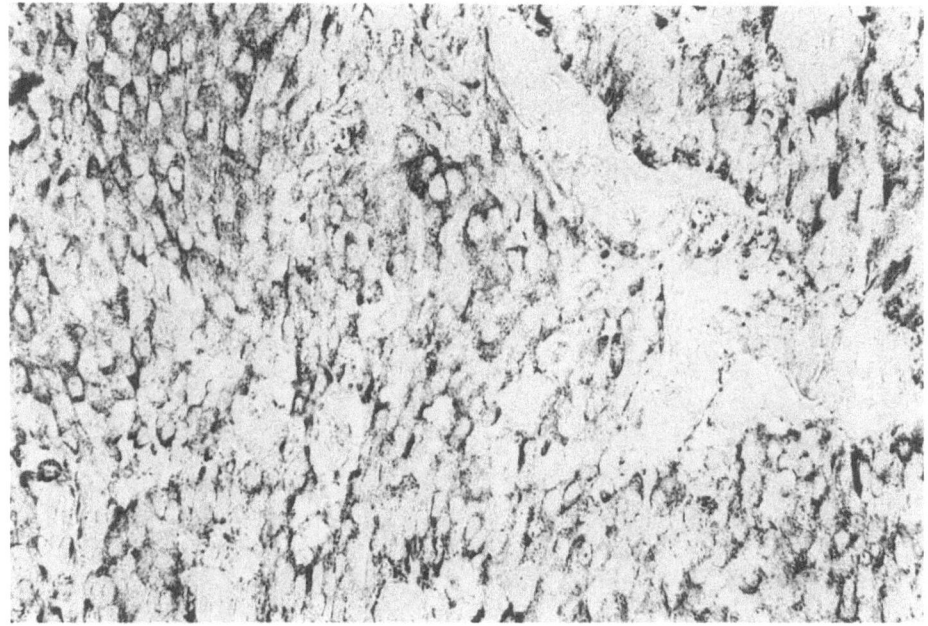

Figure 13. Endocrine tumor of the pancreas with medullary growth pattern. Most tumor cells are impregnated with silver grains. Gastrinoma (pat. Schm.). Technique as in Fig. 11. ×240. Reproduced at 105%.

The only reliable diagnostic method is immunohistology. Cells reacting with an antigastrin serum were found in 19 of 20 gastrinomas investigated in the author's laboratory. The one negative tumor was an undifferentiated pancreatic carcinoma with a very low gastrin content. However, the number of cells reacting with antigastrin serum was much smaller than the Grimelius silver-positive cells and varied considerably from area to area in the same tumor, and from case to case (Figs. 2,3,and 14). Therefore, one has to be careful when interpreting ultrastructural findings and the results of hormone extractions. It must be stressed that with the same immunohistological technique gastrin-producing cells could not be demonstrated in human pancreatic islets in this laboratory.[79] This is in agreement with recent observations[80] and in contradiction with other reports.[45,81,82] Gastrin has been demonstrated immunohistologically in gastrinomas by other groups.[30,45,78] The production of hormones other than gastrin by gastrinomas was also demonstrated frequently by immunohistology (see below).

Reports about the ultrastructural appearance of gastrinomas are contradictory. The identity of their secretory granules with those of A cells,[37] D cells,[83] antral G cells,[79] abnormal islet D cells (similar to gastrointestinal D_1 cells),[45] and type IV cells[84] has been claimed. These different conclusions were based on the study of only a few cases. Two larger series have been studied recently.[30,43] The results do not correspond. Greider *et al.*[30] found in 18 ulcerogenic tumors secretory granules which were indistinguishable from the granules of four

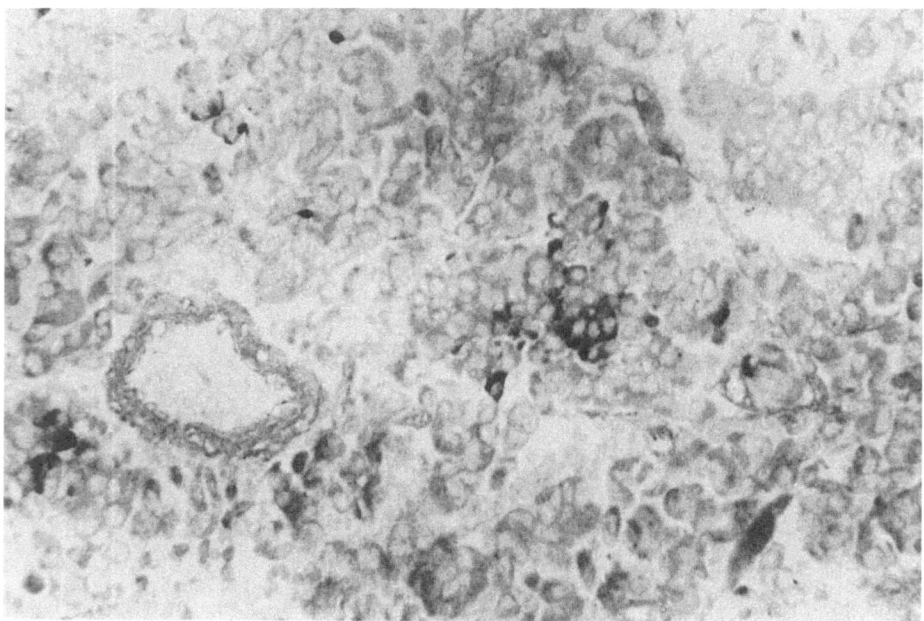

Figure 14. Area from a gastrinoma (pat. Klau.) in which only a few cells react with antigastrin serum. Technique as in Fig. 2. ×240. Reproduced at 105%.

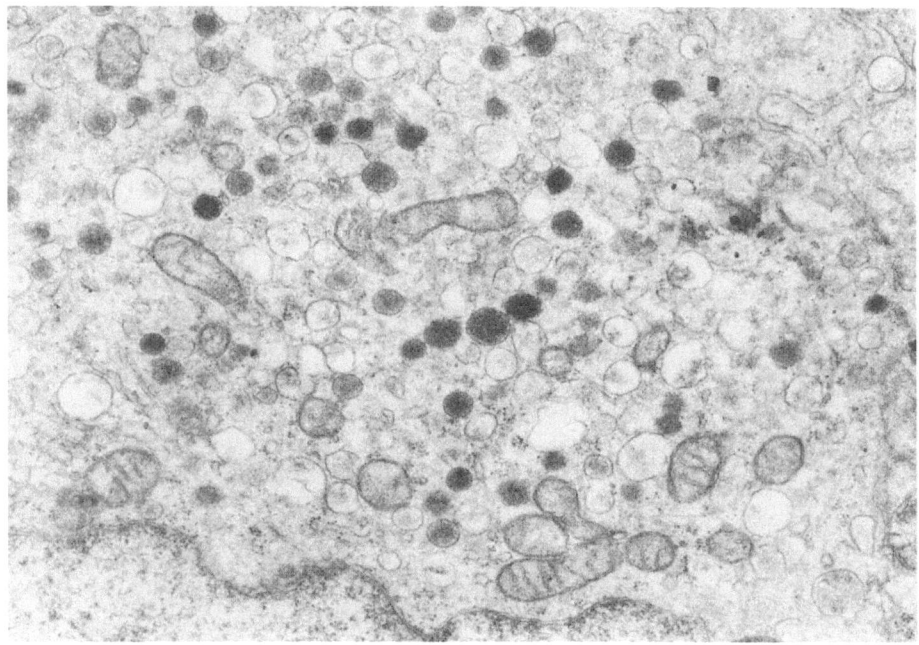

Figure 15. Part of a gastrinoma cell with secretory granules of the type occurring in antral G-cells (pat. Schm.). Technique as in Fig. 5. ×24,000. Reproduced at 75%.

diarrheogenic tumors. They identified a population of round homogeneous small (diameter 150 to 200 nm) granules (type I) and a population of pleomorphic granules with a diameter ranging up to 350 nm (type II). Type I granules predominated in 15 of 22 tumors. Type II granules were occasionally also present; in seven cases type II granules only were noted. No correlation was found between these granule types and the functional activity of the tumors (ulcerogenic or diarrheogenic).

It is difficult to explain why the observations in the author's laboratory[43] are so different. Our material comprises 19 gastrinomas studied ultrastructurally, immunohistologically, and immunochemically. The analysis of tumor pieces which contained gastrin and cells reacting with antigastrin serum showed that the ultrastructural appearance was not uniform. Even in individual cases, the cells sometimes differed considerably in different areas of the tumor. These differences concerned the frequency of cells with or without secretory granules and also the type of secretory granules. Tumors containing virtually agranular cells only were not observed.

In the majority of tumors (14 of 19) some cells were found which contained secretory granules identical to those of the antral G cells, as defined in the Wiesbaden classification.[78,85] These granules show a broad scale of varying electron density. The limiting membranes of some granules are only partially filled with gray filamentous material. Figure 15 demonstrates a tumor cell with typical G cell granules. However, in only 3 of 19 gastrinomas were all granulated tumor cells of the G type. The majority of gastrinomas contained, in addition, cells with atypical granules. The frequency of these cells varied considerably. Their secretory granules were electron dense and round, they were usually smaller than the granules of the well-defined pancreatic islet cells, and they had only tightly fitting or no discernible membranes. The size of these granules varies considerably from area to area and tumor to tumor. Both secretory granules of the G cell type and atypical granules were impregnated with silver grains when the Grimelius technique was applied.[43]

The relative number of either cells with typical G cell granules or cells with atypical granules did not correspond to the gastrin concentration of the respective tumor (Table 4). From this it may be concluded that gastrin can be stored not only in cells with typical G cell granules.

The virtually agranular cells which were found in all gastrinomas in varying number often showed signs of high functional activity with well-developed rough endoplasmic reticulum, Golgi zones, and numerous cytoplasmic vesicles and, in addition, many lysosomes. In analogy to similar findings in insulinomas,[38,72] one can conclude that these cells have a reduced capacity to store their secretory product. In two gastrinomas, besides cells with typical G cell granules and atypical granules, cells were found which contained secretory granules characteristic for other well-defined pancreatic islet cells. In one of these tumors at least five different cells with characteristic secretory granules could be distinguished: G cells, cells with atypical granules, A cells, B cells, and EC cells.

The patients who developed Cushing's syndrome due to ACTH production by the pancreatic gastrinoma showed, in the tumor typical G cells, cells with atypical granules and agranular cells. According to their ultrastructure, gastrinomas have been categorized into the following four types (Fig. 16)[43], (I) tumors with cells containing secretory granules typical for human antral G cells; (II) tumors with cells containing typical G cell granules and cells with atypical secretory granules; (III) tumors with cells containing only atypical secretory granules; and (IV) multihormone-producing tumors with cells containing the characteristic secretory granules of additional gastrointestinal endocrine cells.

The diagnosis of a gastrinoma is not possible on ultrastructural grounds in type III and is not conclusive in types II and IV, if only few typical cells with G cell granules are present in the investigated area. Therefore, hormone extraction and immunohistology should always support the diagnosis.

The occurrence of at least some typical G cells in most gastrinomas studied in the author's laboratory has now been confirmed by Polak and Solcia (personal communication). A possible explanation of the discrepancy between our series and that of Greider *et al.*[30] may be the low number of cases with immunochemical gastrin confirmation (6 of 18) and immunohistological demonstration of gastrin-producing cells (1 of 18) in their material. The type 1 cells of these authors seem to be identical with the cells containing atypical granules and demonstrated by us in insulinomas, gastrinomas, and diarrheogenic tumors. Also, their type 2 cells (pleomorphic granules) have been observed by us in insulinomas (Fig. 10), gastrinomas, and diarrheogenic tumors (Fig. 19).

Table 4. Distribution of Immunoreactivity in Gastrin Components (%) in Sera and Tumor Extracts from 13 Patients with Gastrinoma (extended from Creutzfeldt et al.[43])

Patient	Gastrin source	IRG concentration	>G-45	G-45	G-34	G-17	G-13	Ultrastructural type
Bau.	Serum	1900 pg/ml	—	6.0	56.0	37.0	1.0	
	Tumor	4.2 µg/g	—	—	9.0	91.0	—	II
Be.	Serum	2100 pg/ml	—	—	65.7	26.9	7.4	
	Tumor	0.3 µg/g	—	—	72.7	27.3	—	Insulinoma!
Braun.	Serum	310 pg/ml	—	—	82.0	10.0	—	
	Tumor[a]	75.2 µg/g	—	—	100.0	—	—	II
Brei.	Serum	1300 pg/ml	—	—	62.0	38.0	—	
	Tumor	25.6 µg/g	—	—	10.3	76.1	13.6	II
Bru.	Serum	500 pg/ml	23.2	23.8	37.8	15.1	—	I
	Tumor	400.0 µg/g	13.3	24.8	52.2	14.5	—	
Do.	Serum	84000 pg/ml	—	14.0	38.0	48.0	—	
	Tumor	271.0 µg/g	—	7.0	42.0	51.0	—	II
Dus.	Serum	491 pg/ml	—	1.8	66.0	29.0	5.0	
	Tumor[a]	12.0 µg/g	—	—	17.1	78.4	2.7	III
Hil.	Serum	1000 pg/ml	—	10.4	63.7	36.3	—	
	Tumor[a]	6.4 µg/g	—	—	25.3	64.3	—	I
Kac.	Serum	3100 pg/ml	—	—	56.3	33.9	9.8	
	Tumor	0.48 µg/g	—	—	28.0	64.9	7.1	IV
Klau.	Serum	3700 pg/ml	—	—	25.9	57.3	16.8	
	Tumor	0.07 µg/g	6.4	33.8	31.9	27.9	—	II
Sei.	Serum	177 pg/ml	—	—	—	—	—	
	Tumor[a]	142.9 µg/g	—	10.0	73.0	17.0	—	II
Stei.	Serum	26800 pg/ml	—	4.0	55.0	37.0	4.0	
	Tumor	173.0 µg/g	—	5.6	21.7	72.7	—	I
Stu.	Serum	683 pg/ml	—	4.3	16.3	65.6	13.8	
	Tumor	8.0 µg/g	—	—	4.2	71.3	24.5	II

[a]Primary tumor located in the *duodenal* wall.

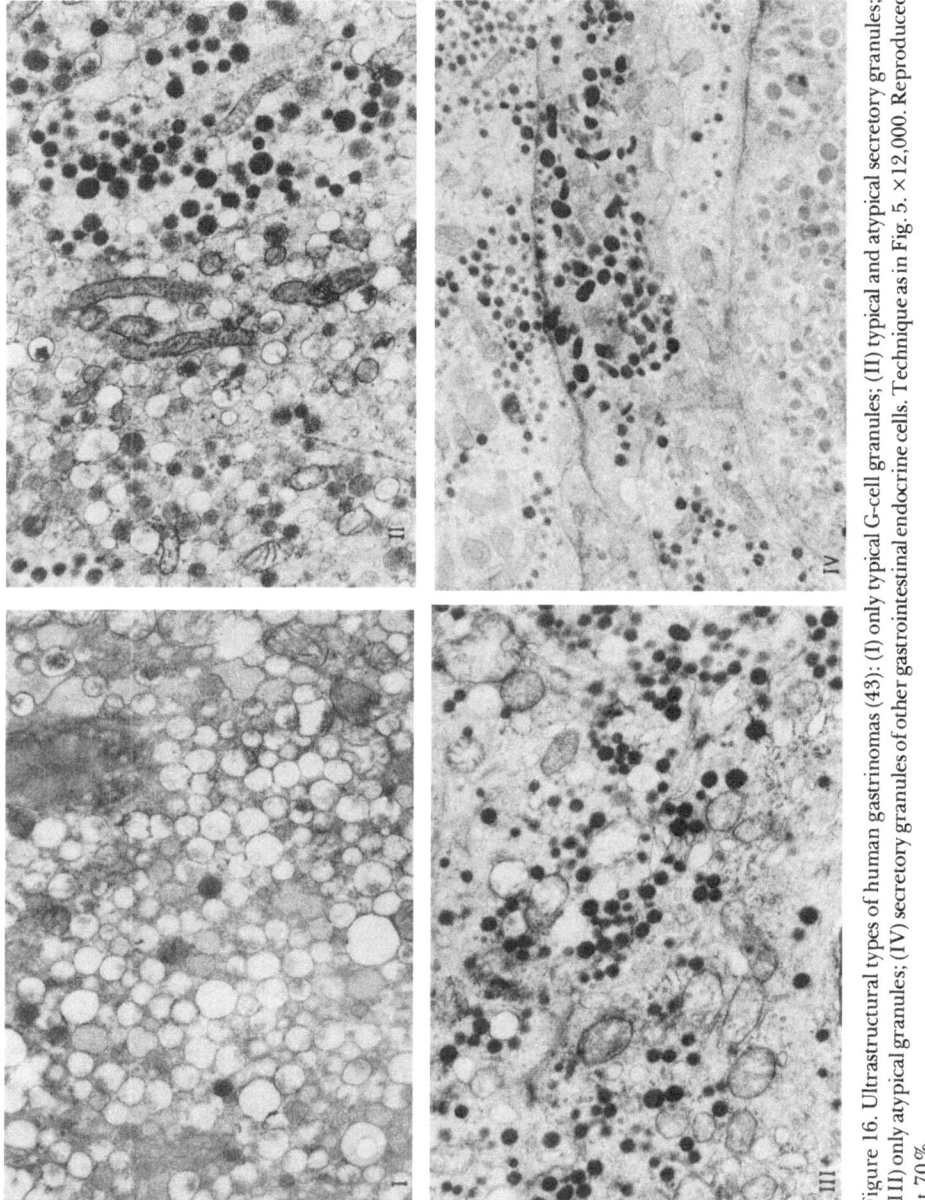

Figure 16. Ultrastructural types of human gastrinomas (43): (I) only typical G-cell granules; (II) typical and atypical secretory granules; (III) only atypical granules; (IV) secretory granules of other gastrointestinal endocrine cells. Technique as in Fig. 5. ×12,000. Reproduced at 70%.

The occurrence of pleomorphic granules can be interpreted as a sign of cellular dedifferentiation. Both cell types, however, are nondiagnostic. Thus, we agree with Greider *et al.*[30] regarding the occurrence of their types I and II cells in gastrinomas (and other endocrine tumors); we do not, however, understand why these authors do not find typical G cells in at least some cells of most of their gastrinomas.

Gastrin in Serum and Tissue

Different from insulinoma patients, who rarely have elevated fasting serum insulin levels, fasting immunoreactive gastrin (IRG) levels 20- to 10,000-fold higher than in normals are typical for gastrinoma patients. As demonstrated in Table 4, the IRG concentration of the tumors varied greatly but rarely exceeded the IRG concentration of normal antral mucosa (15.9 ± 2.6 μg/g)[86] which contains only 1 to 3% G cells. From this follows that most gastrinoma cells have reduced storage capacity, as has been demonstrated for insulinomas.[38]

Sephadex G-50 gel filtration studies have demonstrated gastrin (IRG) heterogeneity in the sera of ZES patients[43,87,88] and a comparable heterogeneity in gastrinoma tissue.[43,88]

Dockray *et al.*[88] investigated the gastrin components in serum and tumor extracts of 10 gastrinoma patients. They found in all cases that in serum G-34 was the major form of gastrin, whereas G-17 was a minor component. In the tumors, however, the opposite was true: G-17 was the major, and G-34 a minor component. The authors concluded that differences in the half-lives of the two gastrin components may partly explain their relative abundance in serum and tumor tissue.

The results in the author's laboratory[43] are presented in Table 4. Since the antigastrin serum used in these studies has different affinities for the gastrin components,[89] the percentage distribution given in Table 4 does not correspond to absolute values. The percentages reported for G-34 are clearly underestimations of the real values. No obvious relationship was found between the distribution of IRG components in the tumor tissue and sera of the individual gastrinoma patients. In 7 of 11 patients the serum percentages of G-34 were higher than the G-17 values. In the tumor extracts the G-34 fraction was extremely high in 3 patients, while in 9 of 13 cases G-17 predominated. However, the percentage of G-34 was, in 10 of 13 cases, still in the range found normally in duodenal extracts, and only in 3 was the percentage in the range of antral extracts.[86] No obvious relationship existed with the morphological data and the origin of the tumor (pancreatic or duodenal). Thus, our findings are similar to the data of Dockray *et al.*[88] but not as uniform.

The interpretation of these findings is much more difficult than that of the proinsulin data in insulinomas. The reasons for this are, firstly, the uncertainty about the roles of the different gastrin components in the physiological synthesis and release of gastrin, and secondly, the methodological problems related to the quantitative estimation of these components.[43] It appears that the storage capacity of gastrinomas is even more impaired than that of insulinomas. Otherwise, the enormous efflux or leakage of gastrin into the blood (reaching 20- to 10,000-fold normal hormone levels) could not be understood. *In vitro* studies have demonstrated that gastrinoma cells have a much faster hormone turnover than insulinoma cells.[90] Possibly, also the abnormal localization of the tumor G cell next to capillaries and not to a luminal surface (like in the antral or duodenal mucosa) contributes to these enormous blood levels. Different from the islet B cell, the G cell under physiological conditions secretes its hormonal product only partially into the blood stream and loses major parts into the surrounding tissue ("paracrine" secretion according to Feyrter) and also into the lumen of the stomach and of the duodenum.[91,92] In the case of a tumor, gastrin is quantitatively secreted into the blood and not wasted into the lumen. This could explain the extremely high blood levels of gastrin found in gastrinoma patients compared with the only slightly elevated insulin levels in insulinoma patients.

Glucagonoma

Glucagon-producing tumors have been observed much less frequently than insulinomas and gastrinomas. In 1966, the first case with radioimmunological hormone estimation and histochemical and ultrastructural investigation of the tumor was published.[11] In 1974, 9 more patients with pancreatic endocrine tumors were described, who also had necrolytic migratory erythema with anemia and diabetes (7 of 9 patients).[12] Elevated plasma glucagon levels could be estimated and glucagon could be extracted from the tumors. Identical cases were described recently.[93,95] One patient's diabetes and skin disease were cured by extirpation of the pancreatic tumor.[12,95]

In addition to these patients with the complete clinical syndrome of skin disease, diabetes, and anemia, several glucagon-producing tumors have been described in combination with diabetes[96-98] or as incidental findings.[96] Also, in the author's laboratory glucagonomas found incidentally have been encountered in four patients. All patients clinically had Zollinger–Ellison's syndrome and elevated serum gastrin levels. Multiple adenomas (diam 2 to 15 mm) were found in the resected pancreas of two patients; they reacted with antiglucagon serum. One patient had a pancreatic tumor with liver metastases reacting strongly with antiglucagon serum. The plasma glucagon levels of these patients were grossly elevated.

There is complete agreement about the morphology of these tumors. The cells react with Bodian's and Grimelius' silver impregnation and with antiglucagon antibodies. Ultrastructually, secretory granules are found revealing the characteristic structure of α granules: a round eccentric highly electron-dense core separated from the limiting membrane by a halo of medium dense material (Fig. 17). In addition, cells with atypical secretory granules (type IV) can be found in glucagonomas. The majority of the proven glucagonomas were malignant.[11,12,93,94,98]

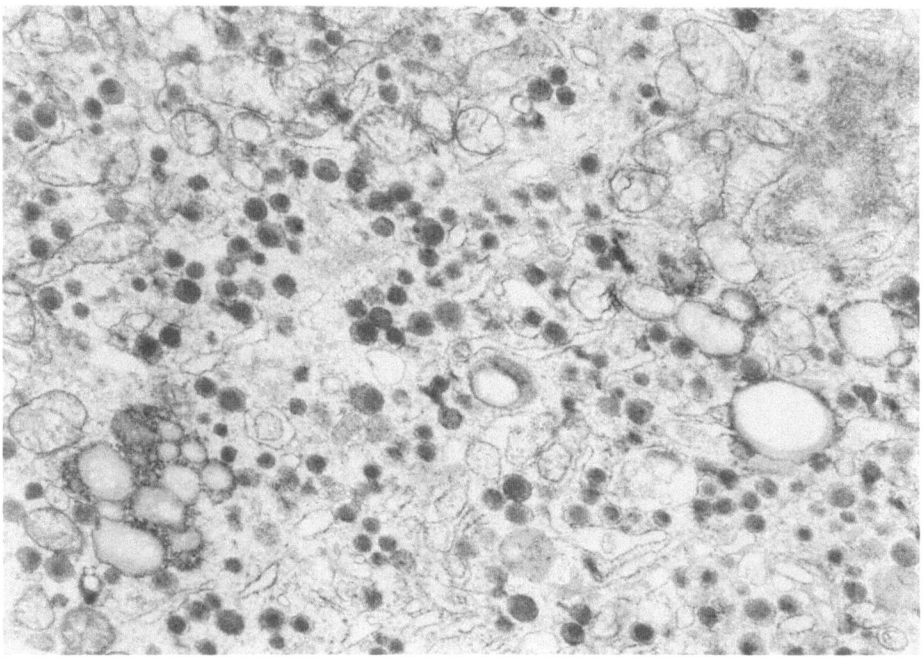

Figure 17. Parts of tumor cells with numerous secretory granules with an electron-dense central core separated from the limiting membrane by a halo of medium dense material. Glucagonoma (pat. Sche.). Technique as in Fig. 5. ×24,000. Reproduced at 75%.

Diarrheogenic Tumors

Since Verner and Morrison, in 1968, described the syndrome of watery diarrhea, hypokalemia, and hypochlorhydria in a patient with endocrine tumor of the pancreas,[10] more than 60 cases of this syndrome have been published.[27,99] It has not yet been decided if one single hormone is responsible for the syndrome or if the same disease can be produced by different hormones or a combination of different hormones which stimulate fluid and electrolyte secretion of the jejunum and perhaps of the pancreas and at the same time inhibit gastric secretion.[76,99] VIP (vasoactive intestinal peptide) has been found to be elevated in plasma, and the peptide has been demonstrated in the pancreatic tumors immunohistologically and by extraction in several cases.[100,101] Also, by immunohistology, GIP (gastric inhibitory polypeptide) was demonstrated in one tumor[102] and secretin in another.[103] All these peptides are chemically closely related. (See also note added in proof.)

About 50% of the published cases with diarrheogenic tumors were malignant.[99] The cells were argyrophil with the Grimelius silver impregnation, but not with the Hellerström–Hellman method.[27]

Ultrastructurally, the tumor cells contain relatively small electron-dense

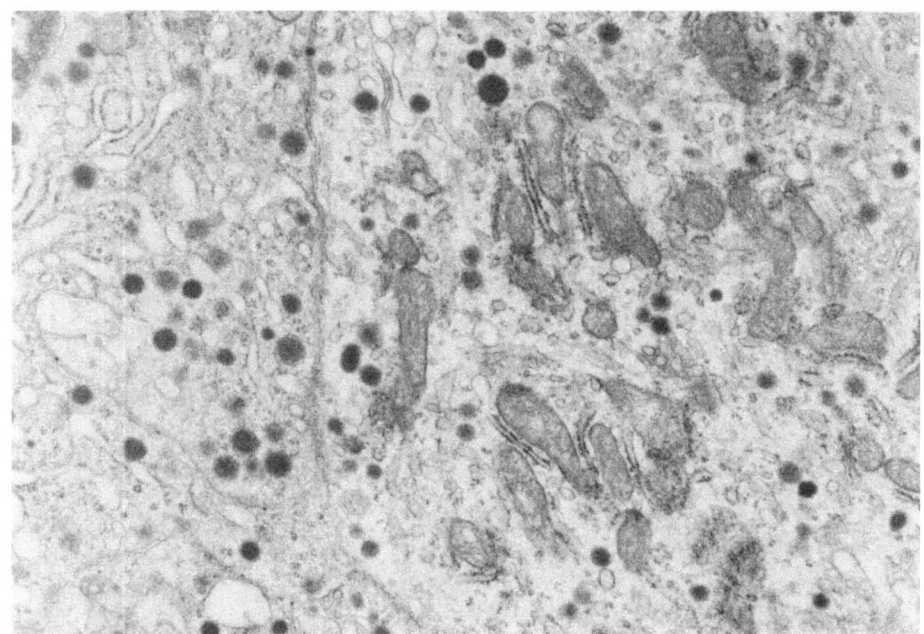

Figure 18. Parts of tumor cells with electron-dense, mostly round granules of different sizes ("atypical" granules), with or without encompassing membranes. Diarrheogenic tumor (pat. Det.). Technique as in Fig. 5. ×24,000. Reproduced at 75%.

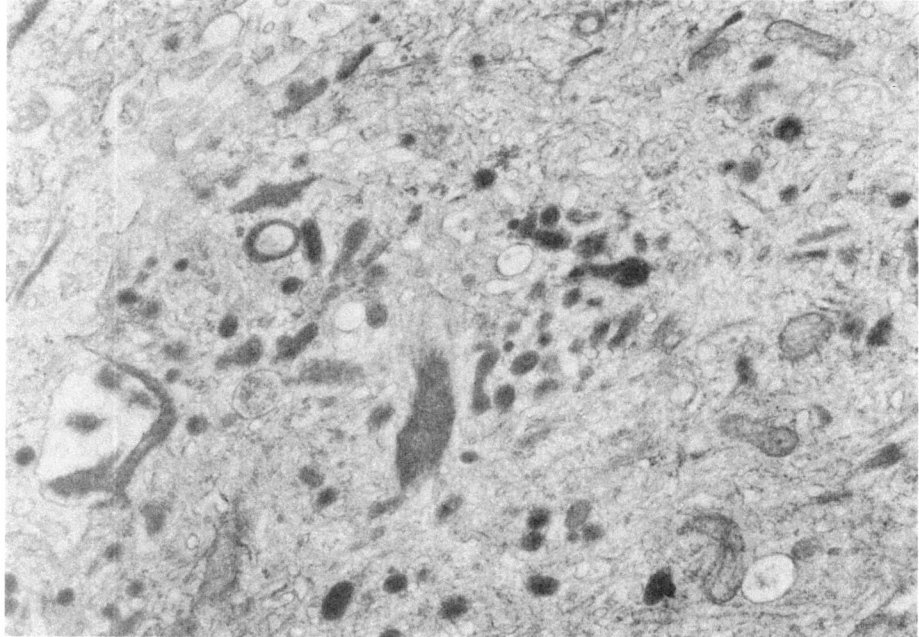

Figure 19. Part of tumor cell with pleomorphic secretory granules and distinctive parallel fibrils similar to tonofibrils. Diarrheogenic tumor (pat. Det.). Technique as in Fig. 5. ×24,000. Reproduced at 75%.

secretory granules closely resembling the type IV or D_1 cells.[27,30,104,105] The four diarrheogenic tumors investigated ultrastructurally in the author's laboratory revealed secretory granules which were indistinguishable from the "atypical granules" observed in insulinomas and gastrinomas of the ultrastructural types II and III (Fig. 18). Also, pleomorphic granules, as described in diarrheogenic and ulcerogenic tumors,[30] were frequently found (Fig. 19).

Hyperplasia of the pancreatic islets has been observed in the watery diarrhea syndrome and regarded as the cause of the diarrhea in some cases.[99] However, it has not been decided if these islet changes are secondary to the clinical disease.

Multiple Hormone Production

Definition and Frequency

The production of more than one hormone by single or multiple endocrine tumors of the pancreas has been known for some time (cf. Bonfils[106]) but has been regarded as an extremely rare event, as long as the diagnosis was based on clinical symptoms alone. This is because only few multiple-hormone-producing tumors give rise to a combination of clinical syndromes. In most cases only one syndrome, e.g., gastric hypersecretion or organic hypoglycemia, predominates, and further hormone elaboration is detected only by special investigation. Ever since immunochemical, immunohistological, and ultrastructural methods have routinely been applied to each endocrine pancreatic tumor, it has become apparent that the majority of these tumors produce more than one hormone.[19,21,43] It is beyond the scope of this article to review the literature on the multiple endocrine neoplasia syndrome (MEN),[23] especially the nonfamilial disease. Ellison and Wilson[26] found, in a collective review of 249 gastrinoma patients, further endocrine tumors in 21%, of which only 3% were of the familial variety. This figure includes tumors of the pituitary and of the parathyroids. Careful investigation of the resected pancreases of 22 patients with Zollinger–Ellison syndrome in the author's laboratory revealed in 5 out of 22 such patients multiple endocrine tumors in the pancreas.[19] These were in addition to one gastrinoma, two insulinomas, four glucagonomas, and two tumors with unidentified hormone production.

Multiple Hormone Production by a Single Pancreatic Tumor

Several authors have demonstrated by hormone extraction and immunohistology the presence of more than one peptide hormone in an endocrine tumor of the pancreas.[18–22,33,43,103,107–114,140] In gastrinomas the following have been found besides gastrin: insulin, glucagon, pancreatic polypeptide, VIP, secretin, ACTH, and MSH; in insulinomas, besides insulin: gastrin, glucagon, somatostatin, and pancreatic polypeptide; in diarrheogenic tumors: VIP, secretin, pancreatic and enteroglucagon, and pancreatic polypeptide; in glucagonomas, besides glucagon: insulin, somatostatin, and pancreatic polypeptide. In

*Table 5.   Frequency of Multiple Hormone Production within Gastrinomas, Insulinomas,
and Glucagonomas as Proved by Immunohistology and/or Hormone Estimation*[19]

	Gastrinoma (n = 18)	Insulinoma (n = 30)	Glucagonoma (n = 3)
Insulin	4/18	30/30	3/3
Gastrin	18/18	1/15	0/3
Glucagon	0/18	0/30	3/3
ACTH	8/14	n.t.	n.t.
Pancreatic polypeptide	5/8	3/15	3/3
Somatostatin	0/18	0/30	3/3

addition, serotonin and prostaglandins have been demonstrated in most of these tumors. In Table 5 are listed the recent results from the author's laboratory.[19] It has been postulated that multiple hormone production can occur in two ways[33]: (1) tumors composed of a homogeneous cell population synthesize more than one hormonal substance (monocellular–multihormonal type); and (2) tumors composed of a heterogeneous cell population produce in different cells different hormones (multicellular–multihormonal type). So far, immu-

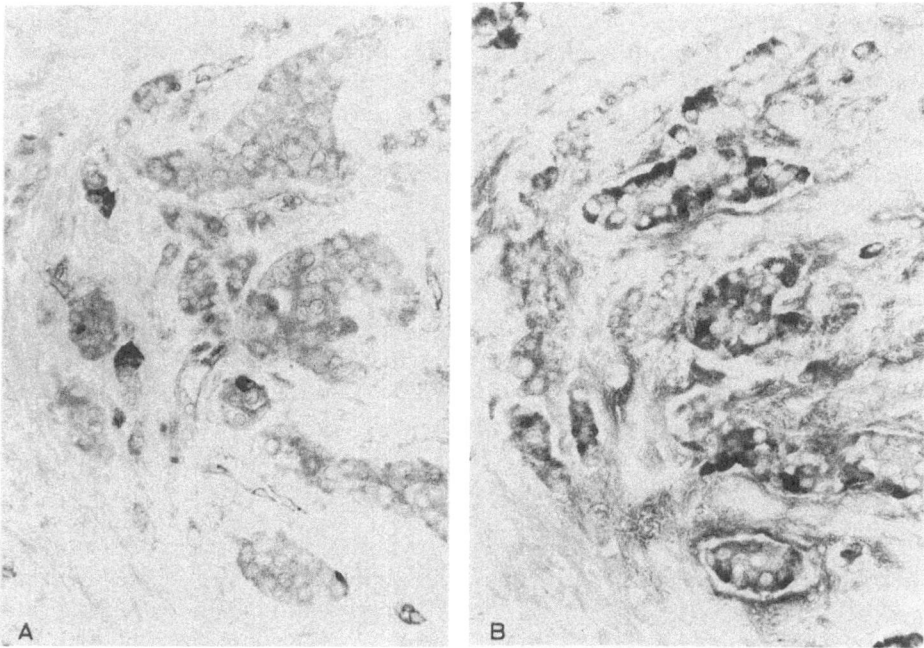

Figure 20. Immunohistologic demonstration of (A) insulin- and (B) gastrin-producing tumor cells (black) in consecutive serial sections of a gastrinoma (pat. Kac.). (A) technique as in Fig. 1; (B) technique as in Fig. 2. × 400. Reproduced at 75%.

nohistological and ultrastructural analyses have provided no support for the existence of a monocellular–multihormonal type.

Figure 20 demonstrates, in serial sections of a multihormonal gastrinoma, that gastrin and insulin are produced in different cells. Ultrastructurally, the tumor cells rarely contain secretory granules characteristic for the hormones demonstrated by immunohistology (Fig. 16). The usual ultrastructural findings are cells with atypical secretory granules (type IV or D_1) which are known to occur in all types of endocrine tumors of the pancreas (see above).

A surprise was the recent finding of Polak *et al.*[18] that pancreatic polypeptide is frequently present in all types of endocrine tumors of the pancreas (Table 5). The hormone which now can be estimated by radioimmunoassay in the blood[18,115,116] and may become a diagnostic marker for some pancreatic endocrine tumors[18] is easily demonstrated immunohistologically in distinct tumor cells (Fig. 21).

Recently, somatostatin-producing cells have also been found immunohistologically in three glucagonomas but not in other endocrine tumors of the pancreas.[19]

Until now, tumors producing exclusively or mainly pancreatic polypeptide or somatostatin have not been observed. Also, clinical symptoms cannot as yet be related to an overproduction of these peptides. (See note added in proof.)

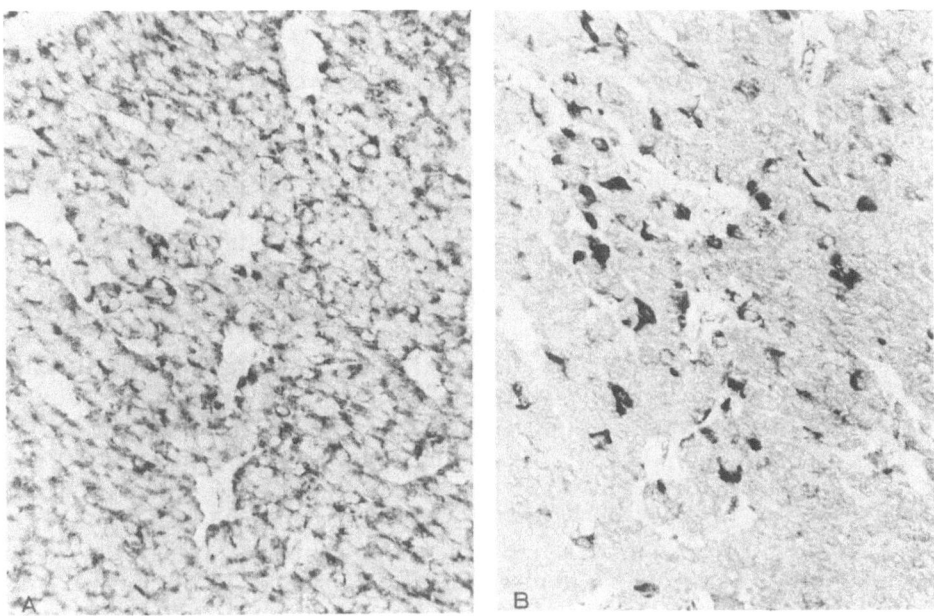

Figure 21. Immunohistologic demonstration of (A) gastrin- and (B) pancreatic polypeptide-producing tumor cells (black) in consecutive serial sections of a gastrinoma (pat. Stei.). (A) Technique as in Fig. 2. (B) Incubation with 1/20 diluted antipancreatic polypeptide serum (gift of Dr. R. E. Chance). × 240. Reproduced at 75%.

However, it has to be pointed out that an additional hormone production is usually not followed by corresponding clinical symptoms. This has been documented in the literature in 14 patients with gastrinomas and additional insulin-producing cells, in 9 patients with gastrinomas and additional glucagon-producing cells, and in 14 patients with gastrinomas and ACTH production. Only in 4 of 14 gastrinoma patients with insulin-producing tumor cells could transitory hypoglycemic states be observed; the majority of the patients were symptom free. Probably, the presence of hypoglycemia does not depend exclusively upon the amount of B cells within a gastrinoma. This could be demonstrated in 2 patients with the Zollinger–Ellison syndrome, where in addition to gastrinomas large insulinomas were resected during laparotomy. Only 1 of these patients on one occasion had low blood glucose levels. Insulin antagonism of gastrin could explain this observation.[19]

Glucagon was found in 9 gastrinoma patients. However, in only 1 of these cases could diabetes mellitus be detected. Increased ACTH production was demonstrable in 14 gastrinoma patients. Out of these 14 patients, 8 had clinical symptoms of hypercorticism. It is quite evident from these data that interactions by different gastrointestinal hormones in the case of excess secretion need further clarification and may be the key to an understanding of the multiple endocrine neoplasia syndrome.[108] Thus, the occurrence of multiple hormone production in endocrine pancreatic tumors—either as orthotopical or ectopical secretion—leads to the problem of the origin of these tumors.

Cellular Origin of Endocrine Tumors of the Pancreas

Any theory explaining the cellular origin and histogenesis of endocrine tumors of the pancreas has to consider the biochemical and morphological findings described in the preceeding sections, namely:

(1) Endocrine tumors of the pancreas can produce hormones which are not found in the normal adult pancreas. The production of such hormones is best explained in terms of dedifferentiation. The tumor cells are in an early stage of pluripotentiality like a precursor or stem cell.

(2) Ontogenetically, the islet and acinar tissues originate from the ductular system which had once budded out from the foregut.[118,119] Ductular or tubular structures can be found in practically all endocrine tumors of the pancreas,[1,29,38–41,43] both in the center and in the periphery of the tumor tissue (Fig. 7). Sometimes tumors are located in an area of the pancreas showing marked fibrosis or even chronic pancreatitis where proliferation of ducts and budding of islets are a normal finding. In other cases, ductular proliferation and budding islets are found without any signs of fibrosis or inflammation. This occurs in the pancreas of patients with insulinomas (Fig. 22) and with gastrinomas. Of special interest is the finding of ductular and islet proliferation in patients with duodenal gastrinomas[43,77,78] or with multiple endocrine neoplasia.[120] In the author's laboratory 3 cases of multiple pancreatic tumors and ductular proliferation have been found incidentally during the investigation of

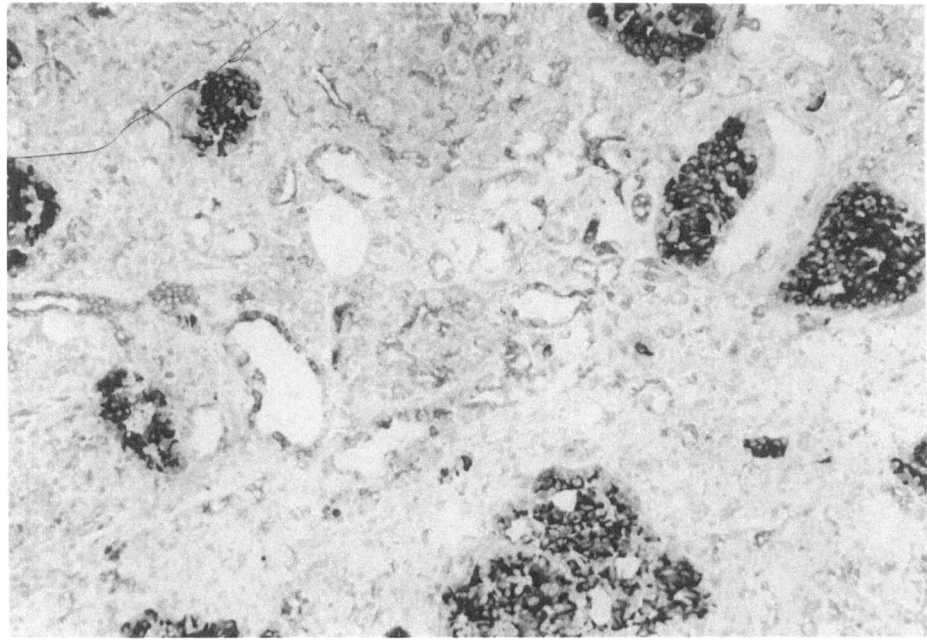

Figure 22. Proliferation of pancreatic ducts with budding islets containing mainly insulin-producing B cells (black) in the pancreas of a patient with insulinoma (pat. Mie.). Technique as in Fig. 1. ×160. Reproduced at 105%.

the resected pancreas of gastrinoma patients (Fig. 23). As in ontogenesis of the pancreas, it is difficult to assess whether the ductular structures consist of nonendocrine ductules or immature endocrine cells. This is because regenerating, phylogenetically primitive, and ontogenetically immature islet tissue tends to form tubular structures.[119,121] This suggests that they originate from cells which are not yet differentiated.

It has to be pointed out, however, that the proliferation of ductular elements and budding of endocrine cells from the ductular epithelium leading to islet hyperplasia is not autonomous tumor growth. For example, islet proliferation is well known from newborns of diabetic mothers but does not persist. In cases of spontaneous or reactive hypoglycemia in newborns diffuse islet hyperplasia has been found in the resected pancreas. Typical insulinomas are rare in the newborn. However, a link between islet hyperplasia and true insulinoma is the so-called "focal adenomatosis" in cases of neonatal hypoglycemia.[122] Here, in a circumscribed area of the pancreas (usually measuring 3 to 10 mm in diam) islet cell clusters and ductular structures are packed together, separated and encapsulated by small cords of acinar tissue and distinct fibrous septa. However, no coherent adenoma is formed. Two such cases of neonatal focal adenomatosis have been investigated in the author's laboratory. In one case the endocrine tissue was palpated as a hard area and suspected because of

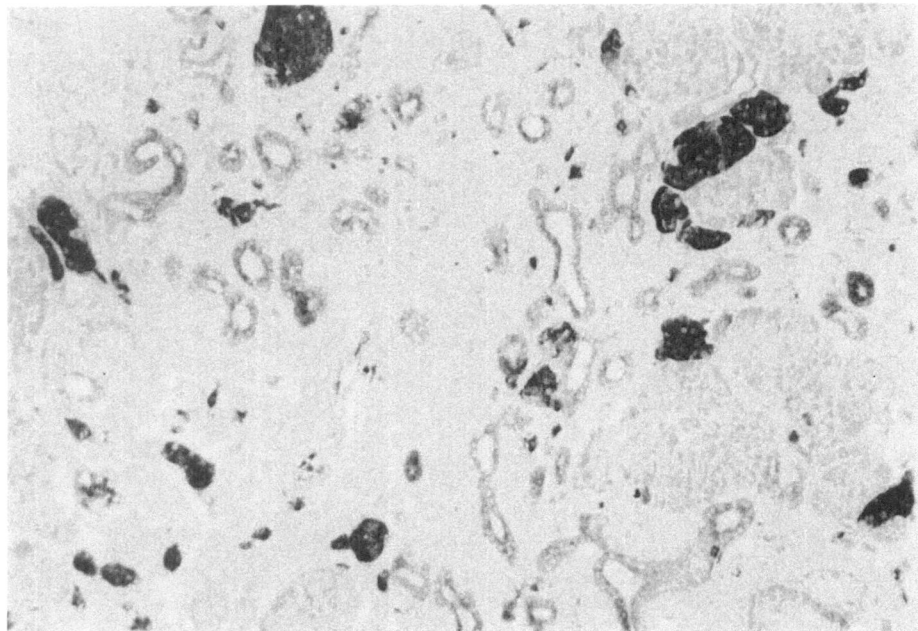

Figure 23. Extreme proliferation of pancreatic ducts with budding islets in fibrotic areas of the pancreas of a patient with multiple endocrine neoplasia syndrome [gastrinoma, insulinoma, gluca-gonoma (pat. Sche.)]. Technique as in Fig. 1. ×160. Reproduced at 105%.

its reddish color, especially after cutting. In the other case, focal adenomatosis was found only during microscopic investigation. The decisive difference between focal adenomatosis as a cause for spontaneous hypoglycemia and insulinoma is the different histological appearance of the tissue. Immunohisto-logical and ultrastructural investigation in focal adenomatosis reveals normal cellular composition of the islet clusters. A, B, D, and PP cells occur in nearly normal relative frequency (Fig. 24). The only difference from normal islet tissue is the frequent finding of poorly granulated (or sometimes even agranu-lar) B cells (Fig. 25). The insulin concentration measured in one of our cases confirmed this: 0.5 U/g was found in the surrounding pancreas and 55.3 U/g were found in the area of focal adenomatosis. The insulin concentration in normal islet tissue is about 200 U/g. Also, the proinsulin percentage was higher in the area of focal adenomatosis than in the normal pancreas.

(3) The only cell which occurs in all types of endocrine tumors of the pancreas is the cell containing atypical secretory granules. This cell is argyrophil by the Grimelius procedure[43,58] and identical with the type IV (D$_1$) cell. It can also be found in islet hyperplasia of persistent neonatal hypoglycemia[123–125] and in lower vertebrates[121] and may well be a precursor or stem cell for the endocrine cells of the foregut and their tumors.[58,75,120–122] This precursor or stem cell theory is incompatible with names like "islet cell" tumors, "nesidioblas-tomas,"[1,108] or "carcinoid islet cell" tumors[126] for the endocrine tumors of the

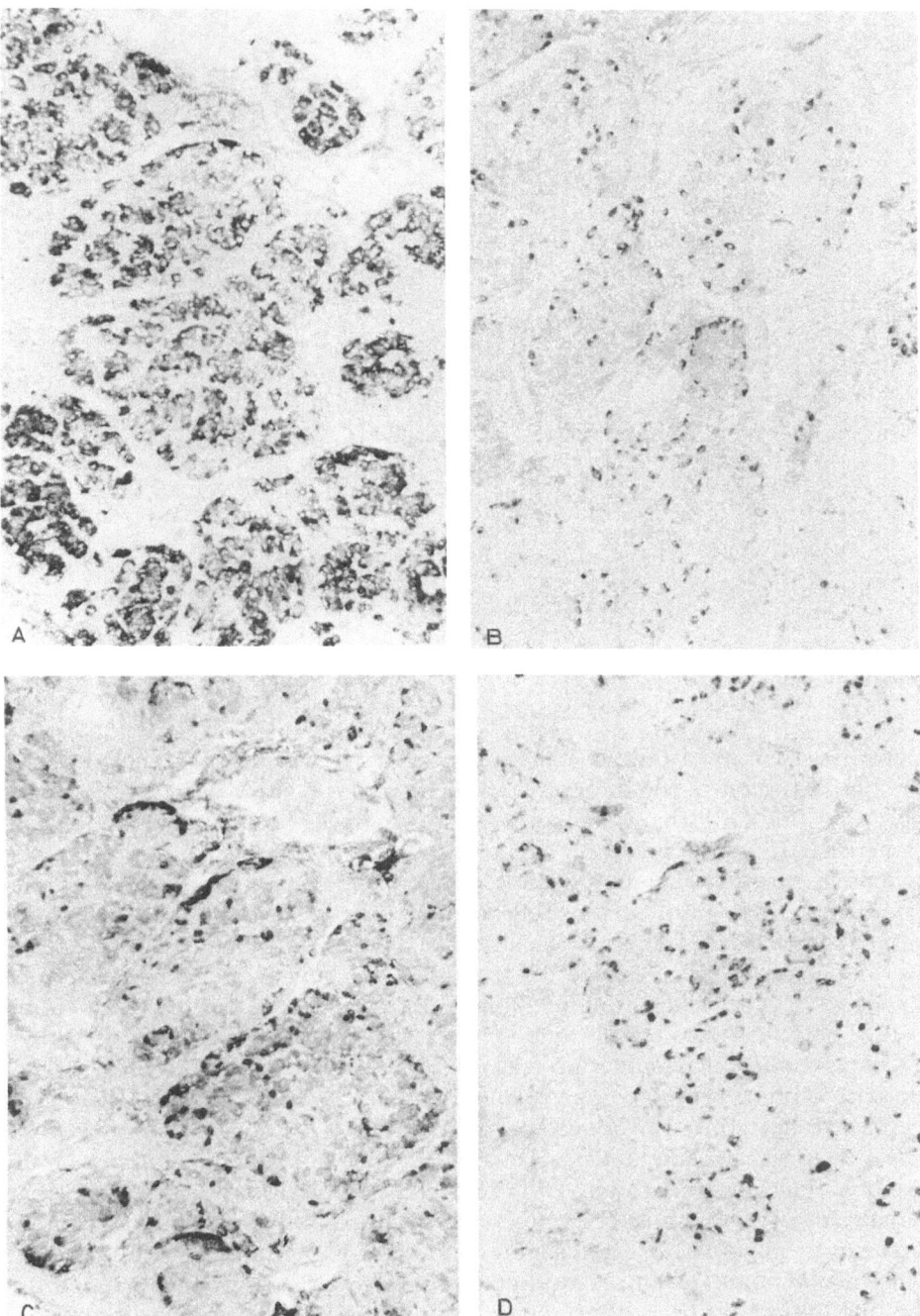

Figure 24. Immunohistological demonstration of the cellular composition of the endocrine tissue in focal adenomatosis in a patient with neonatal hypoglycemia (pat. Sul.). (A) antiinsulin serum; (B) antisomatostatin serum; (C) antiglucagon serum; (D) antipancreatic polypeptide serum. A, C, and D are consecutive serial sections; B is a section of a neighboring area. ×160. Reproduced at 75%.

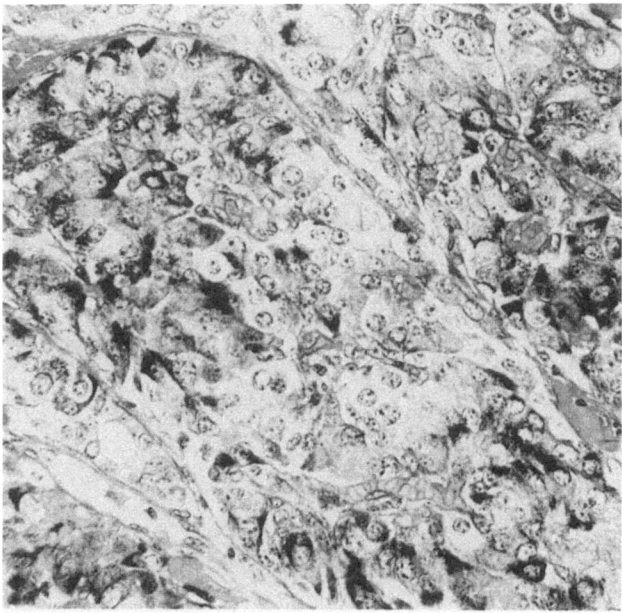

Figure 25. Many poorly granulated or even virtually agranular B cells in the islet tissue of focal adenomatosis in neonatal hypoglycemia (pat. Sul.). Technique as in Fig. 7. ×400.

pancreas. Desirable would be a more general name which should include other endocrine tumors of the foregut. It has been proposed by Weichert,[127] Pearse *et al.*,[48] and Friesen[110] that polypeptide-producing cells of the gut (including the pancreas) are neuroendocrine cells of ectodermal origin which migrate to the primitive gut during embryogenesis. They mature later into the polypeptide-producing cells (apud series of Pearse). If by genetic or individual reasons precursor cells with multiple biochemical potencies become neoplastic, any hormone production (single or multiple) as discussed before must be expected.[128] The term "apudoma" has been used for all tumors of the apud cells. This is an etymologically odd term. If the still-debated[129] neurocrest origin of all gastrointestinal endocrine cells will be finally proven, the term "neuroendocrine" tumors (of the pancreas, duodenum, etc.) would be appropriate. The respective hormone(s) produced could be added.

(4) A last argument for a common origin of endocrine tumors of the pancreas (and the gut) derives from clinical therapeutic studies. Streptozotocin, a naturally occurring oncogenic and oncolytic nitrosourea compound, produces diabetes in mammals by destruction of the islet B cells and, if given together with nicotinamide, produces insulinomas in rats.[130,131] Intravenous streptozotocin application has been effective in malignant insulinomas, regarding regression of liver metastasis and survival of the patients.[132] More recently, it has been found that streptozotocin is also effective (especially if injected not intravenously but into the celiac artery) in malignant gastrinoma,[133,134] metastasizing diarrheogenic tumors (Verner–Morrison syndrome),[135] glucagonoma,[93,94,126]

and malignant carcinoids.[137-139] Since streptozotocin had no effect in nonendocrine gastrointestinal carcinomas, this general effect on malignant endocrine tumors of the pancreas with different hormone production can be interpreted as the response of closely related cells to a special agent.

Note Added in Proof

Since this manuscript went into press a pancreatic tumor with liver metastasis has been described in a patient with the watery diarrhea syndrome who had normal serum VIP levels. The tumor contained only 1% VIP cells, while 90% of the tumor cells were reactive with the antiserum against human pancreatic polypeptide (PP).[141]

Also a pancreatic tumor with liver metastasis producing exclusively somatostatin has been observed.[142] Ultrastructurally, the tumor cells contained secretory granules indistinguishable from those of normal pancreatic D cells. Clinically the patient had steatorrhea, achlorhydria, and impaired glucose tolerance.

References

1. Laidlaw, G. F.: *Amer. J. Pathol.* **14**:125, 1938.
2. Nicholls, A. G.: *J. Med. Res.,* **8**:385, 1902.
3. Heiberg, K. A.: *Die Krankheiten des Pankreas.* J. F. Bergmann, Wiesbaden, 1914, p. 179.
4. Wilder, R. M., Allan, F. N., Power, M. H., and Robertson, H. E.: *J. Amer. Med. Assoc.,* **89**:348, 1927.
5. Spencer, H.: *J. Pathol. Bacteriol.* **69**:259, 1955.
6. Seifert, G., and Berdrow, J.: *Ärztl. Wochenschr.,* **13**:829, 1958.
7. Warren, S., LeCompte, P. M., and Legg, M. A.: *The Pathology of Diabetes Mellitus.* Lea & Febiger, Philadelphia, 1966, p. 377.
8. Becker, V.: *Langenbecks Arch.,* **88**:329, 1971.
9. Zollinger, R. M., and Ellison, E. H.: *Ann. Surg.,* **142**:709, 1955.
10. Verner, J. V., and Morrison, A. R.: *Amer. J. Med.,* **25**:374, 1958.
11. McGavran, M. H., Unger, R. H., Recant, L., Polk, H. C., Kilo, C., and Levin, M. E.: *N. Engl. J. Med.,* **274**:1408, 1966.
12. Mallinson, C. N., Bloom, S. R., Warin, A. P., Salmon, P. R., and Cox, B.: *Lancet,* **2**:1, 1974.
13. Luft, R., Efendic, S., Hökfelt, T., Johansson, O., and Arimura, A.: *Med. Biol.,* **52**:428, 1974.
14. Dubois, M. P.: *Proc. Nat. Acad. Sci.,* **72**:1340, 1975.
15. Orci, L., Baettens, D., Dubois, M. P., and Rufener, C.: *Horm. Metab. Res.,* **7**:400, 1975.
16. Polak, J. M., Grimelius, L., Pearse, A. G. E., Bloom, S. R., and Arimura, A.: *Lancet,* **1**:1220, 1975.
17. Larsson, L.-I., Sundler, F., and Hakanson, R.: *Diabetologia,* **12**:211, 1976.
18. Polak, J. M., Bloom, S. R., Adrian, T. E., Heitz, P., Bryant, M. G., and Pearse, A. G. E.: *Lancet,* **1**:328, 1976.
19. Arnold, R., Creutzfeldt, C., and Creutzfeldt, W.: In: *Endocrinology.* Edited by V. H. T. James, Vol. 2, Excerpta Medica Foundation, Amsterdam, 1977, p. 448.
20. O'Neal, L. W., Kipnis, D. M., Luse, S. A., Lacy, P. E., and Jarett, L.: *Cancer,* **21**:1219, 1968.
21. Larsson, L.-I., Grimelius, L., Hakanson, R., Rehfeld, J. F., Stadil, F., Holst, J., Angervall, L., and Sundler, F.: *Amer. J. Pathol.,* **79**:271, 1975.

22. Dettos, L. J., McMillan, P. J., Sartiano, G. P., Abuid, J., and Robinson, A. G.: *Metabolism,* **25**:543, 1976.

23. Wermer, P.: *Clin. Gasteroenterol.,* **3**:671, 1974.

24. Howard, J. M., Moss, N. H., and Rhoads, J. E.: *Int. Abst. Surg.,* **90**:417, 1950.

25. Stefanini, P., Carboni, M., Patrassi, N., and Basoli, A.: *Surgery,* **75**:597, 1974.

26. Ellison, E. H., and Wilson, S. D.: *Ann. Surg.,* **160**:512, 1964.

27. Burkhardt, A., and Mitschke, H.: *Virchows Arch. Pathol. Anat.,* **364**:145, 1974.

28. Warren, S.: *Amer. J. Pathol.,* **2**:335, 1926.

29. Frantz, V. K.: *Tumors of the Pancreas.* Armed Forces Institute of Pathology, Washington, 1959, p. 79.

30. Greider, M. H., Rosai, J., and McGuigan, J. E.: *Cancer,* **33**:1423, 1974.

31. Porta, E. A., Yerry, R., and Scott, R. F.: *Amer. J. Pathol.,* **41**:623, 1962.

32. Steiner, H.: *Virchow's Arch. Pathol. Anat.,* **342**:170, 1969.

33. Heitz, Ph., Steiner, H., Halter, F., Egli, F., and Kapp, J. P.: *Virchow's Arch. Pathol. Anat.,* **353**:312, 1971.

34. Pearse, A. G. E., Ewen, S. W. B., and Polak, J. M.: *Virchow's Arch. Zellpath.,* **10**:93, 1972.

35. Bargmann, W.: *Z. Zellforsch.,* **29**:562, 1939.

36. Ferner, H.: *Das Inselzellsystem des Pankreas.* Georg Thieme, Stuttgart, 1952.

37. Greider, M. H., and Elliott, D. W.: *Amer. J. Pathol.,* **44**:663, 1964.

38. Creutzfeldt, W., Arnold, R., Creutzfeldt, C., Deuticke, U., Frerichs, H., and Track, N.S.: *Diabetologia,* **9**:217, 1973.

39. Lazarus, S. S., and Volk, B. W.: *Lab. Invest.,* **11**:1279, 1962.

40. Bencosme, S. A., Allen, R. A., and Latta, H.: *Amer. J. Pathol.,* **42**:1, 1963.

41. Suzuki, H. and Matsuyama, M.: *Cancer,* **28**:1302, 1971.

42. Sieracki, J., Marshall, R. B., and Horn, Jr.,R. C.: *Cancer,* **13**:347, 1960.

43. Creutzfeldt, W., Arnold, R., Creutzfeldt, C., and Track, N. S.: *Human Pathol.,* **6**:47, 1975.

44. Cavallero, C., Solcia, E., and Sampietro, R.: *Gut,* **8**:172, 1967.

45. Vassallo, G., Solcia, E., Bussolati, G., Polak, J. M., and Pearse, A. G. E.: *Virchow's Arch. Zellpath.,* **11**:66, 1972.

46. Martin, E. D. and Potet, F.: *Clin. Gastroenterol.,* **3**:511, 1974.

47. Pearse, A. G. E.: *J. Histochem. Cytochem.,* **17**:303, 1969.

48. Pearse, A. G. E., Polak, J. M., and Heath, C. M.: *Virchow's Arch. Zellpath.,* **16**:95, 1974.

49. Paget, G. E.: *Stain Technol.,* **95**:223, 1954.

50. Hellerström, C., and Hellman, B.: *Acta Endocrinol.,* **35**:518, 1960.

51. Grimelius, L: *Acta Soc. Med. Upsal.,* **73**:243, 1968.

52. Arnold, R., Deuticke, U., Frerichs, H., and Creutzfeldt, W.: *Diabetologia,* **8**:250, 1972.

53. Lacy, P. E., and Williamson, J. R.: *Anat. Rec.,* **136**:227, 1960.

54. Lacy, P. E.: *Amer. J. Med.,* **31**:851, 1961.

55. Georgsson, G., and Wessel, W.: *Z. Krebsforsch.,* **69**:70, 1964.

56. Deconinck, J. F., Potvliege, P. R., and Gepts, W.: *Diabetologia,* **7**:266, 1971.

57. Creutzfeldt, W., Creutzfeldt, C., and Arnold, R.: *Rend. Gastroenterol.,* **7**:93, 1975.

58. Creutzfeldt, W., Creutzfeldt, C., Track, N. S., and Arnold, R.: In: *Hypoglycemia.* Edited by D. Andreani, P. Lefèbvre, and V. Marks. Georg Thieme, Stuttgart, 1976, p. 7.

59. Vassallo, G., Capella, C., and Solcia, E.: *Stain Technol.,* **46**:7, 1971.

60. Floyd, J. C., Fajans, S. S., Knopf, R. F., and Conn, J. W.: *J. Clin. Endocrinol.,* **24**:747, 1964.

61. Gepts, W.: *Symposium Deutsche Gesellschaft für Endokrinologie.* Springer Verlag, Berlin, 1968, p. 101.

62. Pi-Sunyer, F. X., van Itallie, and Zintel, H. A.: *Amer. J. Surg.,* **118**:95, 1969.

63. Steinke, J., Soeldner, J. S., and Renold, A. E.: *J. Clin. Invest.,* **42**:1322, 1963.

64. Goldsmith, S., Yalow, R., and Berson, S. A.: *Diabetes,* **18**:834, 1969.

65. Gorden, P., and Roth, J: *Arch. Int. Med.,* **123**:237, 1969.

66. Gorden, P., Sherman, B., and Roth, J.: *J. Clin. Invest.,* **50**:2113, 1971.

67. Gutman, R., Lazarus, N. R., Penhos, J., Recant, L., and Fajans, S. S.: *N. Engl. J. Med.,* **284**:1003, 1970.

68. Melani, F., Ryan, W. G., Rubenstein, A. H., and Steiner, D. F.: *N. Engl. J. Med.,* **283**:713,

69. Lindall, A. W., Wong, E. T., Sorenson, R. L., and Steffes, M. W.: *J. Clin. Endocrinol.,* **34**:718, 1972.

70. Rubenstein, A. H., Block, M. B., Starr, J., Melani, F., and Steiner, D. F.: *Diabetes,* (Suppl. 2) **21**:661, 1972.

71. Kemmler, W., Peterson, J. D., Rubenstein, A. H., and Steiner, D. F.: *Diabetes,* (Suppl. 2) **21**:572, 1972.

72. Creutzfeldt, C., Track, N. S., and Creutzfeldt, W.: *Eur. J. Clin. Invest.,* **3**:371, 1973.

73. Track, N. S., Creutzfeldt, C., and Creutzfeldt, W.: In: *Hypoglycemia.* Edited by D. Andreani, P. Lefèbvre, and V. Marks. Georg Thieme, Stuttgart, 1976, p. 19.

74. Turner, R. C., and Harris, E.: *Lancet,* **2**:188, 1974.

75. Suzuki, H.: *Nagoya Med. J.,* **19**:85, 1974.

76. Isenberg, J. I., Walsh, J. H., and Grossman, M. I.: *Gastroenterology,* **65**:140, 1973.

77. Oberhelman, H. A.: *Arch. Surg.,* **104**:447, 1972.

78. Larsson, L.-I., Ljungberg, O., Sundler, F., Hakanson, R., Svensson, O., Rehfeld, J., Stadil, F., and Holst, J.: *Virchow's Arch. Pathol. Anat.,* **360**:305, 1973.

79. Creutzfeldt, W., Arnold, R., Creutzfeldt, C., Feurle, G., and Ketterer, H.: *Eur. J. Clin. Invest.,* **1**:461, 1971.

80. Lotstra, F., van der Loo, W., and Gepts, W.: *Diabetologia,* **10**:291, 1974.

81. Greider, M. H., and McGuigan, J. E.: *Diabetes,* **20**:389, 1971.

82. Lomský, R., Langr, F., and Vortel, V.: *Nature (London),* **223**:618, 1970.

83. Thiery, J. P., and Bader, J. P.: *Ann. Endocrinol.* **27**:625, 1966.

84. Munger, B. L.: In: *Handbook of Physiology.* Vol. I. *Endocrine Pancreas.* Edited by D. F. Steiner and N. Freinkel, Williams & Wilkins, Baltimore 1972, p. 305.

85. Solcia, E., Pearse, A. G. E., Grube, D., Kobayashi, S., Bussolati, G., Creutzfeldt, W., and Gepts, W.: *Rend. Gastroenterol.,* **5**:13, 1973.

86. Creutzfeldt, W., Arnold, R., Creutzfeldt, C., and Track, N. S.: *Gut,* **17**:745, 1976.

87. Rehfeld, J. F., and Stadil, F.: *Gut,* **14**:369, 1973.

88. Dockray, G. J., Walsh, J. H., and Passaro, Jr., E.: *Gut,* **16**: 353, 1975.

89. Mayer, G., Arnold, R., Feurle, G., Fuchs, K., Ketterer, H., Track, N. S., and Creutzfeldt, W.: *Scand. J. Gastroenterol.,* **9**:703, 1974.

90. Track, N. S., Creutzfeldt, C., Junge, U., and Creutzfeldt, W.: In: *Gastrointestinal Hormones.* Edited by J. C. Thompson. Univ. of Texas Press, Texas, 1975, p. 403.

91. Andersson, S., and Nilsson, G.: *Scand. J. Gastroenterol.,* **9**:619, 1974.

92. Uvnaes-Wallensten, K.: *Acta Physiol. Scand. (Suppl. 438),* 1976.

93. Case Record No. 20-1975. *N. Engl. J. Med.,* **292**:1117, 1975.

94. Danforth, Jr., D. N., Triche, T., Doppman, J. L., Beazley, R. M., Perrino, P. V., and Recant, L.: *N. Engl. J. Med.,* **295**:242, 1976.

95. Lightman, S. L., and Bloom, S. R.: *Brit. Med. J.,* **1**:367, 1974.

96. Lomský, R., Langr, F., and Vortel, V.: *Amer. J. Clin. Pathol.,* **51**:245, 1969.

97. Grimelius, L., Petersson, B., Lundquist, G., Dahlgren, S., and Parrow, A.: *Acta Soc. Med. Upsal.,* **76**:49, 1971.

98. Larsson, L.-I., Sundler, F., Grimelius, L., Hakanson, R., and Holst, J.: *Experientia,* **29**:698, 1973.

99. Verner, J. V., and Morrison, A. B.: *Clin. Gastroenterol.,* **3**:595, 1974.

100. Bloom, S. R., Polak, J. M., and Pearse, A. G. E.: *Lancet,* **2**:14, 1973.

101. Said, S. I., and Faloona, G. R.: *N. Engl. J. Med.,* **293**:155, 1975.

102. Elias, E., Polak, J. M., Bloom, S. R., Pearse, A. G. E., Welbourn, R. B., Booth, C. C., Kuzio, M., and Brown, J. C.: *Lancet,* **2**:791, 1972.

103. Schmitt, Jr., M. G., Soergel, K. H., Hensley, G. T., and Chey, W. Y.: *Gastroenterology,* **69**:206, 1975.

104. Rambaud, J.-C., Modigliani, R., Matuchansky, C., Bloom, S., Said, S., Pessayre, D., and Bernier, J.-J.: *Gastroenterology,* **69**:110, 1975.

105. Martin, E., Dubois, F., Lacourbe, R., Duchesne, G., and Bonfils, S.: *Arch. Fr. Mal. App. Dig.,* **63**:229, 1974.

106. Bonfils, S.: *Clin. Gastroenterol.,* **3**:477, 1974.

107. Creutzfeldt, W., Arnold, R., Creutzfeldt, C., Frerichs, H., and Track, N. S.: In: *Diabetes.* Edited by W. J., Malaisse, J. Pirart, and J. Vallance-Owen. Excerpta Medica Amsterdam, 1974, p. 683.

108. Vance, J. E., Stoll, R. W., Kitabchi, A. E., Buchanan, K. D., Hollander, D., and Williams, R. H.: *Amer. J. Med.,* **52**:211, 1972.

109. Shieber, W.: *Surgery,* **54**:448, 1963.

110. Friesen, S. R., Hermreck, A. S., and Mantz, F. A.: *Amer. J. Surg.,* **127**:90, 1974.

111. Geokas, M. C., Chun, J. Y., Dinan, J. J., and Beck, I. T.: *Canad. Med. Assoc. J.,* **93**:137, 1965.

112. Law, D. H., Liddle, G. W., Scott, H. W., and Tauber, S. D.: *N. Engl. J. Med.,* **273**:292, 1965.

113. Aronson, K. F., Boquist, L., Falkmer, S., Hägerstrand, I., Steiner, H., and von Studnitz, W.: *Acta Pathol. Microbiol. Scand.,* **78**:265, 1970.

114. Block, M. A., Kelly, A. R., and Horn, R. C.: *Arch. Surg.,* **98**:734, 1969.

115. Floyd, J. C., Chance, R. E., Bayashi, R., Moon, N. E., and Fajans, S. S.: *Clin. Res.,* **25**:535 A, 1975.

116. Schwartz, T. W., Rehfeld, J. F., Stadil, F., Larsson, L.-I., Chance, R. E., and Moon, N.: *Lancet,* **2**:1102, 1976.

117. Frerichs, H., and Creutzfeldt, W.: *Clin. Endocrin. Metabol.,* **5**:747, 1976.

118. Pictet, R., and Rutter, W. J.: In: *Endocrinology.* Edited by D.F. Steiner and N. Freinkel. Amer. Physiol. Soc., Washington, 1972, p. 40.

119. Like, A. A., and Orci, L.: *Diabetes, (Suppl. 2)* **21**:511, 1972.

120. Creutzfeldt, W.: *Israel J. Med. Sci.,* **11**:762, 1975.

121. Falkmer, S., and Boquist, L.: In: *Hypoglycemia.* Edited by D., Andreani, P. Lefèbvre, and V. Marks. Georg Thieme, Stuttgart, 1976, p. 55.

122. Klöppel, G., Altenähr, E., and Menke, B.: *Virchow's Arch. Pathol. Anat. Histol.,* **366**:223, 1975.

123. Misugi, K., Misugi, N., Sotos, J., and Smith, B.: *Arch. Pathol.,* **89**:208, 1970.

124. Klöppel, G., Altenähr, E., Reichel, W., Willig, R., and Freytag, G.: *Diabetologia,* **10**:245, 1974.

125. Søvik, O., Vidnes, J., and Falkmer, S.: *Acta Pathol. Microbiol. Scand.,* **83A**:155, 1976.

126. Weichert, R., Reed, R., and Creech, O.: *Ann. Surg.,* **165**:660, 1967.

127. Weichert, R. F.: *Amer. J. Med.,* **49**:232, 1970.

128. Hedinger, C.: In: *Diabetes.* Edited by W.J. Malaisse, J. Pirart, and J. Vallance-Owen. Excerpta Medica Amsterdam, 1974, p. 728.

129. Pictet, R. E., Rall, L. B., Phelps, P., and Rutter, W. J.: *Science,* **191**:191, 1976.

130. Rakieten, N., Gordon, B. S., Beaty, A., Cooney, D. A., Davis, R. D., and Schein, P. S.: *Proc. Soc. Exp. Biol. Med.,* **137**:280, 1971.

131. Volk, B. W., Wellman, K. F., and Brancato, P.: *Diabetologia,* **10**:37, 1974.

132. Broder, L. E., and Carter, S. K.: *Ann. Int. Med.,* **79**:108, 1973.

133. Hayes, J. R., O'Connell, N., O'Neill, T., Fennelly, J. J., and Weir, D. G.: *Gut,* **17**:285, 1976.

134. Stadil, F., Stage, G., Rehfeld, J. F., Efsen, F., and Fischerman, K.: *N. Engl. J. Med.,* **294**:1440, 1976.

135. Lennon, J. R., Sircus, W., Bloom, S. R., Mitchell, S. J., Polak, J. M., Besser, G. M., Hall, R., Coy, D. H., Kastin, A. J., and Schally, A. V.: *Gut,* **16**:821, 1975.

136. Murray-Lyon, I. M., Eddleston, A. L. W. F., Williams, R., Brown, M., Hogbin, B. M., Bennett, A., Edwards, J. C., and Taylor, K. W.: *Lancet,* **2**:895, 1968.

137. Iweze, F. I., Owen-Smith, M., and Polak, J. M.: *Proc. Roy. Soc. Med.,* **65**:2, 1972.

138. Feldman, J. M., Quickel, Jr., K. E., Maracek, R. L., and Lebovitz, H. E.: *South. Med. J.,* **65**:1325, 1972.

139. Carter, S. K., and Broder, L. E.: *Clin. Gastroenterol.,* **3**:733, 1974.

140. Hammar, S., and Sale, G.: *Hum. Pathol.,* **6**:349, 1975.

141. Larsson, L.-I., Schwartz, T., Lundqvist, G., Chance, R. E., Sundler, F., Rehfeld, J. F., Grimelius. L., Fahrenkrug, J., Schaffalitzky de Muckadell, O., and Moon, N.: *Amer. J. Path.,* **85**:675, 1976.

142. Larsson, L.-I., Hirsch, M. A., Holst, J. J., Ingemansson, S., Kühl, C., Lindkaer Jensen, S., Lundqvist, G., Rehfeld, J. F., and Schwartz, T. W.: *Lancet,* **1**:666, 1977.

Index